B. Hamm · R. Forstner (Eds.)

MRI and CT of the Female Pelvis

With Contributions by

E. Beinder · D. Chardonnens · T. Fischer · R. Forstner · K. A. Frei Bonel
H. Fritsch · B. Hamm · G. Heinz-Peer · K. Kinkel · C. Klüner · T. J. Kröncke
R. Kubik-Huch · A. Lienemann · P. Rogalla · J. Roos · A. Schneider · M. Taupitz
U. Zaspel

Foreword by

A. L. Baert

With 312 Figures in 693 Separate Illustrations, 27 in Color and 25 Tables

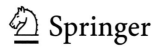 Springer

BERND HAMM, MD
Professor and Chairman
Institut für Radiologie (Campus Mitte)
Klinik für Strahlenheilkunde
(Campus Virchow-Klinikum und Campus Buch)
Charité - Universitätsmedizin Berlin
Charitéplatz 1
10117 Berlin
Germany

ROSEMARIE FORSTNER, MD
PD, Universitätsinstitut für Radiodiagnostik
Salzburger Landeskliniken
Paracelsus Medizinische Privatuniversität
Müllner Hauptstrasse 48
5020 Salzburg
Austria

ISSN   0942-5373
ISBN   978-3-642-06089-2   e-ISBN 978-3-540-68212-7
DOI 10.1007/978-3-540-68212-7

Springer Heidelberg Dordrecht London New York

Library of Congress Control Number: 2005935453

© 2007 Springer-Verlag Berlin Heidelberg

Cover design: Verlagsservice Teichmann, Mauer, Germany

Printed on acid-free paper

9 8 7 6 5 4 3 2 1

Springer is part of Springer Science + Business Media (www.springer.com)

MEDICAL RADIOLOGY

Diagnostic Imaging

Editors:
A. L. Baert, Leuven
M. Knauth, Göttingen
tor, Heidelberg

Foreword

Cross-sectional imaging methods such as ultrasound, computed tomography and magnetic resonance imaging have a different and specific role in diagnostic and interventional imaging of the female pelvis.

Continuing technical progress in CT and MRI explains the need for a volume dedicated to these modalities in our series, Medical Radiology -- Diagnostic Imaging.

This volume offers a very comprehensive but detailed up-to-date review of our current knowledge in the field. The very readable text is complemented by numerous superb illustrations.

I am very much indebted to the editors of this book: Professor Bernd Hamm and Dr. Rosemarie Forstner, both internationally recognized experts in modern radiological imaging of the female pelvis who have lectured and published widely on the topic. Together, they developed the concept of this volume and judiciously selected the various authors of individual chapters on the basis of their outstanding personal knowledge in specific pathological disorders.

I would like to thank and congratulate most sincerely the editors and authors for their superb efforts which have resulted in this excellent work.

This book will be of great value to radiologists, gynecologists and obstetricians. I am also confident that it will meet with the same success among readers as the previous volumes published in this series.

Leuven   ALBERT L. BAERT

Preface

Imaging plays an ever increasing role in the diagnostic evaluation of women with gynecologic disease. While ultrasonography comes to mind first, computed tomography and, of course, magnetic resonance imaging definitely contribute important information to proper diagnosis and therapeutic decision-making.

The focus of this book is on diagnostic imaging of the female pelvis using CT and MRI. We deliberately excluded ultrasonography since ample literature is already available on the subject. Other reasons for focusing on CT and MRI of the female pelvis are the different roles these two diagnostic tools play in different indications and the dramatic technical advances both modalities have seen in recent years.

This book is intended to provide the reader with a comprehensive review of the applications of CT and MRI in gynecology. While it is primarily intended for radiologists, both in training and in daily practice, it also addresses gynecologists and obstetricians. Each author has written their contribution according to their own "how-I-do-it" approaches. It is not meant to be encyclopedic, but rather to provide the reader with the current, up-to-date approaches in clinical practice.

With this practical application in mind, we arranged the chapters mainly according to the different disorders of the female pelvis and not with regard to technical aspects of the imaging modalities or strictly anatomic considerations. The main chapters dealing with the different disorders are preceded by an interesting presentation of a new interpretation of the anatomy of the female pelvis and a general introduction to state-of-the-art CT and MRI techniques.

Besides presenting a kind of "cookbook" with tips on practical imaging strategies and protocols, we aim to provide clear guidelines for indications and procedures, including a description of important differential diagnoses and possible pitfalls of both imaging modalities.

In the course of working on this book, we also came to realize how difficult it may be to achieve timely publication of what constitutes the state of the art in this field. The reader should therefore be aware that what the authors described as state-of-the-art while writing their chapters may already have become outdated by new insights at the time the book finally appears.

All of the co-authors have provided excellent contributions, representing their broad experience and the current clinical applications in their own practices. Without their contributions, this book would not have been possible, and we would like to express our deep-felt gratitude to all of them.

We also wish to thank the co-workers of Springer-Verlag for their cooperation in preparing this book.

It is our hope that this book will prove useful to all our colleagues interested in CT and MRI of the female pelvis and that our patients may benefit from an optimal use of these diagnostic tools.

Berlin   BERND HAMM
Salzburg   ROSEMARIE FORSTNER

Contents

Clinical Anatomy of the Female Pelvis

1

Helga Fritsch

This chapter is dedicated to my friend Harald Hötzinger who was an excellent radiologist and a good co-worker.

H. Fritsch, MD
Professor, Division of Clinical and Functional Anatomy, Department of Anatomy, Histology and Embryology, Medical University of Innsbruck, Müllerstrasse 59, 6020 Innsbruck, Austria

1.1
Introduction

The pelvic floor constitutes the caudal border of the human's visceral cavity. It is characterized by a complex morphology because different functional systems join here. A clear understanding of the pelvic anatomy is crucial for the diagnosis of female pelvic diseases, for female pelvic surgery as well as for fundamental mechanisms of urogenital dysfunction and treatment.

Modern imaging techniques are used for the diagnosis of pelvic floor or sphincter disorders. Furthermore, they are employed to determine the extent of pelvic diseases and the staging of pelvic tumors. In order to be able to recognize the structures seen on CT and MRI as well as on dynamic MRI, a detailed knowledge of the relationship of the anatomical entities within the pelvic anatomy is required.

The *Terminologia Anatomica* [15] contains a mixture of old and new terms describing the different structures of the pelvis. Throughout this chapter the actual anatomical terms are used and compared with clinical terms. Furthermore, they are defined and illustrated (see Table 1.1).

1.2
Morphological and
Clinical Subdivision of the Female Pelvis

The anatomy of the female pelvis and perineum shows a lack of conceptual clarity. These regions are best understood when they are clearly described and subdivided according to functional and clinical requirements: The actual clinical subdivision discerns an anterior, a middle and a posterior compartment. Whereas an anterior and posterior compartment may be found in the male as well as in the female, a middle compartment can only be found in the latter. The

Table 1.1. Box of terms and definitions

Term	Figure	Terminologia Anatomica (TA)		Clinical term	Definition	Renaming (according to our results)	Existence
		English	Latin				
1. Anococcygeal body		Anococcygeal body; anococcygeal ligament	Corpus anococcygeum; corpus anococcygeum	–	TA: The term corpus, rather than ligamentum, is used in TA because it is a stratified non-ligamentous structure in which fleshy muscle attachments underlie a tendon	Not necessary	+
2. Perineal body		Perineal body	Corpus perineale; centrum perinei	–	TA: The perineal body is fibromuscular rather than tendinous and quite unlike the centrum tendineum of the diaphragm. Our option: The perineal body itself is tendinous, nevertheless it cannot be compared with the flat centrum tendineum of the diaphragm	Though tendinous, not necessary	+
3. Perineal membrane		Perineal membrane	Membrana perinea	–	Dense connective tissue between external urethral sphincter (and transverse perineal muscle in male) and pubic bone	Not necessary	+
4. Anorectum		Rectum and anal canal	Rectum et canalis analis	Anorectum	Our option: The clinical term includes both, the rectum and the anal canal, not taking into account that they are of different origin	Necessary to pick up in TA	+
5. Presacral (sub)compartment		–	–	–	Our option: Small space between presacral fascia and sacral and coccygeal vertebrae containing vessels	Necessary to pick up in TA	+
6. Presacral fascia		Presacral fascia	Fascia presacralis	Waldeyer's fascia (?)	Caudal part of the parietal pelvic fascia		+

Term	Figure	Terminologia Anatomica (TA)		Clinical term	Definition	Renaming (according to our results)	Existence
		English	Latin				
7. Perirectal compartment		–	–	Mesorectum	Our option: Compartment filled by the rectal adventitia including nerves, vessels, lymph nodes	Necessary to pick up in TA	+
8. Rectal fascia or "Grenzlamelle"		–	–	Waldeyer's fascia (?)	Our option: Outer connective tissue lamella of the rectal adventitia, bordering the perirectal compartment	Necessary to pick up in TA	+
9. Inferior hypogastric plexus		Inferior hypogastric plexus; pelvic plexus	Plexus hypogastricus inferior; plexus pelvicus	Pelvic plexus	Autonomic nerve plexus within the recto-uterine or recto-vesical fold	Exclusively into the old and clinical term: pelvic plexus	+
10. Uterosacral ligament		Uterosacral ligament or recto-uterine ligament	Li. rectouterinum	–	Dense connective tissue running from the edges of the cervix uteri to the region of the sacrospinous ligament, then ascending and joining the pelvic parietal fascia	Exclusively into the utero-sacral ligament	+
11. Rectovaginal fascia		Rectovaginal fascia; rectovaginal septum (female)	Fascia rectovaginalis; septum rectovaginale	–	Our option: Plate of dense connective tissue, smooth muscle cells and nerves, locally arranged between rectum and vagina	Exclusively into the term rectovaginal/rectogenital septum	+

Table 1.1. Box of terms and definitions (*Continued*)

Term	Figure	*Terminologia Anatomica* (TA) English	*Terminologia Anatomica* (TA) Latin	Clinical term	Definition	Renaming (according to our results)	Existence
12. Anal sphincter complex		–	–	–	Includes all muscle layers of the anal canal: internal (smooth) sphincter, longitudinal (smooth) muscle, external (striated) sphincter	Necessary to pick up in TA	+
13. Pubovesical ligament		Medial pubovesical ligament, pubovesicalis, lateral pubovesical ligament	Lig. mediale pubovesicale, m. pubovesicalis, lig. laterale pubovesicalis	–	Most confusing structure! Our option: there is only one structure running from the pubic bone to the vesical neck. It mainly consists of smooth muscle cells intermingled with strands of dense connective tissue	Exclusively into the term pubovesical muscle	+
14. Levator ani muscle		Levator ani	M. levator ani	–	Muscle that constitutes the main part of the pelvic diaphragm and is composed of the Mm. pubococcygei, iliococcygei, and puborectales of each side		+
15. Tendinous arch of the pelvic fascia		Tendinous arch of the pelvic fascia	Arcus tendineus fasciae pelvis	–	Our option: This structure originates from the pubic bone laterally, it is connected with the superior fascia of the pelvic diaphragm "white line" laterally and with the pubovesical ligament medially. It may falsely be called Lig. laterale puboprostaticum or Lig. laterale pubovesicale		+

Term	Figure	Terminologia Anatomica (TA)		Clinical term	Definition	Renaming (according to our results)	Existence
		English	Latin				
16. Para-visceral fat pad		–	–	–	Our option: Fat pad at the lateral side of the bladder that develops in situ. Functionally necessary for the movements of bladder	Necessary to pick up in TA	+
17. Broad ligament		Broad ligament of the uterus	Lig. latum uteri	–	Peritoneal fold between the uterus and the lateral wall of the pelvis		+
18. Recto-uterine fold		Recto-uterine fold	Plica recto-uterina	–	Peritoneal fold passing from the cervix uteri on each side of the rectum to the posterior pelvic wall		+
19. Recto-uterine pouch		Recto-uterine pouch	Excavatio rectouterina	Space of Douglas	Deep peritoneal pouch situated between the recto-uterine folds of each side		+
20. Vesico-uterine fold		Vesico-uterine fold	Plica vesicouterina	–	Peritoneal fold between bladder and uterus on each side		+
21. Vesico-uterine pouch		Vesico-uterine pouch	Excavatio vesicouterina	–	Slight peritoneal pouch between the vesico-uterine folds of each side		+
22. Transverse cervical ligament or cardinal ligament		Transverse cervical ligament, cardinal ligament	Lig. transversum cervicis, lig. cardinale	Cardinal ligament	Connective tissue structures that should extend from the side of the cervix to the lateral pelvic wall. Our option: The cardinal ligament does not exist	Necessary to omit	0
23. Meso-salpinx		Mesosalpinx	Mesosalpinx	Identical	Double fold of peritoneum at the upper margin of the broad ligament		+
24. Mesovarium		Mesovarium	Mesovarium	Identical	Double fold of peritoneum attached at the dorsal portion of the broad ligament		+
25. Meso-metrium		Mesometrium	Mesometrium	–	So-called meso of the uterus, greatest portion of broad ligament	According to Höckel is morphogenetic unit of cervix and proximal vagina. Necessary to redefine	+

term "compartment" is routinely used by radiologists and all surgeons operating on the pelvic floor. This term is not identical with the term "space". According to former literature a lot of spaces are supposed to be arranged in the region of the pelvis: retrorectal, pararectal, rectoprostatic, rectovaginal, retropubic, paravesical, etc. [35, 43, 56]. From the point of view of the surgeon, "spaces" are empty [45]. They are only filled with loose connective tissue and neither contain large vessels nor nerves. Some years ago, we already proposed dropping the term "space" and speaking of compartments instead, taking into account that a compartment may be filled by different tissue components [19].

Within the following chapter we first present the posterior compartment and then the anterior one. This is in accordance with the viewpoint of the radi-

ologists and with the course of the vessels and nerves. An "extra" middle compartment that is characteristic for the female is presented in detail at the end of this chapter.

What is our common knowledge about the borders of the different pelvic compartments and what do we know about their content?

Posterior compartment

The borders of the posterior compartment are the skeletal elements of the sacrum and the coccyx dorsally. They are completed by the anococcygeal body (see Table 1.1) dorsocaudally and by the components of the levator ani muscle laterally and caudally (Fig. 1.1a). The rectovaginal fascia constitutes an incomplete border ventrocranially. The ventro-

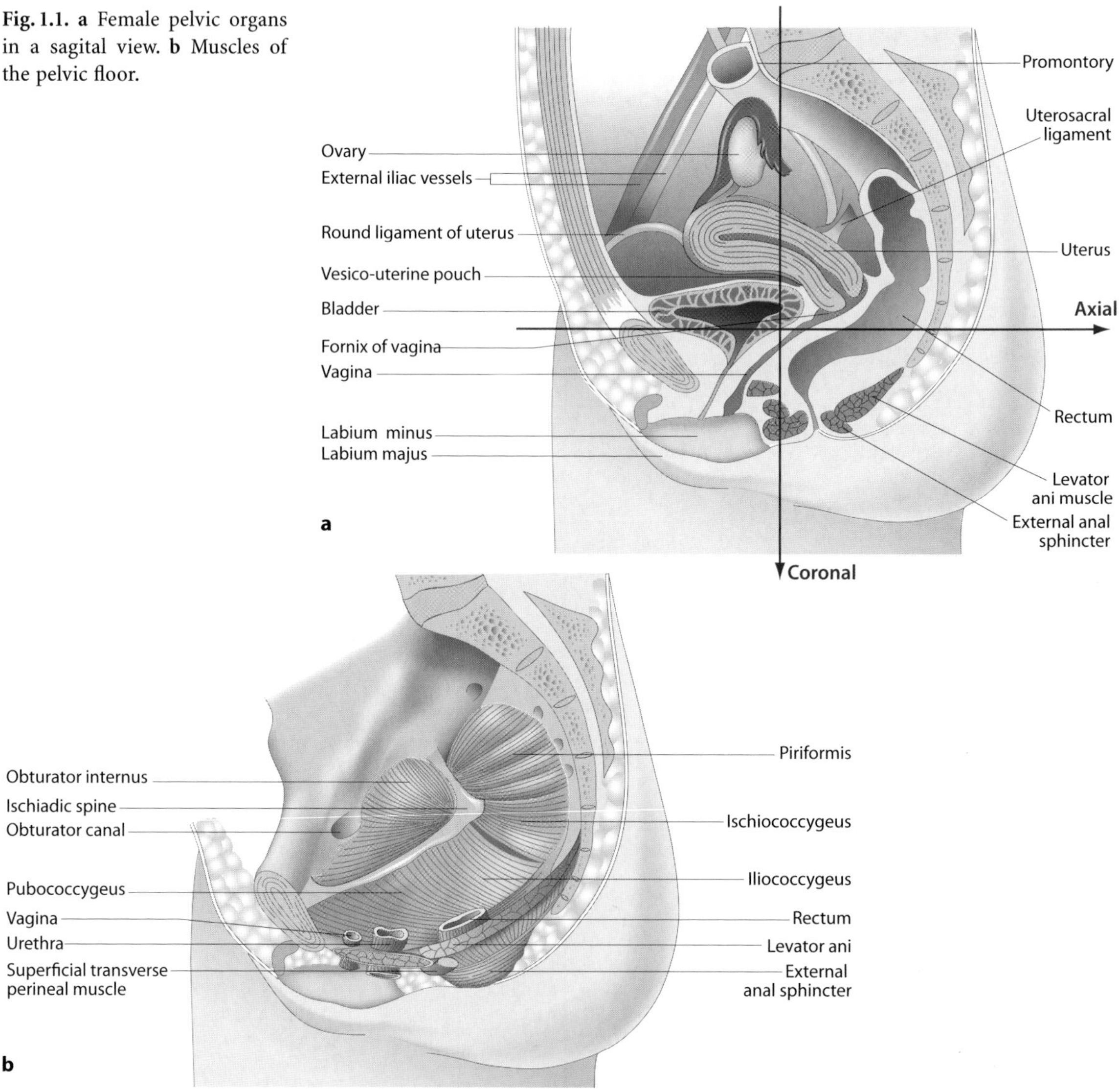

Fig. 1.1. a Female pelvic organs in a sagital view. b Muscles of the pelvic floor.

caudal border is composed of the perineal body (see Table 1.1). The only organ of the posterior compartment is the anorectum (see Table 1.1) (Fig. 1.1a,b).

Anterior compartment

The borders of the anterior compartment are the pubic symphysis ventrally, the components of the levator ani muscle laterally (Fig. 1.1b) and the perineal membrane (see Table 1.1) caudally. There is no distinct border between the anterior and middle compartment in the female. The contents of the anterior compartment are bladder and urethra (Fig. 1.1b).

Middle compartment

The borders are the components of the levator ani muscle laterally and the perineal body caudally (Fig. 1.1b). No distinct borders can be described ventrally, whereas the rectovaginal fascia/septum constitutes the dorsal border. The middle compartment contains the female genital organs that are arranged in a more or less coronal plane. In more detail the ovaries, the uterine tubes, the uterus and the vagina are situated in this compartment (Fig. 1.1a).

Perineal body

The perineal body is part of the perineum. It is situated between the genital organs and the anus and may be considered as a central or meeting point because a number of different structures join here.

1.3
Compartments

1.3.1
Posterior Compartment

1.3.1.1
Connective Tissue Structures

In macroscopic dissection of embalmed cadavers it is nearly impossible to distinguish subcompartments within the connective tissue of the posterior compartment. Our comparative study of adult and fetal pelves shows that two subcompartments can be distinguished within the posterior compartment:

A small presacral subcompartment (see Table 1.1) is situated in front of the sacrum and coccyx. It is bordered by the caudal segments of the vertebral column dorsally and ventrolaterally, it is clearly demarcated by the pelvic parietal fascia (see Table 1.1) (Fig. 1.2), which is called presacral fascia (see Table 1.1) at this position. In fetuses, the presacral subcompartment contains loose connective tissue, but it is predominated by large presacral veins.

The major part of the posterior pelvic compartment is filled by the anorectum and its accompanying tissues, constituting the perirectal subcompartment (see Table 1.1). This perirectal tissue is identical with the rectal adventitial tissue [17, 24] (see Table 1.1), which develops along the superior rectal vessels. In the adult, it mainly consists of adipose tissue subdivided by several connective tissue septa (Fig. 1.3a, b). Within this perirectal tissue the supplying structures of the rectum are enclosed: the superior rectal vessels, stems and branches, the branches of the variable medial rectal vessels, rectal nerves and rectal lymphatics, vessels and nerves. The localization of these lymphatic nodes is strikingly different from that of the other lymph nodes of the posterior compartment that are situated laterally in the neighborhood of the iliac vessels [40, 50].

The rectal adventitia develops from a layer of condensed mesenchymal tissue, which – later on – forms a dense connective tissue in fetuses (Fig. 1.3c). In the newborn child it is remodeled by small fat lobules occurring between the connective tissue lamellae. The outer lamella covers the perirectal subcompartment and is called "rectal fascia" [17, 23] or "Grenzlamelle" [49, 50] (see Table 1.1). It constitutes the morphological border of the perirectal subcompartment. The craniocaudal extent of the perirectal subcompartment depends on the branching pattern of the superior rectal vessels, thus the perirectal compartment is broad laterally and dorsally and it is often rather thin ventrally where it is only composed of some connective tissue lamellae. As can be seen in sagittal sections the extent of the perirectal subcompartment decreases in size in a craniocaudal direction (Fig. 1.2c).

What is situated outside the rectal fascia and therefore outside the perirectal subcompartment? Dorsally, the presacral subcompartment is loosely attached to the perirectal compartment (see above). Laterally the supplying structures (autonomic nerves and branches of the iliac vessels) of the urogenital organs constitute a nerve-vessel plate (Fig. 1.3c). The latter is accompanied by connective tissue and fills the remaining space between the perirectal compartment

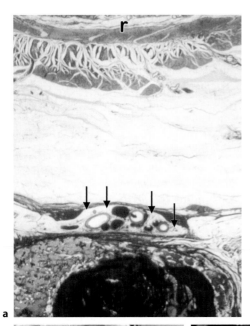

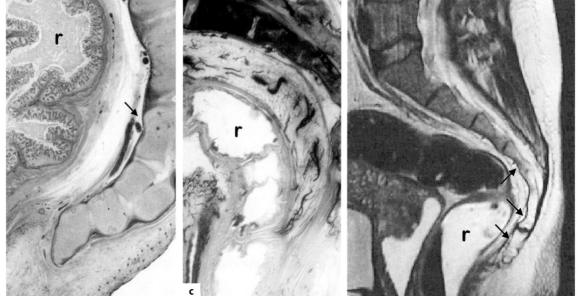

Fig. 1.2a–d. Presacral space (*arrows*). **a** Axial section (500 μm) of an adult. ×4. **b** Sagittal section (400 μm) of a 24-week-old female fetus. ×9. **c** Sagittal section (5 mm) of an adult female. ×0.45. **d** Mid-sagittal MR image of an adult female. *r*, rectum

and the lateral pelvic wall. In the female, the nerves of the inferior hypogastric plexus (see Table 1.1) are attached to the uterosacral ligament (see Table 1.1) that is directly situated between the rectal fascia and the inferior hypogastric plexus (Fig. 1.3a,c) [18].

The ventral border of the perirectal compartment represents the border between posterior and middle compartment. It differs in a craniocaudal direction, i. e. to the peritoneum of the recto-uterine pouch at a level with the cervix uteri and the fornix vaginae and to the posterior wall of the vagina more caudally. As we have recently shown [1, 24, 36] a two layered recto-vaginal fascia/septum (see Table 1.1) develops in the female and is identical to the male's rectoprostatic fascia/septum or Denonvillier´s fascia [53]. At a level with the anorectal flexure, additional bundles of longitudinal smooth muscles are situated at the anterior rectal wall forming the muscular portion of the rectovaginal fascia ventrally (Fig. 1.4). The smooth muscle bundles are accompanied by nerves, some of them crossing the midline and they are connected to the smooth muscle layer of the rectal wall. Caudally these additional smooth muscle bundles are attached to the connective tissue of the perineal body (Fig. 1.4).

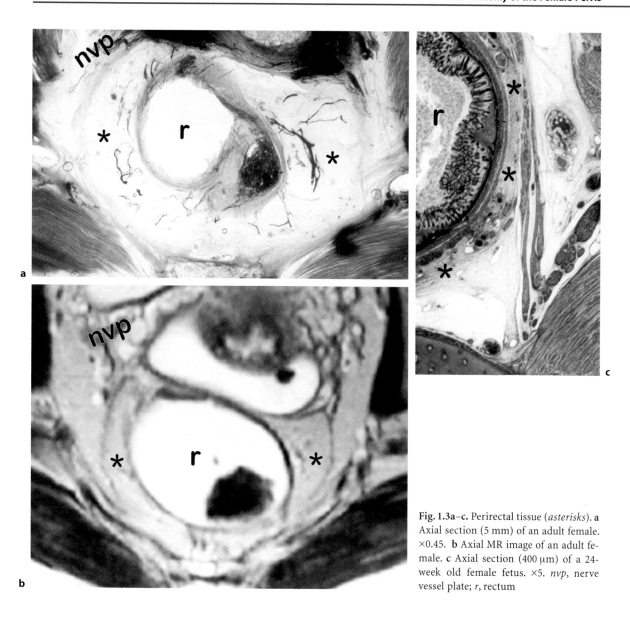

Fig. 1.3a–c. Perirectal tissue (*asterisks*). a Axial section (5 mm) of an adult female. ×0.45. b Axial MR image of an adult female. c Axial section (400 μm) of a 24-week old female fetus. ×5. *nvp*, nerve vessel plate; *r*, rectum

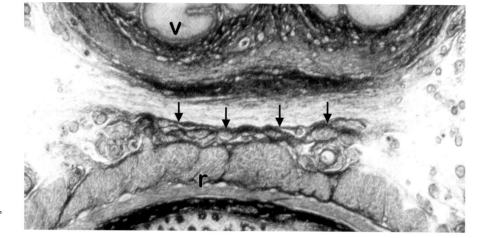

Fig. 1.4. Rectovaginal fascia (*arrows*). Axial section (400 μm) of a 24-week-old female fetus. X 28. *v*, Vagina; *r*, rectum

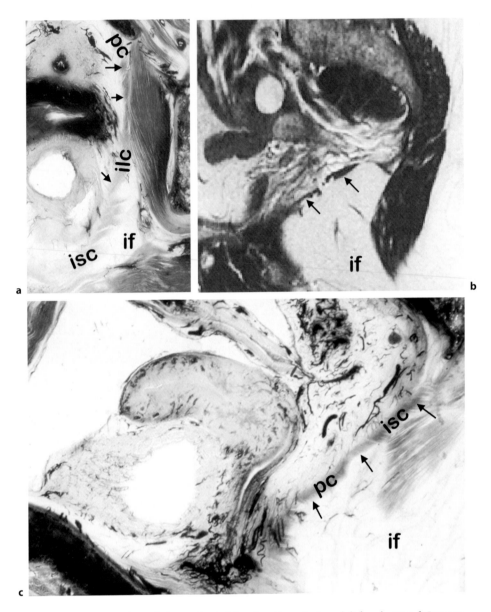

Fig. 1.5a–c. Levator ani muscle (*arrows*). **a** Axial section (5 mm) of an adult female. ×0.6. **b** Parasagittal MR image of an adult female. **c** Sagittal section (5 mm) of an adult female. ×1.0. *isc*, ischiococcygeal muscle; *if*, ischioanal fossa; *ilc*, iliococcygeal muscle; *pc*, pubococcygeal muscle

1.3.1.2
Muscles

Within the posterior pelvic compartment all components of the levator ani muscle are to be found: the pubococcygeus muscles and the iliococcygeus muscles constitute an irregular plate and insert into the coccyx where they overlap each other in a staggered arrangement (Fig. 1.5). The inferior component, the puborectalis muscles, do not insert into any skeletal structure. Behind the rectal wall the fiber bundles of each puborectalis muscle criss-cross, thus constituting a muscular sling around the anorectal flexure (Fig. 1.6). In the craniocaudal direction the pubococcygeus muscle and the puborectalis muscle are more or less continuous. In sectional anatomy they can be differentiated by the different directions of their fiber bundles, those of the pubococcygeus taking a slightly descending course, those of the puborectalis exclusively situated in the horizontal plane. The different

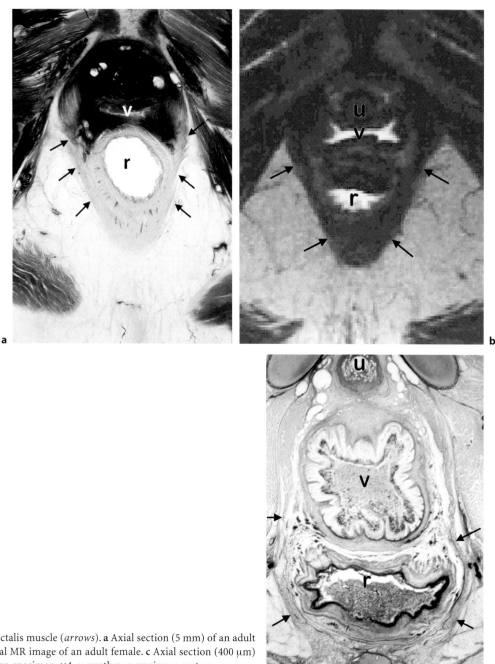

Fig. 1.6a–c. Puborectalis muscle (*arrows*). **a** Axial section (5 mm) of an adult female. ×0.8. **b** Axial MR image of an adult female. **c** Axial section (400 μm) of a female newborn specimen. ×4. *u*, urethra; *v*, vagina; *r*, rectum

components of the levator ani muscle can already be distinguished in early fetal life [21]. Sexual differences found in the levator ani muscle of the adult are already marked in late fetal life: the levator ani constitutes a thick and well developed muscle in the male fetus whereas it is thinner and already intermingled with connective tissue in the female fetus (Fig. 1.6b). This is particularly true of its puborectalis portion.

The puborectalis muscle is continuous with the external anal sphincter caudally (Fig. 1.7). The macroscopic distinction between both muscles is provided by the anococcygeal body. The puborectalis has no skeletal attachment dorsally, but the deep portion of the sphincter ani externus is indirectly fastened to the coccyx by the anococcygeal body.

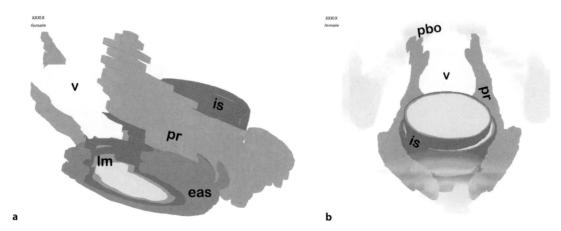

Fig. 1.7a,b. Computer-assisted reconstructions of a female fetus. **a** Oblique ventrolateral view. **b** Descending dorsoventral view. *v*, vagina; *lm*, longitudinal muscular layer; *pr*, puborectalis muscle; *eas*, external anal sphincter; *is*, internal sphincter; *pbo*, pubic bone

The sphincter ani externus is the outer part of the anal sphincter complex (see Table 1.1). The other components are the smooth internal sphincter and the longitudinal muscle layer of the anorectum, the latter is interposed between the sphincters. Whereas macroscopically the external anal sphincter presents itself as a continuous sheet covering the anal canal (Fig. 1.8a), it can be subdivided into a deep, anorectal portion and a superficial, subcutaneous portion in sectional anatomy (see Fig. 1.8b). This deep portion is a clearly demarcated layer of circularly arranged striated muscle fibers; the superficial portion is characterized by an intermingling of the striated muscle fibers with the smooth longitudinal muscle (also called "intersphincteric space"). The form of the external anal sphincter can be best studied in three dimensional reconstructions of histological or anatomical orthogonal sections [20]: At an anorectal level above the perineum where the external anal sphincter is continuous with the puborectalis muscle dorsally (Fig. 1.8c), it is missing in the midline ventrally, but it is thickened ventrolaterally where it becomes part of the anterior compartment in males and the middle compartment in females. At a level of the perineum the external anal sphincter is complete ventrally (see Fig. 1.15a), but it turns inwards and forms a muscular continuum with the smooth internal sphincter and the longitudinal muscle dorsally. As can be seen from the fetal sections, sexual differences in the anal sphincter complex are already present prenatally: the sphincter complex as a whole is thicker in the male than in the female, the anterior portion, however, is thick in the female and thinner and more elongated in the male.

1.3.1.3
Reinterpreted Anatomy and Clinical Relevance

The posterior compartment is predominated by the rectum and its surrounding connective tissue. The morphological demarcation of this compartment is formed by the rectal fascia. In CT the rectal fascia may be discriminated as a slightly hyperdense sheath [27, 47] and in MRI it is visible as a thin, hypointense structure. It is important for the diagnosis and staging of rectal tumor [4, 7, 28]. According to our results the macroscopic borders of the perirectal compartment are clearly demarcated in the adult female where the sacrouterine ligaments constitute the lateral borders and where the posterior border is marked by the pelvic parietal fascia. The perirectal adipose tissue constitutes functional fat that adapts to the different filling volumes of the rectum and constitutes a gliding sheath for the movements of that organ. In contrast to prior literature [43, 46] we did not find any ligament or even ligamentous structures binding the rectum to the lateral pelvic wall. Thus, there is neither a "rectal stalk" nor a dense "paraproctium".

The most common surgically correctable cause of fecal incontinence in woman is childbirth with injury of the sphincter. External sphincter injuries occur in 6%–30% of woman [51]. It should be differentiated between complete or incomplete sphincter disruptions. Our morphological investigation [20] supports the fact that the external anal sphincter is not a totally circular muscle. We have thoroughly described the parts of the sphincter complex, in order to help the pelvic radiologists and surgeons to identify these structures and, if possible, to reconstruct them in a meticulous way.

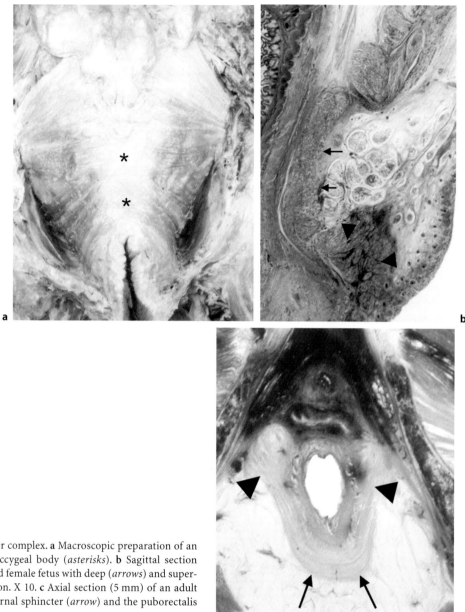

Fig. 1.8a–c. Anal sphincter complex. **a** Macroscopic preparation of an adult female with anococcygeal body (*asterisks*). **b** Sagittal section (500 µm) of a 20-week-old female fetus with deep (*arrows*) and superficial (*arrowheads*) portion. X 10. **c** Axial section (5 mm) of an adult female, fusion of the external sphincter (*arrow*) and the puborectalis (*arrowhead*). ×0.6

Rectoceles are hernial protrusions of the anterior rectal wall and the posterior vaginal wall into the vagina and/or throughout the vaginal introitus. The size of the rectocele does not correlate with symptoms and it is often diagnosed in a population without symptoms. Trauma or obstetrical injuries weaken the rectovaginal fascia/septum. Rectoceles occur with laxity of the connective tissue in advancing years, multiparity, poor bowel habits, perineal relaxation and increased intra-abdominal pressure in constipation [31, 59]. In the successful repair of a rectocele the rectovaginal fascia/septum seems to be the key structure [8, 44].

1.3.1.4
Important Vessels, Nerves and Lymphatics of the Posterior Compartment:

- Superior rectal artery
- Rectal nerves
- Rectal lymph nodes
- Inferior hypogastric plexus
- Superior hypogastric plexus
- Common iliac artery
- Internal iliac artery
  (Veins have a corresponding course.)

1.3.2
Anterior Compartment

1.3.2.1
Connective Tissue Structures

When dissecting along the lateral and ventral wall in embalmed cadavers, it is easy to isolate the bladder including the embedding tissues and all the adjacent structures. During dissection, no lateral stalks are found that might be responsible for the fixation of the bladder or the urethra. Ventrally a cord can be identified. It takes an ascending course from the pubic bone to the neck of the bladder and it is usually called the pubovesical ligament (see Table 1.1) (Fig. 1.9a). It is connected to the tendinous arch of the pelvic fascia (see Table 1.1). Together, both structures incompletely subdivide the retropubic region into a prevesical subcompartment and a preurethral subcompartment. From the comparative sectional study of fetal and adult pelves we learned the detailed composition of the connective tissue structures within the anterior compartment.

With the exception of its neck and its posterior wall the bladder is covered by adipose tissue (Fig. 1.9b). The latter constitutes a semicircular pad that fills the gap between the lateral pelvic wall and the ventral and lateral wall of the bladder. The fat pad is not subdivided by ligaments or any other dense connective tissue septa, but sometimes may be crossed by variable branches from the obturator vessels. It develops in situ (Fig. 1.9c) from a large paravisceral fat pad (see Table 1.1) in human fetuses [22] and neither contains large vessels, nerves nor lymphatics. The latter derive from the internal iliac vessels and join the dorsolateral edge of the bladder. Their branches, which are always accompanied by a sheath of dense connective tissue, embrace the bladder and urethra. Thus nerves, vessels and lymphatics are directly situated at the lateral and dorsal wall of the bladder and medially to the fat pad. Ventrocranially, both fat pads join in the midline. Their dorsal edge nearly abuts at the perirectal compartment and their caudal border abuts the levator ani laterally and the pubovesical or puboprostatic ligament ventrally. Thus they are not part of the preurethral subcompartment that is filled by connective tissue accompanying the deep dorsal vessels of the clitoris.

Within the anterior compartment two structures are found that are composed of dense connective tissue: the tendinous arch of the pelvic fascia that originates from the pubic bone and that is connected to the pelvic parietal fascia covering the levator ani muscle on its visceral side (superior fascia of the pelvic diaphragm; see Table 1.1) and the semicircular fibrous sheath that covers the ventral and lateral

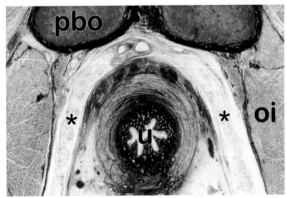
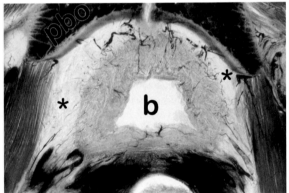
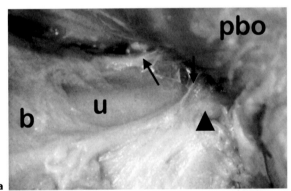

Fig. 1.9a–c. Anterior compartment. **a** Macroscopic preparation of a 23-week-old female fetus with the pubovesical ligament (*arrow*) and the tendinous arch (*arrowhead*). ×9. **b** In an axial section (5 mm) of an adult female with the paravisceral fat pad (*asterisks*). ×. **c** Axial section (400 μm) of a 24-week-old female fetus with the developing paravisceral fat pad (*asterisks*). ×8. *b*, bladder; *u*, urethra; *pbo*, pubic bone; *oi*, obturator internus muscle

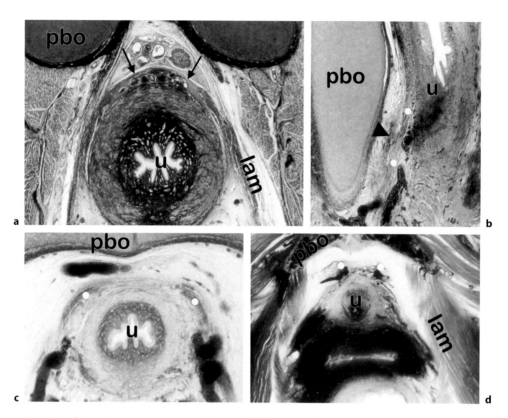

Fig. 1.10a–d. Anterior compartment and the so-called ligaments of the urethra. **a** Axial section (400 μm) of a 24-week-old female fetus with the semicircular urethral sheath (*arrows*). ×12. **b** Sagittal section (500 μm) of a 13- to 14-week-old female fetus with the pubovesical ligament (*white spots*) and the origin of the tendinous arch (*arrowhead*). ×25. **c** Axial section (400 μm) of a 17-week-old female fetus with the pubovesical ligaments (*white spots*). ×12. **d** Axial section (5 mm) of an adult female with the pubovesical ligaments (*white spots*). ×7.5. *pbo*, pubic bone; *u*, urethra; *lam*, levator ani muscle

wall of the bladder and the urethra. As the sheath is strong ventrally it can be considered as an incomplete ventral vesical or urethral fascia. Whereas the ventral vesical fascia has absolutely no fixation to the lateral pelvic wall, at a level of the urogenital hiatus the ventral urethral fascia, but not the urethra [37], is attached to the fascia of the levator ani muscle laterally (Fig. 1.10a). Thus, within the hiatus a fibrous bridge connects the fasciae of the levator ani muscles of both sides. To summarize: the fibrous structures of the anterior compartment build up a hammock-like [12] construction for bladder and urethra. These findings can most clearly be shown in fetuses and are matching but not so evident in the adult. It is important to know that there is absolutely no kind of a lateral bony fixation for bladder or urethra. In a dorsocranial direction, the ventral fascia of bladder and urethra is continuous with the connective tissue sheath of the internal iliac vessels. Ventrally, the hammock-like construction is indirectly fixed to the pu-

bic bone by means of the tendinous arch and by the so-called pubovesical ligament (Fig. 1.10b–d). The latter is composed of cholinergic innervated smooth muscle cells [57] and is connected to the vesical neck cranially (see above).

An additional fibrous structure can be found to close the hiatus ventrally: a plate of dense connective tissue fills the space between pubic bone and urethral sphincter, thus constituting the perineal membrane (Fig. 1.11a).

1.3.2.2
Muscles

The striated muscles of the anterior compartment are the ventral parts of the levator ani muscle (see Table 1.1), i.e. the pubococcygeus and puborectalis muscle of each side. As they are covered by the superior fascia of the pelvic diaphragm, they are clearly separated by the adjacent organs (Fig. 1.10a,d and

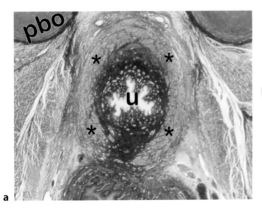

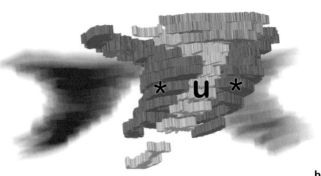

Fig. 1.11a,b. External urethral sphincter (*asterisks*). **a** Axial section (400 μm) of a 24-week-old female fetus, embedded in the transverse perineal membrane. ×9. **b** Computer-assisted three-dimensional reconstruction of a female fetus. *pbo*, pubic bone; *u*, urethra

Fig. 1.11a) and the external urethral sphincter. As has been reported previously [37], this muscle is horseshoe- or omega-shaped during fetal development and incompletely covers the urethra (Fig. 1.11). The dorsal ends of this muscle are connected by a plate of dense connective tissue that is small in the female where it is firmly attached to the ventral wall of the vagina (Figs. 1.10d, 1.11a). Whereas most of the fibers of the external urethral sphincter run semicircular, the most caudal fibers nearly run in a transverse plane. This portion predominates in the male and therefore has been considered as the male's deep transverse perineal muscle. However, it does not exist in the female [42].

As has been described above, smooth muscles are found outside the walls of the urogenital organs constituting parts of the pubovesical ligament in front of the ventral wall of the urethra.

1.3.2.3
Reinterpreted Anatomy and Clinical Relevance

The extent of the fat pad described here is identical to the anterior portion of the paravisceral space as reported by GASPARRI and BRIZZI [25]. It is obvious that the main function of the semicircular, paravisceral fat pad is to constitute a gliding pad for the bladder [33]. The fat pad accompanies the bladder whenever moving.

DORSCHNER et al. [14] pointed out the fact that the smooth muscle bundles of the pubovesical ligaments are continuous with longitudinal muscle fibers of the neck of the bladder that they call dilatator urethrae. Maybe again there is a similarity to the anorectum, where we also found smooth muscle bundles and autonomic nerves outside the ventral wall, which we

think work in functional coactivity to the longitudinal internal bundles [1]. Nevertheless, it seems to be sure that the function of the so-called pubovesical ligaments which receive a presumptive cholinergic innervation [57] is not fixing the urethra to the pubic bone but maintaining its position relative to the bone during micturition [26]. In contrast the contraction of the levator ani muscle and the external urethral sphincter leads to a narrowing of the preurethral space and to an ascending movement of the urethra as can be seen in dynamic MRI [16, 48].

Due to our results that in principle support the hammock hypothesis of DELANCEY [12], an operative "refixation" of the urethra and the bladder neck should result in an ascending dorsocranial traction (nerve guiding plate), as well as a descending ventrocaudal traction (tendinous arch of the pelvic fascia). Though there are innovative ideas regarding the surgical reconstruction of the female urinary tract [55], most procedures are not performed according to the morphological needs, because they mostly consider only one part of the so-called fixation system.

1.3.2.4
Important Vessels, Nerves and Lymphatics of the Anterior Compartment:

- Inferior vesical artery
- Branches to the ureter
- Superior vesical artery
- Vesical lymph nodes
- Internal iliac lymph nodes
- Internal iliac artery
- Inferior hypogastric plexus
- Paravesical fat pad
  (Veins have a corresponding course.)

1.3.3
Middle Compartment

1.3.3.1
Connective Tissue Structures

In macroscopic dissections of the adult female pelvis it is impossible to isolate ligaments fastening the cervix uteri or the vagina to the lateral pelvic wall and thus separating the middle compartment from the anterior or the posterior one laterally. In a refined macroscopic dissection performed with a binocular dissecting microscope it is possible – as well as in any other part of the pelvic subperitoneal tissue – to isolate connective tissue septa within the adipose tissue surrounding uterus and vagina [9, 10]. Our study of female fetal and adult pelvic sections reveals the true nature of the connective tissue structures surrounding uterus and vagina. The only connective tissue belonging to the middle compartment accompanies the vessels of uterus and vagina thus running parallel to the lateral walls of these organs. In fetuses, the connective tissue is still loose and without a differentiated structure, in the adult it mainly consists of adipose tissue with regular connective tissue septa (Fig. 1.12a–d) and it is continuous with the broad ligaments (see Table 1.1) laterally. The paracervical connective tissue abuts to the paravesical adipose tissue laterally and the paravaginal connective tissue abuts to the pelvic parietal fascia caudally (Fig. 1.12a,b). The broad ligaments themselves are part of the recto-uterine and the vesico-uterine folds (see Table 1.1) that tangentially cover the anterior and posterior uterine walls [18]. Apart from dense subperitoneal connective tissue that covers the recto-uterine pouch (see Table 1.1) (Fig. 1.12e) and mainly consists of collagenous fibers, no supportive ligaments are found for the female fetal uterus. In the adult, this condensation of subperitoneal connective tissue has developed to the uterosacral ligaments (see Table 1.1). They are visible in the transparent sections as well as on MRI and form semicircular cords varying in thickness individually. They originate from the lateral margin of the cervix uteri and the vaginal vault and course dorsocranially where they are connected to the pelvic parietal fascia covering the sacrospinous ligaments and the sacrum. As they are part of the recto-uterine ligaments they cover the perirectal tissue laterally. Our study undoubtedly confirmed the existence of the round ligaments as well as their course and their components. However, ligamentous structures constituting cardinal or transverse ligaments (see

Table 1.1) [34, 38] that are to be supposed to fasten the cervix uteri and the vaginal vault with the lateral pelvic wall can not be found in the adult pelvis. Our findings that have been taken from anatomic sections of elder specimens unrestrictedly correlate with the results of the MRI taken from young adult female pelves (Fig. 1.13).

Subperitoneally, the middle compartment and its organs abut the anterior compartment ventrally. This area is predominated by the dense connective tissue bridge intimately connecting the ventral vaginal wall with the dorsal urethral wall (Fig. 1.12b) (see also Sect. 1.3.2).

Dorsomedially, the middle compartment abuts the posterior compartment. The border between these compartments is demarcated by the rectovaginal fascia/septum (see also Sect. 1.3.1), that is composed of dense connective tissue, elastic fibers [44] and smooth muscle cells that belong to the longitudinal layer of the rectal wall.

The uterine tubes lie on each side of the uterus in the upper margin of the broad ligament (see Table 1.1; broad ligament). Each tube is attached on its inferior surface to a double fold of peritoneum called mesosalpinx (see Table 1.1). The lateral and superior part of the tube is the ampulla that opens into the funnel-shaped infundibulum with its fimbria at the abdominal orifice. The ovaries lie in the ovarian fossa, i.e. close to the lateral pelvic wall and are suspended by a double fold of peritoneum, the mesovarium (see Table 1.1). The latter is attached to the broad ligament posteriorly. Behind the ovarian fossa are extraperitoneal structures, especially the ureter and the internal iliac vessels as well as the origin of the uterine artery (Fig. 1.14).

1.3.3.2
Muscles

The middle compartment does not have any specific striated muscles. The lateral vaginal wall comes in close contact to the puborectalis portion of the levator ani muscle. Both structures are always separated by the superior fascia of this muscle (Fig. 1.6b).

1.3.3.3
Reinterpreted Anatomy and Clinical Relevance

Though there are a lot of anatomical and clinical terms describing the tissue surrounding uterus and vagina, neither their definitions nor their origins are clear. The mesometrium (see Table 1.1) for example may be considered to be the largest part of the broad ligament extending from the pelvic floor to the

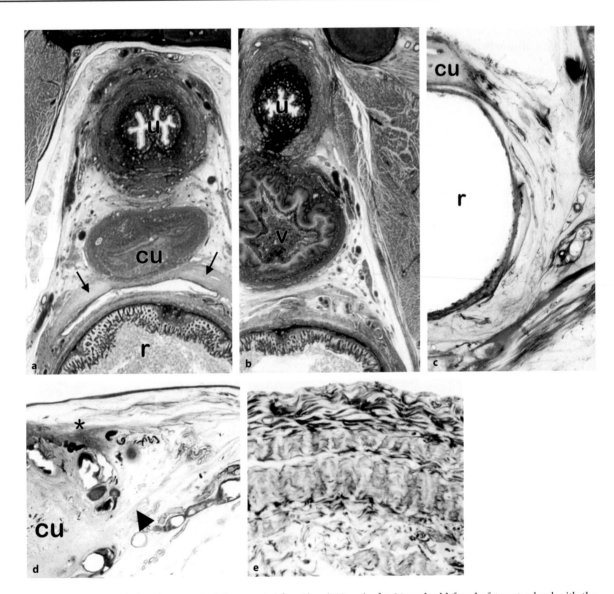

Fig. 1.12a–e. Paracervical and paravaginal tissue. **a** Axial section (400 µm) of a 24-week-old female fetus at a level with the recto-uterine pouch covered by dense connective tissue (*arrow*). ×8. **b** Axial section (400 µm) of the same fetus at a level with the vagina embedded in loose paravaginal tissue. Vagina and urethra are intimately connected. ×8. **c** Axial section (3 mm) of an adult female with the paracervical tissue. ×0.8. **d** Enlargement of an axial section (3 mm) of the same specimen with origin of the round ligament (*asterisk*) and the uterosacral ligament (*arrowhead*). ×3.5. **e** Enlargement of (**a**) with parallel oriented connective tissue fibers constituting the subperitoneal part of the uterosacral ligament. ×40. *u*, urethra; *cu*, cervix uteri; *r*, rectum; *v*, vagina

uterine body enclosing the uterine artery or the connective tissue lying directly beneath the peritoneal covering of the uterus. As has been re-emphasized by HÖCKEL et al. [29] the knowledge of the possible extent of local tumour spread is essential for the planning of surgery and radiotherapy, especially in the female pelvis. Like the posterior compartment with its mesorectum, the "mesometrium" (see Table 1.1) has been redefined and was identified to

be the anatomical territory derived from common precursor tissues. Thus a new operation technique was proposed to operate carcinoma of the uterine cervix (stages IB–IIA). It is termed total mesometrial resection and is identified as the morphogenetic unit for the cervix and the proximal vagina including its neurovasculature.

Surgical techniques for the fixation of uterus and vagina are numerous. They all depend on the idea

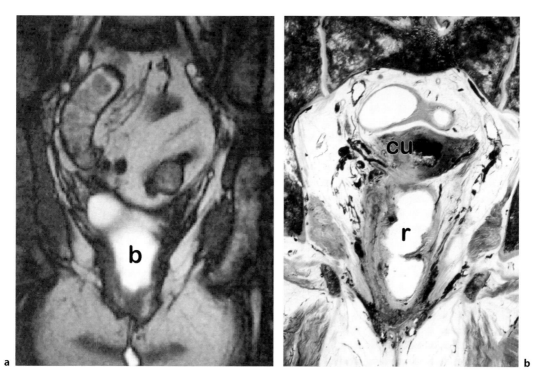

Fig. 1.13a,b. Subperitoneal connective tissue and nerve vessel guiding plate. **a** Coronal section (3 mm) of an adult female with pararectal and paracervical tissue. ×0.4. **b** Coronal MR image of an adult female with paravesical and paracervical tissue

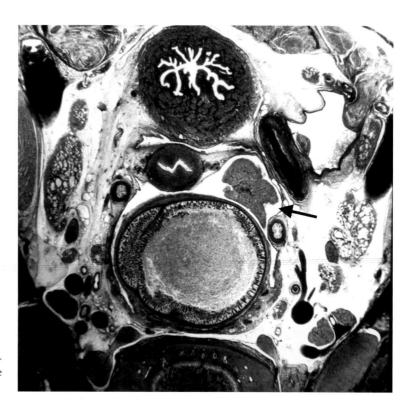

Fig. 1.14. Axial section (400 µm) of a 24-week-old female fetus at a level with the ovarian fossa (*arrow*). ×4

that there are sheath-like condensations within the pelvic cavity that are commonly called fascia. Moreover, these fasciae are thought to be responsible for acting as supportive structures to the uterus and vagina and thus they need to be reconstructed during operation. We think this point is one of the most critical to be discussed in this chapter.

Our reinterpreted anatomy of the connective tissue surrounding uterus and vagina is:

- In accordance with former Anglo-American authors [5, 32, 54] we do not find any visceral fascia covering uterus and vagina. Both organs are accompanied by adventitial connective tissue. The rectovaginal fascia/septum develops in situ [36] and is connected to the uterosacral ligaments, to the longitudinal muscular layer of the rectum and to the perineum (see Sects. 1.3.1 and 1.4).
- As has been clearly summarized by BASTIAN and LASSAU [2] various ligaments are supposed to exist in the pelvis of the adult female. Our results show that – apart from the uterosacral and the round ligaments – no ligaments of the uterus can be found in conventional anatomical specimens, sections or by MRI. We showed, however, that the paracervical and paravaginal region contains adipose tissue, numerous vessels, nerves and connective tissue septa. All together these components may be confounded with a ligamentous structure, especially in the older female. The connective tissue septa have carefully been described by new morphological approaches [10, 13], but they have been over-interpreted as to their functional meaning. There is no doubt that some of these connective tissue septa are connected to the fascia of the levator ani muscle and the contraction of this muscle is directly transferred to the septa and thus also to the vagina. But due to their morphological characteristics they are not supposed to act as supportive structures.

Our results are still in disagreement with the classical descriptions found in clinical and anatomical textbooks. We are aware of the fact that the variability of nomenclature is also misleading. But, nevertheless, the only fixation of the uterus is provided by the sacrouterine ligaments running in a dorsocranial direction. These ligaments are connected to the pelvic parietal fascia at a level with the sacrospinous ligaments, thus producing an upward traction for the whole uterovaginal complex.

There are various surgical procedures to reconstruct the so-called supportive ligaments in patients with genital prolapse. Due to our morphological data, it is useful to carry out a sacral fixation of the uterovaginal complex in terms of prolapse [39, 52], taking into account that the pudendal vessels and the pudendal nerve are not injured during operation [41]. New techniques include meshes that are suggested to support all female pelvic organs [6]. The results of these techniques seem to open the field of female hernia surgery.

1.3.3.4
Important Vessels, Nerves and Lymphatics of the Middle Compartment:

- Uterine artery
- Inferior hypogastric plexus. (Veins have a corresponding course)

1.4
Perineal Body

1.4.1
Connective Tissue Structures and Muscles in the Female

The perineal body separates the urogenital and anal hiatus. It is situated between rectum and vagina, i. e. between the posterior and middle compartments. Within the region of the perineal body the skin is firmly attached to the underlying connective tissue. The perineal body consists of dense connective tissue. It does not possess its own musculature, but it serves muscles of the perineal region to originate or to attach (Fig. 1.15a). Whereas the external anal sphincter is attached to it dorsally (Fig. 1.15a), the muscles of the cavernous tissue are attached ventrally (Fig. 1.15b). A deep transverse perineal muscle that may be attached ventrally does not exist in the female [42]. As has already been pointed out above (see Sect. 1.3.1) the additional smooth rectal muscle bundles that are situated in the rectovaginal fascia/septum are integrated and attached to the connective tissue of the perineal body (Fig. 1.15c). As the region of the female's perineal body is of high clinical interest in terms of damage during childbirth and/or episiotomies [58], again it is described according to the gynecologist's point of view, i.e. from outside (inferior) to the inside (superior): At a level below the orifice of the vagina the external anal sphincter is attached to the perineal body (Fig. 1.15a), whereas at a level with the orifice

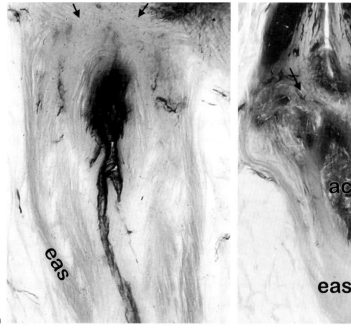

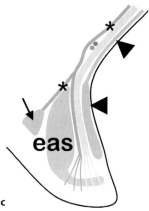

Fig. 1.15a–c. Perineal body (*arrows*) and attached muscles. **a** Axial section (5 mm) of an adult female at a level with the anal cleft. ×2.2. **b** Axial section of the same specimen (**a**) at a level with the vaginal hiatus. ×1.2. **c** The sagittal plane pointing out the ventral anorectal wall (*arrowheads*) and the different muscle layers including the longitudinal muscle cells (*asterisks*). *eas*, external anal sphincter

of the vagina and above the internal sphincter abuts the perineal body and thus indirectly the dorsal wall of the vagina (Fig. 1.15b). At these levels the external sphincter embraces the anal canal, the perineal body and the dorsal wall of the vagina laterally.

The intralevatoric side of the perineal body is connected with connective tissue septa of the ischioanal fossa [11] that are also connected to the inferior fascia of the levator ani muscle [30].

1.4.2
Reinterpreted Anatomy and Clinical Relevance

A detailed knowledge of the anatomy of the perineal body has become of interest since transperineal or even dynamic transperineal ultrasound [3] have been carried out. With the help of these techniques, the infralevatoric viscera, the soft tissues and the puborectalis can be viewed and defined.

For a long time there has been no doubt about the existence of the fibrous components of this region. However, defined in the actual *Terminologia Anatomica* [15], the perineal body should be a fibromuscular rather than a tendinous structure. We categorically disagree with this opinion. The perineal body itself is a fibrous structure, but it is intermingled with all originating and inserting muscles. It has to be considered as a tendinous center for all the muscles that do not have a bony origin or attachment. There is no doubt that it is an important region for absorbing part of the intrapelvic (intraabdominal) pressure. A stretched or even destroyed perineal body may be the cause for urogenital or rectal prolapse [59].

From a morphological as well as a functional point of view there is need for discussion as to how and whether a surgical approach through an intact perineal body should be performed.

The discussion of pelvic floor damage during vaginal delivery and/or after episiotomies has been kindled through the remarkable statistics of SULTAN et al. [51], who showed that episiotomies do not prevent tearing. We think that the indication for episiotomies should clearly be defined by an international committee and it should be restricted to special cases. Perineal damage

may occur not only spontaneously but also iatrogenically through the execution of an episiotomy. It is not at all "old-fashioned" to protect the perineum during vaginal delivery by hands-on methods.

We recommend not carrying out median and lateral episiotomies and being careful with mediolateral ones: As can be seen from a pathological specimen in Fig. 1.16, a perineal tear and/or a lateral episiotomy has led to a scar of the perineal body and the external anal sphincter. The connective tissue septa of the ischioanal fossa are irregular (Fig. 1.16a). At the border between

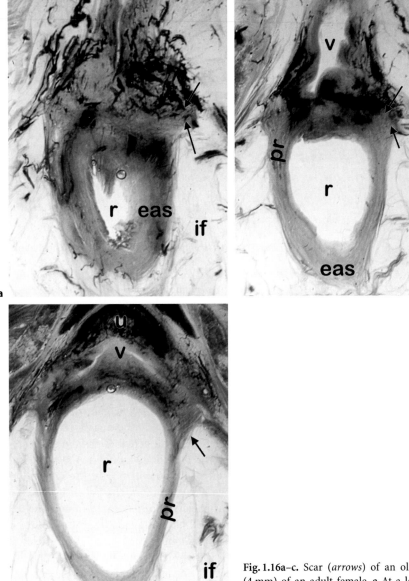

Fig. 1.16a–c. Scar (*arrows*) of an old perineal rupture in axial sections (4 mm) of an adult female. **a** At a level with the perineum. ×0.8. **b** At a level with the fusion of external anal sphincter and puborectalis muscle. ×0. **c** At a level with the rectal ampulla. ×0.8. *r*, rectum; *eas*, external anal sphincter; *if*, ischioanal fossa; *pr*, puborectalis muscle; *v*, vagina

the infralevatoric and levatoric level, it becomes visible that the vaginal wall is slightly displaced, the puborectalis is rather thin and the ischioanal fossa is not symmetric with the contralateral side (Fig. 1.16b), a diagnosis that still remains on supralevatoric levels (Fig. 1.16c). Refined and functional surgical treatment of perineal tears seems to be necessary to avoid such situations. As modern imaging techniques allow a fast and reliable examination, it is the gynecologists´ task to improve the surgical treatment.

References

1. Aigner F, Zbar AP, Kovacs P, Ludwikowski B, Kreczy A, Fritsch H (2004) The rectogenital septum: morphology, function and clinical relevance. Dis Colon Rectum 47:131–140
2. Bastian D, Lassau JP (1982) The suspensory mechanism of the uterus. Surg Radiol Anat 4:147–160
3. Beer-Gabel M, Teshler M, Barzilai N, Lurie Y, Malnick S, Bass D, Zbar A (2002) Dynamic transperineal ultrasound in the diagnosis of pelvic floor disorders. Dis Colon Rectum 45:239–248
4. Beets-Tan RGH, Beets GL, Vliegen RFA, Kessels AGH, Van Boven H, De Bruine A, von Meyenfeldt MF Baeten CGMI, van Engelshoven JMA (2001) Accuracy of magnetic resonance imaging in prediction of tumour-free resection margin in rectal cancer surgery. Lancet 357:497–505
5. Berglas B, Rubin IC (1953) Histologic study of the pelvic connective tissue. Surg Gynecol Obstet 97:277–289
6. Berrocal J, Clave H, Cosson M, Dedodinance Ph, Garbin O, Jacquetin B, Rosenthal C, Salet-Lizee D, Villet R (2004) Conceptual advances in the surgical management of genital prolapse. J Gynecol Obstet Biol Reprod 33:577–587
7. Brown G, Radcliffe AG, Newcombe RG, Dallimore NS, Bourne MW, Williams GT (2003) Preoperative assessment of prognostic factors in rectal cancer using high resolution magnetic resonance imaging. Br J Surg 90:355–364
8. Cundiff GW, Weidner AC, Visco AG, Addison A, Bump RC (1998) An anatomic and functional assessment of the discrete defect rectocele repair. Am J Obstet Gynecol 179:1451–1457
9. DeBlok S (1982) The connective tissue of the female fetal pelvic region. Acta Morphol Neerl Scand 20:65–92
10. DeBlok S (1982) The connective tissue of the adult female pelvic region. Acta Morphol Neerl Scand 20:325–346
11. DeBlok S, DeJong E (1980) The fibrous tissue architecture of the female perineal region. Acta Morphol Neerl Scand 18:181–194
12. DeLancey JO (1994) Structural support of the urethra as it relates to stress urinary incontinence: The hammock hypothesis. Am J Obstet Gynecol 170:1713–1723
13. DeLancey JO (1996) Standing anatomy of the pelvic floor. J Pelvic Surg 2:260–263
14. Dorschner W, Stolzenburg JV, Neuhaus J (2001) Structure and function of the bladder neck. Adv Anat Embryol Cell Biol 159:III–XII, 1–109
15. Federative Committee on Anatomical Terminology (1998) Terminologia Anatomica: International Anatomical Terminology. Georg Thieme Verlag, Stuttgart
16. Fielding JR, Griffiths DJ, Versi E, Mulkern RV, Lee ML, Jolesz FA (1998) MR imaging of pelvic floor continence mechanisms in the supine and sitting positions. AJR Am J Roentgenol 171:1607–1610
17. Fritsch H (1990) Development of the rectal fascia. Anat Anz 170:273–280
18. Fritsch H (1992) The connective tissue sheath of uterus and vagina in the human female fetus. Ann Anat 174:261–266
19. Fritsch H (1994) Topography and subdivision of the pelvic connective tissue. Surg Radiol Anat 16:259–265
20. Fritsch H, Brenner E, Lienemann A, Ludwikowski B (2002) Anal sphincter complex. Dis Colon Rectum 45:188–194
21. Fritsch H, Fröhlich B (1994) Development of the levator ani muscle in human fetuses. Early Hum Dev 37:15–25
22. Fritsch H, Kühnel W (1992) Development and distribution of adipose tissue in the pelvis. Early Hum Dev 28:79–88
23. Fritsch H, Kühnel W, Stelzner F (1996) Entwicklung und klinische Anatomie der Adventitia recti. Langenbecks Arch Chir 381:237–243
24. Fritsch H, Lienemann A, Brenner E, Ludwikowski B (2004) Clinical anatomy of the pelvic floor. Adv Anat Embryol Cell Biol 175:1–64
25. Gasparri F, Brizzi E (1961) Significato anatomo-chirurgico delle formazioni connecttivali del piccolo bacino. Arch Ital Anat Embriol 66:151–169
26. Gosling J (1999) Gross anatomy of the lower urinary tract. In: Abrams P, Khoury S, Wein AJ (eds) Incontinence. Plymbridge Distributors Ltd, Plymouth, pp 21–56
27. Grabbe E, Lierse W, Winkler R (1982) Die Hüllfascien des Rektums. Fortsch Röntgenstr 136:653–659
28. Heald RJ (1995) Total mesorectal excision is optimal surgery for rectal cancer. Br J Surg 82:1297–1299
29. Höckel M, Horn L-Ch, Fritsch H (2005) Association between the mesenchymal compartment of uterovaginal organogenesis and local tumour spread in stage IB–IIB cervical carcinoma: a prospective study. Lancet Oncol 6:751–756
30. Janssen U, Lienemann A, Fritsch H (2001) Die Bedeutung des M. levator ani – Fossa ischioanalis-Glutaeus maximus (LFG) – Komplexes für den weiblichen Beckenboden. Ann Anat Suppl 183:11
31. Khubchandani IT, Sheets JA, Stasik JJ, Hakki AR (1983) Endorectal repair of rectocele. Dis Colon Rectum 26:792–796
32. Koster H (1933) On the supports of the uterus. Am J Obstet Gynecol 25:67–74
33. Kux M, Fritsch H (2000) On the extraperitoneal origin of hernia. Hernia 4:259–263
34. Kocks J (1880) Normale und pathologische Lage und Gestalt des Uterus sowie deren Mechanik. Cohen, Bonn, pp 1–60
35. Lierse W (1984) Becken. In: von Lanz T, Wachsmuth W (eds) Praktische Anatomie, Bd 2, Teil 8A. Springer, Berlin Heidelberg New York Tokio
36. Ludwikowski B, Oesch-Hayward I, Fritsch H (2002) Rectovaginal fascia: an important structure in pelvic visceral surgery? About its development, structure, and function. J Pediatr Surg 37:634–638
37. Ludwikowski B, Oesch-Hayward I, Brenner E, Fritsch H (2001) The development of the external urethral sphincter in humans. BJU International 87:565–568
38. Mackenrodt A (1895) Ueber die Ursachen der normalen und pathologischen Lage des Uterus. Arch Gynaekol 48:393–421

39. Niemen K, Heinonen PK (2001) Sacrospinous ligament fixation for massive genital prolapse in women aged over 80 years. BJOG 108:817–821

40. Nobis A (1988) Untersuchungen zur feineren Struktur des retrorektalen Raumes beim Menschen. Inaugural Dissertation, Bonn

41. Occelli B, Narducci F, Hautefeuille J, Francke JP, Querleu D, Crepin G, Cosson M (2001) Anatomic study of arcus tendineus fasciae pelvis. Eur J Obstet Gynecol Reprod Biol 97:213–219

42. Oelrich TM (1983) The striated urogenital sphincter in the female. Anat Rec 205:223–232

43. Pernkopf E (1941) Topographische Anatomie des Menschen. Urban & Schwarzenberg, Berlin; Bd 2, Teil 1: Bd 2, Teil 2

44. Richardson AC (1993) The rectovaginal septum revisited: Its relationship to rectocele and its importance in rectocele repair. Clin Obstet Ggynecol 36:976–983

45. Richter K, Frick H (1985) Die Anatomie der Fascia pelvic visceralis aus didaktischer Sicht. Geburtsh Frauenheilk 45:282–287

46. Richter K (1998) Gynäkologische Chirurgie des Beckenbodens. Heinz F, Terruhn V (eds) Georg Thieme Verlag, Stuttgart New York

47. Roediger WEW, Tucker WG (1986) Thickening of the pelvic fascia in carcinoma of the rectum. Dis Colon Rectum 29:117–119

48. Sprenger D, Lienemann A, Anthuber C, Reiser M (2000) Funktionelle MRT des Beckenbodens: Normale anatomische und pathologische Befunde. Radiologe 40:458–464

49. Stelzner F (1989) Die Begründung, die Technik und die Ergebnisse der knappen transabdominalen Kontinenzresektion. Langenbecks Arch Chir 374:303–314

50. Stelzner F (1998) Chirurgie an vizeralen Abschlusssystemen. Georg Thieme, Stuttgart New York

51. Sultan AH, Kamm MA, Hudson CN, Thomas JM, Bartram CI (1993) Anal sphincter disruption during vaginal delivery. N Engl J Med 329:1905–1911

52. Thakar R, Stanton S (2002) Management of genital prolapse. BMJ 324:1258–1262

53. Tobin CE, Benjamin JA (1945) Anatomical and surgical study of Denonvilliers fascia. Surg Gynecol Obstet 80:373–

54. Uhlenhuth E, Nolley GW (1957) Vaginal fascia, a myth? Obstet Gynecol 10:349–358

55. Ulmsten U (2001) The basic understanding and clinical results of tension-free vaginal tape for stress urinary incontinence. Urologe 40:269–273

56. Waldeyer W (1899) Das Becken. Cohen, Bonn

57. Wilson PD, Dixon JS, Brown ADG, Gosling JA (1983) Posterior pubo-urethral ligaments in normal and genuine stress incontinent women. J Urol 130:802–805

58. Woodmann PJ, Graney DO (2002) Anatomy and physiology of the female perineal body with relevance to obstetrical injury and repair. Clin Anat 15:321–334

59. Zbar AP, Lienemann A, Fritsch H, Beer-Gabel M, Pescatori M (2003) Rectocele: pathogenesis and surgical management. Int J Colorectal Dis 29:1–11

MR and CT Techniques

Mathias Taupitz and Patrik Rogalla

CONTENTS

M. Taupitz, MD; P. Rogalla, MD
Institut für Radiologie, Charité – Universitätsmedizin Berlin,
Campus Mitte, Charitéplatz 1, 10117 Berlin, Germany

2.1
Magnetic Resonance Imaging

2.1.1
Introduction

With its intrinsic high soft tissue contrast, magnetic resonance imaging (MRI) has been the imaging modality of first choice for dedicated examinations of the female pelvis since the early 1990s. MRI is superior to CT in examinations of the true pelvis where CT is susceptible to beam-hardening artifacts due to adjacent bony structures which degrade image quality with regard to soft tissue detail. When MRI was first used for pelvic examinations, its spatial resolution was still limited. At that time, only the integrated whole-body resonator was available for abdominal imaging because coil systems such as a Helmholtz arrangement or flexible one-element surface coils had proved to be inadequate. Initially, abdominal imaging was performed exclusively with spin echo sequences, which enabled imaging only with a coarse matrix due to their rather long acquisition time. Important advances in abdominal MR imaging have been made since the mid-1990s through an improved signal-to-noise ratio (SNR) achieved with the newly introduced body phased-array coils. While the early phased-array coil systems with only few elements (e.g. four) improved pelvic imaging, the expanded phased-array coil systems available today have eight or more coil elements and allow high-resolution imaging of the entire abdomen. The earlier spin echo sequences have since been completely replaced with turbo spin echo sequences for the acquisition of both T1- and T2-weighted images. These techniques enable pelvic MRI studies with an excellent image quality when combined with suitable techniques for reducing motion artifacts. Motion artifacts continue to be a challenge in pelvic MRI. Respiratory and peristaltic motion is fast relative to the scan time necessary to obtain a morphologic sequence with a high spatial resolution (approximately 2–5 min). These motions can blur the abdominal organs and cause the well-known double contour artifacts in the phase-encoding direction. This is why special measures are needed to suppress motion artifacts. Fast imaging techniques with scan times of about 1 s per image are not sensitive to motion and can be used to obtain fast scout views or to image dynamic processes such as motion or contrast medium inflow. So-called whole-body MRI using whole-body phased-array coil systems is especially useful to combine the examination of the pelvis with imaging of the upper abdomen and chest in the staging of patients with pelvic malignancy. Pelvic MRI is performed at field strengths of 1.0–1.5 T with 1.5 T probably yielding the best results. Whole-body MR imagers operating at 3.0 T have recently become available for routine clinical use. Whether this higher field strength with its better SNR will actually improve the diagnostic yield of pelvic exams remains to be determined.

In this chapter, the most important general aspect of pelvic MRI will be discussed with regard to imaging hardware and technical aspects of the examination. The specific MR protocols used for different indications will be presented in the respective chapters.

2.1.2
Patient Preparation, Positioning, and Scan Planes

No special patient preparation is necessary for pelvic MRI in most cases, unless otherwise stated in the respective chapters. When making an appointment for a pelvic MRI, the patient should be informed about the most important aspects of an MR examination. This also includes questions regarding contraindications to MRI or to IV contrast agent administration. In this way, the patient may be spared a trip to the MRI center and an effective workflow in the MRI department is ensured. Moreover, the patient should be informed beforehand that a spasmolytic agent will be given to reduce artifacts due to bowel peristalsis, which would degrade image quality. Patients who will receive butyl scopolamine should be told that vision may be transiently impaired immediately after the examination. Finally, the patient should be asked about claustrophobia. If a patient is likely to need sedation, she has to be warned about possible adverse effects.

The standard position for pelvic MRI is the comfortable supine position with a bolster placed under the knees. Respiratory movement of the internal organs or abdominal wall will degrade pelvic MR

examinations though their effect is less pronounced as compared with MRI of the upper abdomen. A spatial presaturation slab should be positioned appropriately in a sagittal scout view to reduce signal intensity from moving anterior abdominal wall. However, this presaturation slab should not cover the inguinal region where enlarged lymph nodes might be present (Fig. 2.1). When imaging a patient on a scanner without a phased-array body coil, a belt should be used to minimize respiratory motion artifacts by restricting respiratory excursions. Before a patient is examined without breath-hold – i.e. during free breathing – she should be carefully instructed to breathe regularly and shallowly to minimize respiratory excursions of the abdominal wall. When a fast imaging technique is used, the patient should be carefully advised about the breathing instructions to be given when she should hold her breath. In patients in whom a contrast-enhanced examination is planned, a flexible indwelling line should be placed, ideally in an antecubital vein, and connected to an NaCl-filled syringe with a tube or, where available, to an MR-compatible injection pump.

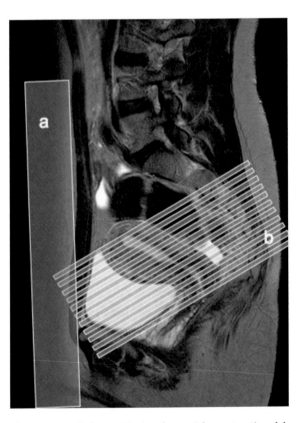

Fig. 2.1. Example for positioning the spatial presaturation slab (**a**) and the imaging slices (**b**) for an MRI examination of the uterine cervix. The specific MR protocols used for different indications are presented in the respective chapters

For optimal evaluation of the target organs (especially the uterine corpus and cervix, vagina, and adnexa), images need to be obtained in at least two scan planes perpendicular to each other. Typically, this is a sagittal plane angled parallel with the main organ axis and a second, paraxial image oriented perpendicular to the first plane. Evaluation of congenital anomalies or of the pelvic floor requires imaging in strict coronal or paracoronal planes. Images in strictly axial orientation are necessary for lymph node evaluation in oncologic patients. In these patients, the stack should extend from the region of the infrarenal abdominal aorta to the pelvic floor. The MR protocols for these indications are presented in the respective chapters. As a general rule, the diagnostic yield of all pelvic MRI examinations crucially relies on the careful planning of imaging planes used.

2.1.3
Coils

Nearly all vendors offer body or torso phased-array coils for abdominal MRI. These additional coils improve the SNR compared with standard body coils [2]. The gain in signal can be used to acquire fast sequences or, when conventional sequences are used, to acquire thinner slices compared with the whole-body resonator or simple surface coils. A relative disadvantage is that subcutaneous fatty tissue is depicted with a very high signal intensity, which may accentuate motion artifacts in images obtained without breath-hold. For this reason, imaging with a body phased-array coil without breath-hold should always be performed with presaturation to reduce the signal from the moving abdominal wall. However, care is required not to unduly saturate the inguinal region and its lymph nodes. Another option to reduce motion artifacts is fat suppression (see below). Apart from improving the SNR, a body phased-array coil with multiple elements (at least four) is a prerequisite for performing so-called parallel imaging (e.g. SENSE, sensitivity encoding; PAT, parallel acquisition technique), which reduces scan time relative to conventional sequences. Hence, parallel imaging can be used either to shorten the scan time of a given sequence or to improve resolution. Parallel imaging can be performed with T1- and T2-weighting but the SNR will be reduced [6]. Intracavitary coils yield a better image quality by improving the local SNR. The true pelvis, in particular the cervix, can be examined with an endorectal or endovaginal coil [1, 3, 5]. Intra-cavitary coils can be used alone or in combination with surface coil elements (phased array) as with MRI of the prostate.

2.1.4
Pulse Sequences

The standard protocol for pelvic imaging comprises unenhanced T1- and T2-weighted sequences. The high soft tissue contrast of MRI is a prerequisite for the reliable detection and characterization of pathology in the female pelvis. Spatial resolution and good visualization of anatomic detail are often equated with a high image quality. The latter, however, is predominantly determined by the absence of motion artifacts and a high SNR. As a general rule, the SNR increases with the acquisition time assuming there is efficient elimination of motion artifacts. This is why the best results in terms of image quality are achieved when using T1- and T2-weighted TSE sequences with multiple signal averages and a scan time of up to about 5 min. With these sequences, images with a matrix of up to 512 pixels in the frequency-encoding direction can be acquired. Only some general principles are discussed below while the specific MR protocols will be presented in the individual chapters.

2.1.4.1
T1-Weighted Imaging

T1-weighted images with good image quality and morphologic detail resolution are obtained by using TSE sequences with a short echo train (e.g. three) and an echo time of about 10 ms. A repetition time of approximately 400–600 ms will generate heavily T1-weighted images. Repeated image averaging (e.g. four) will average out motion artifacts. In cases where differentiation of blood or fat in a lesion is required (e.g. ovarian pathology, endometriosis), the T1-weighted TSE sequence can be combined with spectral fat suppression without unduly lengthening scan time.

In cases where a short scan time is a primary concern and excellent morphologic detail recognition is less important, T1-weighted gradient echo sequences can be used, e.g. multislice GRE sequences (FLASH or FFE) for breath-hold imaging. Depending on the performance of the gradient system available, between 5 and 25 slices can be acquired during a breath-hold of 15–25 s. In this way, the pelvis can be imaged with high contrast and good image quality in one plane during 1–3 breath-holds, depending on the number of slices and the slice thickness selected. Instead of a multislice GRE sequence with TRs of around 150 ms and TEs of about 5 ms, one can acquire sequential single slices with very short TRs and TEs (10–20 ms and 2–7 ms, respectively). To improve the low contrast associated with short TRs and TEs, these sequences are combined with an inversion prepulse (e.g. turbo FLASH or turbo FFE). Instead of the 2D GRE sequences, a 3D GRE sequence with fat suppression can be used (e.g. VIBE, volumetric interpolated breath-hold examination) [4]. The 3D GRE sequence has the advantage that thinner slices can be acquired. For instance, one can acquire 32 slices with a slice thickness of 5.0 mm in about 20–23 s and these can be interpolated to 64 slices of 2.5 mm. However, this 3D technique has a lower signal yield and contrast when used without contrast administration than the above-mentioned T1-weighted 2D sequence. The 3D GRE technique is most suitable to perform dynamic studies after IV injection of a gadolinium-based contrast medium. When a GRE technique is used, specific diagnostic information can be obtained by acquiring images under in-phase (IP) and opposed-phase (OP) conditions. The corresponding echo times needed to obtained IP and OP images vary with the field strength used. At 1.5 T, OP images are obtained at TEs of about 2.4 and 7.2 ms, IP images at TEs of 4.8 and 9.6 ms. Different image effects result from the addition or subtraction of signal contributions in the same voxel. As a rule, interfaces between tissues that differ in water or fat contents appear dark on the resulting image. This effect can provide diagnostic information, for example in differentiating lesions with a high fat content such as ovarian dermoid cysts.

2.1.4.2
T2-Weighted Imaging

T2-weighted pelvic imaging is nearly exclusively performed using turbo or fast spin echo (TSE or FSE) sequences, either with classical TSE sequences with the patient breathing freely or with single-shot TSE sequences during breath-hold (e.g. HASTE). With free breathing, the pelvic region can be scanned in 2–5 min as opposed to about 15–20 s with the single-shot breath-hold sequence. An examiner using a single-shot TSE sequence must be aware, however, that two tissues with very similar T2 relaxation times may be more difficult to differentiate than on images obtained with a standard T2-weighted TSE sequence. The usual echo times range from 90–130 ms. Another

fast T2-weighted sequence uses fast imaging with steady-state free precession (e.g. true FISP) and is employed in cardiac imaging and evaluation of other fast dynamic processes. Fat suppression is not routinely used for T2-weighted pelvic imaging but only to answer specific questions. The reason is that there is better delineation of intra-abdominal organs and of the pelvic wall on pelvic images acquired without fat suppression. As with T1-weighted sequences, the fat signal can be suppressed using spectral fat saturation. Alternatively, the fat signal can be nulled on T2-weighted images using the short time inversion recovery (STIR) technique. With this technique, the time from the inversion pulse to the point at which fat crosses through zero is used as inversion delay (100–170 ms). The STIR technique is not very susceptible to magnetic field inhomogeneities but scan time will be longer. This drawback can be compensated for by combining STIR with a TSE or FSE sequence (so-called turbo inversion recovery, TIR). STIR images combine T1 and T2 contrast with the T2 contribution being small at short TEs (< 30 ms) and somewhat greater at longer TEs (60 ms or more).

2.1.5
Spasmolytic Medication

The routine administration of a spasmolytic agent (Buscopan or Glucagon) is recommended for all pelvic MR examinations to reduce peristalsis-related motion artifacts, unless patients have contraindications to these agents. A longer-lasting effect is achieved with the IM injection of 40 mg Buscopan as compared with IV administration of this spasmolytic.

2.1.6
Contrast Agents

So-called unspecific IV contrast agents such as Magnevist (Gd-DTPA) or Dotarem (Gd-DOTA) are well established in the routine clinical setting. More recently, various nonionic or low-osmolar agents have become available. These include, Omniscan (gadodiamide, Gd-DTPA-BMA), Prohance (gadoteridol, Gd-HP-DO3A), and Optimark (gadoversetamide). All of these agents rapidly distribute in the extracellular space after injection and are eliminated renally. Hence, their pharmacokinetic behavior is comparable to that of iodine-based X-ray contrast agents as they are also used in CT. These contrast agents mainly act by markedly shortening T1 relaxation time. This effect is best appreciated on strongly T1-weighted sequences. The standard contrast medium dose for soft tissue imaging is 0.1 mmol Gd/kg body weight. If an additional MR angiography is planned, the contrast agent is administered at a dose of 0.2 mmol Gd/kg. In these cases, the contrast-enhanced morphologic MR examination may be performed after MR angiography. The contrast medium may be injected manually or automatically. A strict injection protocol is not required when static contrast-enhanced images are acquired. However, a standardized injection protocol with use of an MR-compatible, automatic injector is recommended when dynamic studies are performed. In both cases, contrast medium injection should be followed by a saline flush of 20 ml to ensure that all of the rather small amount of contrast medium of about 10–20 ml reaches the central veins.

2.2
CT Scanning Technique

There have been considerable technical advances in computed tomography in recent years. The most important technical development was the introduction of multislice scanners. The option to acquire and reconstruct more than one slice per gantry rotation offers new diagnostic potential for many applications. The diagnostic gain resulting from the advent of multislice CT is of special significance in examining organs that are often depicted with blurred contours due to respiratory motion on conventional spiral CT scans. The gain in speed can be exploited in one of two ways:

- On the one hand, overall scan time can be shortened as more slices are acquired per rotation. This reduces motion artifacts and enables better exploitation of intravenous contrast enhancement because there is only little change of the perfusion phase during the scan. In other words, the entire scan can be acquired during a defined phase of perfusion.
- On the other hand, thinner slices can be used. This has the advantage of reducing partial volume effects and, if a very small slice thickness, e.g. 1 mm, is used, offers the option of performing secondary image reconstruction that is comparable to the axial source images in terms of spatial resolution.

Depending on the scanner used, both advantages of multislice CT can be combined by finding a compromise between slice thickness and speed.

2.2.1
Spiral CT

With the advent of spiral CT scanners, it has become possible for the first time to continuously scan an anatomic region without having to interrupt data acquisition. This new technique has therefore almost completely eliminated the problem of misregistration of small anatomic or abnormal structures [7]. Incremental CT, the predecessor of spiral CT, was limited in the diagnostic evaluation of round pulmonary lesions, focal liver lesions, and lymph nodes because this technique might either miss such lesions or depict them twice when the patient moved between acquisitions [8]. This is why protocols for incremental CT are not presented here.

CT of the female pelvis can be performed alone but patients typically undergo CT scans of the upper abdomen and pelvis, especially when CT is done for staging of malignancy. Other indications include determination of the extent of thrombotic disease, evaluation of vascular supply, and diagnostic evaluation of other gynecologic conditions or follow-up of therapy.

Liver metastases from malignant tumors of the female pelvis are typically hypovascularized. These metastases can be most reliably detected during the portal venous phase of enhancement after contrast medium administration [9–11] while scanning during the arterial perfusion phase provides little additional diagnostic information, unless surgical resection or alternative therapy is planned and knowledge of the vascular supply is important for therapeutic decision-making [12, 13]. This means that examination of the upper abdomen should be performed with a scan delay of 50–70 s after the start of intravenous contrast medium administration in order to scan the liver while contrast between the enhancing normal liver and focal lesions is highest. The slice thickness should not be greater than 5 mm while the table increment per rotation (pitch factor) can be increased to 1.7 on spiral CT scanners. Care must be taken to scan the entire liver during a single breath-hold. The reconstruction interval should be smaller than the slice thickness, and reconstruction with an overlap of up to 50% of the slice thickness has been shown to be advantageous [8].

Depending on the speed and slice thickness selected, it may be possible to scan the liver and pelvis in a single breath-hold. A continuous scan has the advantage of an uninterrupted transition in the mid-abdomen but not all patients may be able to hold their breath that long. A scan impaired by respiratory motion degrades diagnostic quality more than does a planned interruption in mid-abdomen. Moreover, use of a thinner slice thickness is preferable to a continuous scan of the liver and pelvis.

If one plans to perform two scans, the liver can be scanned from bottom to top. In this way, there is better venous enhancement at the end of the scan, which reduces the risk of mistaking unfilled veins of the venous confluence above the liver for focal liver lesions. Another advantage of this direction is that one can continue to scan where required. Subsequently, the pelvis is examined during a second breath-hold.

In patients scheduled for a pelvic scan only, the start delay should be at least 60 s; practical experience suggests that 70–90 s are optimal. With this start delay, there is contrast enhancement of the iliac, external, internal, and common veins already at the beginning of the scan and it is thus possible to exclude venous thrombosis or tumor infiltration of the veins. Since perfusion of the pelvic organs such as the uterus is not a major diagnostic concern, it is not necessary to perform a scan of the early arterial phase.

2.2.2
Multislice CT

The higher speed of multislice CT scanners allows for performing a complete abdominal examination during one breath-hold. Two generations of multislice CT scanners can be distinguished: scanners which acquire four slices per gantry rotation (4-slice CT) and scanners which typically acquire 16 slices or more (16-slice CT). The 6-slice scanners also offered by some manufacturers can be classified as 4-slice scanners while the 10-slice scanners belong to the family of 16-slice scanners although there are slight differences.

2.2.2.1
4-Slice CT

With 4-slice CT scanners, the entire abdomen can be scanned continuously with slices as thin as 2–3 mm. When scanning from top to bottom, the liver should be imaged during the portal venous phase and the pelvis in a late phase (70 s). A scan of the abdomen and pelvis taking about 20–30 s, both the liver and the pelvis are imaged during the optimal imaging window when a start delay of 60 s is used.

In patients in whom the chest should be included in the scan for staging of cancer, it is recommended to perform a spiral chest scan prior to imaging of the liver. The preferred scan direction for the chest is from bottom to top; in this way the upper portions of the chest, which are least impaired by inadvertent respiratory motion, are scanned last. For the chest, a start delay of 30 s is recommended.

2.2.2.2
16-Slice to 64-Slice CT

A 16-slice scanner reduces the overall scan time to less than 15 s even when very thin slices are used. With most 16-slice CT scanners, the operator can only choose from two primary slice thicknesses, depending on detector width. In contrast, the pitch factor is variable; however, a pitch factor of 1 or slightly less than 1 provides optimal results on most CT scanners in terms of signal-to-noise ratio and slice sensitivity profile (SSP). Since effective scan time is not an issue on 16-slice scanners, there is no need to use a higher pitch factor.

As with other scanners, the liver should be scanned during the portal venous phase, immediately followed by scanning of the pelvis. When a continuous scan from top to bottom is performed with a delay of 60 s, the pelvis tends to be scanned too early. Here, the examiner must decide whether the advantage of an uninterrupted scan with the option of creating continuous coronal reconstructions is more important than scanning of the pelvis during the optimal imaging window.

Scanning on a 64-slice CT scanner requires only some minor adjustments of the scanning protocol. A continuous examination of the chest, abdomen, and pelvis may be beneficial in individual cases. When scanning from top to bottom, the scan delay for the chest should be between 50 and 55 s in order to scan the liver during the portal venous phase. However, with this delay, one will miss the phase of maximum enhancement of the pulmonary arteries.

For all multislice CT protocols, the reconstructed slice thickness for liver and pelvic scans should be 3–5 mm in all orientations. Thinner slices contain more noise and are less suitable for primary image interpretation. Thin slices are mostly acquired to generate multiplanar reformations with a comparable spatial resolution.

2.2.3
Positioning of the Patient

The patient should be positioned as comfortably as possible for any examination. For this purpose, special headrests, arm supports (particularly for supporting the arms in the above-head position), and cushion-like supports for the knees are available. The patient must be positioned on a soft surface, which should in addition be heat-insulated. Because most CT scanners are no longer water-cooled but dissipate their heat directly into the room air and because the scanner rooms must normally be fully air-conditioned for this reason, the patient should be covered with a protective sheet. None of the materials employed should contain silicate, glass or other absorbing substances, since the presence of these substances in the scan field can lead to artifacts or increased image noise as a result of beam hardening.

Most manufacturers assume that the patient will be in the "head-first" position, and the preset protocols are designed accordingly. A "head-first" position has the following disadvantages:

- The patient's head always moves through the gantry, which may not be tolerated by claustrophobic patients.
- The tube for intravenous contrast medium administration must be connected from behind the CT scanner; after being inserted, the venous access must first be closed and the reopened and connected to the contrast medium tube once the arms have been repositioned. Unfortunately, blood quite often drips onto the gantry during this procedure.
- If it suddenly becomes necessary to interrupt the examination and withdraw the patient from the gantry, the patient is "hanging" on the contrast medium tube, which is now drawn through the gantry and can become overstretched.
- The staff can talk to the patient only from behind his or her head or through the gantry.

With most CT scanners, the patient can be positioned "foot-first" as an alternative. This has the following advantages:

- The patient almost always lies with his or her head outside the gantry, can observe the procedure better and does not perceive the scanner as a tube.
- The contrast medium tube can be connected to the patient immediately after insertion of the venous access and before positioning of the arms.

- If the examination has to be interrupted (e.g. because the patient becomes nauseous), the radiographer or physician has direct access to the patient, and bringing the patient's arms down does not lead to tension on the contrast medium tube.
- Communication with the patient is face-to-face.

A disadvantage of the foot-first position is that most CT tables need to be extended for patients to be positioned comfortably without their legs dangling; the extension may prevent the table from being lowered far enough, and alterations are necessary if a head-first position is required (e.g. for additional head CT). The patient's direction must, without fail, be entered correctly in the examination protocol, since the left side may otherwise be taken for the right and some scanners do not allow later correction of the side identifiers.

2.2.4
Oral and Rectal Contrast Media

Two kinds of contrast media are available for oral and rectal administration: iodinated, aqueous solutions and barium sulfate suspensions. Both substances are used alike, and no serious side effects have so far been reported when properly dosed. Nevertheless, iodinated solutions have some pharmacological and physical properties that make them superior to barium sulfate suspensions:

- Iodinated solutions have a moderately positive effect on intestinal peristalsis, resulting in faster transit to distal loops of the ileum within 30–60 min after oral administration. Disadvantage: Mild diarrhea in rare cases.
- Iodinated solutions spread evenly through the bowel and, unlike barium sulfate, do not tend to flocculate. Large lumps of barium can become so radiodense that artifacts result and mural processes are obscured.
- In some patients, the use of barium sulfate causes circular thickening of the bowel wall – mainly in distal small bowel segments – which closely resembles the appearance of enteritis and can be misinterpreted. This effect may be attributable to edematous swelling of the mucosa due to the hydrophilic nature of the barium sulfate suspension.
- Only iodinated and, sometimes, no oral contrast medium at all should be given if the potential differential diagnosis includes bowel perforation.

Administering a liter of contrast medium over a period of 1 h before the examination has proved its value. Some radiologists add 20 mg of metoclopramide (MCP, 2 tablets) to the first beaker of contrast medium in order to speed up transit, which typically shortens patient preparation to 30 min. Side effects of metoclopramide – diarrhea and muscle tremor – are unlikely on single administration.

The same substances are available as rectal contrast media. Rectal contrast administration is a troublesome, time-consuming procedure for both the examiner and the patient. With some patients, the doctor must overcome a considerable sense of embarrassment, apart from the sometimes painful introduction of the rectal tube owing to hemorrhoids. An enema should nevertheless be given for every pelvic examination as long as there are no contraindications such as anal carcinoma or deep rectal carcinoma. In these cases, and if the presence of such a disease is suspected, a digital examination must be performed beforehand in order to avoid iatrogenic perforation by forceful, uncontrolled introduction of the rigid tube.

Despite the diagnostic advantages of complete rectal opacification, some radiologists still hesitate to use it routinely. "Mini-contrasting" using a disposable enema set has proved to be an excellent alternative. After removal of the cap on the enema syringe, the fluid contained in it is made up to 200 ml with tap water and about 10 ml iodinated contrast medium (300 mg/ml) is then added to it. The syringe can be inserted either by the physician or by the patient. It is more comfortable for the patient if the enema is warmed up to body temperature beforehand (in the warming cabinet for intravenous contrast medium).

The use of pure tap water without the addition of radiopaque substances is a fundamentally different approach to oral and rectal opacification. It is almost impossible to achieve complete filling of the small intestine and certainly not of the large intestine with water, since normal enteral absorption prevents retention of water in the bowel lumen. Water absorption is effectively inhibited by the addition of mannitol. The best effect is achieved with 250 ml mannitol (5%) in 750 ml of water or juice. Administration of "negative" oral and rectal contrast medium is required only for differentiation of the mucosa and intestinal lumen if adequate intravenous contrast enhancement can be achieved.

2.2.5
Intravenous Contrast Media

An unenhanced scan is not required for most pelvic indications, the only exception being patients with suspected calcifications, for example when there are tumor implants from ovarian cancer. Nonionic, iodine-based contrast media are used for intravenous contrast. They are typically injected into an antecubital vein using a power injector. In contrast to CT of the lung or heart, the contrast medium concentration is irrelevant for pelvic examinations. A saline flush following contrast medium injection, which is useful for chest scans, is not required for pelvic examinations. A dose of 90–120 ml contrast medium with a concentration of 300–370 mg iodine/ml administered at a rate of 2–3 ml/s is sufficient. For CT angiography of the pelvic arteries, it is advisable to determine individual circulation time by using a bolus-tracking program, to choose a faster injection rate (3–5 ml/s), and to scan the pelvis during the arterial phase.

An additional late scan 120–180 s after intravenous contrast administration may be helpful to exclude deep pelvic vein thrombosis or if there is poor visualization of pelvic veins on the arterial phase scans (Fig. 2.2). Depending on the patient's pelvic circumference, the late scan may be acquired with a reduced tube current, e.g. 50 mAsec. Late scans obtained after 3–5 min are also suitable for evaluation of the bladder, which, at this time, contains part of the renally eliminated contrast medium. Even filling of the bladder with contrast medium is achieved by rotating the patient about her longitudinal axis.

2.2.6
Image Postprocessing

Since workstations have different user surfaces, it is next to impossible to give general guidelines on how to postprocess CT data sets. However, some clues as to what kind of postprocessing is useful for specific diagnostic purposes are included with the individual protocols. Some general recommendations can be given to obtain postprocessed images of a high quality:

- Use of the thinnest slice thickness justifiable (isotropic voxels where needed).
- Slice reconstruction with an overlap of 30%–60% for spiral CT and 10%–20% for multislice CT.
- For 3D reconstructions, use of a reconstruction filter that does not highlight the edges too much (soft tissue filter).

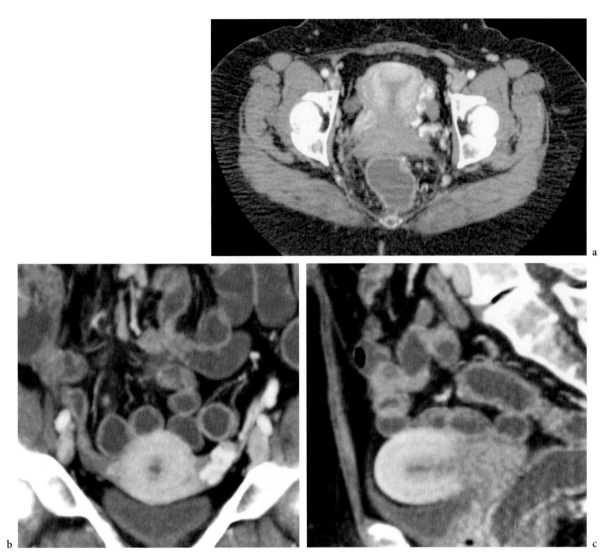

Fig. 2.2a-c. A 47-year-old, obese patient. Pelvic scan obtained 70 s after intravenous contrast medium administration. Note that there is still incomplete opacification of the pelvic veins. There is strong perfusion of the myometrium and the zonal anatomy of the uterus is clearly seen in all three planes: axial (**a**), coronal (**b**), sagittal (**c**). The ovarian vein on the left is dilated by varicosis and shows more pronounced enhancement due to reflux from the left renal vein. The intestinal tract was opacified with water and mannitol

- Scanning with a minimum of artifacts due to patient motion and other causes.

2.2.7
Image Documentation

Many users of spiral and multislice CT scanners have switched from conventional image interpretation to primary digital interpretation on the monitor. The interactive options have numerous advantages and digital processing also offers long-term savings on film cost. However, only very few hospitals and departments are completely digitalized and have the facilities for digital image transfer to all departments or referring physicians. This is why it is still necessary to document image data on X-ray films or in the form of normal paper printouts.

Depending on the film and technical prerequisites, 16 on 1 or 20 on 1 documentation using a 42*35 cm format appears to be sufficient for diagnostic purposes. Reconstructed images, in particular color images, can be printed out on DICOM-capable ink jet or laser printers. For documentation of reconstructed thin-slice data sets, the number of films required can be reduced by regularly skipping images.

The author advises against individual adjustment of window levels for documentation because it reduces the comparability of gray-scale values. Based on our practical experience, we recommend window levels of 400/50 for soft tissue, 1300/–500 for the lung, and 1700–2300/300 for bone.

2.2.8
Summary

CT of the pelvis is predominantly performed for cancer staging, which means that the CT examination should include the upper abdomen. Scanning of the pelvis during a specific perfusion phase is less critical than for the liver, which should be scanned during the portal venous phase 50–70 s after intravenous contrast medium injection. If the scans are obtained too early, there is the risk of overlooking thromboses due to incomplete enhancement of the pelvic veins.

When planning the CT scan, care should be taken to include the entire pelvis to below the pubic bone. The field of view should be chosen such that all pelvic bone structures and the gluteal muscles are depicted. Too small a field of view impairs spatial resolution if the reconstructed images are optically magnified for better documentation.

For examinations on a multislice scanner, thin slices should be used to compute high-quality multiplanar reformations. However, for interpretation of the source images, the reconstruction slice thickness should not be less than 3–5 mm, regardless of the slice orientation.

As for all CT examinations, radiation protection is a critical concern, especially for pelvic scans. It is highly recommended to use tube modulation in all cases and in particular in women with very oval pelvic shape (extensive subcutaneous fat). Here, tube modulation will improve image quality and reduce predominantly horizontal artifacts.

For oral and rectal contrast, radiopaque substances are available or water or a mixture of water and mannitol can be used. The latter should be used only when there is good intravenous enhancement. Only nonionic contrast media should be used for intravenous contrast. For routine clinical administration, a total dose of 90–120 ml of a contrast medium with a concentration of 300–370 mg injected at a rate of 2–3 ml/s is recommended.

2.2.9
Summary of CT Protocols

2.2.9.1
Pelvis

Anatomic region	From pelvic inlet/lower kidney pole to below pubic bone	
Scout image	350 mm, 120 kV, 10–50 mA	
Contrast medium	IV:	90–120 ml nonionic CM, iodine content of 300–370 mg/ml
	Oral:	1000 ml over 60 min
	Rectal:	500 ml or "mini enema"
Injection rate	2–3 ml/s	
Scan delay	70–90 s after start of bolus	
CT parameters	120 kV, 100–200 mAsec, inspiration	
	Spiral:	8 mm slice thickness, 8–12 mm table feed
	MS-CT:	2 mm slice thickness, pitch factor of 1–1.5:1
		1 mm slice thickness, pitch factor of 1–1.5:1
		Top-to-bottom scan direction
Reconstruction	Spiral:	4 mm interval, soft tissue filter
	MS-CT:	5 mm slice thickness, 4 mm interval,
		soft tissue filter
		1 mm slice thickness, 0.8–1 mm interval, soft tissue filter
Documentation	12–20 on 1	
	Patient information, scout image with/without scan lines, all images (MS-CT), every other image (spiral) in soft tissue window from top to bottom	

2.2.9.2
Abdomen and Pelvis

Anatomic region	From diaphragm to pubic bone
Scout image	500 mm, 120 kV, 10–50 mA
Contrast medium	IV: 90–120 ml nonionic CM, iodine content of 300–370 mg/ml
	Oral: 1000 ml over 60 min
	Rectal: 500 ml or "mini edema"
Injection rate	2–3 ml/s
Scan delay	50–60 s *For continuous scan from top to bottom*
	50–60 s for bottom-to-top scan of upper abdomen, break, followed by bottom-to-top pelvic scan
CT parameters	120 kV, 100–200 mAsec, inspiration
	Spiral: 8 mm slice thickness, 8–12 mm table feed
	1. Abdominal spiral, from tip of liver to diaphragm
	2. Pelvic spiral, from pubic bone to tip of liver
	MS-CT: 2 mm slice thickness, pitch factor of 1–1.5:1
	1 mm slice thickness, pitch factor of 1–1.5:1
	Top-to-bottom scan direction
Reconstruction	Spiral: 4 mm interval, soft tissue filter
	MS-CT: 5 mm slice thickness, 4 mm interval
	soft tissue filter, lung portions with lung filter
	1 mm slice thickness, 0.8–1 mm interval, soft tissue filter
Documentation	12–20 on 1
	Patient information, scout image with/without scan lines, all images (MS-CT), every other image (spiral) in soft tissue window from top to bottom, lung portions in lung window

2.2.9.3
Chest, Abdomen, and Pelvis

Region	From above clavicle to below pubic bone
Scout image	800 mm, 120 kV, 10–50 mA
Contrast medium	IV: 100–120 ml nonionic CM, iodine content of 300–370 mg/ml
	Oral: 1000 ml over 60 min
	Rectal: 500 ml or "mini edema"
Injection rate	2–3 ml/s
Scan delay	25–30 s *For bottom-to-top scan of chest, break, followed by top-to-bottom scan of abdomen and pelvis*
	25–30 s For continuous top-to-bottom scan (MS-CT only)
	50–60 s For bottom-to-top scan (abdomen and chest), break, followed by pelvic scan
CT parameters	120 kV, 50–100 mAs (chest), inspiration
	120 kV, 100–200 mAsec (abdomen, pelvis), inspiration
	Spiral: 8 mm slice thickness, 8–12 mm table feed
	1. Abdominal spiral, from tip of liver to diaphragm
	2. Chest spiral, from recesses to above clavicle
	3. Pelvic spiral, from pubic bone to tip of liver
	MS-CT: 2 mm slice thickness, pitch factor of 1–1.5:1
	1 mm slice thickness, pitch factor of 1–1.5:1
	1. Chest spiral, from recesses to above clavicle
	2. Abdominal spiral, diaphragm to pubic bone
Reconstruction	Spiral: 4 mm interval
	1st spiral with soft tissue filter
	2nd spiral with lung filter
	3rd spiral with soft tissue filter
	MS-CT: 5 mm slice thickness, 4 mm interval
	soft tissue filter (all), lung portions with lung filter
	1 mm slice thickness, 0.8–1 mm interval, soft tissue filter
Documentation	12–20 on 1
	Patient information, scout image with/without scan lines, all images (MS-CT), every other image (spiral) in soft tissue window from top to bottom, lung portions in lung window

References

1. Corn BW, Schnall MD, Milestone B, King S, Hauck W, Solin LJ (1996) Signal characteristics of tumors shown by high-resolution endorectal coil magnetic resonance imaging may predict outcome among patients with cervical carcinoma treated with irradiation. A preliminary study. Cancer 78:2535–2542

2. Helmberger T, Holzknecht N, Lackerbauer CA, Muller Lisse U, Schnarkowski P, Gauger J, Reiser M (1995) Array-Oberflachenspule und Atemanhaltetechnik bei der MRT der Leber. Vergleich konventioneller Spinechosequenzen mit schnellen, fettunterdruckenden Gradientenecho- und Turbospinechosequenzen. Radiologe 35:919–924

3. Kinkel K, Chapron C, Balleyguier C, Fritel X, Dubuisson JB, Moreau JF (1999) Magnetic resonance imaging characteristics of deep endometriosis. Hum Reprod 14:1080–1086

4. Rofsky NM, Lee VS, Laub G, Pollack MA, Krinsky GA, Thomasson D, Ambrosino MM, Weinreb JC (1999) Abdominal MR imaging with a volumetric interpolated breath-hold examination. Radiology 212:876–884

5. Soutter WP, Hanoch J, D'Arcy T, Dina R, McIndoe GA, DeSouza NM (2004) Pretreatment tumour volume measurement on high-resolution magnetic resonance imaging as a predictor of survival in cervical cancer. Bjog 111:741–747

6. Vogt FM, Antoch G, Hunold P, Maderwald S, Ladd ME, Debatin JF, Ruehm SG (2005) Parallel acquisition techniques for accelerated volumetric interpolated breath-hold examination magnetic resonance imaging of the upper abdomen: assessment of image quality and lesion conspicuity. J Magn Reson Imaging 21:376–382

7. Bluemke D, Fishman E (1993) Spiral CT of the liver. AJR Am J Roentgenol 160:787–792

8. Urban B, Fishman E et al. (1993) Detection of focal hepatic lesions with spiral CT: comparison of 4- and 8-mm interscan spacing. Am J Roentgenol 160:783–785

9. Bluemke D, Soyer P et al. (1995) Helical (spiral) CT of the liver. Radiol Clin North Am 33:863–886

10. Foley WD, Mallisee TA, et al. (2000) Multiphase hepatic CT with a multirow detector CT scanner. Am J Roentgenol 175:679–685

11. Tempany C, Zou K, et al. (2000) Staging of advanced ovarian cancer: comparison of imaging modalities – report from the Radiological Diagnostic Oncology Group. Radiology 215:761–767

12. Valls C, Andia E, et al. (2001) Hepatic metastases from colorectal cancer: preoperative detection and assessment of resectability with helical CT. Radiology 218:55–60

13. Kopka L, Rogalla P, et al. (2002) Multislice CT of the abdomen – current indications and future trends. Fortschr Geb Röntgenstr Neuen Bildgeb Verfahr 174:273–282

Normal Imaging Findings of the Uterus

Claudia Klüner and Bernd Hamm

CONTENTS

3.1
Embryonic Development and Normal Anatomy of the Uterus

During embryonal life, fusion of the two Müllerian ducts gives rise to the uterine corpus, isthmus, cervix, and the upper third of the vagina. The Müllerian ducts are of mesodermal origin and arise in the 4th week of gestation. They course on both sides lateral to the ducts of the mesonephros (Wolffian ducts). The lower two thirds of the vagina arise from the sinovaginal bulb, which develops from the posterior portion of the urogenital sinus. The vaginal epithelium arises from the cellular lining of the urogenital sinus [1].

The uterus is composed of three distinct anatomic regions, namely the corpus, the isthmus (or lower uterine segment), and the cervix. In women of reproductive age, the uterus usually is 6–9 cm long and weighs 40–60 g. The longitudinal axis is flexed forward (anteversion) with the corpus and cervix forming a blunt angle (anteflection) (Fig. 3.1a). The uterus straightens with increasing bladder filling and the anteversion angle becomes smaller (Fig. 3.1b).

The wall of the uterine corpus differs from that of the cervix in that it mostly consists of myometrium, the strong muscle coat forming the mass of the organ. The myometrium is mostly comprised of spindle-shaped smooth muscle cells and additionally contains reserve connective tissue cells, which give rise to additional myometrial cells in pregnancy through hyperplasia. The uterine cavity is only a thin cleft and is lined by endometrium (Fig. 3.2). Functionally, the endometrium consists of basal and functional layers.

The isthmus of uterus (lower uterine segment), together with the internal os, forms the junction between the corpus and cervix. In nonpregnant women the isthmus is only about 5 mm high and is less muscular than the corpus. Unlike the uterine cervix, the isthmus becomes overproportionally large in the course of pregnancy and serves as a kind of reserve for fetal development in addition to the uterine corpus. The endometrium of the isthmus consists of a single layer of columnar epithelium and only undergoes abortive cyclic transformation.

The uterine cervix consists of the supravaginal cervical canal (endocervix) and the vaginal portion that projects into the vagina (Fig. 3.3). The wall of the cervix is primarily made up of firm connective tissue. In contrast to the uterine corpus, the muscular portion accounts for less than 10% of the cervical wall and primarily consists of smooth muscle cells in circular arrangement. The cervical canal is coated with mucus-producing columnar epithelium and contains numerous gland-like units, the crypts. The squamocolumnar junction is the transition from the columnar epithelium of the endocervix to the nonkeratinizing squamous epithelium of the ectocervix and is situated at the level of the external os.

The uterus is supplied with blood through the uterine and ovarian arteries. The uterine arteries course to the organ through the cardinal ligaments and, at the level of the uterine isthmus (internal os of the cervical canal), divide into an ascending and a descending branch. Lymphatic drainage from the corpus is through the broad ligament into the para-aortic lymph nodes and from the cervix into parametrial and iliac lymph nodes.

C. KLÜNER, MD
Institut für Radiologie (Campus Mitte), Charité – Universitäts-medizin Berlin, Charitéplatz 1, 10117 Berlin, Germany
B. HAMM, MD
Professor and Chairman, Institut für Radiologie (Campus Mitte), Klinik für Strahlenheilkunde (Campus Virchow-Klinikum und Campus Buch), Charité – Universitätsmedizin Berlin, Charitéplatz 1, 10117 Berlin, Germany

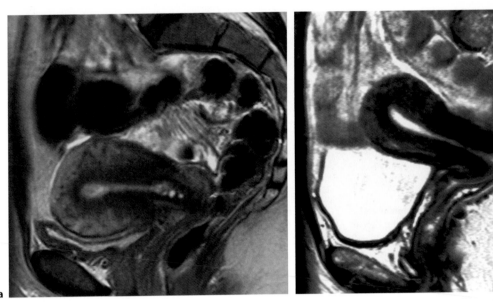

a   b

Fig. 3.1a,b. T2-weighted TSE images of two different healthy premenopausal women in sagittal orientation

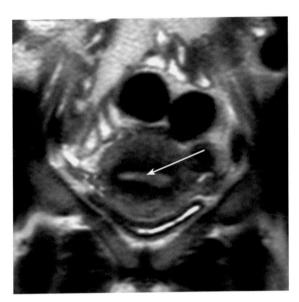

Fig. 3.2. T2-weighted TSE image of a 40-year-old healthy woman in coronal orientation. The uterine cavity is marked by the *white arrow*

Besides the pelvic floor, the normal topography of the uterus is primarily ensured by the parametria, a kind of suspension system primarily consisting of connective tissue. In addition, the parametria contain large amounts of fatty tissue, especially in their lateral portions near the pelvic sidewall and a dense network of lymphatic and blood vessels. About 2 cm lateral to the uterine cervix, both ureters course through the parametria and cross the uterine arteries (Fig. 3.4).

Below, the parametria extend to the cardinal ligament, which passes from the uterine cervix to the pelvic sidewall and separates the parametrium from the paravaginal connective tissue (paracolpium). A total of eight ligaments contribute to the support of the uterus. Diagnostically, which primarily pertains to the evaluation of the local extent of cervical cancer, the vesicouterine and the sacrouterine ligaments are most important. The vesicouterine ligament extends from the cervix to the posterior wall of the urinary bladder and only has a minor role in supporting the uterus. The sacrouterine ligament has a more important supportive function and originates on the anterior aspect of the sacral bone, arches around the rectum and attaches at the level of the uterine isthmus.

Most of the uterus is covered by peritoneum (Fig. 3.5). The peritoneum contributes only little support but ensures adequate mobility of the uterus relative to the urinary bladder and rectum, which is necessary to adjust to the variation in bladder filling and especially during pregnancy. The peritoneum extends from the roof of the urinary bladder to the anterior uterine wall, forming the vesicouterine pouch in between. Below this fold, there is the vesicouterine ligament. The posterior peritoneal coat of the uterus extends downward to form the rectouterine pouch (Douglas space) that reaches to the level of the posterior vaginal fornix and from there extends to cover the anterior rectal wall.

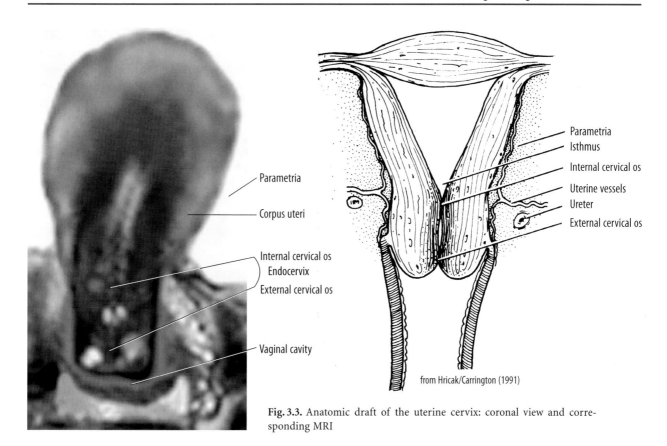

Parametria

Corpus uteri

Internal cervical os
Endocervix

External cervical os

Vaginal cavity

Parametria
Isthmus

Internal cervical os

Uterine vessels
Ureter

External cervical os

from Hricak/Carrington (1991)

Fig. 3.3. Anatomic draft of the uterine cervix: coronal view and corresponding MRI

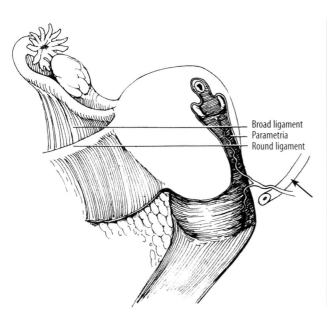

Broad ligament
Parametria
Round ligament

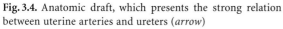

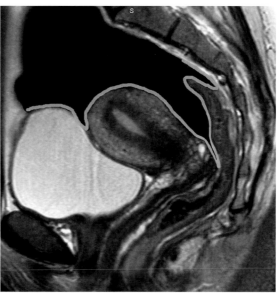

Fig. 3.4. Anatomic draft, which presents the strong relation between uterine arteries and ureters (*arrow*)

Fig. 3.5. T2-TSE image in sagittal orientation. The extension of the peritoneum is marked by the *grey line*

3.2
Imaging Findings: Uterine Corpus

The imaging appearance of the uterine corpus varies widely with the age and hormonal status of the patients examined [2–7].

On unenhanced CT scans, the layered anatomy of the wall cannot be distinguished. After administration of contrast medium, the myometrium can be distinguished in most cases during the arterial phase as it shows early and strong enhancement while the junctional zone/endometrium is of relatively low density (Fig. 3.6). As with MRI, the endometrium and junctional zone cannot be differentiated in most cases on the basis of their morphologic appearance on CT. In most cases, venous plexuses can be identified within the parametria on the basis of their strong enhancement. However, reliable differentiation of myometrium from parametrial portions is usually not possible while the peripheral fatty portions of the parametrium can be distinguished from the pelvic wall with an adequate degree of accuracy.

Unenhanced T1-weighted MRI depicts the uterine corpus with a low and homogeneous signal intensity similar to that of skeletal muscle (Fig. 3.7a and b).

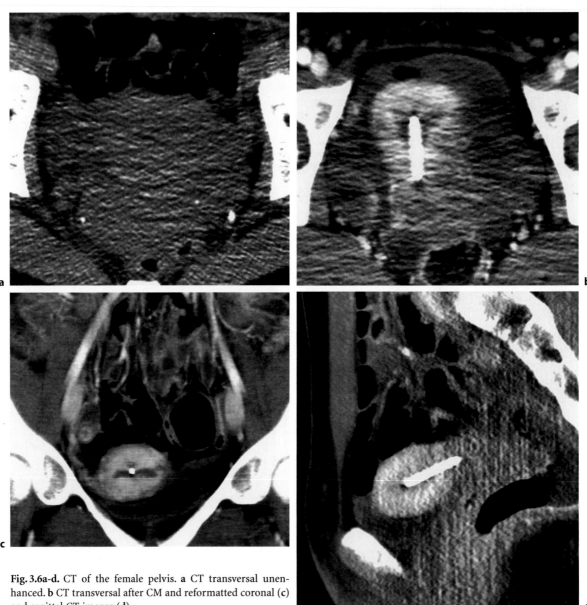

Fig. 3.6a-d. CT of the female pelvis. **a** CT transversal unenhanced. **b** CT transversal after CM and reformatted coronal (**c**) and sagittal CT images (**d**)

Thus, it is not possible to differentiate the individual layers.

On the other hand, T2-weighted MR images in women of reproductive age clearly depict the three layers of the uterine corpus: the endometrium, the junctional zone, and the myometrium (Fig. 3.7c and d) [8].

The endometrium always has a high signal intensity on T2-weighted images regardless of the hormonal state and age while its thickness clearly varies in the course of the menstrual cycle [9]. The thickness ranges from 1–3 mm in the early proliferative phase (Fig. 3.7 and 3.8) and 5–10 mm in the middle of the secretory phase (Fig. 3.9 and 3.10). The endometrium is thickest under the effect of estradiol (follicular phase) on days 8 through 16 of the cycle [10]. After day 16, when the effect of progesterone becomes stronger (luteal phase), there is hardly any further increase in thickness but primarily a transformation of the mucosa with increased formation of glands and ingrowth of vessels. During menstruation, a blood clot may occasionally be present in the uterine cavity (Fig. 3.9), which must not be mistaken for a foreign body, polyp, or submucosal myoma.

The layer adjacent to the endometrium that can be distinguished on MRI is the junctional zone, which corresponds to the inner part of the myometrium and is hypointense on T2-weighted images relative to the outer portion of the myometrium. The lower signal is primarily attributable to a lower water content, the higher nucleus-to-cytoplasm ratio, and the smaller extracellular space of the inner myometrium [11, 12].

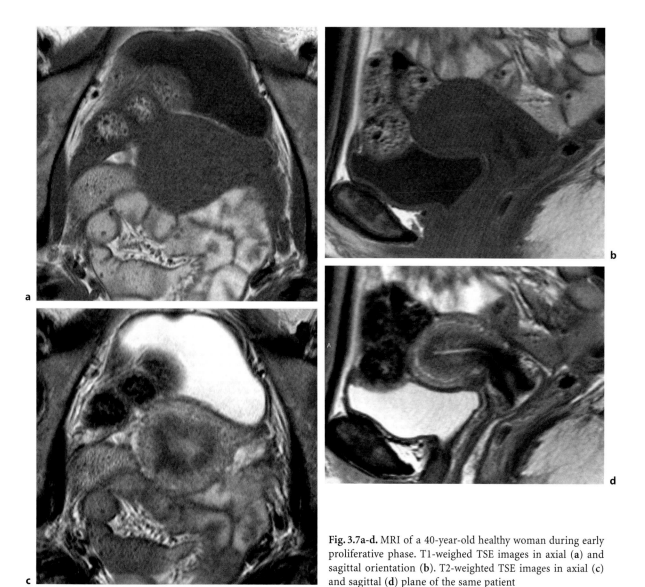

Fig. 3.7a-d. MRI of a 40-year-old healthy woman during early proliferative phase. T1-weighed TSE images in axial (**a**) and sagittal orientation (**b**). T2-weighted TSE images in axial (**c**) and sagittal (**d**) plane of the same patient

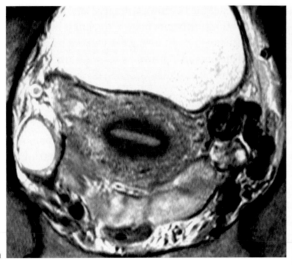

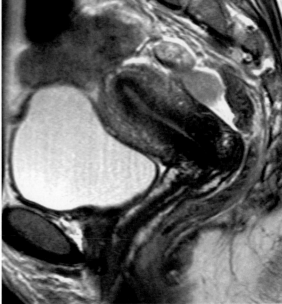

Fig. 3.8a,b. MRI of a healthy woman during early proliferative phase (T2-weighted TSE in axial and sagittal plane)

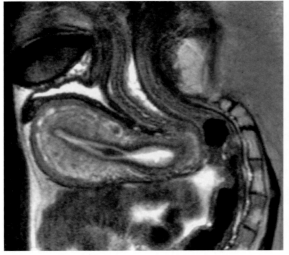

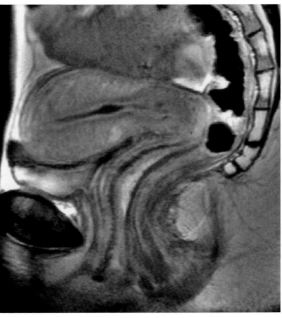

Fig. 3.9a,b. MRI of a healthy woman during secretory phase. The T2-weighed TSE image (a) as well as the contrast-enhanced T1-weighted TSE image (b), both in sagittal orientation demonstrate a blood clot (*arrow*) in the uterine cavity

Similar to the endometrium, the junctional zone also varies over the menstrual cycle and is thickest around the 24th day. The mean thickness of the junctional zone does not exceed 5 mm under normal conditions. A focal thickness of over 12 mm of the junctional zone can be interpreted as a sign of adenomyosis. However, a focal pathologic thickening of the junctional zone has to be differentiated from uterine contractions. Uterine contractions may be diagnosed by a repeated T2-weighted sequence a view minutes later, showing a normal appearance of the former thickened junctional zone in contrast to unchanged appearance of adenomyosis. By using cine MRI sequences (SSFSE: single-shot half-Fourier fast spin echo) it was furthermore shown that the junctional zone maintains cervicofundal contractions that vary with the phase of the cycle [13] and are assumed to have a role in transporting sperm and in maintaining early pregnancy.

The normal outer myometrium is of an intermediate signal intensity on T2-weighted images. Its signal intensity is slightly higher during the secretory phase due to an increased fluid content, which improves the differentiation from the junctional zone as compared with other phases of the cycle (comparison of Figs. 3.7 and 3.10). Vessels in the myometrium are also highly prominent during this phase of the cycle. Ultrasonography likewise depicts three uterine layers but the thickness of the junctional zone and of the endometrium determined by ultrasound and MRI clearly differ, especially during the luteal phase [14]. This discrepancy is attributed to the fact that ultrasound does not demonstrate the three layers in the same way as MRI [15].

Following intravenous administration of a paramagnetic contrast medium, the zonal anatomy of the uterus is also depicted on T1-weighted images (Fig. 3.9b). Both the endometrium and the outer myometrium are characterized by pronounced contrast enhancement while the junctional zone is of low signal intensity. This is attributed to the denser tissue and smaller extracellular volume of distribution of the contrast medium [12, 16].

The uterus of newborns still shows good differentiation of the myometrium, junctional zone, and endometrium as a result of the effect of maternal estrogen. Before the onset of menstruation, the endometrium is merely seen as a very thin stripe of high signal intensity or not at all and the junctional zone is not distinguishable from the low-signal-intensity myometrium. The corpus is smaller than the cervix during this phase while in adult women the length ratio of the cervix to the corpus is 1:2.

After menopause the uterine corpus as a whole is markedly smaller (Figs. 3.11 and 3.12) with a length ratio of nearly 1:1. On T2-weighted images the endometrium is seen as a thin central stripe of high signal intensity. The myometrium has a markedly lower signal intensity as compared with women of reproductive age and is therefore difficult to distinguish from the junctional zone, which also has a low signal intensity. The endometrium decreases in thickness to about 3–5 mm. However, in women on external hormone replacement therapy, the premenopausal signal pattern and zonal anatomy may be preserved. In this situation the endometrium may be up to 10 mm thick.

Exogenous hormonal replacement may considerably alter the MRI appearance of the uterus and vagina. In premenopausal women taking oral contraceptives, the signal intensity of the myometrium is increased [17]. Moreover, the junctional zone appears thinner and is more difficult to differentiate.

Long-term use of oral contraceptives is also associated with marked thinning of the endometrium. In women on GnRH analogues, the uterus is comparable to the premenopausal uterus in terms of size and signal intensities with depiction of the endometrium as a very thin stripe of high signal intensity that is clearly delineated from the low-intensity myometrium. The junctional zone is not seen or very difficult to distinguish. Despite its anti-estrogen activity,

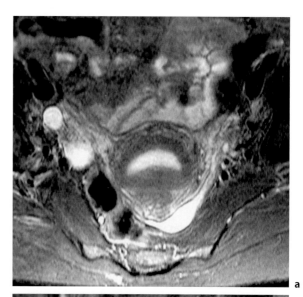

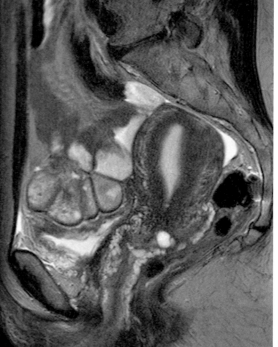

Fig. 3.10a,b. MRI of a healthy woman during secretory phase (T2-weighted TSE)

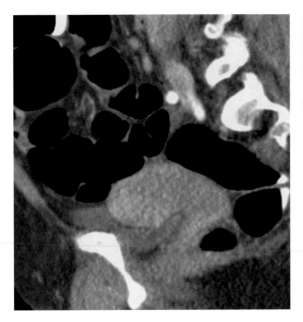

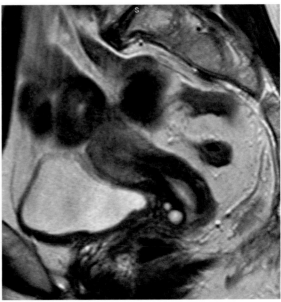

Fig. 3.11. Reformatted sagittal CT image of a 55-year-old woman, who underwent MSCT for polyp detection of the colon

Fig. 3.12. T2-weighted MRI of a healthy 58-year-old woman

tamoxifen treatment in postmenopausal women has an effect that is comparable to that of oral contraceptives: There is a clear increase in the thickness of the endometrium. Moreover, the endometrium becomes increasingly heterogenous, which may be misinterpreted as endometrial cancer [18].

3.3
Imaging Findings: Uterine Cervix

In contrast to the uterine corpus, the uterine cervix shows only little variation of its zonal anatomy as depicted by MRI with age, phase of the menstrual cycle, hormone replacement therapy, or use of oral contraceptives.

On CT scans the individual layers of the wall of the cervix cannot be distinguished. The same holds true for unenhanced T1-weighted MR images, which depict the uterine cervix as a homogeneous cylinder-shaped structure of intermediate signal intensity without distinction of individual layers (Fig. 3.13a,b). The orientation of the longitudinal axis of the cervix is highly variable.

T2-weighted images depict three layers in most cases: an inner layer of high signal intensity, a fairly wide middle layer of low signal intensity, and an outer layer of intermediate signal intensity (Fig. 3.13c,d). The inner layer of high signal intensity corresponds to the endocervical mucosa. Sometimes an additional central area of very high signal intensity can be seen, which corresponds to the mucous within the cervical canal (Fig. 3.14).

On high resolution T2-weighted images palmate folds of the cervical canal can be depicted as normal findings (Fig. 3.15).

Often, nabothian cysts are seen. These are benign cysts of the uterine cervix that are assumed to result from obstruction of the cervical mucous glands [19]. The cysts are depicted on T2-weighted images as round to oval lesions with a smooth margin (Fig. 3.16).

The low-signal-intensity middle layer corresponds to the cervical stroma and mostly consists of connective tissue. The outer layer has a signal intensity that is comparable to that of the myometrium and is characterized by a more loose tissue structure [20] and may not always be distinguishable from the parametria even on T2-weighted images. The mucosa in the cervical canal shows the strongest enhancement and is thus clearly distinct from the less enhancing stromal layer. The outer stromal layer of the cervix and the portio also show contrast enhancement.

The differentiation of the cervix versus the paracervical tissue of the parametria is best on T2-weighted images compared to pre- or postcontrast T1-weighted images or CT scans.

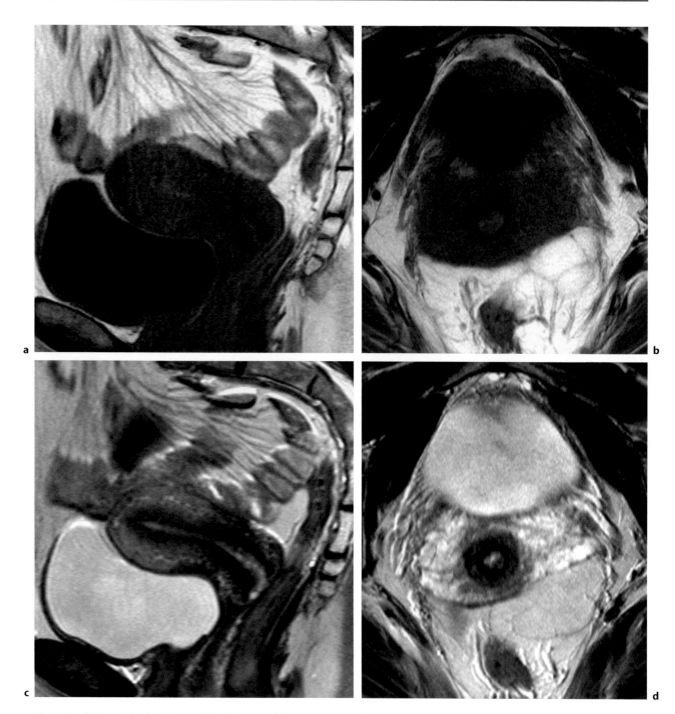

Fig. 3.13a–d. T1-weighted and T2-weighted images of the cervix uteri of a 36-year-old woman

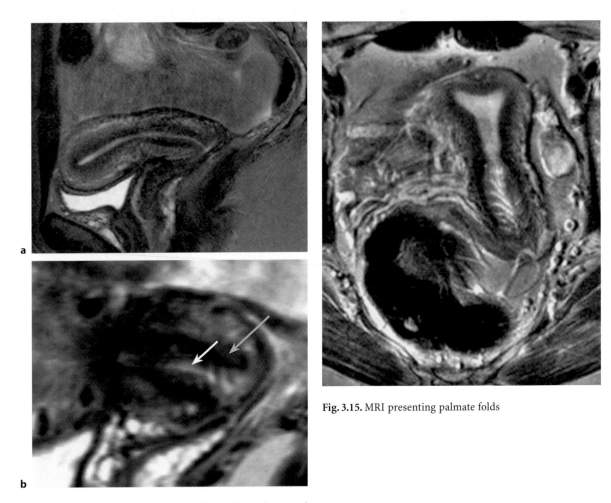

Fig. 3.14a,b. T2-weighted TSE image detect the endocervical mucosa (*white arrow*) and cervical stroma (*grey arrow*) from the outer tissue

Fig. 3.15. MRI presenting palmate folds

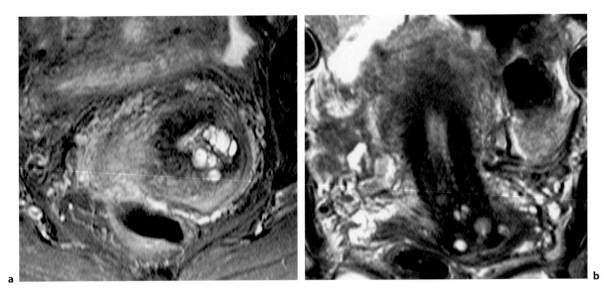

Fig. 3.16a,b. Transversal and coronal MR images of a 40-year-old asymptomatic woman depicting Nabothian (cervical) cysts

References

1. Martius G, Breckwoldt M, Pfleiderer A (1996) Lehrbuch der Gynäkologie und Geburtshilfe. Thieme, Stuttgart
2. Cunha TM, Felix A, Cabral I (2001) Preoperative assessment of deep myometrial and cervical invasion in endometrial carcinoma: comparison of magnetic resonance imaging and gross visual inspection. Int J Gynecol Cancer 11:130–136
3. Haynor D, Mack L, Soules M et al. (1986) Changing appearance of the normal uterus during the menstrual cycle: MR studies. Radiology 161:459–462
4. Hötzinger H, Spätling L (1994) MRI in der Gynäkologie und Geburtshilfe. Springer, Berlin
5. Lee JK, Gersell DJ, Balfe DM, Worthington JL, Picus D (1985) The uterus: in vitro MR anatomic correlation of normal and abnormal specimens. Radiology 157:175–179
6. Masui, T, Katayama M, Kobayashi S, et al. (2001) Changes in myometrial and junctional zone thickness and signal intensity: demonstration with kinematic T2-weighted MR imaging. Radiology 221:75–85
7. Togashi K, Nakai A, Sugimura K (2001) Anatomy and physiology of the female pelvis: MR imaging revisited. J Magn Reson Imaging 13:842–849
8. Bartoli JM, Moulin G, Delannoy L, Chagnaud C, Kasbarian M (1991) The normal uterus on magnetic resonance imaging and variations associated with the hormonal state. Surg Radiol Anat 13:213–220
9. Hoad CL, Raine-Fenning NJ, Fulford J, Campbell BK, Johnson IR, Gowland PA (2005) Uterine tissue development in healthy women during the normal menstrual cycle and investigations with magnetic resonance imaging. Am J Obstet Gynecol 192:648–654
10. Janus CL, Wiczyk HP, Laufer N (1988) Magnetic resonance imaging of the menstrual cycle. Magn Reson Imag 6:669–674
11. McCarthy, S., G. Scott, S. Majumdar et al. (1989) Uterine junctional zone: MR study of water content and relaxation properties. Radiology 171:241–243
12. Scoutt, LM, Flynn SD, Luthringer DJ, McCauley TR, McCarthy SM (1991) Junctional zone of the uterus: correlation of MR imaging and histologic examination of hysterectomy specimens. Radiology 179:403–407
13. Masui T, Katayama M, Kobayashi S, Nakayama S, Nozaki A, Kabasawa H, Ito T, Sakahara H (2001) Changes in myometrial and junctional zone thickness and signal intensity: demonstration with kinematic T2-weighted MR imaging. Radiology 221:75–85
14. Togashi K, Nakai A, Sugimura K (2001) Anatomy and physiology of the female pelvis: MR imaging revised. J Magn Res Imag 13:842-849
15. Mitchell DG, Schonholz L, Hilpert PL et al. (1990) Zones of the uterus: Discrepancy between US and MR images. Radiology 174:827–831
16. Brown HK, Stoll BS, Nicosia SV et al. (1991) Uterine junctional zone: correlation between histologic findings and MR imaging. Radiology 179:409–413
17. McCarthy S, Tauber C, Gore J (1986) Female pelvic anatomy: MR assessment of variations during the menstrual cycle and with use of oral contraceptives. Radiology 160:119–123
18. Ascher SM, Johnson JC, Barnes WA, Bae CJ, Patt RH, Zeman RK (1996) MR imaging appearance of the uterus in postmenopausal women receiving tamoxifen therapy for breast cancer: histopathologic correlation. Radiology 200:105–110
19. Li, H., Sugimura K, Okizuka H et al. (1999) Markedly high signal intensity lesions in the uterine cervix on T2-weighted imaging: differentiation between mucin-producing carcinomas and nabothian cysts. Radiat Med 17:137-143de
20. Souza NM, Hawley IC, Schwieso JE, Gilderdale DJ, Soutter WP (1994) The uterine cervix on in vitro and in vivo MR images: a study of zonal anatomy and vascularity using an enveloping cervical coil. AJR Am J Roentgenol 163:607–612

Congenital Malformations of the Uterus

Justus Roos and Rahel Kubik-Huch

4.1
Clinical Background

4.1.1
Epidemiology

Congenital malformations of the uterus, also termed Müllerian duct anomalies (MDA) are an uncommon, but often treatable cause of infertility. Estimates of its frequency vary widely owing to different patient populations, non-standardized classification systems, and differences in diagnostic data acquisition. Because normal pregnancies can occur in women with MDA and the anomalies are discovered in most cases of patients presenting with infertility, the reported prevalence of MDA in the general population is probably underestimated. The overall published data suggest a prevalence range of uterovaginal anomalies of around 1%–3% [1–7] in the general population among women with normal and abnormal fertility. While conceiving is a minor problem for the majority of women with MDA, the risk of pregnancy loss is truly associated with MDA and its prevalence in women with repeated miscarriage is considered to be around 3% [3, 4, 8–10]. No racial predilection is noted in the literature.

4.1.2
Clinical Presentation

MDA may become clinically evident at different ages depending on their specific characteristics and associated disorders. The distribution among the different classes of MDA and their clinical presentations are summarized in Table 4.1. In the newborn/infant age, an initial presentation of a palpable abdominal or pelvic mass due to a utero or/and vaginal obstruction causing intraluminal fluid retention can be discovered. In the adolescent age group a delayed menarche or primary amenorrhea with/without a fluid retention in the uterus (hematometra) and/or vagina (hematocolpos) may present as a painful intraabdominal tumor. Some patients also have cyclical pain. In the childbearing age, MDA can present with various problems of infertility, repeated spontaneous abortions, premature delivery, fetal intrauterine growth retardation, and difficulties during delivery. By understanding the defective embryological development one can understand the potential for the presence of associated congenital malformations of other organ systems. Most frequently,

J. Roos, MD
Department of Radiology, Medical Center Stanford University, 300 Pasteur Drive, Room S-072, CA 94305 Stanford, USA
R. Kubik-Huch, MD, MPH
PD, Institute of Radiology, Kantonsspital Baden AG, CH-5404 Baden, Switzerland

Table 4.1. Distribution among the different classes of MDA and their clinical presentations

Müllerian duct anomalies (MDA)	Influence on reproductive/obstetric outcome			Other major associations
	Spontaneous abortion	Premature delivery	Fetal survival rate	
Class I: Dysplasia (4%–10%)	No potential for reproduction			Mayer-Rokitansky-Kuster-Huser syndrome
Class II: Unicornuate uterus (5%–20%)	50%[a] (41%–62%)	15% (10%–20%)	40% (38%–57%)	Renal agenesis 67%
Class III: Uterus didelphys (5%–11%)	45% (32%–52%)	38% (20%–45%)	55% (41%–61%)	Longitudinal vaginal septum 75%
Class IV: Bicornuate uterus (10%–39%)	30% (28%–35%)	20% (14%–23%)	60% (57%–63%)	High cervical incompetence 38%
Class V: Septate uterus (34%–55%)	65% (26%–94%)	20% (9%–33%)	30% (10%–75%)	Vaginal septum 25%
Class VI: Arcuate uterus (7%)	Mostly compatible with normal-term gestation			
Class VII: DES-exposed uterus	Increased	Increased	Decreased	Cervical anomalies 44%

[a] All percentage data are pooled and form the current literature [6, 7, 9, 33]; values in brackets represent percentage ranges.

renal malformations like renal agenesis or ectopia can occur. Much less frequent are bony malformations – most of them occur in a complex of varying symptoms – like abnormal scapula, supernumerary or fused ribs, vertebral malsegmentation, fusion of the vertebral column (i.e. Klippel-Feil syndrome) and radio-carpal hypoplasia. The non-random association of MDA, renal agenesis/ectopia, and cervicothoracic somite dysplasia are subsumed under the so-called MURCS associations [11]. Although other malformations such as cardiac defects have been described, it remains unclear if some of the associated malformations are caused in the same development field or if early exposure to teratogenic agents were causative [11]. The literature does not show increased mortality for patients carrying an MDA compared to the general population, whereas the morbidity may be increased in some specific types of MDA causing obstructed Müllerian systems with the presence of hematosalpinx (retention of blood in the fallopian tubes), hematocolpos (retention of blood in the vagina), retrograde menses causing the potential problem of endometriosis.

Once an MDA is suggested based on evidence from the patient history and physical examination, the next diagnostic step includes an imaging work-up, which often detects the underlying anomaly and guides further (surgical) interventions.

4.1.3
Embryology

The understanding of the embryogenesis of the urogenital female tract is of paramount importance to understand the pathogenesis of the different types of MDA. The female reproductive system develops from the two paired Müllerian ducts (synonym: paramesonephric duct) that start off in the embryonal mesoderm lateral to each Wolffian duct (synonym: mesonephric duct). The paired Müllerian ducts develop in medial and caudal directions, the cranial part remains non-fused and forms the fallopian tubes. The caudal part fuses to a single canal forming the uterus and the upper two thirds of the vagina. This is called lateral fusion. In a process called vertical fusion, the intervening midline septum of both ducts undergoes regression. The caudal part of the vagina arises from the sinovaginal bulb and fuses with the lower fused Müllerian ducts. The ovaries originate from the gonadal ridge, a completely different tissue than the mesoderm forming both the urinary and genital systems. Hence, associated malformations of the kidney, but not of the ovaries are frequently observed together with MDA. Pathogenesis of MDA (MDA) can be basically classified into the presence of agenesis, hypoplasia, and defects in vertical and lateral fusion of the paired ducts. In 1988, the AMERIcan FERTILITY SOCIETY (AFS) [12] presented a consensus in classification of uterovaginal anomalies and published a schematization system that is widely accepted among specialists. Other used classification systems are referenced [13–15]. Most Müllerian duct anomalies occur sporadically and some reports give descriptions of the patterns of inheritance or of exposure to teratogenic agents such as di-ethyl-stilbestrol (DES) and thalidomide [16].

4.1.4
Pathology

Whatever steps in embryogenesis are defective different types of MDA can occur. The AFS introduced a classification system in 1988 [12] that stratifies MDA into seven different classes of uterine anomalies (Fig. 4.1). It is based on a previous classification system introduced by BUTTRAM et al. [13]. Other classification systems followed and included broader collections of anomalies in order to avoid conflicting observations and over simplicity [15]. With all classification systems, one must emphasize that with the overlap of associated cervical and vaginal anomalies, the classifications describe primarily the uterine defects whereas the cervicovaginal defects as well as the associated malformations must be added separately

in the form of a subset. The distribution among the different classes of MDA and their clinical presentations are summarized in Table 4.1. The diagnosis of MDA is based upon the clinical presentation, physical examination and subsequent imaging workup with different imaging methods available, of which MR imaging takes a leading role, especially in complex uterine malformation [17]. For the following descriptions of the specific pathologies, we use the AFS classification system and provide definitions of the different types of MDA in the imaging section.

4.2
Imaging

4.2.1
Technique

Once an MDA is suggested based on evidence from the patient history and physical examination, the next diagnostic step includes different imaging workups in order to detect and specify MDA and to guide further treatment options. Before US and MRI were capable of visualizing MDA with a high accuracy, imaging of MDA was limited to hysterosalpingography (HSG)

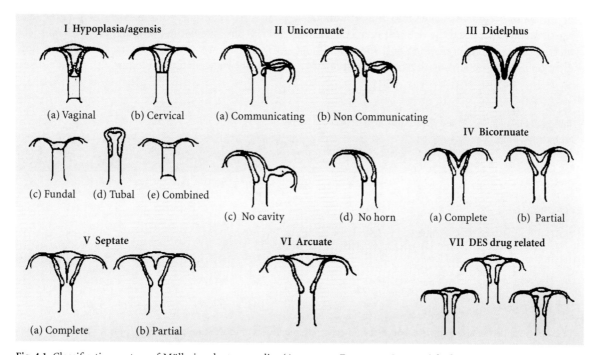

Fig. 4.1. Classification system of Müllerian duct anomalies (AMERICAN FERTILITY SOCIETY) [12]

[18], a fluoroscopic spot film technique in combination with endoluminal filling of the uterine cavity with radioopaque contrast agent. Since the diagnostic imaging properties of MDA include mainly the configuration of the endometrial cavity and the external uterine contour, HSG is able to depict only certain types of MDA, whereas it fails in other cases and stays non-specific for precise diagnosis, the latter mainly due to the lack of the visualization of the outer uterine contour. Because of this drawback, HSG did not provide diagnoses with high degrees of confidence and US and MRI soon began to play a larger role in assessment and treatment of patients. As HSG provides, besides the morphological, also the functional information of tubal patency, it is still used in the primary imaging work-up in case of infertility clarification. A newer technique using MR for the visualization of the tubal patency, so called 3D MR-HSG, is a promising imaging alternative, although still in the development stage, to the conventional HSG and avoids exposure of the ovaries to ionizing radiation.

Nowadays, the first imaging modality in the MDA assessment includes pelvic US [19, 20]; (1) transabdominal US (performed with a 2.5- to 5-Mhz probe) for evaluation of the entire abdomen, especially for associated renal malformations, and (2) transvaginal US (performed with a 5- to 8-Mhz endovaginal probe) for better delineation of the uterus, vagina and ovaries. Hysterosonography, a technique consisting of endovaginal US with prior infusion of saline or ultrasound contrast agent into the endometrial canal, further increased the delineation of the endometrial cavity and is performed only for selected indications, i.e., in patients with a history of infertility.

US is highly accurate for the detection of MDA [21]. Newer techniques, such as 3D US [22], even further improved the imaging diagnostics by giving better information about the external contour of the uterus and its volume.

Magnetic resonance imaging (MRI) is today considered standard in the evaluation of MDA and accepted as the leading imaging modality for further surgical planning. MRI provides high resolution images of the entire uterine anatomy (internal and external contour), as well as of secondary findings like renal malformations. Among the three major imaging methods, MRI has the best accuracy in the evaluation of uterine anomalies and accuracies of up to 100% have been reported [21, 23]. According to the author's institution's imaging protocol (Siemens, Sonata, 1.5-Tesla MR unit, Siemens Medical; Erlangen, Germany) for the assessment of congenital uterine anomalies, MRI of the uterus includes six native sequences without intravenous contrast using a bodyflex phased array MR surface coil as shown in Table 4.2. If possible, patients should be scheduled in the second half of the menstrual cycle, since the thickness of the endometrial stripe increases during the follicular and secretory phase and thus the normal zonal anatomy of the uterus can be better appreciated. No specific patient preparation is necessary; however, the application of a tampon by the patient prior to the examination can be helpful to delineate the vaginal lumen. An axial T1-weighted as well as an axial STIR sequences are standard techniques for the assessment of the female pelvis. In this patient population with suspected MDA, they are mainly performed in order not to miss any associated pathologies, e.g. ovarian disease.

Table 4.2. MR imaging protocol for assessment of MDA

Sequence	Slice thickness	Slice spacing	Matrix	TR (ms)	TE (ms)	TI (ms)	Flip angle	Field of view (mm)
STIR axial	7 mm	10%	256×256	6650	74	150	150	350×245
T1 TSE axial	7 mm	20%	512×256	500	11		150	350×245
T2 TSE sagittal	5 mm	20%	512×256	4900	113		180	180×180
T2 TSE coronal oblique	5 mm	10%	512×256	3770	114		150	180×180
T2 TSE axial oblique	5 mm	20%	512×256	3860	114		150	180×180
TRUFISP coronal	6 mm	25%	256×220	3.86	1.93		80	Including kidney

TSE, turbo spin echo; also known as FSE, fast spin echo; TR, repetition time; TE, time to echo; TI, time for inversion; coronal oblique, parallel to the long axis of the uterus; axial oblique, parallel to the short axis of the uterus; TRUFISP, 'fast induction steady state potential' gradient sequence (Siemens Medical, Germany).

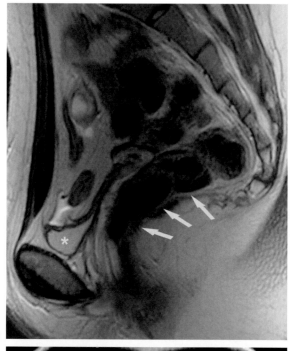

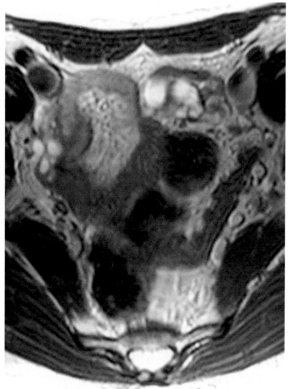

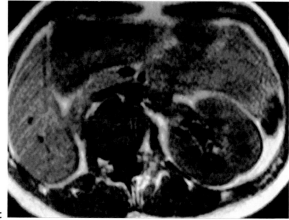

Fig. 4.2a–c. An 18-year-old female patient with primary amenorrhea. Sagittal T2-weighted (**a**) and axial T2-weighted (**b**) MR image confirms the diagnosis of Mayer-Rokitansky-Kuster syndrome consisting of agenesis of uterus and vagina. Note absence of uterus and upper two thirds of vagina (*asterisk*, bladder; *arrows*, rectum) and the associated renal agenesis depicted on an additional acquired axial T1-weighted image (**c**)

In addition, the demonstration of hemorrhage within the endometrial cavity (hematometra) and/or vagina (hematocolpos) benefits from T1-weighted imaging. T2-weighted images are most important for the assessment of the uterus. Sagittal sections are best suited to image the uterus. Additional axial oblique sections parallel to the endometrial cavity results in a long-axis view being most helpful for imaging the fundal contour. Whereas an oblique sequence obtained perpendicular to the cervical results in a short-axis view allows accurate assessment of the cervix, i.e., the diagnosis of duplication or septation. The protocol further includes a fast sequence of the upper abdomen to diagnose or exclude renal pathology.

4.2.2
Classes of Müllerian Duct Anomalies (MDA)

The percentage distribution of the different MDA classes and their influence on reproductive and obstetric outcome, as well as their major associations, is summarized in Table 4.1.

4.2.2.1
Class I Anomalies: Dysgenesis

Definition: Dysgenesis (segmental agenesis and variable hypoplasia) of the Müllerian ducts (uterus and upper 2/3 vagina) [11, 24] (Fig. 4.2).

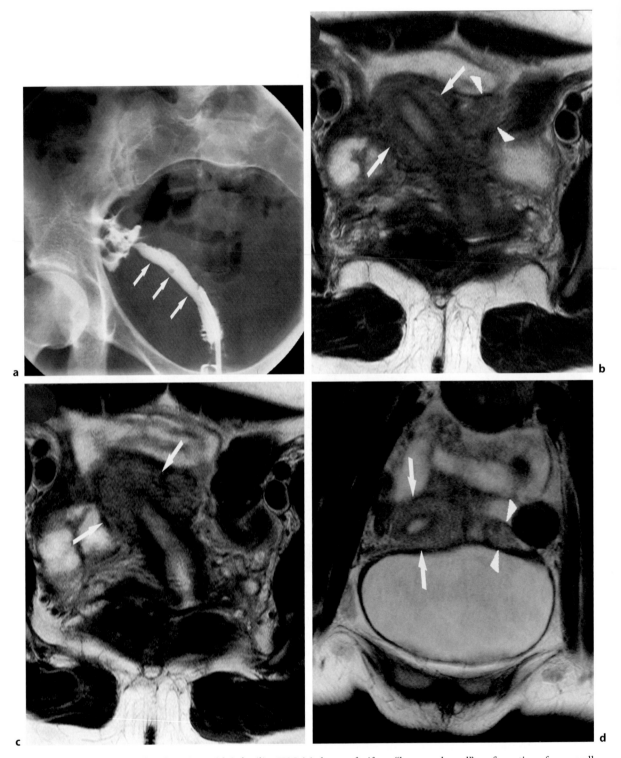

Fig. 4.3a–d. A 28-year-old female patient with infertility. HSG (**a**) shows a fusiform "banana-shaped" configuration of one small endometrial cavity (*arrows*) that is deviated to the right and drains into one fallopian tube. Note the absence of the normal triangular appearance of the fundal cavity. This configuration is highly suggestive of the presence of a unicornuate uterus. Iatrogenic filling defects in the uterine cavity by air bubbles. Oblique T2-weighted MR images (**b,c**) and coronal T2-weighted MR image (**d**) confirm the diagnosis of a unicornuate uterus with the presence of a small elongated uterus that shows normal zonal anatomy (*arrows*). A rudimentary horn with low signal intensity and no zonal anatomy – thus corresponding to a rudimentary horn with no endometrium – can be depicted on the right side (*arrowheads*). No surgical resection is needed in this case

Mayer-Rokitansky-Kuster syndrome is the most common form of Class I anomaly and includes agenesis of uterus and vagina.

4.2.2.2
Class II Anomalies: Unicornuate Uterus

Definition: Unicornuate uterus as a result of partial or complete hypoplasia of one Müllerian duct [25] (Fig. 4.3).

Unicornuate uterus may be isolated (35%) or associated with a contralateral rudimentary horn. The rudimentary horns present with or without communication to the endometrial cavity and may be associated with or without endometrium, which is also called no cavity rudimentary horn. In patients with cavity non-communicating rudimentary horn, dysmenorrhea and hematometra may occur. Surgical resection to either relieve symptomatic pain or to reduce the risk of potential ectopic pregnancy is justified. As with every obstructed system, the risk of endometriosis is also increased with a non-communicating rudimentary horn. Renal malformations are common with unicornuate uterus and occur mostly

on the same side as the rudimentary horn could be found.

4.2.2.3
Class III Anomalies: Uterus Didelphys

Definition: Uterus didelphys as a result of complete non-fusion of the Müllerian ducts forming a complete uterine duplication with no communication between each other [23, 26, 27] (Fig. 4.4).

Uterus didelphys may be associated with a longitudinal (75%) or, more rarely, with a transverse vaginal septum, the latter causing obstructive hematometrocolpos. Endometriosis as a result of retrograde menstruation may also occur in these conditions. A non-obstructive uterus didelphys is usually asymptomatic.

4.2.2.4
Class IV Anomalies: Bicornuate Uterus

Definition: Bicornuate uterus is the result of incomplete fusion of the cranial parts of the müllerian ducts [21, 28] (Fig. 4.5).

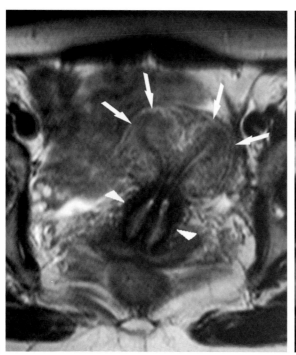 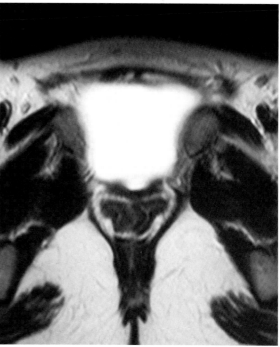

a   b

Fig. 4.4a,b. A 33-year-old female patient with a history of partially resected longitudinal vaginal septum. Transverse oblique T2-weighted MR images (**a**) show complete duplication of the uterine horns (*arrows*), as well as two duplicated cervices (*arrowheads*). The cavities show their normal zonal anatomy. Note the longitudinal vaginal septum (**b**) which appears in 75% of uterus didelphys

Two uterine cavities with normal zonal anatomy can be depicted. The leading imaging feature is a fundal cleft greater than 1 cm of the external uterine contour that helps to distinguish bicornuate uterus from septate uterus.

Bicornuate uterus occurs with wide variability. Extension of the intervening fundal cleft to the internal cervical os characterizes the complete bicornuate uterus with a single cervix (bicornuate, unicollis uterus), whereas variants of partial bicornuate uterus exist if the cleft is of variable length. Bicornuate uterus may be associated with a duplicated cervix (bicornuate bicollis uterus), as well as with a longitudinal vaginal septum that coexists in up to 25% of bicornuate uterus. Nevertheless, a degree of communication is always present between both uterine cavities. Still controversial is the need for surgical intervention and this is probably only necessary in specific cases. A higher rate of cervical incompetence seems to be associated with bicornuate uterus.

4.2.2.5
Class V Anomalies: Septate Uterus

Definition: Septate uterus is a result of partial or complete non-regression of the midline uterovaginal

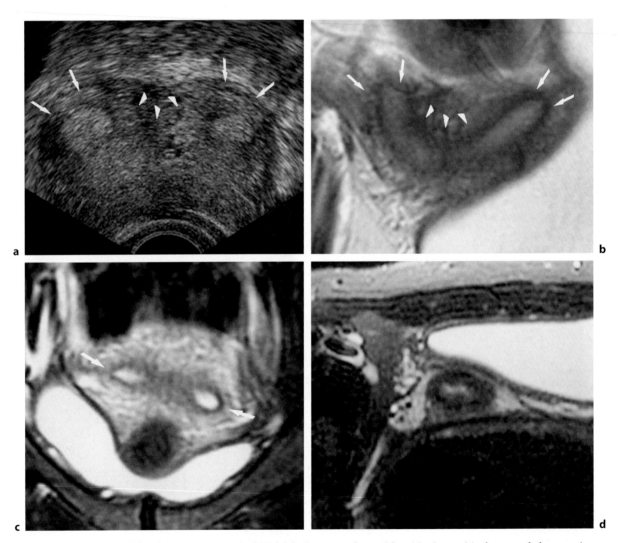

Fig. 4.5a–d. A 17-year-old female patient. Transvaginal US (**a**) depicts two endometrial cavities (*arrows*) in the coronal plane consisting of a hyperechogenic endometrial stripe and a hypoechogenic myometrial layer. A intervening external fundal cleft was visible during the examination by interactively turning the image plane (*arrowheads*). The highly suspected presence of a bicornuate uterus was confirmed by MR with a coronal T2-weighted image (**b**) showing two uterine cavities (*arrows*) separated by a deep external fundal cleft (*arrowheads*). In the same image plane, the separation of both cavities (*arrows*) are visible to the level of the internal cervical os (**c**) before they conjoin to one single cervix (**d**) as shown in a T2-weighted axial image (bicornuate, unicollis uterus)

septum [21, 23, 29–32] (Fig. 4.6). The main imaging feature is that the external contour of the uterine fundus may be either convex of mildly concave (<1 cm) and not with a cleft greater than 1 cm, the latter defining a bicornuate or didelphic uterus [3, 23].

Septate uterus is the most common Müllerian duct anomaly and is unfortunately associated with the poorest reproductive outcome. Because of different treatment options, septate uterus must be differenti-ated from bicornuate and didelphic uterus. A widely accepted definition therefore – empirically invented during laparoscopy procedures – states that a uterus is septate if the outer contour of the uterine fundus is only mildly concave in the presence of a septum. The cut-off of concavity is 1 cm; deeper concavity is associated with bicornuate uterus and uterus didelphys. In a complete septate uterus, the septum extends to the external cervical os. In 25% of septate uteri, the

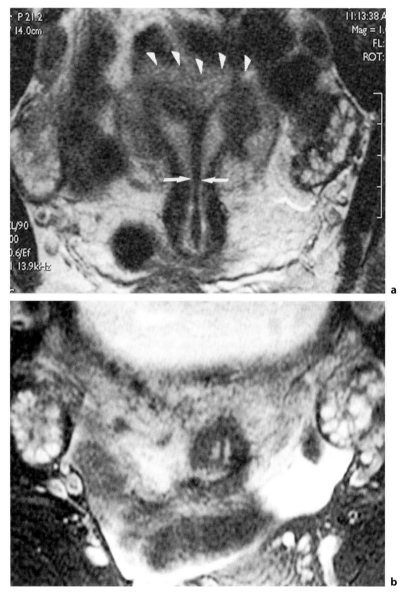

Fig. 4.6a,b. A 29-year-old female patient with infertility. Coronal T2-weighted MR image (**a**) demonstrates an external uterine contour with mild external cleft (*arrowheads*), as well as a hypointense thin septum dividing the endometrial cavity at the level of the uterine body and cervix (*arrows*). **b** Axial T2-weighted image show the extension of the longitudinal septum to the external cervix os

septum extends even further into the upper part of the vagina.

Obstetric outcome seems not to be correlated with the length of the septum. The septum may be composed of muscle or fibrous tissue and is not a reliable means of distinguishing septate and bicornuate uteri. Resection of the septum by hysteroscopic metroplasty is indicated and may improve the reproductive outcome significantly.

4.2.2.6
Class VI Anomalies: Arcuate Uterus

Defintion: Arcuate uterus is the result of a near complete regression of the uterovaginal septum forming a mild and broad saddle-shaped indentation of the fundal endometrium [13].
Differentiation from bicornuate uterus is based on the complete fundal unification; however, a broad-based septate uterus is difficult to distinguish from an arcuate uterus. There is much controversy as to whether an arcuate uterus should be considered a real anomaly or an anatomic variant. Fact is that MRI may detect this abnormality but, typically, it is not clinically significant because arcuate uterus has no significant negative effects on pregnancy outcome.

4.2.2.7
Class VII Anomalies

DES-exposed uterus. DES (synthetic estrogen, diethyl-stilbestrol, 1948-1971) may induce abnormal myometrial hypertrophy in the fetal uterus forming small T-shaped endometrial cavities [33], as well as increase the risk of developing a clear cell carcinoma of the vagina [34]. The characteristic uterine abnormalities must be categorized in the group of complex uterine anomalies and may occur with or without the exposure of DES.

References

1. Acien P (1997) Incidence of Mullerian defects in fertile and infertile women. Hum Reprod 12:1372–1376
2. Ashton D, Amin HK, Richart RM, Neuwirth RS (1988) The incidence of asymptomatic uterine anomalies in women undergoing transcervical tubal sterilization. Obstet Gynecol 72:28–30
3. Homer HA, Li TC, Cooke ID (2000) The septate uterus: a review of management and reproductive outcome. Fertil Steril 73:1–14
4. Raga F, Bauset C, Remohi J, Bonilla-Musoles F, Simon C, Pellicer A (1997) Reproductive impact of congenital Mullerian anomalies. Hum Reprod 12:2277–2281
5. Saleem SN (2003) MR imaging diagnosis of uterovaginal anomalies: current state of the art. Radiographics 23:e13
6. Simon C, Martinez L, Pardo F, Tortajada M, Pellicer A (1991) Mullerian defects in women with normal reproductive outcome. Fertil Steril 56:1192–1193
7. Troiano RN, McCarthy SM (2004) Mullerian duct anomalies: imaging and clinical issues. Radiology 233:19–34
8. Clifford K, Rai R, Watson H, Regan L (1994) An informative protocol for the investigation of recurrent miscarriage: preliminary experience of 500 consecutive cases. Hum Reprod 9:1328–1332
9. Nahum GG (1998) Uterine anomalies. How common are they, and what is their distribution among subtypes? J Reprod Med 43:877–887
10. Raziel A, Arieli S, Bukovsky I, Caspi E, Golan A (1994) Investigation of the uterine cavity in recurrent aborters. Fertil Steril 62:1080–1082
11. Pittock ST, Babovic-Vuksanovic D, Lteif A (2005) Mayer-Rokitansky-Kuster-Hauser anomaly and its associated malformations. Am J Med Genet A 135:314–316
12. The American Fertility Society (1988) The American Fertility Society classifications of adnexal adhesions, distal tubal occlusion, tubal occlusion secondary to tubal ligation, tubal pregnancies, mullerian anomalies and intrauterine adhesions. Fertil Steril 49:944–955
13. Buttram VC Jr., Gibbons WE (1979) Mullerian anomalies: a proposed classification. (An analysis of 144 cases). Fertil Steril 32:40–46
14. Rock JA, Schlaff WD (1985) The obstetric consequences of uterovaginal anomalies. Fertil Steril 43:681–692
15. Rock JA, Adam RA (2000) Surgery to repair disorders of development. In: Nichols DH, Clark-Pearson DL (eds) Gynecologic, obstetric and related surgery, 2nd edn. Mosby, St Louis, pp 780–813
16. Kaufman RH, Adam E, Hatch EE, Noller K, Herbst AL, Palmer JR, Hoover RN (2000) Continued follow-up of pregnancy outcomes in diethylstilbestrol-exposed offspring. Obstet Gynecol 96:483–489
17. Minto CL, Hollings N, Hall-Craggs M, Creighton S (2001) Magnetic resonance imaging in the assessment of complex Mullerian anomalies. Bjog 108:791–797
18. Krysiewicz S (1992) Infertility in women: diagnostic evaluation with hysterosalpingography and other imaging techniques. AJR Am J Roentgenol 159:253–261
19. Byrne J, Nussbaum-Blask A, Taylor WS, Rubin A, Hill M, O'Donnell R, Shulman S (2000) Prevalence of Mullerian duct anomalies detected at ultrasound. Am J Med Genet 94:9–12
20. Goldberg JM, Falcone T, Attaran M (1997) Sonohysterographic evaluation of uterine abnormalities noted on hysterosalpingography. Hum Reprod 12:2151–2153
21. Pellerito JS, McCarthy SM, Doyle MB, Glickman MG, DeCherney AH (1992) Diagnosis of uterine anomalies: relative accuracy of MR imaging, endovaginal sonography, and hysterosalpingography. Radiology 183:795–800
22. Wu MH, Hsu CC, Huang KE (1997) Detection of congenital mullerian duct anomalies using three-dimensional ultrasound. J Clin Ultrasound 25:487–492
23. Carrington BM, Hricak H, Nuruddin RN, Secaf E, Laros RK Jr., Hill EC (1990) Mullerian duct anomalies: MR imaging evaluation. Radiology 176:715–720

24. Strubbe EH, Willemsen WN, Lemmens JA, Thijn CJ, Rolland R (1993) Mayer-Rokitansky-Kuster-Hauser syndrome: distinction between two forms based on excretory urographic, sonographic, and laparoscopic findings. AJR Am J Roentgenol 160:331–334

25. Brody JM, Koelliker SL, Frishman GN (1998) Unicornuate uterus: imaging appearance, associated anomalies, and clinical implications. AJR Am J Roentgenol 171:1341–1347

26. Fedele L, Dorta M, Brioschi D, Massari C, Candiani GB (1989) Magnetic resonance evaluation of double uteri. Obstet Gynecol 74:844–847

27. Fedele L, Ferrazzi E, Dorta M, Vercellini P, Candiani GB (1988) Ultrasonography in the differential diagnosis of „double" uteri. Fertil Steril 50:361–364

28. Toaff ME, Lev-Toaff AS, Toaff R (1984) Communicating uteri: review and classification with introduction of two previously unreported types. Fertil Steril 41:661–679

29. Fedele L, Bianchi S (1995) Hysteroscopic metroplasty for septate uterus. Obstet Gynecol Clin North Am 22:473–489

30. Fedele L Bianchi S, Marchini M, Franchi D, Tozzi L, Dorta M (1996) Ultrastructural aspects of endometrium in infertile women with septate uterus. Fertil Steril 65:750–752

31. Reuter KL, Daly DC, Cohen SM (1989) Septate versus bicornuate uteri: errors in imaging diagnosis. Radiology 172:749–752

32. Valle RF (1996) Hysteroscopic treatment of partial and complete uterine septum. Int J Fertil Menopausal Stud 41:310–315

33. Rennell CL (1979) T-shaped uterus in diethylstilbestrol (DES) exposure. AJR Am J Roentgenol 132:979–980

34. Herbst AL, Ulfelder H, Poskanzer DC (1971) Adenocarcinoma of the vagina. Association of maternal stilbestrol therapy with tumor appearance in young women. N Engl J Med 284:878–881

Benign Uterine Lesions

5

Thomas J. Kröncke

CONTENTS

5.1
Uterine Leiomyomas: Background

5.1.1
Epidemiology

Leiomyomas, or fibroids, are the most common benign tumors of the uterus. The incidence of fibroids is difficult to estimate and frequencies reported in the literature range between 25% and 50%. In autopsy studies, leiomyomas of the uterus have been found in up to 77% of women [2, 21, 30]. Only about one third of affected women have fibroids that become clinically apparent before menopause. Fibroids may cause abnormal menstrual bleeding (menorrhagia with secondary anemia, dysmenorrhea) or pelvic pressure due to their mass effect (urinary frequency, constipation, pelvic pain, dyspareunia). Finally, leiomyomas of the uterus are also implicated in female infertility and are the most common indication for hysterectomy in western industrialized countries. In the USA 200,000 hysterectomies are performed for uterine fibroids each year [42, 47, 170].

Fibroids are smooth muscle tumors of the uterus that are influenced by steroid hormones and develop in women of reproductive age. They do not occur before puberty and fibroid-related symptoms become less severe or resolve altogether with the onset of menopause as a result of decreasing levels of steroid hormones (estrogen, progesterone) and cessation of the menstrual cycle. However, women on hormone replacement therapy may suffer from fibroid-related

T. J. Kröncke, MD
Institut für Radiologie (Campus Mitte), Charité – Universitätsmedizin Berlin, Charitéplatz 1, 10117 Berlin, Germany

complaints even after the sixth decade of life [153]. Hormonal stimulation during pregnancy can lead to considerable growth of fibroids and spontaneous infarction [29, 59]. Uterine fibroids are more common in black women compared with Caucasians or Asians. A black woman has a two to three times higher relative risk of developing fibroids than a white woman [114]. Reproductive factors also play a role. Fibroids are two times more common in nulliparous women as compared with women who have given birth and multiple pregnancies reduce the risk further [134, 162, 166]. Other factors associated with an increased risk (early menarche and late menopause, obesity, tamoxifen therapy) or reduced risk of leiomyoma development (smoking, low-meat diet) have been described [41, 47].

5.1.2
Pathogenesis

Our knowledge of the pathogenesis of uterine fibroids is still inadequate. Both genetic factors, steroid hormones and growth factors play a role in their development and growth. Two mechanisms involved in the development of fibroids can be distinguished: the initial neoplastic transformation of normal myocytes and the further increase in size under the influence of hormones and growth factors [47, 170]. While only little is known about the initial stimulus, it is undisputed that leiomyomas exhibit a variety of characteristic changes of the karyotype which give rise to a similar phenotype whose further growth occurs via clonal expansion [60, 198].

Estrogen and progesterone promote the development of leiomyomas whereas growth factors are assumed to act as mediators or effectors of these steroid hormones in leiomyomas [47, 48]. Estrogens are assigned a central role both in the development of leiomyomas and with regard to local effects resulting from a so-called leiomyoma-related hyperestrogenic environment. Compared to normal myometrium, fibroid tissue is more sensitive to estradiol, has more estrogen receptors, and an increased aromatase activity, which enhances the synthesis of estrogens within the fibroids [108, 164, 172, 192]. Finally, glandular hyperplasia of the endometrium has been demonstrated in the immediate vicinity of submucosal leiomyomas and is attributed to the effect of local hyperestrogenism [21]. Traditionally, estrogens were assumed to have the most important role in fibroid growth. Alternatively, it has been hypothesized that

progesterones have a crucial role as it has been observed that the highest progesterone levels that occur during the secretory phase of the uterus coincide with the highest mitotic rate in leiomyomas [85, 154]. Many cytokines and growth factors stimulate fibroid growth [177]. These include transforming growth factor-ß (TGF-β), insulin-like growth factors 1 and 2 (IGF-1/2), basic fibroblast growth factor (bFGF), platelet-derived growth factor (PDGF), and epidermal growth factor (EGF) [176]. The expression of these factors is modulated by steroid hormones, suggesting that these factors are the ultimate effectors of the steroid hormones [207].

5.1.3
Histopathology

Leiomyomas are benign tumors arising from uterine smooth muscle cells. They typically develop in the uterine corpus or fundus but may also originate in the cervix (<8%) or rarely in the supporting structures of the uterus such as the broad ligament. So-called parasitic leiomyomas are no longer contiguous with the uterus and develop an atypical blood supply [88, 109, 217]. Two thirds of affected women have multiple fibroids. The majority of fibroids are seen as round lesions with a well-defined margin (Fig. 5.1). Growing fibroids displace the surrounding tissue, giving rise to a pseudocapsule of condensed myometrium, which allows surgical enucleation of the tumors. Macroscopically, the cut surface of leiomyomas has a whorl-like appearance. Histologically, leiomyomas are made up of intertwined smooth muscle cells arranged in fascicles forming whorl-like patterns (Fig. 5.2). These smooth muscle cells are embedded in a stroma of collagen fibers. Microscopically, the uniform cells have cigar-shaped nuclei and an eosinophilic fibrillary cytoplasm. The majority of fibroids show higher cell density than the surrounding myometrium. Mitosis and atypia are not found in fibroids. Histologically, different subtypes are distinguished, of which cellular and myxoid leiomyoma as well as lipoleiomyoma can also be differentiated by magnetic resonance imaging. Rare manifestations are diffuse leiomyomatosis of the uterus and forms that extend beyond the uterus. The latter comprise benign metastatic leiomyomatosis, peritoneal disseminated leiomyomatosis, and intravenous leiomyomatosis [62, 160, 189, 203]. Diffuse leiomyomatosis (Fig. 5.3) is characterized by the presence of many small ill-defined leiomyomas that may be confluent. The tumors are found

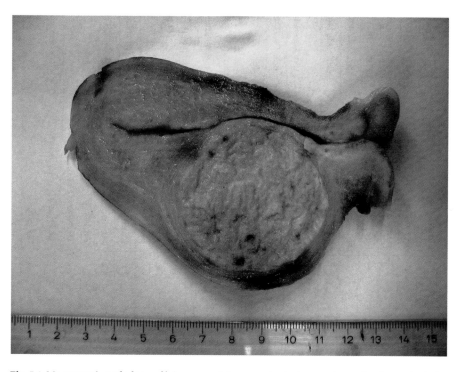

Fig. 5.1. Macroscopic pathology of leiomyoma. Macroscopic uterine specimen showing a single intramural leiomyoma in the wall of the uterine corpus abutting the endometrial cavity and deforming the outer contour of the uterus. A surrounding pseudocapsule of compressed myometrium can also be depicted

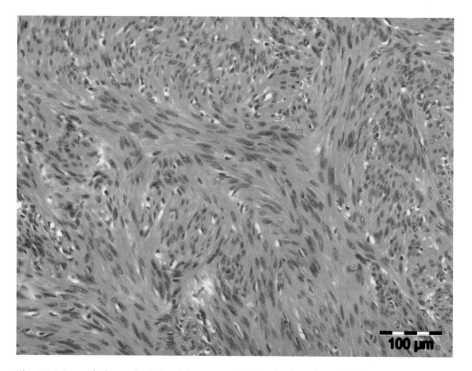

Fig. 5.2. Histopathology of uterine leiomyoma. H&E stained section of a leiomyoma specimen showing monomorphic smooth muscle cells arranged in fascicles forming whorl-like patterns

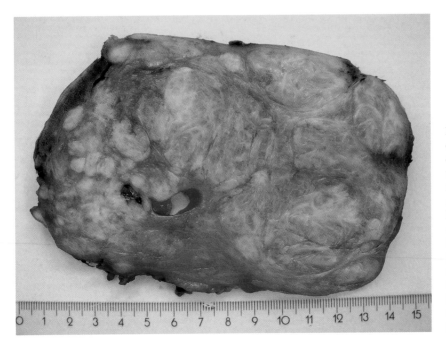

Fig. 5.3. Macroscopic pathology of diffuse leiomyomatosis of the uterus. Macroscopic uterine specimen showing multiple ill-defined leiomyomas throughout all uterine layers ranging from millimeters to several centimeters in size. The leiomyomas are partially confluent and have replaced almost the entire normal myometrium, a condition also known under the term of (diffuse) leiomyomatosis

throughout the myometrium and cause symmetrical enlargement of the uterus [125, 161].

Another factor contributing to the very heterogeneous imaging appearance of uterine fibroids is the presence of degenerative changes. Fibroids undergo degeneration when the tumors outgrow their blood supply. Typical degenerative changes such as hyaline degeneration, which is present in over 60% of leiomyomas, as well as hemorrhagic (red), myxoid, and (rare) cystic degeneration (4%) can be differentiated by MRI [220]. Other typical changes are amorphous or plaque-like calcifications, which are present in 3%–8% of leiomyomas [24]. Most of the fibroid subtypes that can be distinguished histologically or by imaging as well as the degenerative changes outlined above have no clinical relevance for therapeutic decision-making. An exception is hemorrhagic infarction of a fibroid during pregnancy, which is identified by MRI in a straightforward manner [59]. Criteria that are used for the differentiation of a leiomyosarcoma from fibroids include an increased mitosis rate, the presence of cytologic atypia as well as the presence of coagulation necrosis with or without intralesional hemorrhage [11, 54, 77, 87]. Hemorrhage and necrosis within leiomyomas only occur in the rare cases of spontaneous or pregnancy-related hemorrhagic infarction but are common early after interventional therapy by means of uterine artery embolization (UAE). Postinterventional hemorrhage and necrosis may in this setting affect large portions or the whole leiomyoma [211].

5.1.4
Clinical Presentation

Leiomyomas of the uterus are rare under the age of 30; they typically become manifest during the fourth to sixth decades of life. Typical symptoms are excessive and/or prolonged menstrual bleeding (hypermenorrhea and menorrhagia). Bleeding between periods or irregular bleeding may be observed in patients with pedunculated submucosal fibroids but is not characteristic and therefore requires diagnostic evaluation of the endometrium (endometrial biopsy, dilatation and curettage). Women with heavy periods frequently develop iron deficiency anemia. Other frequently reported complaints are bulk symptoms manifesting as a premenstrual sensation of fullness (increased abdominal/pelvic girth), urinary urgency, and indigestion. Affected women usually complain of painful periods (dysmenorrhea), less common is unspecific pain radiating into the flank or the back, or pain during intercourse (dyspareunia). These symptoms alone are not characteristic of uterine fibroids and must be interpreted in conjunction with a patient's history and imaging findings.

A patient's symptoms vary with the location and size of the fibroids. For example, submucosal fibroids can cause severe menstrual bleeding even when they are very small. In women with this type of fibroid, abnormal menstrual bleeding is attributed to ulceration and rarefaction of the endometrium over the fibroid due to compression, reduced uterine contractility, and congestion of endometrial veins. Intramural fibroids are associated with an especially high incidence of abnormal and painful menstrual bleeding.

In patients presenting with dysmenorrhea as the leading clinical symptoms, the examiner should always consider uterine adenomyosis and endometriosis in the differential diagnosis [219]. Subserosal fibroids can become very large without causing any symptoms. Compression of the intestine and urinary bladder with urinary frequency or urgency, and abdominal bloating around periods are more commonly associated with subserosal fibroids. Moreover, there is increasing evidence suggesting that symptoms are not only due to merely mechanical local effects, but that additional factors associated with specific biological activities of the fibroids also play a considerable role. Such functional factors influence the subendometrial vascular bed through dysregulation of growth and angiogenic factors and are primarily implicated to cause fibroid-related abnormal menstrual bleeding [32, 187].

The impairment of quality of life caused by fibroid-related problems and the measurable loss of economic productivity due to absence from work are considerable. For the US it has been estimated that at least 5 million workdays are lost per year due to fibroids and that the annual treatment cost amounts to US$ 3 billion [56]. The high incidence of fibroids and its socio-economic implications as well as individual loss of quality of life are in sharp contrast to our still limited understanding of the pathogenesis of uterine fibroids and inadequate therapeutic options. A lack of research into the epidemiology, pathogenesis, and pathophysiology of leiomyomas of the uterus as well as their "benign nature" are the most important factors that have so far inhibited the search for alternative therapeutic options to replace the radical surgical approach of hysterectomy [126]. Surgical removal of the uterus continues to be the most widely used therapeutic approach in patients with symptomatic fibroids. In Western industrialized countries, uterine fibroids are the most frequent indication for removal of the uterus, accounting for 200,000 hysterectomies per year in the US alone [42, 47, 170]. One in five women in Great Britain will undergo hysterectomy before the age of 55 with 90% of all hysterectomies being performed for uterine leiomyomas [40, 206]. Only recently – and not least of all because more and more affected patients are asking for alternative nonsurgical, uterus-sparing therapies – has research interest in this area focused on the stratification of therapy and the scientific evaluation of alternative therapeutic options such uterine artery embolization [3].

5.1.5
Therapy

5.1.5.1
Indications

Treatment of uterine fibroids is indicated when they cause symptoms [3] while a wait-and-see approach is in order in women without symptoms. Whether treatment is indicated or not does not depend on the size of the uterus or that of individual fibroid tumors since there is no evidence that marked enlargement of the uterus is associated with an increased surgical morbidity. Traditionally, rapid growth of a fibroid has been interpreted as a sign of malignancy (leiomyosarcoma), while the results of larger studies do not confirm this assumption [106, 137]. When deciding about hysterectomy for exclusion of potential leimyosarcoma (prevalence: 1:2000), one has to critically weigh the benefit against the surgical mortality rate (1.0–1.6:1000) [3]. More recent studies suggest that transcervical needle biopsy in combination with enzyme marker determination (LDH) and MRI can contribute to therapeutic decision-making [87]. A relative indication for treating asymptomatic leiomyomas exists in women who want to conceive and have a history of miscarriage and proven fibroid-related deformity of the uterine cavity. In these cases treatment is indicated because the fibroids can interfere with placentation and pregnancy is associated with additional risks [59, 143, 146, 159].

5.1.5.2
Medical Therapy and Ablation

Medical therapy is usually symptomatic and aims to relieve fibroid-related abnormal menstrual bleeding (hypermenorrhea, menorrhagia), dysmenorrhea, and bulk symptoms. Oral contraceptives of different hormonal composition and nonsteroidal anti-inflammatory drugs with analgesic and antifibrinolytic effects are used, although evidence for their long-term effectiveness in treating uterine fibroids is not available [126, 186]. Moreover, there is no data demonstrating a growth-reducing effect of oral contraceptives. These therapeutic options are used in the routine clinical setting to bridge the time until definitive therapy is performed. Treatment with GnRH analogues improves fibroid-related symptoms and leads to a transient reduction of fibroid size. Maximum size reduction is seen after about 3 months of treatment. Once GnRH analogues are discontinued, however, leiomyomas will again increase in size. This is why

GnRH analogues are given only to reduce leiomyoma size prior to surgery [218]. GnRH administration is also beneficial to minimize blood loss in case of larger fibroids or for the transient treatment of anemia resulting from heavy menstrual bleeding. However, GnRH treatment causes softening of fibroids, which is a disadvantage for surgical enucleation.

The severity of menstrual bleeding can be reduced by insertion of a *levonorgestrel-releasing intrauterine device* (IUD) [123, 213]. The effect of such IUDs is based on the local activity of continuously released progesterone, which effectively suppresses the endometrium. While data from larger studies regarding risks, adverse events and the long-term effectiveness in patients with multiple leiomyomas of the uterus is lacking, it is known that an IUD for the treatment of hypermenorrhea has a higher failure rate in the presence of submucosal fibroids [213].

Endometrial ablation is a permanent and invasive therapeutic option which relieves excessive menstrual bleeding in 62%–79% of cases [175]. Thermoablation of the endometrium is performed using a balloon or roller ball technique and a hysteroscopic access. The success of endometrial ablation in the presence of fibroids is small since not the entire endometrium is accessible in women with multiple leiomyomas because of enlargement and deformity of the uterine cavity.

5.1.5.3
Surgical Therapy

Hysterectomy is a definitive cure in patients with a symptomatic multifibroid uterus. Both abdominal and vaginal hysterectomy is associated with a low mortality and morbidity. However, given that uterine leiomyomas are benign lesions, the large number of hysterectomies performed worldwide to treat this condition appears to be disproportionate [16]. As an alternative to hysterectomy, uterus-sparing operative, ablative, and interventional radiological procedures are available, depending on location and size of fibroids present, the patient's age, desire to have children, and personal preferences.

Depending on their location, leiomyomas can be resected or enucleated using a hysteroscopic or laparoscopic access or open laparotomy. Hysteroscopic resection is suitable to remove submucosal leiomyomas. Hysteroscopic resection is generally considered unsuitable for submucosal leiomyomas larger than 5 cm in size, if more than three fibroids are present, or if the uterine cavity is very large (length of uterine probe > 12 cm). Moreover, the size of the intramural

component is a risk factor of the hysteroscopic resection because the risk of perforation increases when the residual myometrium is thin [210]. The rate of repeat interventions necessary after hysteroscopic fibroid resection is reported to range from 16%–21% for a follow-up period of 4–9 years [31, 58]. Fewer repeat interventions are required (8%) when hysteroscopic fibroid resection is combined with ablation of the endometrium [205].

A laparoscopic access is used to remove visible subserosal and intramural leiomyomas in combination with reconstruction of the uterus. This approach is unsuitable in the presence of very large fibroids or a markedly enlarged uterus because these factors limit the use of the laparoscope and visibility. Using the laparoscopic approach, multiple fibroids can be enucleated in one session. Visible fibroids can be removed while intramural tumors are not easily accessible to laparoscopic removal. Incision of the uterine cavity necessary for the removal of transmural fibroids is considered a disadvantage because it is associated with the risk of synechia. Adhesions are observed in 33%–54% of patients following laparoscopic interventions [35, 61, 110]. The risk of recurrence after laparoscopic fibroid removal is up to 50% in women followed up for up to 5 years [34, 127]. Laparotomy is primarily used in patients with one or more large fibroids, which are removed using an adjusted abdominal incision. The perioperative risks of laparotomy are comparable to those of hysterectomy while the rate of adhesions may be as high as 90% [167, 202]. The recurrence rate after abdominal myomectomy is 10% within 5 years and up to 27% after 10 years. One third of the patients with recurrent leiomyomas will ultimately undergo hysterectomy [23, 43].

5.1.5.4
Uterine Artery Embolization (UAE)

Uterine artery embolization (UAE) is an established technique that has been used to stop life-threatening vaginal hemorrhage in women with malignancy, postpartum uterine atony, or traumatic injury since the mid-1970s [8, 18, 52, 64, 112]. The first successful treatment of symptomatic fibroids of the uterus by UAE was reported by Ravina et al. in 1994 [150].

Embolization of the uterine artery induces infarction of fibroids while uterine perfusion is maintained [84, 119]. Infarction leads to coagulation necrosis and subsequent complete hyalinization of the fibroids [27, 119, 211]. Further transformations cause softening and shrinkage of the tumors. Follow-up for 3–24 months has shown that there is an average size reduction of the uterus of 23%–60%, while the dominant fibroid decreases by 42%–78% on average. Progressive shrinkage of the fibroids has been documented for a period of 12 months [19, 70, 101, 120, 147, 148, 179, 209]. Several studies provide evidence for a relief of bleeding-related symptoms in 80%–100% of patients and a regression of bulk symptoms in 60%–100% of patients followed up for 3–60 months [4, 19, 70, 83, 101, 120, 147, 148, 179, 209]. Studies comparing UAE with hysterectomy and myomectomy in the treatment of symptomatic uterine leiomyomas suggest that UAE has a similar success rate in terms of symptom relief and patient satisfaction, while it has a lower complication rate and shorter recovery period as compared with the surgical procedures [15, 111, 152, 182]. These results are confirmed by two randomized studies [63, 144]. Only few investigators report long-term results after UAE but the available data suggests that permanent improvement of symptoms can be expected in two thirds of women [15, 181]. Complications during the intervention are extremely rare [100, 185]. Following UAE, 5%–10% of the patients report vaginal discharge with or without tissue passage and expulsion of infarcted fibroids may occur [1, 13, 98, 136]. Fibroid expulsion occurs weeks to months after the intervention and may necessitate administration of antibiotics and pain medication if complicated by superinfection and, in rare cases, surgically assisted removal or hysteroscopic resection [70, 120, 179]. Transient amenorrhea persisting for up to three cycles is not unusual while permanent amenorrhea is rare and occurs more commonly in patients over 45 years than in younger ones [26, 200, 209]. UAE can be performed in patients with single or multiple fibroids but, based on current knowledge, patients who wish to preserve their fertility should be treated by UAE only if alternative, uterus-sparing therapeutic approaches have been attempted or are not an option. All uterus-sparing therapeutic approaches share the risk of newly occurring fibroids and may require repeat interventions or hysterectomy due to complications of surgical or interventional treatment.

5.2
Adenomyosis of the Uterus

5.2.1
Epidemiology

Adenomyosis (endometriosis genitalis interna) of the uterus affects premenopausal women and is pre-dominantly seen in multiparous women and women over 30 years of age [9, 135]. Because its symptoms are unspecific, adenomyosis rarely comes to clinical attention, which is why the incidence of this uterine condition is underestimated [9]. Until recently, the diagnosis was established almost exclusively after hysterectomy. Histologic examination of hysterectomy specimens demonstrates adenomyosis in 19%–63% of cases [9]. Adenomyosis often occurs in conjunction with fibroids and endometriosis (endometriosis genitalis externa et extragenitalis) [103, 219].

5.2.2
Pathogenesis

Adenomyosis is a nonneoplastic condition which results from the dislocation of basal endometrial glands and stroma into the underlying myometrium [46]. It has been shown that adenomyosis progresses with age, suggesting that there is continuous progression from superficial to deep myometrial involvement [102]. The dislocated endometrial glands in adenomyosis do not undergo cyclic changes, which has been attributed to the predominance of the zona basalis in these glands [9]. The mechanism underlying the dislocation of basal endometrium is largely unknown. Estrogen-mediated and mechanical effects seem to play a role. Since adenomyosis is seen predominantly in parous women, a breakdown of the basal layer of the endometrium and myometrium due to postpartum endometritis has also been proposed as a possible cause [173].

5.2.3
Histopathology

Adenomyosis presents morphologically as focal areas or diffuse involvement of the uterus. Grossly, the cut surface is characterized by a whorled texture which results from the irregular trabeculations of the thickened myometrium (Fig. 5.4). Another common feature are cyst-like lesions. Hemorrhagic foci within the myometrium may also be seen on gross inspection. The diagnosis is based on the histologic demonstration of dispersed endometrial glandular tissue in the myometrium and requires the presence of at least one glandular nest at a depth of more than 2.5 mm or one-half of a low-power field (×100) within the myometrium measured from the endo-myometrial junction [220]. The islets of glandular tis-

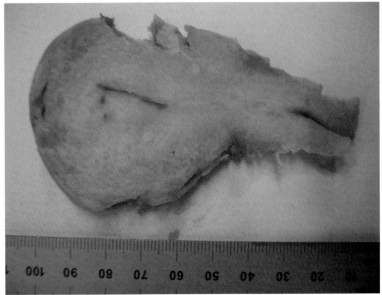

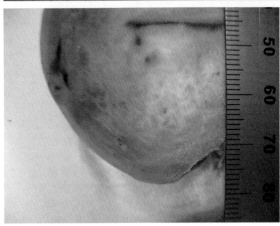

Fig. 5.4a,b. Macroscopic pathology of adenomyosis of the uterus. **a** Macroscopic uterine specimen showing focal adenomyosis. A thickened anterior uterine wall with broadening of the myometrium as well as irregular myometrial trabeculations and multiple micro-cysts are visible. **b** Magnified area of the anterior uterine wall showing coarse trabeculation of the myometrium without a mass lesion and small brownish cysts corresponding to hemorrhagic foci of dislocated endometrial glands

sue are surrounded by hypertrophied myometrium (Fig. 5.5). Pathologically a superficial form of adenomyosis which only involves the inner myometrium can be differentiated from deep-infiltrating adenomyosis which considerably enlarges the uterine wall due to smooth muscle hyperplasia adjacent to deep-infiltrating endometrial glands [46].

5.2.4
Clinical Presentation

The clinical presentation of adenomyosis is unspecific and includes symptoms such as dysmenorrhea, menorrhagia, and pelvic pain, which are also common in disorders like dysfunctional bleeding, leiomyoma, and endometriosis. The uterus is frequently enlarged in women with adenomyosis but not distorted in its shape like with uterine leiomyoma. Women with superficial or focal adenomyosis may be asymptomatic in contrast to women with extensive disease in whom the uterus usually is also markedly enlarged. The depth of involvement of the uterine wall correlates to some degree with clinical symptoms [12, 14, 117]. Dysmenorrhea has been reported to be more frequent when involvement of the myometrium by adenomyosis exceeds 80% of the diameter of the uterine wall [128].

5.2.5
Therapy

Hysterectomy is still considered the definitive treatment in patients with symptomatic adenomyosis. However, initially less invasive therapeutic options

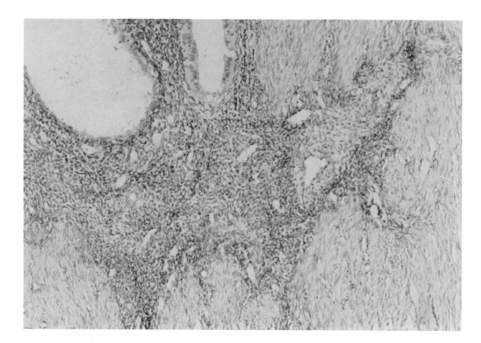

Fig. 5.5. Histopathology of adenomyosis of the uterus. Dislocated endometrial glands are surrounded by hypertrophied myometrium. (Reproduced with permission from [222])

should be considered taking into account the patient's age, symptom severity, and desire of future fertility, as well as the presence of associated disorders such as leiomyomas and endometriosis. Symptom relief can be achieved with nonsteroidal anti-inflammatory drugs, but suppression of the endometrium by hormonal treatment with danazol or gonadotropin-releasing hormones (GnRH) may be needed. Intrauterine devices (IUD) which release levonorgestrel have been shown to be effective in controlling menorrhagia caused by adenomyosis although symptoms return once the IUD is removed [45]. Endometrial ablation or resection denudes the endometrial layer of the uterus and is an option for women with predominantly abnormal uterine bleeding. Adenomyosis of the superficial type with less than 2 mm penetration responds better than deep-infiltrating adenomyosis to endometrial ablation [118].

Uterus-conserving surgery is hampered by the lack of a clearly defined dissection plane but may be of value in the infertile patient [133]. Laparoscopic resection of adenomyosis has been shown to reduce pain, menorrhagia, and dysmenorrhea in small case series with limited follow-up [124, 214]. Recently, uterine artery embolization (UAE) has been reported to be successful in relieving menorrhagia and dysmenorrhea at short-term. The long-term benefit of UAE in patients with adenomyosis is still under investigation [93, 94, 141, 174].

5.3
Imaging

5.3.1
Diagnostic Imaging for Uterine Leiomyomas and Adenomyosis – An Overview

Uterine leiomyomas and adenomyosis cannot be reliably differentiated on clinical grounds because both conditions cause similar symptoms.

Leiomyomas of the uterus, once they have reached a certain size, can be palpated and differentiated from the uterine wall as solid tumors that tend to be mobile. Bimanual palpation is typically supplemented by transvaginal ultrasound (TVUS) or, in patients with a markedly enlarged uterus, transabdominal ultrasound. The ultrasound examination allows assessment of the uterus and especially TVUS provides additional information on the endometrium and ovaries. TVUS is the primary imaging modality in the diagnostic work-up of women with uterine leiomyomas. Ultrasound depicts fibroids as hypoechoic round lesions which are sharply demarcated from the remainder of the uterus (Fig. 5.6). Anechoic cystic portions and degenerative changes with a heterogeneous echo pattern within the lesions are quite common. US enables reliable assessment of the location of fibroids and their topographic

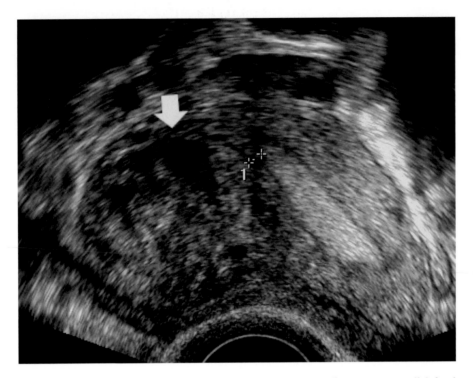

Fig. 5.6. Transvaginal ultrasound (TVUS) of uterine leiomyoma. TVUS demonstrates a well defined subserosal leiomyoma (*arrow*) distorting the outer contour of the uterine wall. The leiomyoma shows a heterogenous echotexture and is hypoechoic compared to the adjacent myometrium and endometrium. The endometrium is seen as a hyperechoic stripe

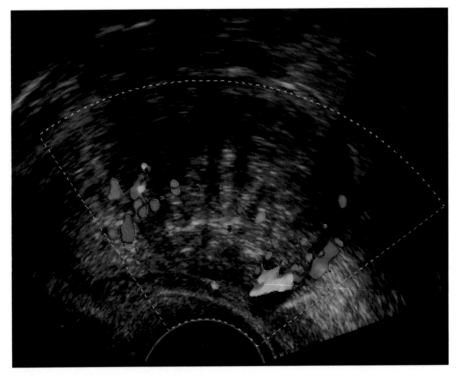

Fig. 5.7. Transvaginal ultrasound of leiomyoma. Transvaginal color-coded duplex ultrasound demonstrates the perifibroid plexus vessels surrounding the leiomyoma

relationship to surrounding structures, and in particular the uterine cavity, in most cases. Additional color-coded duplex ultrasound will depict tumor vascularity and demonstrate typical features such as a central vessel or a marginal vascular network (Fig. 5.7). Hysterosonography with the instillation of fluid into the uterine cavity improves the diagnostic accuracy of TVUS in detecting submucosal fibroids, differentiation from endometrial polyps, and determining depth of myometrial (uterine wall) involvement [38].

Endoscopic procedures such as laparoscopy or hysteroscopy have a role in patients with suspected fibroids and inconclusive US findings. Moreover, hysteroscopy is performed in conjunction with endometrial sampling in women with abnormal menstrual bleeding and for specific diagnostic purposes such as evaluation of the uterine cavity and tubes in infertile women with fibroids. In patients with known uterine leiomyomas, laparoscopy and hysteroscopy have their main role as therapeutic procedures for the uterus-sparing resection of known uterine fibroids.

Magnetic resonance imaging (MRI) is the most accurate diagnostic modality for assessing uterine leiomyomas [37]. MRI enables assessment of the uterus in multiplanar orientation and without interference from superimposed structures. MRI provides not only accurate information on the number and size of fibroids but also on their location within the uterus (cervix, corpus, fundus) and within the wall (submucosal, intramural,

subserosal), as well as their relationship to neighboring structures such as the tubes and ovaries (Figs. 5.8 and 5.9). The unique soft tissue contrast afforded by MRI enables good delineation of the fibroid tumors from adjacent myometrium, the junctional zone, which is important for the differential diagnosis, and the endometrium and also enables evaluation of the internal make-up of fibroids including secondary degenerative changes. These features thus make MRI superior to all other imaging modalities in characterizing uterine fibroids. MRI is of use in patients with inconclusive US findings with regard to the differential diagnosis of a pelvic lesion or the origin of a lesion from the uterus or the ovary [171, 212]. MRI is increasingly being used to evaluate the feasibility of uterus-sparing surgical therapy or a radiologic intervention [36]. To establish the indication for hysteroscopic or laparoscopic resection, it is necessary to know the number and size of fibroids as well as their precise position, in particular their relationship to the uterine cavity and their depth within the wall [39, 68]. In evaluating potential candidates for UAE, MRI provides information on the size of the individual fibroids, the presence of pedunculated or parasitic leiomyomas, the nature of degenerative changes, the degree of fibroid vascularization and the vascular supply of the uterus.

Computed tomography (CT) with its poor soft tissue contrast is of limited value in diagnosing benign changes of the uterus. CT does not allow adequate differen-

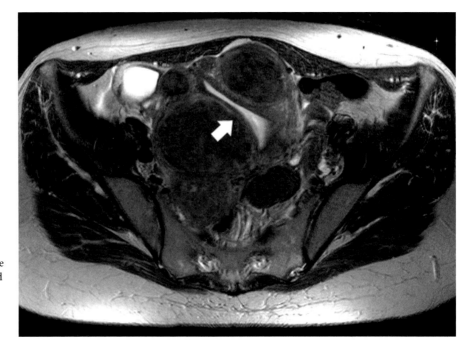

Fig. 5.8. MRI of leiomyoma – locations. Transaxial T2-weighted image depicts multiple, mainly subserosal uterine leiomyoma. There is mild distortion of the uterine cavity by a transmural (full thickness) leiomyoma (*arrow*)

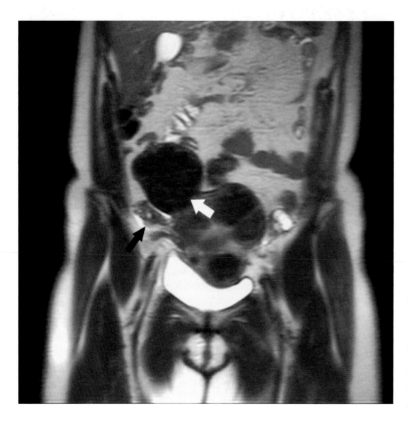

Fig. 5.9. MRI of leiomyoma – locations. T2-weighted coronal image of a polyfibroid uterus. A subserosal pedunculated uterine fibroid (*white arrow*) is easily identified by its low signal intensity and continuity with the right lateral aspect of the uterine fundus while sonographically the lesion could not be separated from the right ovary (*black arrow*). (Reproduced with permission from [223])

tiation of the different uterine layers and hence fails to reliably assign uterine lesions to a specific layer. Intravenous contrast medium administration improves the differentiation of adjacent structures but does not improve the differential diagnosis (Fig. 5.10). On CT scans, uterine fibroids are isodense with muscle and can occasionally be identified by the presence of typical calcifications on unenhanced images. There are no specific CT criteria for the presence of adenomyosis.

Adenomyosis – when severe – causes enlargement of the uterus but differs from fibroid-related enlargement in that the uterus is soft on palpation. TVUS will depict areas of reduced echogenicity or a heterogeneous appearance in about 75% of patients with adenomyosis [17, 44, 155]. Apart from asymmetric thickening of the myometrium in the presence of focal adenomyosis, other morphologic features that are indicative of adenomyosis are a poor definition of the endomyometrial junction, the presence of myometrial cysts (< 5 mm) in up to 50% of affected patients, as well as echogenic lines or spots within the myometrium [44, 72]. Circumscribed lesions are absent in the majority of cases. Good diagnostic performance can be expected if diagnostic criteria as described above are combined and real-time examination is

used. An increased vascularization demonstrated by color duplex US is indicative of adenomyosis [25, 65]. Transvaginal ultrasound has a reported sensitivity of 53%–89% and a specificity ranging from 50%–99% [6, 17, 44, 155]. The wide variation is primarily attributable to the examiner dependence of US. The diagnostic accuracy is limited in the presence of fibroids [10]. Many of the features of adenomyosis seen on US are depicted more clearly on T2-weighted MR images, which clearly show changes in zonal anatomy based on the excellent soft tissue contrast of this imaging modality (Fig. 5.11). Despite its sensitivity of 86%–100% and specificity of 85%–90.5% for the diagnosis of adenomyosis and its high diagnostic accuracy in establishing the differential diagnosis, MRI is rarely used in the routine clinical setting, for two reasons: adenomyosis is rarely suspected as the cause of hypermenorrhea or dysmenorrhea before surgery and reliable pretherapeutic demonstration of adenomyosis as the underlying cause in symptomatic women in the fourth or fifth decades of life was considered irrelevant for therapeutic decision-making (hysterectomy) [6, 113, 156, 195]. MRI is thus not indicated and cost-effective in the initial evaluation of patients with unspecific complaints suggestive of adenomyosis. However, MRI has its place as an ad-

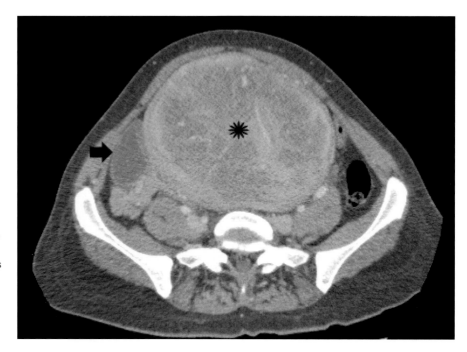

Fig. 5.10. CT of uterine leiomyoma. Contrast-enhanced CT of the pelvis in a 39-year-old women with a known uterine leiomyoma shows a large oval mass within the uterus with heterogenous enhancement (*asterisk*) which displaces the hypodense right ovary (*arrow*) and distends the abdomen

junctive tool in patients with diffusely enlarged uteri of unknown cause, in the work-up of infertile women, and for follow-up of patients receiving GnRH therapy for adenomyosis or prior to uterus-conserving surgical therapy and UAE [71, 90, 93, 133].

5.3.2
Magnetic Resonance Imaging

5.3.2.1
Magnetic Resonance Imaging – Technique

A short clinical history including menstrual status, previous pelvic surgery, clinical symptoms, time point within the menstrual cycle, and current hormonal therapy should be taken prior to an MR examination of the female pelvis. Due to the cyclic changes of the uterus, imaging is best performed in the second half of the menstrual cycle to take advantage of maximum signal differences between the uterine layers. The pelvis should be imaged on a high-field (1.5-T) scanner using a pelvic or torso phased-array coil. Motion artifacts caused by bowel peristalsis can degrade image quality significantly and should be eliminated. Measures to reduce such artifacts include asking the patient to fast for 4–6 h prior to the examination and intramuscular injection of butylscopolamine in patients who have no contraindications. Patients should

also be instructed to void prior to the examination. The standard protocol for pelvic MR imaging should include both T1- and T2-weighted sequences. Breath-hold T2-weighted sequences acquired in the true axial, sagittal, and coronal planes (T2-HASTE, SSFSE) are sufficient to diagnose uterine leiomyomas and adenomyosis in the majority of cases [7, 115]. However, the relationship of a uterine lesion to the uterine cavity may be difficult to recognize on breath-hold images alone. Additional high-resolution (512-matrix) T2-weighted TSE sequences acquired in the axial and sagittal planes in conjunction with presaturation of the anterior abdominal wall are recommended in cases of inconclusive breath-hold images or a severely distorted uterine cavity [215]. T1-weighted pulse sequences with and without fat saturation acquired in the axial plane provide information on fatty components and blood products within a lesion and accentuate areas of calcification otherwise not seen on T2-weighted imaging. Gadolinium-enhanced T1-weighted images can provide additional information on the vascularity of uterine leiomyomas, improve the visualization of the surrounding pseudocapsule, and may help to delineate the uterine origin of a subserosal leiomyoma, but are not necessary to diagnose uterine leiomyomas and adenomyosis [67]. However, additional MRA gradient-echo sequences are recommended in patients with leiomyomas and adenomyosis in whom uterine artery embolization is planned [99].

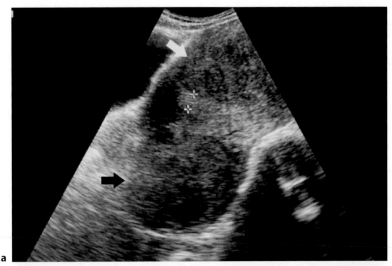

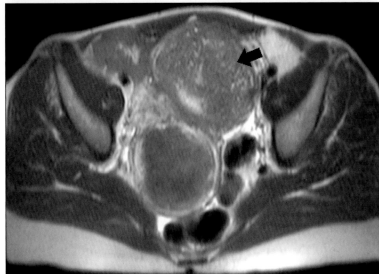

Fig. 5.11a,b. Correlation of transvaginal ultrasound (TVUS) and magnetic resonance imaging (MRI) in a patient with leiomyoma and adenomyosis of the uterus. **a** TVUS of a 48-year-old women with menorrhagia and dysmenorrhea. Two leiomyoma were reported to be present, one in a subserosal location (*black arrow*) of the posterior wall and a second intramurally in the anterior uterine wall (*white arrow*). However, a poor definition of the endomyometrial junction and asymmetric myometrial thickening of the anterior uterine wall rather than a clear mass lesion is seen. Calipers indicate measurement of endometrial thickness. **b** Corresponding T2-weighted transaxial image shows a subserosal leiomyoma of the posterior uterine wall and focal adenomyosis of the anterior uterine wall (*black arrow*) characterized by a broadening of the junctional zone and cyst-like inclusions in the myometrium corresponding to endometrial glands

5.3.2.2
MR Appearance of Uterine Leiomyomas

Leiomyomas of the uterus present as well-defined round or oval low-signal intensity masses on T2-weighted MR images. They are characterized by expansive growth but do not infiltrate surrounding structures and therefore distort the shape of the uterus in relation to their size and location. MRI performed in three orthogonal planes allows one first to accurately localize leiomyomas as submucosal, intramural, transmural (full thickness), subserosal, pedunculated, or (extrauterine) intraligamentous and second to assign them to the cervix (less than 8%), uterine corpus (anterior, posterior, lateral uterine wall), or fundus. Uterine leiomyomas can be single but usually are multiple and may reach considerable size. In a multifibroid uterus normal myometrium often represents only a minor portion of the uterine tissue (Fig. 5.12). Diffuse leiomyomatosis is a rare form where the myometrium is displaced by confluent leiomyomas [89] (Fig. 5.13).

5.3.2.3
Locations, Growth Patterns, and Imaging Characteristics

The localization of leiomyomas by imaging is of clinical importance because symptoms are related to and treatment varies based on the position of a fibroid within the uterus. Whether a submucosal leiomyoma can be resected depends on its size and ingrowth into

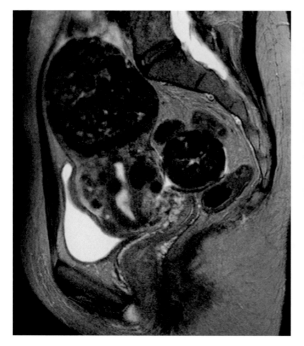
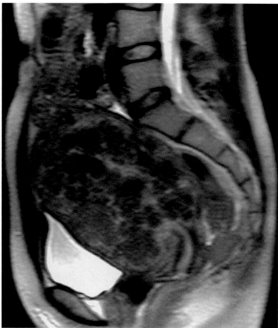

Fig. 5.12. Polyfibroid uterus – MRI appearance. T2-weighted sagittal image of a 44-year-old women shows multiple uterine leiomyoma, the largest extending subserosal from the fundus of the uterus. All leiomyomas are well marginated and show typical hypointense signal intensity with some speckled hyperintense spots. A pedunculated subserosally leiomyoma is present in the posterior cul-de-sac

Fig. 5.13. MRI of diffuse leiomyomatosis of the uterus. T2-weighted sagittal image of a 41-year-old women shows multiple uterine leiomyoma throughout the uterine layers ranging from millimeters to several centimeters in size. The leiomyomas are partially confluent and have replaced almost the entire normal myometrium (compare also with Fig. 5.3)

the uterine wall [210]. A subserosal leiomyoma can be surgically treated by enucleation but opening and surgical reconstruction of the uterine cavity may be necessary if the leiomyoma grows transmurally [188]. Leiomyomas are characterized by expansive growth with displacement of neighboring tissue and therefore already have a mass effect when they are still small. Deformity of the uterine contour is primarily associated with submucosal and subserosal fibroids because they distend neighboring layers such as the endometrium and serosa (Fig. 5.14). In patients with a markedly enlarged uterus due to multiple fibroids, these tumors are often difficult to differentiate from extrauterine or ovarian lesions on ultrasound. The presence of a claw-like extension of myometrium surrounding the lesion and corkscrew-like flow voids at the interface between lesion and normal uterine tissue, which can be detected on T1-weighted images, less commonly on T2-weighted images, indicate uterine fibroids with a high degree of certainty [91, 171, 196, 212]. These flow voids represent the arteries arising from the uterine artery and feeding the

large-caliber vascular plexus of a fibroid (Fig. 5.15). The MR imaging signs of uterine leiomyomas are summarized in Table 5.1.

5.3.2.4
Histologic Subtypes and Forms of Degeneration

Different histologic subtypes of leiomyomas exist, some of them showing characteristic features on MRI. Cellular leiomyomas, a subgroup of leiomyomas characterized by compact smooth muscle cells with little intervening collagen, exhibit a homogenously high signal intensity on T2-weighted images (Fig. 5.16). They are isointense to surrounding myometrium on T1-weighted images and tend to enhance fairly homogenously after gadolinium administration [216]. Lipoleiomyoma is a rare type of leiomyoma which displays a signal intensity similar to subcutaneous fat on all pulse sequences due to the presence of various amounts of fat cells. Chemical shift imaging or spectral fat suppression may be useful to determine the fatty nature of these leiomyomas [201]. While MRI can dis-

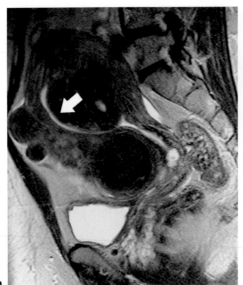

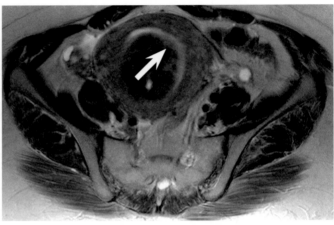

Fig. 5.14a,b. Mass effect of uterine leiomyoma. **a** T2-weighted sagittal image shows a multifibroid uterus with a large submucosal leiomyoma that exerts mass effect on the underlying endometrium (*arrow*). **b** T2-weighted axial image at correspondig level

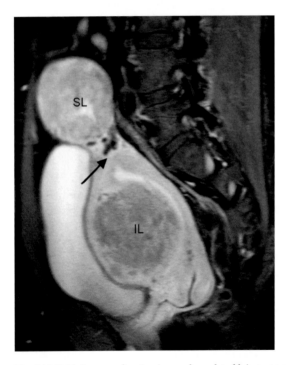

Fig. 5.15. Bridging vascular sign in a pedunculated leiomyoma. T1-weighted contrast-enhanced fat-suppressed sagittal image depicts a large pedunculated subserosal leiomyoma originating from the uterine fundus. Flow-voids are seen within the vessel stalk (*arrow*). A second intramural leiomyoma in the anterior wall is seen displacing the endometrial stripe. (Reproduced with permission from [223])

Table 5.1. MRI criteria for leiomyoma

Location	● Corpus, fundus, less often cervical or within uterine ligaments, subserosal, intramural, transmural, submucous, pedunculated, in statu nascendi
Morphology	● Spherical, sharply marginated, pseudocapsule may be present, mass effect even if small, deforming the uterine outline and/or cavity may be singular but often numerous ● Size range from 0.5 cm - > 20 cm ● Claw-like extension of myometrium surrounding the lesion
Appearance on T1	● Isointense to the myometrium ● Peripheral hypointense rim indicates calcification ● Hyperintense areas related to hemorrhage ● Peripheral high SI rim or homogenous high SI indicates hemorrhagic infarction
Appearance on T2	● Variable, in general hypointense mass relative to myometrium but different SI seen in individual leiomyomas ● Homogenously high SI often seen in cellular leiomyomas ● High SI rim represents dilated lymphatics in large leiomyoma
Appearance on Gd-enhanced T1	● Can appear hypo-, iso- and hyperintense relative to myometrium Hypervascularity often seen in cellular leiomyomas ● Pseudocapsule more prominent ● Absence of enhancement seen in partially or completely infarcted leiomyoma (bridging-vascular-sign)
Additional findings	● Flow voids in the periphery (best seen on T1-weighted images) indicate the perifibroid plexus vessels ● A vessel stalk may be seen in pedunculated leiomyomas

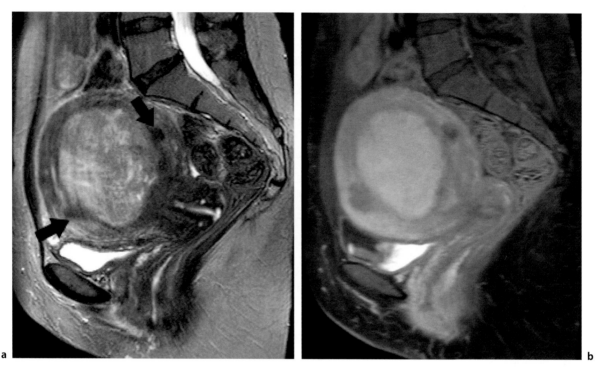

Fig. 5.16a,b. MRI of cellular leiomyoma. **a** T2-weighted sagittal image of the uterus demonstrating a large intramural cellular leiomyoma with homogenous high signal intensity compared to surrounding myometrium. Two small intramural leiomyoma show the typical low intensity signal (*arrows*). **b** T1-weighted contrast-enhanced fat-suppressed sagittal image showing marked enhancement of the intramural cellular leiomyoma which appears hyperintense compared to surrounding myometrium

tinguish among the different subtypes in only 69% of all cases, the method is highly sensitive and specific in identifying simple fibroids without any major degenerative changes, fibroids having undergone hemorrhagic infarction, and fibroids with cystic degenerative changes [169]. Degeneration of uterine leiomyomas is common and is attributed to an inadequate blood supply. It is a sudden event in case of hemorrhagic degeneration or degenerative changes may develop gradually when a tumor outgrows its blood supply.

The typical MRI appearance of a smoothly marginated tumor with a nearly homogeneous low signal intensity relative to surrounding myometrium on T2-weighted images and intermediate signal on T1-weighted images (Fig. 5.17) is attributable to hyalinization [129]. Hyaline degeneration is the predominant form of degeneration and is present in about 60% of all leiomyomas. It is characterized by the accumulation of high-protein eosinophilic substrate in the extracellular spaces between strands of muscle cells. Other types of degeneration that can be differentiated are cystic, myxoid, and hemorrhagic (red) degeneration. Cystic degeneration is characterized by the presence of clearly delineated cystic

lesions with a signal intensity isointense to fluid on T1- and T2-weighted images. Myxoid degeneration is seen as intralesional areas of very high signal intensity on T2-weighted images. These portions represent viable tissue and are of intermediate to low signal on T1-weighted images and typically show enhancement after contrast medium administration (Fig. 5.18). Histology demonstrates gelatinous portions containing hyaluronic mucopolysaccharides. Hemorrhagic or red degeneration is more common during pregnancy or in women on gestagen therapy. It is attributed to sudden infarction of fibroid tissue with secondary intralesional hemorrhage [59]. MRI shows a lesion with an increased internal signal and a low-signal-intensity margin on T2-weighted images while T1-weighted images depict a lesion with a heterogeneous high signal that varies with the amount of blood degradation products present and is often confined to the margin (Fig. 5.19) [86]. Hemorrhagic fibroids typically show no enhancement after contrast medium administration. MRI confirms the diagnosis of acute hemorrhagic degeneration in conjunction with the clinical symptoms comprising acute pain, subfebrile temperature, and leukocytosis [57, 86].

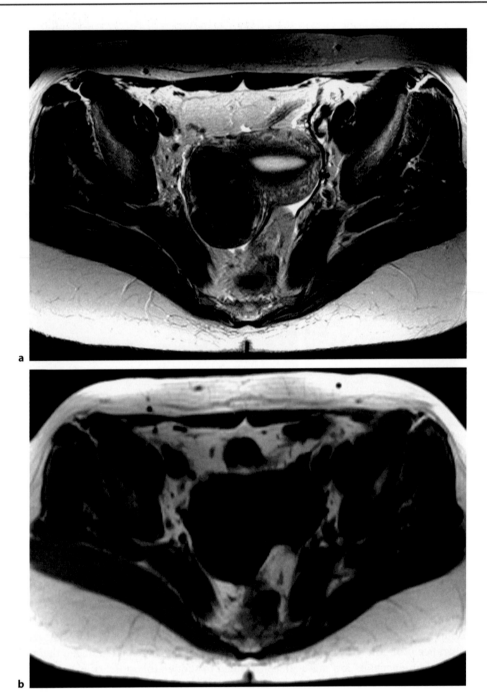

Fig. 5.17a,b. Signal intensity characteristics of leiomyoma. **a** T2-weighted transaxial image of the uterus (secretory phase of menstrual cycle) showing a subserosal leiomyoma with typical low signal intensity compared to adjacent myometrium. Note the bright signal of the endometrium and intermediate signal intensity of the junctional zone. **b** Corresponding T1-weighted transaxial image of the uterus showing intermediate signal intensity of the leiomyoma which can hardly be differentiated from the adjacent myometrium

Fig. 5.18a–c. a,b MRI of myxoid leiomyoma. **a** T2-weighted transaxial image of the uterus showing also heterogenous signal intensity of the leiomyoma and a c-shaped area at the left border of the leiomyoma (*arrow*) of high signal intensity corresponding to myxoid degeneration. Note high signal intensity stripe of the endometrium is displaced laterally. **b** On the corresponding T1-weighted fat suppressed transaxial image the whole leiomyoma has a heterogenous intermediate signal intensity and the c-shaped area shows no low signal as expexted if liquification had occured. **c** Contrast-enhanced T1-weighted fat suppressed transaxial image shows heterogenous enhancement of the leiomyoma including septations of myxoid tissue, Note enhancement of endometrial stripe (*arrow*)

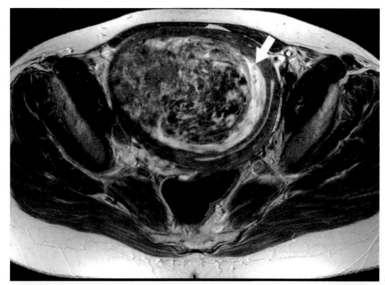

a

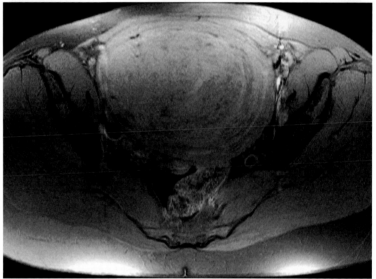

b

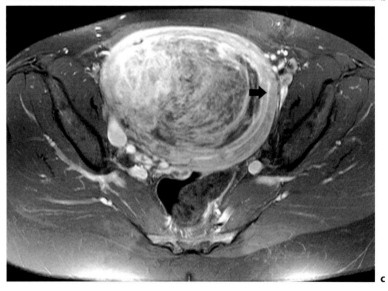

c

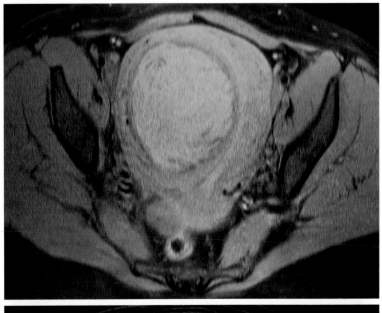

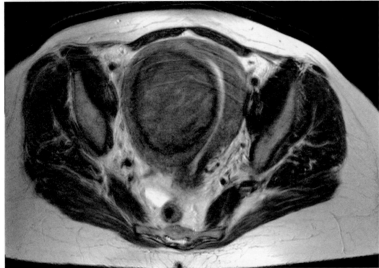

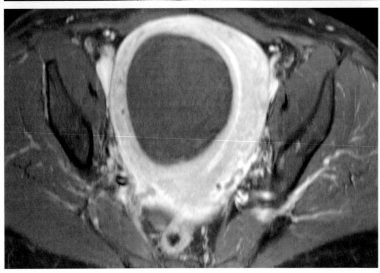

Fig. 5.19a–b. MRI of spontaneously infarcted leiomyoma. **a** T1-weighted fat-suppressed transaxial image of a spontaneously infarcted submucosal leiomyoma. The central portion shows an slightly hyperintense signal intensity compared to the surrounding myometrium. **b** T2-weighted transaxial image of a spontaneous infarcted submucosal leiomyoma. The central portion shows a signal intensity isointense to the myometrium while a marked hypointense rim is seen which corresponds to blood degradation products (hemosiderin) after hemorrhagic infarction. c Contrast-enhanced T1-weighted fat-suppressed transaxial image confirms infarction of the leiomyoma while the surrounding myometrium is well perfused(Reproduced with permission from [223])

MRI is methodologically limited in that it does not reliably show intralesional calcifications, which are frequently identified on conventional radiographs or CT scans by their popcorn-like appearance [169]. Occasionally, calcifications take the form of a peripheral rim after hemorrhagic infarction and can be identified on T1-weighted MR images (Fig. 5.20).

5.3.2.5
Differential Diagnosis

In evaluating lesions in close topographic relationship to the uterus, the examiner must consider ovarian masses in the differential diagnosis. If it is not possible to definitely assign the lesion to the uterus, an intraligamentous or ovarian fibroid may be present if the lesion shows homogeneous low signal intensity on T2-weighted images and an intermediate signal on T1-weighted images relative to the signal intensity of the myometrium of the uterus. However, an inhomogeneous intermediate, or high signal relative to the myometrium may indicate both a fibroid with degenerative changes or an extrauterine benign or malignant tumor.

Myometrial contractions can mimic submucosal leiomyomas or focal adenomyosis [193]. Uterine contractions involve the endo- and myometrium but spare the outer uterine contour (Fig. 5.21). They are characterized by band- or stick-like low-signal-intensity areas on T2-weighted images [116]. These signal changes are transient and changing appearances can be noted on sequential images obtained with a delay of 30–45 min [193, 194].

Endometrial polyps, seen most frequently in perimenopausal and postmenopausal women, are usually asymptomatic but may cause uterine bleeding, especially in postmenopausal women [33]. In 20% of the cases polyps are multiple. They can be broadbased or pedunculated and may occur in conjunction with endometrial hyperplasia. On T2-weighted images a central fibrous core or intratumoral cysts may be visible [55]. On T1-weighted images endometrial polyps show an intermediate signal while they exhibit a slightly hypointense or isointense signal intensity relative to the endometrium on T2-weighted images and present as localized endometrial thickening (Fig. 5.22). Small polyps enhance and become more conspicuous after gadolinium administration, especially on early enhanced scans while large polyps exhibit a heterogenous enhancement pattern [55, 67]. Submucosal leiomyomas are best distinguished from endometrial polyps by their rather spherical shape, their obvious connection to the myometrium, and lower signal intensity on T2-weighted images.

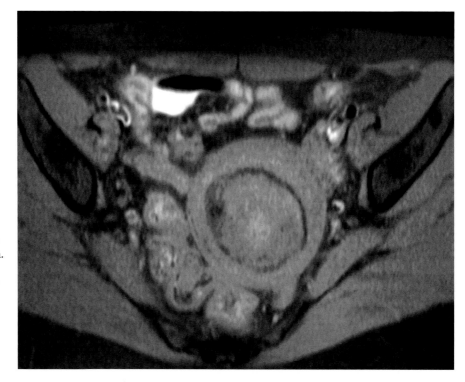

Fig. 5.20. MRI of rim calcification of a leiomyoma. T1-weighted fat-suppressed transaxial image showing a leiomyoma with a discontinuous, markedly hypointense rim corresponding to asymmetrical calcification

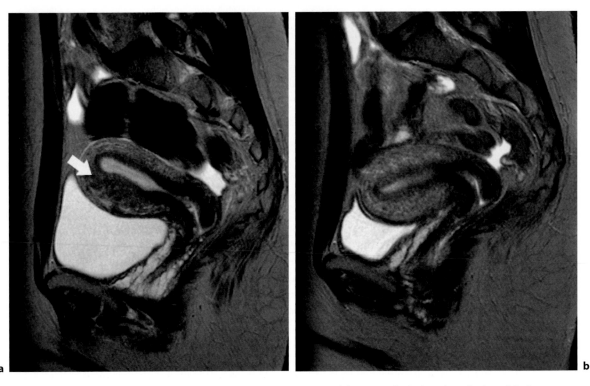

a   b

Fig. 5.21a,b. Transient uterine contraction. **a** T2-weighted sagittal image of the uterus depicting a broadening of the inner myometrium of the anterior uterine wall with bulging into the uterine cavity (*arrow*). **b** T2-weighted sagittal image of the uterus obtained 5 min before (**a**) shows absence of any structural abnormality, a finding consistent with myometrial contraction

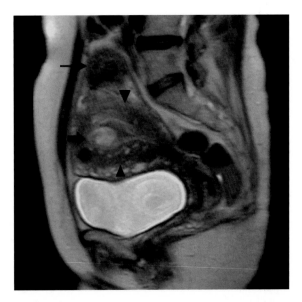

Fig. 5.22. Leiomyoma, diffuse adenomyosis and endometrial polyp on MRI. T2-weighted sagittal image of a patient depicts diffuse adenomyosis (*arrowheads*) with symmetrical broadening of the junctional zone. An endometrial polyp exhibiting similar high signal intensity as the endometrium can be clearly identified within the uterine cavity (*short arrow*). A fibroid is present in the fundus (*long arrow*)

Leiomyosarcomas of the uterus are rare with a frequency of incidentally discovered tumors of 1:2000 while large series of hysterectomy specimen quote a frequency of 2–5:1000 [3, 149]. It is felt that leiomyosarcomas arise de novo and may be unrelated to benign leiomyomas [107]. They are predominantly observed in older women (6th decade of life) as compared to women with leiomyoma (4th decade of life) [149]. While rapid growth is not an indicator of malignancy in premenopausal women, it is always suspicious in postmenopausal women although not specific [130, 137]. The imaging appearance does not enable reliable differentiation of leiomyosarcoma from benign leiomyoma [73, 137, 169, 190]. Besides frank signs of invasiveness or metastatic disease, an irregular contour, inhomogeneous appearance with pockets of high signal intensity on T2, as well as hemorrhagic changes with high signal intensity on T1 have been proposed to suggest a leiomyosarcoma rather than a leiomyoma [54, 138, 165, 169]. Recently, early enhancement on dynamic scans after administration of contrast medium together with serum determination of LDH and its isoenzymes was reported to be highly sensitive and specific in differentiating leiomyosarcoma from degenerated leiomyoma [54].

5.3.2.6
MR Appearance of Uterine Adenomyosis

Adenomyosis of the uterus is diagnosed on T2-weighted images where it is characterized by ill-defined low-signal-intensity areas representing diffuse or focal broadening of the junctional zone as a result of smooth muscle hyperplasia associated with heterotopic endometrial glands [132, 156]. A junctional zone thickness of ≥ 12 mm (Fig. 5.23) is the threshold for which a high degree of accuracy in the diagnosis of adenomyosis has been reported [79, 158]. Adenomyosis can be excluded if the junctional zone thickness is 8 mm or less [156]. Bright foci and cyst-like inclusions may be seen on T2-weighted images in up to 50% of patients and represent heterotopic endometrial glands, cystic dilatations, or hemorrhagic foci [156, 195]. Corresponding high signal on T1-weighted images is less frequently observed but highly suggestive of adenomyosis (Fig. 5.24). Additionally, striations of high signal intensity extending from the endometrium into the myometrium as a result of direct invasion of the myometrium may be seen and result in pseudo-widening of the endometrium [157]. These high-signal-intensity changes associated with adenomyosis may fluctuate during the menstrual cycle. The MR imaging signs of adenomyosis are summarized in Table 5.2.

Table 5.2. MRI criteria for adenomyosis

Location	• Focal or diffuse widening of junctional zone (JZ) > 12 mm • More often found in the posterior uterine wall • Not seen in the cervix • Seldom seen as focal lesion without contact to JZ (adenomyoma)
Morphology	• Either diffusely involving the uterus or presenting as a lesion with ill-defined margins blending with the surrounding myometrium • Poor definition of endomyometrial junction • If focal, may be globular, elliptical but usually not round, spherical • Significant mass effect missing, even if large lesion present • Mild distortion of endometrium but marked enlargement of the uterus in diffuse adenomyosis • Adenomyoma may rarely present as round lesion located away from JZ • Lesion may include large cystic areas (cystic adenomyosis)
Appearance on T1	• Mostly isointense to the myometrium • May show hyperintense foci corresponding to small areas of hemorrhage
Appearance on T2	• Low SI uterine lesion with or without punctuate high SI foci scattered throughout the lesion or high SI linear striations extending from the edometrium that may lead to a pseudowidening of the endometrium • High SI (micro) cysts may be seen (< 5 mm) • Rarely large cystic spaces within a lesion (cystic adenomyosis)
Appearance on Gd-enhanced T1	• Can appear hypo-, iso- and hyperintense relative to myometrium • Perfusion abnormalities may be seen on dynamic contrast-enhanced MRI
Additional findings	• No pseudocapsule • Adenomyosis frequently seen in combination with findings of endometriosis

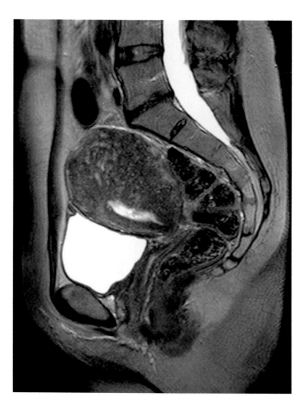

Fig. 5.23. Focal adenomyosis of the uterus. T2-weighted sagittal image of a patient with focal adenomyosis of the uterus. There is enlargement with only mild deformity of the uterus. The fundus and posterior uterine wall is thickened due to marked broadening of the junctional zone. Hyperintense foci are seen within the lesion. (Reproduced with permission from [223])

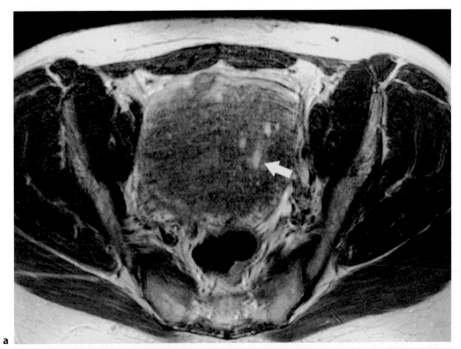

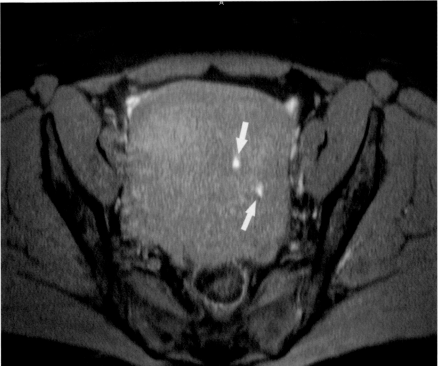

Fig. 5.24a,b. MRI of diffuse adenomyosis of the uterus. **a** T2-weighted transaxial image of a patient with diffuse adenomyosis of the uterus. The uterine wall is thickened, there is poor definition of the endomyometrial junction and the junctional zones blend with the myometrium. No focal mass is present. Cyst-like inclusions of hyperintense signal intensity are present (*arrow*). **b** Corresponding fat-suppressed T1-weighted transaxial image showing hyperintense spots within the myometrium indicating fresh blood related to the dislocated endometrial glands (*arrows*)

5.3.2.7
Locations, Growth Patterns, and Imaging Characteristics

Uterine adenomyosis is found more often in the posterior than in the anterior wall of the uterus and the fundus [22]. Adenomyosis does not involve the uterine cervix. A focal type can be differentiated from a diffuse type of thickening of the junctional zone. Diffuse adenomyosis (Fig. 5.25) may lead to a markedly enlarged uterus with a surprisingly small or disproportional mass effect on the uterine contour and cavity. Focal adenomyosis (Fig. 5.26) manifests as an oval or round lesion which leads to thickening of the uterine wall but differs from leiomyoma in that there is only little distortion of the uterine cavity or serosal surface. The lesion shows poorly defined margins and blends with surrounding myometrium. It lacks the pseudocapsule that may be seen with uterine leiomyoma. Signal voids at the periphery of the lesion are rare in focal adenomyosis [22]. Gadolinium-enhanced T1-weighted imaging does not increase the accuracy in diagnosing adenomyosis of the uterus although perfusion abnormalities may be seen [67]. Unusual growth patterns include adenomyoma of the uterus which represents a localized form that manifests as a myometrial or subserosal mass without a direct connection to the junctional zone [50, 191]. Another

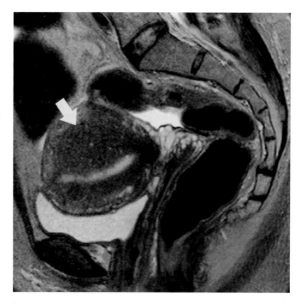

Fig. 5.26. MRI of focal adenomyosis of the uterus. T2-weighted sagittal image of the uterus. The posterior wall of the uterus is thickened and a focally broadened junctional zone with hyperintense foci appearing as a globular lesion is seen (*arrow*). The uterus is enlarged but no mass effect is seen

rare variant is cystic adenomyosis which is thought to result from extensive hemorrhage within adenomyotic implants, leading to a well circumscribed cystic myometrial lesion which may show different stages of blood product degradation such as a low intensity rim on T2-weighted images corresponding to hemosiderin and areas of high signal intensity on T1-weighted images representing fresh blood [157, 191, 199]. Treatment of adenomyosis by GnRH agonists may also alter its appearance on MR imaging and a decrease in junctional zone thickness and a better lesion demarcation may be observed [71].

5.3.2.8
Differential Diagnosis

Leiomyomas of the uterus are part of the differential diagnosis for adenomyosis and differentiation is especially important since therapeutic options differ for both entities. Imaging features that favor adenomyosis are poorly defined lesion borders, minimal mass effect, an elliptical instead of a globular shape, and high-signal-intensity spots, cysts, and striations on T2-weighted imaging. Adenomyoma and cystic adenomyosis, however, may be indistinguishable from degenerated leiomyomas at MR imaging or may resemble an aggressive uterine neoplasm [28,

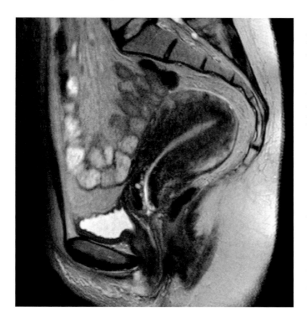

Fig. 5.25. MRI of diffuse adenomyosis of the uterus. T2-weighted sagittal image of the uterus. A broadened junctional zone (> 12 mm) is seen with poor definition of the endomyometrial junction. The junctional zone blends with the myometrium

191]. Myometrial contractions may also mimic focal adenomyosis but are transient phenomena.

Endometrial carcinoma can show some overlap with the imaging features associated with adenomyosis such as an irregular endomyometrial junction, high-signal-intensity linear striations on T2-weighted imaging, as well as pseudowidening of the endometrium. Contrast-enhanced MR imaging has been reported to be useful in the case of endometrial carcinoma invading adenomyosis [204]. Endometrial stroma sarcoma (ESS) must also be considered when both endometrial and myometrial involvement of an apparently infiltrative lesion with cystic changes is detected [97]. A rare differential diagnosis is an adenocarcinoma arising in adenomyosis [96, 104].

5.3.3
Computed Tomography

5.3.3.1
CT Technique

Given the availability and cost-effectiveness of ultrasound as a first-line imaging tool to diagnose benign uterine lesions and the proven benefits of MRI in delineating soft tissue masses of the uterus, little room is left for the use of CT in this setting. With the advent of multislice spiral CT (MSCT) spatial resolution has improved considerably. Current scanner technology allows the acquisition of slices as thin as 0.5 mm. The generation of isotropic voxels allows multiplanar reformations in the desired plane of interest and can aid in determining the exact location of a presumed uterine lesion with respect to surrounding tissues. However, the improvement in spatial resolution is of little benefit for the diagnosis of benign uterine conditions.

5.3.3.2
CT Appearance of
Uterine Leiomyoma and Adenomyosis

While there are no specific CT features of leiomyomas, their presence may be suggested by uterine enlargement, contour deformity, and the depiction of calcifications. Calcification is the most specific sign of a leiomyoma and can be found in up to 10% of cases. Calcifications may be mottled, whorled, or streaked in appearance but can also present as a well-defined peripheral rim surrounding the leiomyoma [24]. Calcifications may be found only in one of multiple leiomyomas and may be only present in a part of a fibroid. On CT leiomyomas usually exhibit a similar density as surrounding myometrium but may show low-density areas that represent degenerative cystic changes (Fig. 5.27). CT cannot reliably identify adenomyosis of the uterus. As with uterine leiomyomas, enlargement of the uterus may be present. In adenomyosis there is enlargement while a clear mass lesion or distortion of the uterine contour is absent.

5.3.3.3
Atypical Appearances on CT and Differential Diagnosis

Leiomyomas may undergo spontaneous infarction, which presents clinically as an acute abdomen. Infarction may be related to rapid growth during pregnancy or may be due to acute torsion (Fig. 5.28)

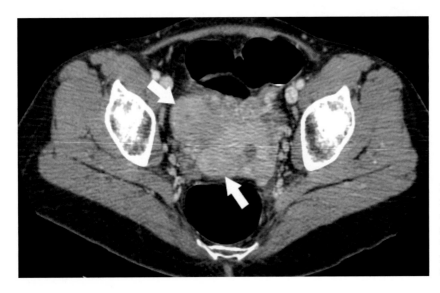

Fig. 5.27. CT of uterine leiomyomas of the uterus. Contrast-enhanced CT shows subserosal leiomyomas distorting the uterine contour (*arrows*). The fibroids show similar enhancement to adjacent myometrium

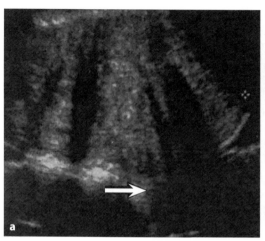

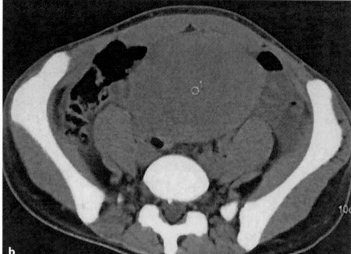

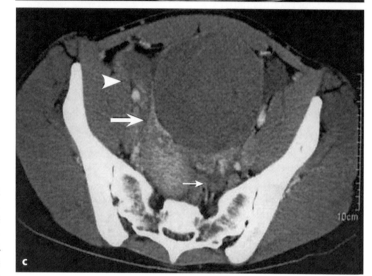

Fig. 5.28a–d. Acute torsion of a uterine leiomyoma. A 30-year-old-woman with torsion of a pedunculated subserosal leiomyoma. **a** Suprapubic US examination in the sagittal plane shows a large (13 cm in diameter), echogenic, heterogeneous mass that compresses the bladder. The uterus is displaced posteriorly (*arrow*). Shadows inside the mass are due to acoustic reflections. **b** Unenhanced CT scan shows a large, slightly heterogeneous, abdominopelvic mass (mean value 45 HU). Some linear parts have a higher value of 55 HU. **c** Contrast-enhanced CT scan shows intense rim enhancement localized against uptake of contrast medium inside tortuous vessels between the upper anterior part of the corpus uteri and the mass (*large arrow*). There is no enhancement inside the mass. The left ovary is normal and far from the mass (*arrowhead*). Note fluid inside the cul-de-sac (*small arrow*). **d** Contrast-enhanced CT scan at a level inferior to that depicted in (c) shows thin rim enhancement that is more intense in contact with persistent uptake of contrast medium against the anterior part of the uterus (*arrow*). No enhancement inside the mass was recorded. The endometrial cavity is normally enlarged during the second part of the menstrual cycle. The right ovary is normal (*arrowhead*). (Reproduced with permission from [224])

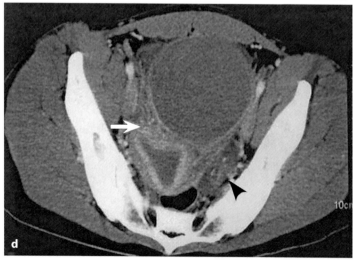

of a pedunculated subserosal leiomyoma [163]. On unenhanced images small areas of high attenuation indicate hemorrhagic infarction, which is confirmed on contrast-enhanced images [163]. Superinfection of leiomyomas may occur secondary to degeneration or hemorrhagic infarction if predisposing factors such as diabetes, adnexitis, or an ascending infection that can spread to leiomyomas with contact to the endometrial cavity are present. Pyomyoma develops slowly over days and weeks, particularly in patients after delivery or abortion [80]. Specific findings are hypodense areas in combination with pockets of gas within the leiomyoma. If perforation into the peritoneal cavity occurs, discontinuity of the uterine wall, intraperitoneal gas and fluid are usually present, and peritoneal enhancement is seen with peritonitis [80].

The differential diagnosis of acute torsion of a pedunculated leiomyoma includes ovarian/adnexal torsion and uterine torsion [49, 74]. The most valuable sign to diagnose acute adnexal torsion is thought to be thickening of the fallopian tube due to venous congestion and edema. Coronal and sagittal reformations from thin section contrast-enhanced MSCT also aid in identifying the ovarian vascular pedicle and confirm the ovarian origin of a pelvic tumor [105]. Uterine torsion has been reported to occur more often during pregnancy and is characterized by torsion along the corpus and cervix uteri. A whorled structure of the uterine cervix or a twisting upper vagina is seen on CT [74].

5.4
UAE for the Treatment of Leiomyoma and Adenomyosis

5.4.1
Indications

UAE is an established treatment for symptomatic fibroids. The gynecologist and interventional radiologist should closely cooperate in establishing the indication for fibroid embolization and carefully weigh the indications and contraindications in light of the range of therapeutic options available for the individual patient [53, 66]. UAE must not be performed without careful pre-interventional diagnostic workup of the patient's symptoms by the gynecologist. UAE is an alternative therapeutic option only in patients with symptomatic leiomyoma who would otherwise undergo surgery. The "ideal" candidate for UAE is a premenopausal woman with a symptomatic multifibroid uterus in whom surgery is indicated and who does not desire to preserve fertility and prefers a minimally invasive intervention. As a rule, both single and multiple fibroids can be treated by UAE. The number and location of the individual tumors (subserosal, intramural, transmural, submucosal) does not affect the approach, technique or outcome of UAE. Nevertheless, one must always thoroughly evaluate the clinical symptoms, imaging findings, and the patient's preferences on an individual basis to decide when UAE should be preferred to uterus-sparing surgical approaches or hysterectomy.

Embolization of subserosal pedunculated and intraligamentous fibroids is considered to be more risky because postprocedural necrosis of the tumors may cause peritoneal adhesions and decomposition of the fibroids into the free abdominal cavity. More recent studies, however, have not demonstrated a higher complication rate of UAE for subserosal pedunculated fibroids [81]. From the interventional radiologist's perspective, there is no size limit above which it becomes technically impossible to perform UAE. Early reports on higher complication rates in fibroids > 10 cm were not confirmed by later studies, which found good clinical results after embolization of large uterine leiomyomas [82, 147]. However, the patient must be aware that a markedly enlarged uterus will persist after UAE despite shrinkage of the fibroids in case of a multifibroid uterus associated with pronounced enlargement before the intervention. UAE is not indicated in patients with contraindications to angiography (clotting disorder, renal insufficiency, manifest hyperthyroidism) and in women with pelvic or urogenital infections (adnexitis, endometritis, urinary tract infection), an adnexal tumor, status post-pelvic radiotherapy, and suspected malignant tumor. An unwillingness to undergo follow-up examinations is a relative contraindication because follow-up is absolutely necessary to evaluate the success of the intervention and to identify and treat possible complications. Since data on the effect of UAE on fertility and the course of pregnancy after UAE is still inadequate, the wish to conceive is considered a contraindication to UAE, while a desire to have further children is a relative contraindication to embolization in those women in whom other therapeutic approaches (e.g. laparoscopic/abdominal leiomyoma resection) are an option [78, 92, 121, 145, 151, 183]. In addition to the gynecologic examination, a recent cervical smear (Papanicolaou's smear) is required, and women with irregular periods (metrorrhagia) should undergo endometrial sampling before UAE. UAE for adenomyosis occurring either alone or in conjunction with uterine leiomyomas is still under investigation. Contrary to previous reports, UAE has been shown to be effective in the midterm for both scenarios [51, 76, 93, 94, 122, 141, 174].

5.4.2
Technique

UAE is performed under local anesthesia, which may be supplemented by sedation where required, using a transfemoral access and standard Seldinger technique. Prior to embolization, patients receive an intravenous line and a bladder catheter. A 4- or 5-F catheter sheath is placed and the internal iliac artery is probed using end-hole catheters. An abdominal aortogram or selective angiographic series of the pelvic arteries is required only in those cases where the road map of the internal iliac artery in left or right anterior oblique projection does not provide adequate information on the origin of the uterine artery. When the uterine artery is strong and its origin takes a straight course, it can be catheterized with the diagnostic catheter. However, coaxial advanced microcatheters should be used liberally to prevent vascular spasm, in particular when the uterine artery has a small caliber or its origin is at a right angle or twisted. The embolic agent is administered with the blood flow in a fractionated manner (free-flow embolization) once the catheter comes to lie in the horizontal segment of the uterine artery and the angiogram shows good flow. Spasm sometimes results in complete cessation of flow and should then be addressed with intra-arterial administration of nitroglycerin or tolazoline. In case of strong spasm, the interventional radiologist should first proceed to embolize the contralateral uterine artery and then try again. Particulate agents are used for UAE in treating both symptomatic uterine leiomyomas and adenomyosis. Well-documented experience is available with polyvinyl alcohol (PVA), Gelfoam, and trisacryl gelatin-coated microspheres (TGM) [69, 83, 93, 101, 120, 141, 142, 174, 178, 180]. Nonspherical particles measuring 350–750 μm and microspheres ranging in size from 500–900 μm are used. The angiographic endpoint using non-sherical PVA is stasis indicating complete occlusion of the uterine arteries while a limited embolization with sluggish antegrade flow but complete

occlusion of fibroid plexus vessels is advocated when using trisaryl-gelantin microspheres [139, 180]. The level of occlusion is documented by last image hold or a final selective series. Following embolization of the contralateral side, the ipsilateral uterine artery is catheterized by formation of a Waltman loop or by simply pulling down a curved catheter such as the Rösch inferior mesenteric catheter which acts like a hook and easily enters the internal iliac artery. When confronted with a difficult anatomic situation on the ipsilateral side, it may become necessary to puncture the other groin for cross-over catherization. A controversy exists regarding the necessity of obtaining a final aortogram at the time of the intervention to exclude relevant collateral flow to the uterus (e.g. ovarian artery). If MR angiography is performed, relevant blood supply to the uterus through the ovarian artery can be identified noninvasively already before embolization [99]. The technical success rate is over 95% for primary bilateral embolization. Postprocedural management during the first 24(–48) h comprises adequate pain relief using intravenous opioid analgesics or placement of a peridural catheter and administration of nonsteroidal anti-inflammatory agents and antiemetic medication.

5.4.3
MR Imaging in the Setting of UAE and Uterus-Conserving Surgery

MR imaging prior to UAE or uterus-conserving surgery offers a comprehensive view of the pelvis without superimposed structures even in patients with a markedly enlarged polyfibroid uterus. It has been demonstrated that MRI affects patient treatment by reducing unnecessary surgery and identifying co-pathologies prior to UAE [131, 168]. MR imaging can aid in the preoperative planning for myomectomy by its ability to accurately determine the size and position of individual leiomyomas within the uterine wall and to differentiate conditions which may mimic leiomyoma both clinically and on ultrasound [212]. Preoperative classification of leiomyomas is of clinical significance since a submucosal tumor with a minor intramural component may be treated by hysteroscopic resection whereas a laparoscopic or transabdominal approach may be required in intramural or subserosal fibroids [36]. Knowing the position of a fibroid and the thickness of the surrounding myometrium helps one to minimize the risk of uterine perforation during hysteroscopic resection and inadvertent entry into the uterine cavity at myomectomy, which is associated with synechia and may require endometrial repair [188]. MR imaging is also useful in monitoring the effect of GnRH therapy on leiomyomas [5, 221].

Besides its high accuracy in the diagnosis of fibroids and additional pathologies of the adnexa prior to UAE, MR imaging enables identification of tumors in which embolization is associated with a higher risk such as subserosal pedunculated fibroids (Fig. 5.15) with a narrow stalk or those which will probably not respond to embolization due to their parasitic blood supply such as intraligamentous leiomyomas. However, the ability of MR imaging to predict a successful clinical outcome based on the location, size, and signal intensity of a leiomyoma is still under investigation [20, 75, 184]. Three-dimensional contrast-enhanced MR angiography can show

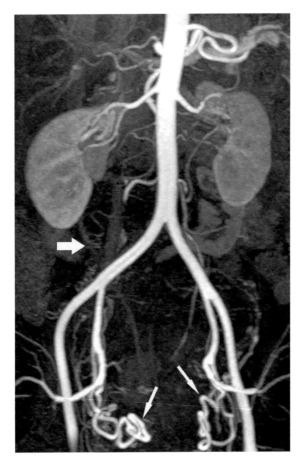

Fig. 5.29. Contrast-enhanced MRA prior to UAE. Maximum intensity projection of a T1-weighted contrast-enhanced MR angiography depicts the uterine arteries (*long white arrows*) as well as an enlarged the right ovarian artery (*thick white arrow*)

the uterine arteries and collateral flow via enlarged ovarian arteries and may serve as a "road map" prior to embolization (Fig. 5.29).

Typical imaging features are observed after fibroid embolization (Fig. 5.30). The tumors show a homogeneous low signal intensity on T2-weighted images after UAE and high signal intensity on T1-weighted images due to hemorrhagic infarction (Fig. 5.31).

MR imaging also depicts morphologic changes such as sloughing of fibroids in contact with the uterine cavity (Fig. 5.32). The latter may be associated with vaginal discharge in patients having undergone UAE but does not require additional treatment in the majority of cases [208]. MRI also identifies side effects and complications associated with UAE such as ongoing fibroid expulsion, endometritis, and uterine necrosis [95, 197]. In cases of ongoing fibroid expulsion a dilated cervical os and leiomyoma tissue pointing towards the cervix may be observed (Fig. 5.33). Endometritis is seen in 0.5% of cases after UAE, is associated with fibroid expulsion, and usually responds well to antibiotics but may spread and result in septicemia if left untreated. At MR imaging tissue within the uterine cavity may be observed together with high-signal-intensity fluid on T2-weighted images indicating retained fluid. Punctuate foci of low signal intensity represent signal voids due to the presence of air on T1- and T2-weighted images. Contrast-enhanced MR images increase the conspicuity of intracavitary fluid collections and also depict hyperperfusion of inflamed adjacent endometrium [95]. Contrast-enhanced MRI is helpful in determining persistent perfusion of fibroids and adenomyosis after UAE. It has been demonstrated that persistent perfusion may lead to regrowth of leiomyoma tissue and recurrence of symptoms [140]. It is important to know that uterine or individual leiomyoma size reduction is not a good indicator of successful embolization since even a partially infarcted leiomyoma undergoes shrinkage while at the same time perfused areas may be present from which the tumor may regrow. The frequency of recurrence of symptoms in cases of persistent perfusion is largely unknown, but it is generally accepted among interventional radiologists that persistent perfusion of leiomyoma tissue in the setting of recurrent symptoms indicates technical failure of UAE, which may be attributable to underembolization (causes: vasospasm during UAE, inadequate choice of level of occlusion or of embolic agent) or collateral supply. Complete infarction of leiomyomas indicates technical success of UAE and is associated with long-term clinical success [140].

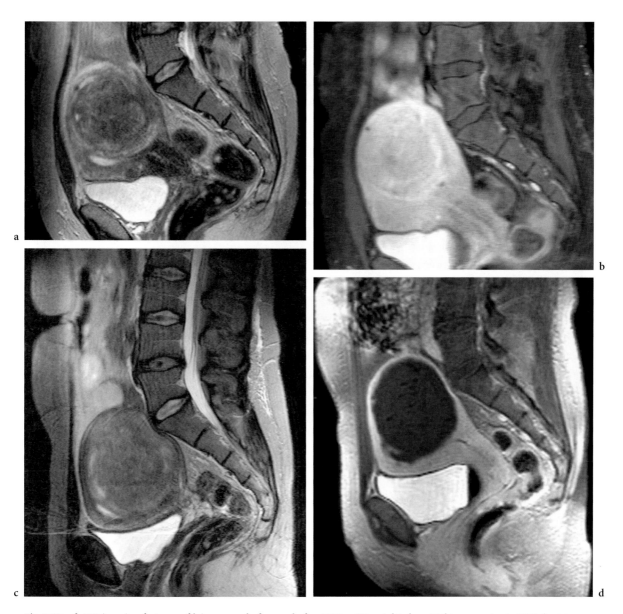

Fig. 5.30a–d. MR imaging features of leiomyoma before and after UAE. **a** T2-weighted sagittal image prior to UAE depicts an intramural leiomyoma with iso- to hypointense signal intensity compared to the adjacent myometrium of the uterus. **b** Contrast-enhanced T1-weighted fat-suppressed sagittal image prior to UAE. Strong enhancement of the uterus and leiomyoma. **c** T2-weighted sagittal image 72 h after UAE. The leiomyoma shows an increased signal intensity due to edema. **d** Contrast-enhanced T1-weighted sagittal image obtained 72 hours after UAE shows complete lack of enhancement of the leiomyoma consistent with infarction. The myometrium shows normal perfusion. (Reproduced with permission from [223])

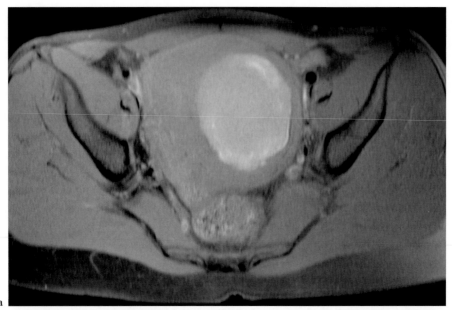

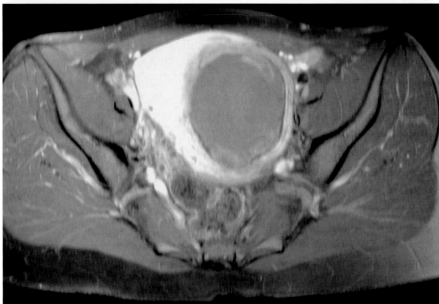

Fig. 5.31a,b. MRI of hemorrhagic leiomyoma infarction: "bag-of-blood-sign". **a** Transaxial T1-weighted fat-suppressed image obtained 3 months after UAE. Peripherally accentuated hyperintense signal intensity of the leiomyoma indicating hemorrhagic transformation of the leiomyoma ("bag-of-blood-sign"). **b** Transaxial contrast-enhanced T1-weighted fat-suppressed image obtained 3 months after UAE. Lack of enhancement of the leiomyoma consistent with infarction. (Reproduced with permission from [223])

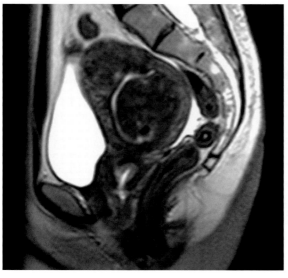

a

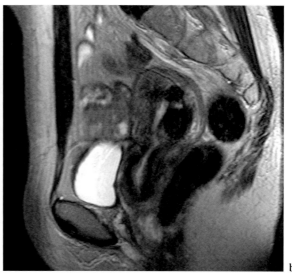

b

Fig. 5.32a,b. Sloughing of uterine fibroids after UAE. **a** Sagittal T2-weighted prior to UAE shows an intramural leiomyoma in the fundus and a submucosal leiomyoma in the posterior uterine wall. **b** Sagittal T2-weighted 24 months after UAE. While the patient reported marked improvement of leiomyoma-associated menorrhagia as early as 3 months after UAE, a late follow-up MRI shows marked decrease in size of the leiomyoma due to ongoing fibroid sloughing

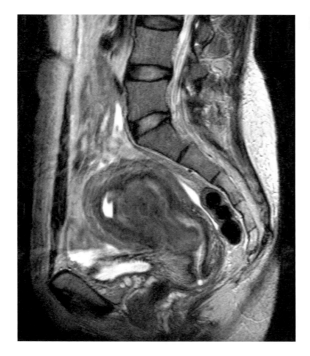

Fig. 5.33. MRI of ongoing leiomyoma expulsion. T2-weighted sagittal image of a patient 72 h after UAE. A submucosal fibroid shows the typical homogenous high signal intensity of edematous change after embolization. The leiomyoma is deformed, mainly within the uterine cavity and points towards the cervix. This finding, together with clinical signs (crampy pain), is indicative of ongoing fibroid expulsion

References

1. Abbara S, Spies JB, Scialli AR, Jha RC, Lage JM, Nikolic B (1999) Transcervical expulsion of a fibroid as a result of uterine artery embolization for leiomyomata. J Vasc Interv Radiol 10:409–411
2. ACOG (1994) Uterine leiomyomata. ACOG technical bulletin Number 192, May 1994. Int J Gynaecol Obstet 46:73-82
3. ACOG (2001) ACOG practice bulletin. Surgical alternatives to hysterectomy in the management of leiomyomas. Number 16, May 2000 (replaces educational bulletin number 192, May 1994). Obstet Gynecol 73:285–293
4. Andersen PE, Lund N, Justesen P, Munk T, Elle B, Floridon C (2001) Uterine artery embolization of symptomatic uterine fibroids. Initial success and short-term results. Acta Radiol 42:234–238
5. Andreyko JL, Blumenfeld Z, Marshall LA, Monroe SE, Hricak H, Jaffe RB (1988) Use of an agonistic analog of gonadotropin-releasing hormone (nafarelin) to treat leiomyomas: assessment by magnetic resonance imaging. Am J Obstet Gynecol 158:903-910
6. Ascher SM, Arnold LL, Patt RH, Schruefer JJ, Bagley AS, Semelka RC, Zeman RK, Simon JA (1994) Adenomyosis: prospective comparison of MR imaging and transvaginal sonography. Radiology 190:803–806
7. Ascher SM, O'Malley J, Semelka RC, Patt RH, Rajan S, Thomasson D (1999) T2-weighted MRI of the uterus: fast spin echo vs. breath-hold fast spin echo. J Magn Reson Imaging 9:384–390
8. Athanasoulis CA, Waltman AC, Barnes AB, Herbst AL (1976) Angiographic control of pelvic bleeding from

treated carcinoma of the cervix. Gynecol Oncol 4:144–150

9. Azziz R (1989) Adenomyosis: current perspectives. Obstet Gynecol Clin North Am 16:221-235

10. Bazot M, Cortez A, Darai E, Rouger J, Chopier J, Antoine JM, Uzan S (2001) Ultrasonography compared with magnetic resonance imaging for the diagnosis of adenomyosis: correlation with histopathology. Hum Reprod 16:2427–2433

11. Bell SW, Kempson RL, Hendrickson MR (1994) Problematic uterine smooth muscle neoplasms. A clinicopathologic study of 213 cases. Am J Surg Pathol 18:535–558

12. Benson RC, Sneeden VD (1958) Adenomyosis: a reappraisal of symptomatology. Am J Obstet Gynecol 76:1044-1057; discussion 1057–1061

13. Berkowitz RP, Hutchins FL, Jr, Worthington-Kirsch RL (1999) Vaginal expulsion of submucosal fibroids after uterine artery embolization. A report of three cases. J Reprod Med 44:373–376

14. Bird CC, McElin TW, Manalo-Estrella P (1972) The elusive adenomyosis of the uterus revisited. Am J Obstet Gynecol 112:583–593

15. Broder MS, Goodwin S, Chen G, Tang LJ, Costantino MM, Nguyen MH, Yegul TN, Erberich H (2002) Comparison of long-term outcomes of myomectomy and uterine artery embolization. Obstet Gynecol 100:864–868

16. Broder MS, Kanouse DE, Mittman BS, Bernstein SJ (2000) The appropriateness of recommendations for hysterectomy. Obstet Gynecol 95:199–205

17. Brosens JJ, de Souza NM, Barker FG, Paraschos T, Winston RM (1995) Endovaginal ultrasonography in the diagnosis of adenomyosis uteri: identifying the predictive characteristics. Br J Obstet Gynaecol 102:471–474

18. Brown BJ, Heaston DK, Poulson AM, Gabert HA, Mineau DE, Miller FJ Jr (1979) Uncontrollable postpartum bleeding: a new approach to hemostasis through angiographic arterial embolization. Obstet Gynecol 54:361–365

19. Brunereau L, Herbreteau D, Gallas S, Cottier JP, Lebrun JL, Tranquart F, Fauchier F, Body G, Rouleau P (2000) Uterine artery embolization in the primary treatment of uterine leiomyomas: technical features and prospective follow-up with clinical and sonographic examinations in 58 patients. AJR Am J Roentgenol 175:1267–1272

20. Burn P, McCall J, Chinn R, Healy J (1999) Embolization of uterine fibroids. Br J Radiol 72:159-161

21. Buttram VC Jr, Reiter RC (1981) Uterine leiomyomata: etiology, symptomatology, and management. Fertil Steril 36:433–445

22. Byun JY, Kim SE, Choi BG, Ko GY, Jung SE, Choi KH (1999) Diffuse and focal adenomyosis: MR imaging findings. Radiographics 19 Spec No, S161–170

23. Candiani GB, Fedele L, Parazzini F, Villa L (1991) Risk of recurrence after myomectomy. Br J Obstet Gynaecol 98:385–389

24. Casillas J, Joseph RC, Guerra JJ Jr (1990) CT appearance of uterine leiomyomas. Radiographics 10:999–1007

25. Chiang CH, Chang MY, Hsu JJ, Chiu TH, Lee KF, Hsieh TT, Soong YK (1999) Tumor vascular pattern and blood flow impedance in the differential diagnosis of leiomyoma and adenomyosis by color Doppler sonography. J Assist Reprod Genet 16:268–275

26. Chrisman HB, Saker MB, Ryu RK, Nemcek AA, Jr., Gerbie MV, Milad MP, Smith SJ, Sewall LE, Omary RA, Vogelzang RL (2000) The impact of uterine fibroid embolization on resumption of menses and ovarian function. J Vasc Interv Radiol 11:699–703

27. Colgan TJ, Pron G, Mocarski EJ, Bennett JD, Asch MR, Common A (2003) Pathologic features of uteri and leiomyomas following uterine artery embolization for leiomyomas. Am J Surg Pathol 27:167–177

28. Connors AM, deSouza NM, McIndoe GA (2003) Adenomyoma mimicking an aggressive uterine neoplasm on MRI. Br J Radiol 76:66–68

29. Coronado GD, Marshall LM, Schwartz SM (2000) Complications in pregnancy, labor, and delivery with uterine leiomyomas: a population-based study. Obstet Gynecol 95:764–769

30. Cramer SF, Patel A (1990) The frequency of uterine leiomyomas. Am J Clin Pathol 94:435–438

31. Derman SG, Rehnstrom J, Neuwirth RS (1991) The long-term effectiveness of hysteroscopic treatment of menorrhagia and leiomyomas. Obstet Gynecol 77:591–594

32. deSouza NM, Williams AD (2002) Uterine arterial embolization for leiomyomas: perfusion and volume changes at MR imaging and relation to clinical outcome. Radiology 222:367–374

33. DeWaay DJ, Syrop CH, Nygaard IE, Davis WA, Van Voorhis BJ (2002) Natural history of uterine polyps and leiomyomata. Obstet Gynecol 100:3–7

34. Doridot V, Dubuisson JB, Chapron C, Fauconnier A, Babaki-Fard K (2001) Recurrence of leiomyomata after laparoscopic myomectomy. J Am Assoc Gynecol Laparosc 8:495–500

35. Dubuisson JB, Fauconnier A, Chapron C, Kreiker G, Norgaard C (1998) Second look after laparoscopic myomectomy. Hum Reprod 13:2102–2106

36. Dudiak CM, Turner DA, Patel SK, Archie JT, Silver B, Norusis M (1988) Uterine leiomyomas in the infertile patient: preoperative localization with MR imaging versus US and hysterosalpingography. Radiology 167:627–630

37. Dueholm M, Lundorf E, Hansen ES, Ledertoug S, Olesen F (2002) Accuracy of magnetic resonance imaging and transvaginal ultrasonography in the diagnosis, mapping, and measurement of uterine myomas. Am J Obstet Gynecol 186:409–415

38. Dueholm M, Lundorf E, Olesen F (2002) Imaging techniques for evaluation of the uterine cavity and endometrium in premenopausal patients before minimally invasive surgery. Obstet Gynecol Surv 57:388–403

39. Dueholm M, Lundorf E, Sorensen JS, Ledertoug S, Olesen F, Laursen H (2002) Reproducibility of evaluation of the uterus by transvaginal sonography, hysterosonographic examination, hysteroscopy and magnetic resonance imaging. Hum Reprod 17:195–200

40. Edozien LC (2005) Hysterectomy for benign conditions. BMJ 330:1457–1458

41. Faerstein E, Szklo M, Rosenshein N (2001) Risk factors for uterine leiomyoma: a practice-based case-control study. I. African-American heritage, reproductive history, body size, and smoking. Am J Epidemiol 153:1–10

42. Farquhar CM, Steiner CA (2002) Hysterectomy rates in the United States 1990-1997. Obstet Gynecol 99:229–234

43. Fauconnier A, Chapron C, Babaki-Fard K, Dubuisson JB (2000) Recurrence of leiomyomata after myomectomy. Hum Reprod Update 6:595–602

44. Fedele L, Bianchi S, Dorta M, Arcaini L, Zanotti F, Carinelli

S (1992) Transvaginal ultrasonography in the diagnosis of diffuse adenomyosis. Fertil Steril 58:94–97

45. Fedele L, Bianchi S, Raffaelli R, Portuese A, Dorta M (1997) Treatment of adenomyosis-associated menorrhagia with a levonorgestrel-releasing intrauterine device. Fertil Steril 68:426–429

46. Ferenczy A (1998) Pathophysiology of adenomyosis. Hum Reprod Update 4:312–322

47. Flake GP, Andersen J, Dixon D (2003) Etiology and pathogenesis of uterine leiomyomas: a review. Environ Health Perspect 111:1037–1054

48. Friedman AJ, Rein MS, Pandian MR, Barbieri RL (1990) Fasting serum growth hormone and insulin-like growth factor-I and -II concentrations in women with leiomyomata uteri treated with leuprolide acetate or placebo. Fertil Steril 53:250–253

49. Ghossain MA, Buy JN, Bazot M, Haddad S, Guinet C, Malbec L, Hugol D, Truc JB, Poitout P, Vadrot D (1994) CT in adnexal torsion with emphasis on tubal findings: correlation with US. J Comput Assist Tomogr 18:619–625

50. Gilks CB, Clement PB, Hart WR, Young RH (2000) Uterine adenomyomas excluding atypical polypoid adenomyomas and adenomyomas of endocervical type: a clinicopathologic study of 30 cases of an underemphasized lesion that may cause diagnostic problems with brief consideration of adenomyomas of other female genital tract sites. Int J Gynecol Pathol 19:195–205

51. Goldberg J (2005) Uterine artery embolization for adenomyosis: looking at the glass half full. Radiology 236:1111–1112; author reply 1112

52. Goldstein HM, Medellin H, Ben-Menachem Y, Wallace S (1975) Transcatheter arterial embolization in the management of bleeding in the cancer patient. Radiology 115:603–608

53. Goodwin SC, Bonilla SM, Sacks D, Reed RA, Spies JB, Landow WJ, Worthington-Kirsch RL (2001) Reporting standards for uterine artery embolization for the treatment of uterine leiomyomata. J Vasc Interv Radiol 12:1011–1020

54. Goto A, Takeuchi S, Sugimura K, Maruo T (2002) Usefulness of Gd-DTPA contrast-enhanced dynamic MRI and serum determination of LDH and its isozymes in the differential diagnosis of leiomyosarcoma from degenerated leiomyoma of the uterus. Int J Gynecol Cancer 12:354–361

55. Grasel RP, Outwater EK, Siegelman ES, Capuzzi D, Parker L, Hussain SM (2000) Endometrial polyps: MR imaging features and distinction from endometrial carcinoma. Radiology 214:47–52

56. Greenberg MD, Kazamel TI (1995) Medical and socioeconomic impact of uterine fibroids. Obstet Gynecol Clin North Am 22:625–636

57. Hamlin DJ, Pettersson H, Fitzsimmons J, Morgan LS (1985) MR imaging of uterine leiomyomas and their complications. J Comput Assist Tomogr 9:902–907

58. Hart R, Molnar BG, Magos A (1999) Long term follow up of hysteroscopic myomectomy assessed by survival analysis. Br J Obstet Gynaecol 106:700–705

59. Hasan F, Arumugam K, Sivanesaratnam V (1991) Uterine leiomyomata in pregnancy. Int J Gynaecol Obstet 34:45–48

60. Hashimoto K, Azuma C, Kamiura S, Kimura T, Nobunaga T, Kanai T, Sawada M, Noguchi S, Saji F (1995) Clonal determination of uterine leiomyomas by analyzing differential inactivation of the X-chromosome-linked phosphoglycerokinase gene. Gynecol Obstet Invest 40:204–208

61. Hasson HM, Rotman C, Rana N, Sistos F, Dmowski WP (1992) Laparoscopic myomectomy. Obstet Gynecol 80:884–888

62. Hayasaka K, Tanaka Y, Fujii M, Himi K, Negishi N (2000) Intravenous leiomyomatosis. J Comput Assist Tomogr 24:83–85

63. Hehenkamp WJ, Volkers NA, Donderwinkel PF, de Blok S, Birnie E, Ankum WM, Reekers JA (2005) Uterine artery embolization versus hysterectomy in the treatment of symptomatic uterine fibroids (EMMY trial): peri- and postprocedural results from a randomized controlled trial. Am J Obstet Gynecol 193:1618–1629

64. Higgins CB, Bookstein JJ, Davis GB, Galloway DC, Barr JW (1977) Therapeutic embolization for intractable chronic bleeding. Radiology 122:473–478

65. Hirai M, Shibata K, Sagai H, Sekiya S, Goldberg BB (1995) Transvaginal pulsed and color Doppler sonography for the evaluation of adenomyosis. J Ultrasound Med 14:529–532

66. Hovsepian DM, Siskin GP, Bonn J, Cardella JF, Clark TW, Lampmann LE, Miller DL, Omary RA, Pelage JP, Rajan D, et al. (2004) Quality improvement guidelines for uterine artery embolization for symptomatic leiomyomata. Cardiovasc Intervent Radiol 27:307–313

67. Hricak H, Finck S, Honda G, Goranson H (1992) MR imaging in the evaluation of benign uterine masses: value of gadopentetate dimeglumine-enhanced T1-weighted images. AJR Am J Roentgenol 158:1043–1050

68. Hurst BS, Matthews ML, Marshburn PB (2005) Laparoscopic myomectomy for symptomatic uterine myomas. Fertil Steril 83:1–23

69. Hutchins FL Jr, Worthington-Kirsch R (2000) Embolotherapy for myoma-induced menorrhagia. Obstet Gynecol Clin North Am 27:397–405

70. Hutchins FL Jr, Worthington-Kirsch R, Berkowitz RP (1999) Selective uterine artery embolization as primary treatment for symptomatic leiomyomata uteri. J Am Assoc Gynecol Laparosc 6:279–284

71. Imaoka I, Ascher SM, Sugimura K, Takahashi K, Li H, Cuomo F, Simon J, Arnold LL (2002) MR imaging of diffuse adenomyosis changes after GnRH analog therapy. J Magn Reson Imaging 15:285–290

72. Iribarne C, Plaza J, De la Fuente P, Garrido C, Garzon A, Olaizola JI (1994) Intramyometrial cystic adenomyosis. J Clin Ultrasound 22:348–350

73. Janus C, White M, Dottino P, Brodman M, Goodman H (1989) Uterine leiomyosarcoma – magnetic resonance imaging. Gynecol Oncol 32:79–81

74. Jeong YY, Kang HK, Park JG, Choi HS (2003) CT features of uterine torsion. Eur Radiol 13[Suppl 4]:L249–250

75. Jha RC, Ascher SM, Imaoka I, Spies JB (2000) Symptomatic fibroleiomyomata: MR imaging of the uterus before and after uterine arterial embolization. Radiology 217:228–235

76. Jha RC, Takahama J, Imaoka I, Korangy SJ, Spies JB, Cooper C, Ascher SM (2003) Adenomyosis: MRI of the uterus treated with uterine artery embolization. AJR Am J Roentgenol 181:851–856

77. Jones MW, Norris HJ (1995) Clinicopathologic study of 28

uterine leiomyosarcomas with metastasis. Int J Gynecol Pathol 14:243–249

78. Kakarla A, Ash AK (2005) Pregnancy after embolisation of a fibroid: emergency caesarean myomectomy. J Obstet Gynaecol 25:300–301

79. Kang S, Turner DA, Foster GS, Rapoport MI, Spencer SA, Wang JZ (1996) Adenomyosis: specificity of 5 mm as the maximum normal uterine junctional zone thickness in MR images. AJR Am J Roentgenol 166:1145–1150

80. Karcaaltincaba M, Sudakoff GS (2003) CT of a ruptured pyomyoma. AJR Am J Roentgenol 181:1375–1377

81. Katsumori T, Akazawa K, Mihara T (2005) Uterine artery embolization for pedunculated subserosal fibroids. AJR Am J Roentgenol 184:399–402

82. Katsumori T, Nakajima K, Mihara T (2003) Is a large fibroid a high-risk factor for uterine artery embolization? AJR Am J Roentgenol 181:1309–1314

83. Katsumori T, Nakajima K, Mihara T, Tokuhiro M (2002) Uterine artery embolization using gelatin sponge particles alone for symptomatic uterine fibroids: midterm results. AJR Am J Roentgenol 178:135–139

84. Katsumori T, Nakajima K, Tokuhiro M (2001) Gadolinium-enhanced MR imaging in the evaluation of uterine fibroids treated with uterine artery embolization. AJR Am J Roentgenol 177:303–307

85. Kawaguchi K, Fujii S, Konishi I, Nanbu Y, Nonogaki H, Mori T (1989) Mitotic activity in uterine leiomyomas during the menstrual cycle. Am J Obstet Gynecol 160:637–641

86. Kawakami S, Togashi K, Konishi I, Kimura I, Fukuoka M, Mori T, Konishi J (1994) Red degeneration of uterine leiomyoma: MR appearance. J Comput Assist Tomogr 18:925–928

87. Kawamura N, Ichimura T, Ito F, Shibata S, Takahashi K, Tsujimura A, Ishiko O, Haba T, Wakasa K, Ogita S (2002) Transcervical needle biopsy for the differential diagnosis between uterine sarcoma and leiomyoma. Cancer 94:1713–1720

88. Kebapci M, Aslan O, Kaya T, Yalcin OT, Ozalp S (2002) Pedunculated uterine leiomyoma associated with pseudo-Meigs' syndrome and elevated CA-125 level: CT features. Eur Radiol 12[Suppl 3]:S127–129

89. Kido A, Monma C, Togashi K, Ueda H, Itoh K, Fujii S, Konishi J (2003) Uterine arterial embolization for the treatment of diffuse leiomyomatosis. J Vasc Interv Radiol 14:643–647

90. Kido A, Togashi K, Koyama T, Yamaoka T, Fujiwara T, Fujii S (2003) Diffusely enlarged uterus: evaluation with MR imaging. Radiographics 23:1423–1439

91. Kim JC, Kim SS, Park JY (2000) "Bridging vascular sign" in the MR diagnosis of exophytic uterine leiomyoma. J Comput Assist Tomogr 24:57–60

92. Kim MD, Kim NK, Kim MH, Lee MH (2005) Pregnancy following uterine artery embolization with polyvinyl alcohol particles for patients with uterine fibroid or adenomyosis. Cardiovasc Intervent Radiol 28:611–615

93. Kim MD, Won JW, Lee DY, Ahn CS (2004) Uterine artery embolization for adenomyosis without fibroids. Clin Radiol 59:520–526

94. Kitamura Y, Allison SJ, Jha RC, Spies JB, Flick PA, Ascher SM (2006) MRI of adenomyosis: changes with uterine artery embolization. AJR Am J Roentgenol 186:855–864

95. Kitamura Y, Ascher SM, Cooper C, Allison SJ, Jha RC, Flick PA, Spies JB (2005) Imaging manifestations of complica-tions associated with uterine artery embolization. Radiographics 25[Suppl 1]:S119–132

96. Koshiyama M, Suzuki A, Ozawa M, Fujita K, Sakakibara A, Kawamura M, Takahashi S, Fujii H, Hirano T, Okagaki A, et al. (2002) Adenocarcinomas arising from uterine adenomyosis: a report of four cases. Int J Gynecol Pathol 21:239–245

97. Koyama T, Togashi K, Konishi I, Kobayashi H, Ueda H, Kataoka ML, Itoh T, Higuchi T, Fujii S, Konishi J (1999) MR imaging of endometrial stromal sarcoma: correlation with pathologic findings. AJR Am J Roentgenol 173:767–772

98. Kroencke TJ, Gauruder-Burmester A, Enzweiler CN, Taupitz M, Hamm B (2003) Disintegration and stepwise expulsion of a large uterine leiomyoma with restoration of the uterine architecture after successful uterine fibroid embolization: case report. Hum Reprod 18:863–865

99. Kroencke TJ, Scheurig C, Kluner C, Taupitz M, Schnorr J, Hamm B (2006) Contrast-enhanced magnetic resonance angiography to predict ovarian artery supply of uterine fibroids – initial experience. Radiology 241:181–189

100. Kroncke TJ, Gauruder-Burmester A, Gronewold M, Lembcke A, Fischer T, Puls R, Juran R, Scheurig C, Neymeyer J, Hamm B (2004) Technical success rate, peri-interventional complications and radiation exposure of the transarterial embolization for leiomyomas of the uterus. Rofo 176:580–589

101. Kroncke TJ, Gauruder-Burmester A, Scheurig C, Gronewold M, Kluner C, Fischer T, Klessen C, Rudolph J, Siara K, Zimmermann E, et al. (2005) Transarterial embolization for uterine fibroids: clinical success rate and results of magnetic resonance imaging. Rofo 177:89–98

102. Kunz G, Beil D, Huppert P, Leyendecker G (2000) Structural abnormalities of the uterine wall in women with endometriosis and infertility visualized by vaginal sonography and magnetic resonance imaging. Hum Reprod 15:76–82

103. Kunz G, Beil D, Huppert P, Noe M, Kissler S, Leyendecker G (2005) Adenomyosis in endometriosis – prevalence and impact on fertility. Evidence from magnetic resonance imaging. Hum Reprod 20:2309–2316

104. Kuwashima Y, Uehara T, Kishi K, Tajima H, Shiromizu K, Matsuzawa M, Takayama S (1994) Intramural adenocarcinoma of the uterus, arisen from adenomyosis uteri, showing unique histologic appearances. Report of two cases. Eur J Gynaecol Oncol 15:418–423

105. Lee JH, Jeong YK, Park JK, Hwang JC (2003) "Ovarian vascular pedicle" sign. AJR Am J Roentgenol 181:131–137

106. Leibsohn S, d'Ablaing G, Mishell DR Jr, Schlaerth JB (1990) Leiomyosarcoma in a series of hysterectomies performed for presumed uterine leiomyomas. Am J Obstet Gynecol 162:968–974; discussion 974–966

107. Levy B, Mukherjee T, Hirschhorn K (2000) Molecular cytogenetic analysis of uterine leiomyoma and leiomyosarcoma by comparative genomic hybridization. Cancer Genet Cytogenet 121:1–8

108. Lumsden MA, West CP, Hawkins RA, Bramley TA, Rumgay L, Baird DT (1989) The binding of steroids to myometrium and leiomyomata (fibroids) in women treated with the gonadotrophin-releasing hormone agonist Zoladex (ICI 118630). J Endocrinol 121:389–396

109. Lurie S, Gorbacz S, Caspi B, Borenstein R (1991) Parasitic leiomyoma: a case report. Clin Exp Obstet Gynecol 18:7–8

110. Malzoni M, Rotond M, Perone C, Labriola D, Ammaturo F, Izzo A, Panariello S, Reich H (2003) Fertility after laparoscopic myomectomy of large uterine myomas: operative technique and preliminary results. Eur J Gynaecol Oncol 24:79–82

111. Mara M, Fucikova Z, Maskova J, Kuzel D, Haakova L (2005) Uterine fibroid embolization versus myomectomy in women wishing to preserve fertility: preliminary results of a randomized controlled trial. Eur J Obstet Gynecol Reprod Biol [Epub ahead of print]

112. Margolies MN, Ring EJ, Waltman AC, Kerr WS Jr, Baum S (1972) Arteriography in the management of hemorrhage from pelvic fractures. N Engl J Med 287:317–321

113. Mark AS, Hricak H, Heinrichs LW, Hendrickson MR, Winkler ML, Bachica JA, Stickler JE (1987) Adenomyosis and leiomyoma: differential diagnosis with MR imaging. Radiology 163:527–529

114. Marshall LM, Spiegelman D, Barbieri RL, Goldman MB, Manson JE, Colditz GA, Willett WC, Hunter DJ (1997) Variation in the incidence of uterine leiomyoma among premenopausal women by age and race. Obstet Gynecol 90:967–973

115. Masui T, Katayama M, Kobayashi S, Sakahara H, Ito T, Nozaki A (2001) T2-weighted MRI of the female pelvis: comparison of breath-hold fast-recovery fast spin-echo and nonbreath-hold fast spin-echo sequences. J Magn Reson Imaging 13:930–937

116. Masui T, Katayama M, Kobayashi S, Shimizu S, Nozaki A, Sakahara H (2003) Pseudolesions related to uterine contraction: characterization with multiphase-multisection T2-weighted MR imaging. Radiology 227:345–352

117. McCausland AM (1992) Hysteroscopic myometrial biopsy: its use in diagnosing adenomyosis and its clinical application. Am J Obstet Gynecol 166:1619–1626; discussion 1626–1618

118. McCausland AM, McCausland VM (1996) Depth of endometrial penetration in adenomyosis helps determine outcome of rollerball ablation. Am J Obstet Gynecol 174:1786–1793; 1793–1784

119. McCluggage WG, Ellis PK, McClure N, Walker WJ, Jackson PA, Manek S (2000) Pathologic features of uterine leiomyomas following uterine artery embolization. Int J Gynecol Pathol 19:342–347

120. McLucas B, Adler L, Perrella R (2001) Uterine fibroid embolization: nonsurgical treatment for symptomatic fibroids. J Am Coll Surg 192:95–105

121. McLucas B, Goodwin S, Adler L, Rappaport A, Reed R, Perrella R (2001) Pregnancy following uterine fibroid embolization. Int J Gynaecol Obstet 74:1–7

122. McLucas B, Perrella R, Adler L (2002) Embolization for the treatment of adenomyosis. AJR Am J Roentgenol 178:1028–1029

123. Mercorio F, De Simone R, Di Spiezio Sardo A, Cerrota G, Bifulco G, Vanacore F, Nappi C (2003) The effect of a levonorgestrel-releasing intrauterine device in the treatment of myoma-related menorrhagia. Contraception 67:277–280

124. Morita M, Asakawa Y, Nakakuma M, Kubo H (2004) Laparoscopic excision of myometrial adenomyomas in patients with adenomyosis uteri and main symptoms of severe dysmenorrhea and hypermenorrhea. J Am Assoc Gynecol Laparosc 11:86–89

125. Mulvany NJ, Ostor AG, Ross I (1995) Diffuse leiomyomatosis of the uterus. Histopathology 27:175–179

126. Myers ER, Barber MD, Gustilo-Ashby T, Couchman G, Matchar DB, McCrory DC (2002) Management of uterine leiomyomata: what do we really know? Obstet Gynecol 100:8–17

127. Nezhat FR, Roemisch M, Nezhat CH, Seidman DS, Nezhat CR (1998) Recurrence rate after laparoscopic myomectomy. J Am Assoc Gynecol Laparosc 5:237–240

128. Nishida M (1991) Relationship between the onset of dysmenorrhea and histologic findings in adenomyosis. Am J Obstet Gynecol 165:229–231

129. Oguchi O, Mori A, Kobayashi Y, Horiuchi A, Nikaido T, Fujii S (1995) Prediction of histopathologic features and proliferative activity of uterine leiomyoma by magnetic resonance imaging prior to GnRH analogue therapy: correlation between T2-weighted images and effect of GnRH analogue. J Obstet Gynaecol 21:107–117

130. Okamoto T, Koshiyama M, Yamamoto K (2004) Rapidly growing leiomyoma in a postmenopausal woman. J Obstet Gynaecol Res 30:316–318

131. Omary RA, Vasireddy S, Chrisman HB, Ryu RK, Pereles FS, Carr JC, Resnick SA, Nemcek AA Jr, Vogelzang RL (2002) The effect of pelvic MR imaging on the diagnosis and treatment of women with presumed symptomatic uterine fibroids. J Vasc Interv Radiol 13:1149–1153

132. Outwater EK, Siegelman ES, Van Deerlin V (1998) Adenomyosis: current concepts and imaging considerations. AJR Am J Roentgenol 170:437–441

133. Ozaki T, Takahashi K, Okada M, Kurioka H, Miyazaki K (1999) Live birth after conservative surgery for severe adenomyosis following magnetic resonance imaging and gonadotropin-releasing hormone agonist therapy. Int J Fertil Womens Med 44:260–264

134. Parazzini F, La Vecchia C, Negri E, Cecchetti G, Fedele L (1988) Epidemiologic characteristics of women with uterine fibroids: a case-control study. Obstet Gynecol 72:853–857

135. Parazzini F, Vercellini P, Panazza S, Chatenoud L, Oldani S, Crosignani PG (1997) Risk factors for adenomyosis. Hum Reprod 12:1275–1279

136. Park HR, Kim MD, Kim NK, Kim HJ, Yoon SW, Park WK, Lee MH (2005) Uterine restoration after repeated sloughing of fibroids or vaginal expulsion following uterine artery embolization. Eur Radiol 15:1850–1854

137. Parker WH, Fu YS, Berek JS (1994) Uterine sarcoma in patients operated on for presumed leiomyoma and rapidly growing leiomyoma. Obstet Gynecol 83:414–418

138. Pattani SJ, Kier R, Deal R, Luchansky E (1995) MRI of uterine leiomyosarcoma. Magn Reson Imaging 13:331–333

139. Pelage JP, Beregi J, LeDref O, Nonent M, Robert YH, Rymer R (2001) Uterine artery embolization for fibroids using a different end-point for embolization: preliminary results using calibrated microspheres. Radiology 221(P):356

140. Pelage JP, Guaou NG, Jha RC, Ascher SM, Spies JB (2004) Uterine fibroid tumors: long-term MR imaging outcome after embolization. Radiology 230:803–809

141. Pelage JP, Jacob D, Fazel A, Namur J, Laurent A, Rymer R, Le Dref O (2005) Midterm results of uterine artery embolization for symptomatic adenomyosis: initial experience. Radiology 234:948–953

142. Pelage JP, Le Dref O, Soyer P, Kardache M, Dahan H, Abitbol

M, Merland JJ, Ravina JH, Rymer R (2000) Fibroid-related menorrhagia: treatment with superselective embolization of the uterine arteries and midterm follow-up. Radiology 215:428–431

143. Phelan JP (1995) Myomas and pregnancy. Obstet Gynecol Clin North Am 22:801–805

144. Pinto I, Chimeno P, Romo A, Paul L, Haya J, de la Cal MA, Bajo J (2003) Uterine fibroids: uterine artery embolization versus abdominal hysterectomy for treatment – a prospective, randomized, and controlled clinical trial. Radiology 226:425–431

145. Price N, Gillmer MD, Stock A, Hurley PA (2005) Pregnancy following uterine artery embolisation. J Obstet Gynaecol 25:28–31

146. Pritts EA (2001) Fibroids and infertility: a systematic review of the evidence. Obstet Gynecol Surv 56:483–491

147. Prollius A, de Vries C, Loggenberg E, du Plessis A, Nel M, Wessels PH (2004) Uterine artery embolisation for symptomatic fibroids: the effect of the large uterus on outcome. Bjog 111:239–242

148. Pron G, Bennett J, Common A, Wall J, Asch M, Sniderman K (2003) The Ontario Uterine Fibroid Embolization Trial. Part 2. Uterine fibroid reduction and symptom relief after uterine artery embolization for fibroids. Fertil Steril 79:120–127

149. Rammeh-Rommani S, Mokni M, Stita W, Trabelsi A, Hamissa S, Sriha B, Tahar-Yacoubi M, Korbi S (2005) Uterine smooth muscle tumors: retrospective epidemiological and pathological study of 2760 cases. J Gynecol Obstet Biol Reprod (Paris) 34:568–571

150. Ravina J, Merland J, Herbetreau D, Houdart E, Bouret J, Madelenat P (1994) Embolisation pré-opératoire des fibromes utérins. Presse Med 23:1540

151. Ravina JH, Vigneron NC, Aymard A, Le Dref O, Merland JJ (2000) Pregnancy after embolization of uterine myoma: report of 12 cases. Fertil Steril 73:1241–1243

152. Razavi MK, Hwang G, Jahed A, Modanloo S, Chen B (2003) Abdominal myomectomy versus uterine fibroid embolization in the treatment of symptomatic uterine leiomyomas. AJR Am J Roentgenol 180:1571–1575

153. Reed SD, Cushing-Haugen KL, Daling JR, Scholes D, Schwartz SM (2004) Postmenopausal estrogen and progestogen therapy and the risk of uterine leiomyomas. Menopause 11:214–222

154. Rein MS, Barbieri RL, Friedman AJ (1995) Progesterone: a critical role in the pathogenesis of uterine myomas. Am J Obstet Gynecol 172:14–18

155. Reinhold C, Atri M, Mehio A, Zakarian R, Aldis AE, Bret PM (1995) Diffuse uterine adenomyosis: morphologic criteria and diagnostic accuracy of endovaginal sonography. Radiology 197:609–614

156. Reinhold C, McCarthy S, Bret PM, Mehio A, Atri M, Zakarian R, Glaude Y, Liang L, Seymour RJ (1996) Diffuse adenomyosis: comparison of endovaginal US and MR imaging with histopathologic correlation. Radiology 199:151–158

157. Reinhold C, Tafazoli F, Mehio A, Wang L, Atri M, Siegelman ES, Rohoman L (1999) Uterine adenomyosis: endovaginal US and MR imaging features with histopathologic correlation. Radiographics 19 Spec No:S147–160

158. Reinhold C, Tafazoli F, Wang L (1998) Imaging features of adenomyosis. Hum Reprod Update 4:337–349

159. Rice JP, Kay HH, Mahony BS (1989) The clinical signifi-cance of uterine leiomyomas in pregnancy. Am J Obstet Gynecol 160:1212–1216

160. Robboy SJ, Bentley RC, Butnor K, Anderson MC (2000) Pathology and pathophysiology of uterine smooth-muscle tumors. Environ Health Perspect 108[Suppl 5]:779–784

161. Robles-Frias A, Severin CE, Robles-Frias MJ, Garrido JL (2001) Diffuse uterine leiomyomatosis with ovarian and parametrial involvement. Obstet Gynecol 97:834–835

162. Ross RK, Pike MC, Vessey MP, Bull D, Yeates D, Casagrande JT (1986) Risk factors for uterine fibroids: reduced risk associated with oral contraceptives. Br Med J (Clin Res Ed) 293:359–362

163. Roy C, Bierry G, Ghali SE, Buy X, Rossini A (2005) Acute torsion of uterine leiomyoma: CT features. Abdom Imaging 30:120–123

164. Sadan O, van Iddekinge B, van Gelderen CJ, Savage N, Becker PJ, van der Walt LA, Robinson M (1987) Oestrogen and progesterone receptor concentrations in leiomyoma and normal myometrium. Ann Clin Biochem 24 (Pt 3):263–267

165. Sahdev A, Sohaib SA, Jacobs I, Shepherd JH, Oram DH, Reznek RH (2001) MR imaging of uterine sarcomas. AJR Am J Roentgenol 177:1307–1311

166. Samadi AR, Lee NC, Flanders WD, Boring JR 3rd, Parris EB (1996) Risk factors for self-reported uterine fibroids: a case-control study. Am J Public Health 86:858–862

167. Sawin SW, Pilevsky ND, Berlin JA, Barnhart KT (2000) Comparability of perioperative morbidity between abdominal myomectomy and hysterectomy for women with uterine leiomyomas. Am J Obstet Gynecol 183:1448–1455

168. Schwartz LB, Panageas E, Lange R, Rizzo J, Comite F, McCarthy S (1994) Female pelvis: impact of MR imaging on treatment decisions and net cost analysis. Radiology 192:55–60

169. Schwartz LB, Zawin M, Carcangiu ML, Lange R, McCarthy S (1998) Does pelvic magnetic resonance imaging differentiate among the histologic subtypes of uterine leiomyomata? Fertil Steril 70:580–587

170. Schwartz SM (2001) Invited commentary: studying the epidemiology of uterine leiomyomata - past, present, and future. Am J Epidemiol 153:27–29; discussion 30

171. Scoutt LM, McCarthy SM, Lange R, Bourque A, Schwartz PE (1994) MR evaluation of clinically suspected adnexal masses. J Comput Assist Tomogr 18:609–618

172. Shozu M, Murakami K, Inoue M (2004) Aromatase and leiomyoma of the uterus. Semin Reprod Med 22:51–60

173. Siegler AM, Camilien L (1994) Adenomyosis. J Reprod Med 39:841–853

174. Siskin GP, Tublin ME, Stainken BF, Dowling K, Dolen EG (2001) Uterine artery embolization for the treatment of adenomyosis: clinical response and evaluation with MR imaging. AJR Am J Roentgenol 177:297–302

175. Soysal ME, Soysal SK, Vicdan K (2001) Thermal balloon ablation in myoma-induced menorrhagia under local anesthesia. Gynecol Obstet Invest 51:128–133

176. Sozen I, Arici A (2002) Interactions of cytokines, growth factors, and the extracellular matrix in the cellular biology of uterine leiomyomata. Fertil Steril 78:1–12

177. Sozen I, Arici A (2006) Cellular biology of myomas: interaction of sex steroids with cytokines and growth factors. Obstet Gynecol Clin North Am 33:41–58

178. Spies JB, Allison S, Flick P, McCullough M, Sterbis K,

Cramp M, Bruno J, Jha R (2004) Polyvinyl alcohol particles and tris-acryl gelatin microspheres for uterine artery embolization for leiomyomas: results of a randomized comparative study. J Vasc Interv Radiol 15:793–800

179. Spies JB, Ascher SA, Roth AR, Kim J, Levy EB, Gomez-Jorge J (2001) Uterine artery embolization for leiomyomata. Obstet Gynecol 98:29–34

180. Spies JB, Benenati JF, Worthington-Kirsch RL, Pelage JP (2001) Initial experience with use of tris-acryl gelatin microspheres for uterine artery embolization for leiomyomata. J Vasc Interv Radiol 12:1059–1063

181. Spies JB, Bruno J, Czeyda-Pommersheim F, Magee ST, Ascher SA, Jha RC (2005) Long-term outcome of uterine artery embolization of leiomyomata. Obstet Gynecol 106:933–939

182. Spies JB, Cooper JM, Worthington-Kirsch R, Lipman JC, Mills BB, Bennenati JF (2004) Outcome of uterine embolization and hysterectomy for leiomyomas: results of a multicenter study. Obstet Gynecol Surv 59:819–820

183. Spies JB, Patel AA, Epstein NB, White AM (2005) Recent advances in uterine fibroid embolization. Curr Opin Obstet Gynecol 17:562–567

184. Spies JB, Roth AR, Jha RC, Gomez-Jorge J, Levy EB, Chang TC, Ascher SA (2002) Leiomyomata treated with uterine artery embolization: factors associated with successful symptom and imaging outcome. Radiology 222:45–52

185. Spies JB, Spector A, Roth AR, Baker CM, Mauro L, Murphy-Skrynarz K (2002) Complications after uterine artery embolization for leiomyomas. Obstet Gynecol 100:873–880

186. Stewart EA (2001) Uterine fibroids. Lancet 357:293–298

187. Stewart EA, Nowak RA (1996) Leiomyoma-related bleeding: a classic hypothesis updated for the molecular era. Hum Reprod Update 2:295–306

188. Stringer NH, Strassner HT, Lawson L, Oldham L, Estes C, Edwards M, Stringer EA (2001) Pregnancy outcomes after laparoscopic myomectomy with ultrasonic energy and laparoscopic suturing of the endometrial cavity. J Am Assoc Gynecol Laparosc 8:129–136

189. Suginami H, Kaura R, Ochi H, Matsuura S (1990) Intravenous leiomyomatosis with cardiac extension: successful surgical management and histopathologic study. Obstet Gynecol 76:527–529

190. Takemori M, Nishimura R, Sugimura K (1992) Magnetic resonance imaging of uterine leiomyosarcoma. Arch Gynecol Obstet 251:215–218

191. Tamai K, Togashi K, Ito T, Morisawa N, Fujiwara T, Koyama T (2005) MR imaging findings of adenomyosis: correlation with histopathologic features and diagnostic pitfalls. Radiographics 25:21–40

192. Tamaya T, Fujimoto J, Okada H (1985) Comparison of cellular levels of steroid receptors in uterine leiomyoma and myometrium. Acta Obstet Gynecol Scand 64:307–309

193. Togashi K, Kawakami S, Kimura I, Asato R, Okumura R, Fukuoka M, Mori T, Konishi J (1993) Uterine contractions: possible diagnostic pitfall at MR imaging. J Magn Reson Imaging 3:889–893

194. Togashi K, Kawakami S, Kimura I, Asato R, Takakura K, Mori T, Konishi J (1993) Sustained uterine contractions: a cause of hypointense myometrial bulging. Radiology 187:707–710

195. Togashi K, Ozasa H, Konishi I, Itoh H, Nishimura K, Fujisawa I, Noma S, Sagoh T, Minami S, Yamashita K, et al.

(1989) Enlarged uterus: differentiation between adenomyosis and leiomyoma with MR imaging. Radiology 171:531–534

196. Torashima M, Yamashita Y, Matsuno Y, Takahashi M, Nakahara K, Onitsuka Y, Ohtake H, Tanaka N, Okamura H (1998) The value of detection of flow voids between the uterus and the leiomyoma with MRI. J Magn Reson Imaging 8:427–431

197. Torigian DA, Siegelman ES, Terhune KP, Butts SF, Blasco L, Shlansky-Goldberg RD (2005) MRI of uterine necrosis after uterine artery embolization for treatment of uterine leiomyomata. AJR Am J Roentgenol 184:555–559

198. Townsend DE, Sparkes RS, Baluda MC, McClelland G (1970) Unicellular histogenesis of uterine leiomyomas as determined by electrophoresis by glucose-6-phosphate dehydrogenase. Am J Obstet Gynecol 107:1168–1173

199. Troiano RN, Flynn SD, McCarthy S (1998) Cystic adenomyosis of the uterus: MRI. J Magn Reson Imaging 8:1198–1202

200. Tropeano G, Di Stasi C, Litwicka K, Romano D, Draisci G, Mancuso S (2004) Uterine artery embolization for fibroids does not have adverse effects on ovarian reserve in regularly cycling women younger than 40 years. Fertil Steril 81:1055–1061

201. Tsushima Y, Kita T, Yamamoto K (1997) Uterine lipoleiomyoma: MRI, CT and ultrasonographic findings. Br J Radiol 70:1068–1070

202. Tulandi T, Murray C, Guralnick M (1993) Adhesion formation and reproductive outcome after myomectomy and second-look laparoscopy. Obstet Gynecol 82:213–215

203. Ueda H, Togashi K, Konishi I, Kataoka ML, Koyama T, Fujiwara T, Kobayashi H, Fujii S, Konishi J (1999) Unusual appearances of uterine leiomyomas: MR imaging findings and their histopathologic backgrounds. Radiographics 19:131–145

204. Utsunomiya D, Notsute S, Hayashida Y, Lwakatare F, Katabuchi H, Okamura H, Awai K, Yamashita Y (2004) Endometrial carcinoma in adenomyosis: assessment of myometrial invasion on T2-weighted spin-echo and gadolinium-enhanced T1-weighted images. AJR Am J Roentgenol 182:399–404

205. Vercellini P, Maddalena S, De Giorgi O, Aimi G, Crosignani PG (1998) Abdominal myomectomy for infertility: a comprehensive review. Hum Reprod 13:873–879

206. Vessey MP, Villard-Mackintosh L, McPherson K, Coulter A, Yeates D (1992) The epidemiology of hysterectomy: findings in a large cohort study. Br J Obstet Gynaecol 99:402–407

207. Walker CL, Stewart EA (2005) Uterine fibroids: the elephant in the room. Science 308:1589–1592

208. Walker WJ, Carpenter TT, Kent AS (2004) Persistent vaginal discharge after uterine artery embolization for fibroid tumors: cause of the condition, magnetic resonance imaging appearance, and surgical treatment. Am J Obstet Gynecol 190:1230–1233

209. Walker WJ, Pelage JP (2002) Uterine artery embolisation for symptomatic fibroids: clinical results in 400 women with imaging follow up. BJOG 109:1262–1272

210. Wamsteker K, Emanuel MH, de Kruif JH (1993) Transcervical hysteroscopic resection of submucous fibroids for abnormal uterine bleeding: results regarding the degree of intramural extension. Obstet Gynecol 82:736–740

211. Weichert W, Denkert C, Gauruder-Burmester A, Kurzeja

R, Hamm B, Dietel M, Kroencke TJ (2005) Uterine arterial embolization with tris-acryl gelatin microspheres: a histopathologic evaluation. Am J Surg Pathol 29:955–961

212. Weinreb JC, Barkoff ND, Megibow A, Demopoulos R (1990) The value of MR imaging in distinguishing leiomyomas from other solid pelvic masses when sonography is indeterminate. AJR Am J Roentgenol 154:295–299

213. Wildemeersch D, Schacht E (2002) The effect on menstrual blood loss in women with uterine fibroids of a novel „frameless" intrauterine levonorgestrel-releasing drug delivery system: a pilot study. Eur J Obstet Gynecol Reprod Biol 102:74–79

214. Wood C, Maher P, Hill D (1994) Biopsy diagnosis and conservative surgical treatment of adenomyosis. J Am Assoc Gynecol Laparosc 1:313–316

215. Yamashita Y, Tang Y, Abe Y, Mitsuzaki K, Takahashi M (1998) Comparison of ultrafast half-Fourier single-shot turbo spin-echo sequence with turbo spin-echo sequences for T2-weighted imaging of the female pelvis. J Magn Reson Imaging 8:1207–1212

216. Yamashita Y, Torashima M, Takahashi M, Tanaka N, Katabuchi H, Miyazaki K, Ito M, Okamura H (1993) Hyperintense uterine leiomyoma at T2-weighted MR imaging: differentiation with dynamic enhanced MR imaging and clinical implications. Radiology 189:721–725

217. Yeh HC, Kaplan M and Deligdisch L (1999) Parasitic and pedunculated leiomyomas: ultrasonographic features. J Ultrasound Med 18:789–794

218. Ylikorkala O, Tiitinen A, Hulkko S, Kivinen S, Nummi S (1995) Decrease in symptoms, blood loss and uterine size with nafarelin acetate before abdominal hysterectomy: a placebo-controlled, double-blind study. Hum Reprod 10:1470–1474

219. Zacharia TT, O'Neill M J (2006) Prevalence and distribution of adnexal findings suggesting endometriosis in patients with MR diagnosis of adenomyosis. Br J Radiol 79:303–307

220. Zaloudek C, Hendrickson MR, Ed. (2002) Mesenchymal tumors of the uterus. In: RJ Kurmann (ed) Blaustein's pathology of the female genital tract. Springer-Verlag, Berlin Heidelberg New York

221. Zawin M, McCarthy S, Scoutt LM, Comite F (1990) High-field MRI and US evaluation of the pelvis in women with leiomyomas. Magn Reson Imaging 8:371–376

222. Keckstein J, Ulrich U (2004) Gynäkologische Endokrinologie. Springer Verlag, Berlin Heidelberg New York, 2:11–18

223. Kröncke TJ, Hamm B (2003) Role of magnetic resonance imaging (MRI) in establishing the indication for planning and following up uterine artery embolization (UAE) for treating symptomatic leiomyomas of the uterus [article in German]. Radiologe 43:624–633

224. Roy C, Bierry G, Ghali SE, Buy X, Rossini A (2005) Acute torsion of uterine leiomyoma: CT features. Abdom Imaging. 30:120-123

Endometrial Carcinoma

Kathrin A. Frei Bonel and Karen Kinkel

CONTENTS

6.1
Introduction and Epidemiology

Worldwide, endometrial carcinoma is the seventh most common malignant disorder, but incidence varies among regions [37]. In less developed countries, risk factors are less common and endometrial cancer is rare, although specific mortality is higher [22, 33]. The incidence is ten times higher in North America and Europe than in less developed countries; in these regions, this cancer is the commonest of the female genital tract and the fourth commonest site after breast cancer, lung, and colorectal cancers [37]. The incidence is rising as life expectancy increases

K. A. Frei Bonel, MD
Department of Obstetrics and Gynecology, University Hospital Bern, Inselspital, Effingerstrasse 102, 3010 Bern, Switzerland
K. Kinkel, MD, PD
Institut de radiologie, Clinique des Grangettes, chemin des Grangettes 7, 1224 Chêne-Bougeries, Switzerland

[1]. The typical age–incidence curve for endometrial cancer shows that most cases are diagnosed after the menopause, with the highest incidence around the seventh decade of life.

The appearance of symptoms early in the course explains why most women with endometrial cancer have early-stage disease at presentation. The cornerstone of treatment for endometrial cancer is surgery, which not only is important for staging purposes but also enables appropriate tailoring of adjuvant treatment modalities that benefit high-risk patients only. Patients with endometrial cancer have a favourable prognosis with a 5-year survival of about 80%.

6.2
Pathology

Pathological examination is very important for diagnosis of endometrial cancer. About 80% of all endometrial carcinomas are of the endometrioid type; this term refers to endometrial-type glands of varying differentiation easily recognisable on microscopy. Several subtypes or variants of endometrioid carcinoma have been described [9] (see Table 6.1).

Squamous differentiation is a common finding in endometrioid carcinoma. Histological grading applies only to the endometrioid carcinoma; serous and clear-cell carcinomas are classified as high-grade by definition. According to the system of the International Federation of Gynecology and Obstetrics (FIGO), an endometrioid carcinoma of grade 1 consists of well-formed glands, with no more than 5% solid non-squamous areas [12]. Carcinoma of grade 2 consist of 6%–50% and those of grade 3 of more than 50% solid non-squamous areas [12, 48]. Most endometrioid carcinomas are well to moderately differentiated and arise on a background of

Table 6.1. WHO histological classification of endometrial carcinoma

Endometrioid adenocarcinoma
Variants: With squamous differentiation
Villoglandular
Secretory
With ciliated cells
Other adenocarcinomas
Mucinous carcinoma
Serous carcinoma
Clear-cell carcinoma
Mixed carcinoma
Squamous-cell carcinoma
Transitional-cell carcinoma
Small-cell carcinoma
Undifferentiated carcinoma

endometrial hyperplasia. These tumours, also known as type 1 (low grade) endometrial carcinomas, have a favourable prognosis [5]. They are associated with long-duration unopposed estrogenic stimulation. About 10% of endometrial cancers are type 2 (high-grade) lesions. Women with such tumours are at high risk of relapse and metastatic disease. These tumours are not oestrogen driven, and most are associated with endometrial atrophy; surgery is commonly followed by adjuvant therapy. The histological type is either poorly differentiated endometrioid or non-endometrioid adenocarcinoma.

Serous carcinoma is the most aggressive type of non-endometrioid endometrial carcinoma. The histological diagnosis is based on the presence of papillae, covered by highly pleiomorphic tumour cells with frequent mitoses and necroses. About 8% of endometrial carcinomas are associated with the simultaneous presence of an ovarian carcinoma with the same histology [14]. In most instances, especially when both tumours are well differentiated and the endometrial tumour is only superficially invasive into the myometrium, these are independent primary tumours [45]. Endometrial carcinosarcoma has lately been considered a special subtype of endometrial cancer. Given a tendency to lymphatic and transperitoneal spread with a 50% recurrence rate, surgical therapy is as for type 2 endometrial cancers.

6.3
Risk Factors

Exposure to unopposed oestrogens is a risk factor for endometrial carcinoma. Unopposed oestrogens should no longer be used to treat postmenopausal symptoms in women who have not had hysterectomy. Excessive fat consumption and overweight [defined as a body-mass index (BMI) of at least 25 kg/m^2] are important risk factors present in almost 50% of women with endometrial cancer [7, 26] (see Table 6.2).

Table 6.2. Risk factors for endometrial cancer

Factors increasing risk
Increasing age
Long-term exposure to unopposed oestrogens
High concentrations of oestrogens postmenopausally
Metabolic syndrome
Years of menstruation
Nulliparity
History of breast cancer
Long-term use of tamoxifen
First-degree relative with endometrial cancer
Hereditary nonpolyposis colon cancer family syndrome (HNPCC)
Factors decreasing risk
Grand multiparity
Smoking
Oral-contraceptive use
Physical activity
Diet of some phyto-oestrogens

Pregnancy with intense placental production of progestogens, protects against endometrial cancer. Nulliparity is a risk factor that is more important if infertility is also present; grand multiparity protects [23]. The use of an intrauterine device and tubal ligation have also been associated with a lower risk [25, 29]. Contraceptive pills containing oestrogens and progestogens lower the endometrial-cancer risk. After menopause for women taking hormone-replacement therapy, addition of progestogens to oestrogen counteracts the adverse effects of oestrogens on the endometrium. Women with breast cancer are at increased risk of endometrial cancer. Breast cancer can rarely metastasise to the endometrium, and primary endometrial cancers are more likely to occur in breast-cancer survivors because of common risk factors [20]. An additional endometrial-cancer risk has been related to the use of tamoxifen for breast cancer treatment. This drug triples the risk of endometrial cancer and also increases the chance of developing benign endometrial lesions [10]. The proportion of cases of endometrial cancer on a background of familial risk is low but having a first-degree relative with this cancer is a risk factor. Endometrial cancer can also be part of a hereditary cancer syndrome such as hereditary nonpolyposis colon cancer (HNPCC). HNPCC is a mendelian-dominant syndrome of right-sided colon, endometrial, and other cancers. Guidelines have been published for selection of HNPCC; endometrial cancer before the age of 45 years is one of the criteria [46].

6.4
Symptoms and Diagnosis

Abnormal uterine bleeding is the most frequent clinical symptom of endometrial cancer although many other disorders give rise to the same symptom. All postmenopausal women with vaginal bleeding and those with abnormal uterine bleeding associated with risk factors for endometrial cancer or hyperplasia (e.g., polycystic ovaries, hormone-replacement therapy, tamoxifen use) should undergo further diagnostic endometrial assessment. Transvaginal ultrasound is considered the first step of choice in the diagnostic work up in any woman presenting with abnormal uterine bleeding [8]. The normal endometrium in post-menopausal women is defined as a thin symmetrical endometrial line of less than 4–5 mm double endometrial thickness. A literature review including almost 6000 women found that the probability of cancer in a postmenopausal women with vaginal bleeding and a 10% pre-test probability of endometrial cancer was 1% following a normal (<5-mm endometrial thickness) transvaginal ultrasound. Given this low risk of endometrial cancer, the authors suggested that endometrial sampling might be unnecessary in women with a negative study [42]. However, one other meta-analysis including nine studies (3483 women without endometrial cancer and 380 with the disease) found that the detection rate for endometrial cancer varied according to the criteria for judging the endometrial thickness as abnormal. The detection rate was 63% when considering an endometrial thickness that resulted in a false positive rate of only 10%; however, the detection rate increased to 96% if a false positive rate of 50% was considered acceptable. The authors concluded that even with a lower threshold for calling

results suspicious, 4% of endometrial cancers would be missed; thus, further invasive diagnostic testing was indicated in all symptomatic women with a thin endometrial thickness. They also noted that median endometrial thickness varied among centres such that 5 mm may not be a universally reliable threshold [43]. Another systematic review consisted of 57 studies with 9031 patients. Only four studies used the >5-mm cutoff level, which was the best-quality criteria. Using the pooled estimates from these four studies only, a positive test result raised the probability of carcinoma from 14% to 31%, while a negative test reduced it to 2.5%. The authors concluded that a negative result (≤5 mm) usually excluded endometrial pathology, but ultrasound measurement of endometrial thickness alone could not be used to reliably exclude cancer [19]. For further investigation of patients with vaginal bleeding an endometrial biopsy should be performed.

Endometrial biopsy is a cost-effective initial approach with a high sensitivity. In some patients dilation and curettage might be necessary as further diagnostic procedures. Because intraperitoneal spillage of endometrial cells may occur during hysteroscopy, this procedure should not be performed in patients with malignant cells at endometrial biopsy or if transvaginal ultrasound strongly suggests endometrial cancer [36].

The value of transvaginal ultrasound in symptomatic premenopausal women and those using hormone-replacement therapy is lower because the "normal" endometrial thickness varies with circulating concentrations of female steroid hormones. A Pap smear is only of value when it is abnormal. A normal result is not sufficient to exclude endometrial cancer in symptomatic women and an abnormal result frequently points to advanced disease [18]. Imaging findings at transvaginal ultrasound are nonspecific and include endometrial thickening or endometrial masses (Figs. 6.1, 6.2) for both benign and malignant endometrial neoplasm and warrant the performance of endometrial biopsy.

6.5
Staging

Endometrial cancer is considered a surgically and histologically staged disease since clinical estimates and preoperative imaging of disease extent were incorrect in over 20% of cases [11]. The depth of myometrial, cervical stroma invasion and extrauterine

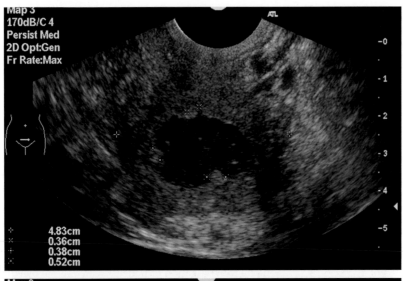

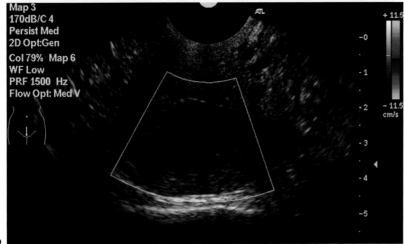

Fig. 6.1a,b. A 67-year-old woman presenting with postmenopausal bleeding. **a** Axial view at transvaginal ultrasound demonstrates a fluid-filled uterine cavity with nodular hyperechoic endometrial lining. **b** Sagittal view at color Doppler transvaginal ultrasound identifies a nonspecific small vessel at the endometrial myometrial interface. Endometrial biopsy and subsequent histology of the hysterectomy specimen diagnosed Stage 1A endometrioid adenocarcinoma of the uterus

Table 6.3. Staging system for endometrial cancer (UICC, TNM Classification of Malignant Tumours, FIGO Staging System)

TNM	FIGO	
TX		**Primary tumour cannot be assessed**
T0		**No evidence of primary tumour**
Tis		**Carcinoma in situ (preinvasive carcinoma)**
T1	**Stage I**	**Limited to corpus**
T1a	IA	Tumor limited to endometrium
T1b	IB	Invasion < ½ of myometrium
T1c	IC	Invasion > ½ of myometrium
T2	**Stage II**	**Involvement of the cervix (invasion not beyond uterus)**
T2a	IIA	Endocervical glandular involvement only
T2b	IIB	Cervical stroma involvement
T3 and/or N1	**Stage III**	**Spread outside of the uterus, confined to pelvis (not including rectal or bladder involvement)**
T3a	IIIA	Involvement of uterine serosa and/or adnexa, and/or positive peritoneal cytology
T3b	IIIB	Spread to vagina (direct extension or metastasis)
N1	IIIC	Metastases to pelvic and/or para-aortic lymph nodes
	Stage IV	
T4	IVA	Spread to the bladder and/or rectal mucosa
M1	IVB	Distant metastasis (excluding metastasis to vagina, pelvic serosa or adnexa)

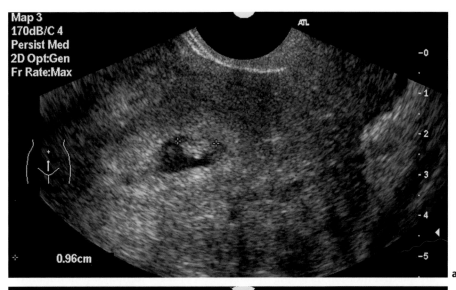

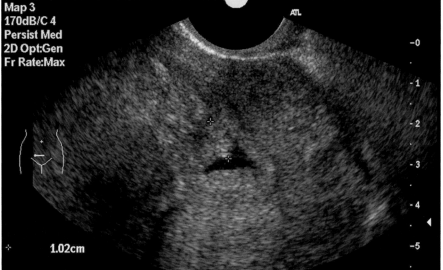

Fig. 6.2a–c. A 36-year-old woman with menorrhagia. **a** Sagittal view of a transvaginal pelvic ultrasound demonstrates fluid within the uterine cavity and irregular thickness of the hyperechoic endometrial lining with a polypoid isthmic mass. **b** The axial view of the transvaginal ultrasound confirms the presence of a right-sided hyperechoic endometrial mass. **c** Sagittal view of the color Doppler transvaginal ultrasound demonstrates nonspecific small vessels within the abnormal aspect of the endometrium. Pathology of the endometrial mass obtained through hysteroscopic resection and curettage confirmed a benign endometrial polyp

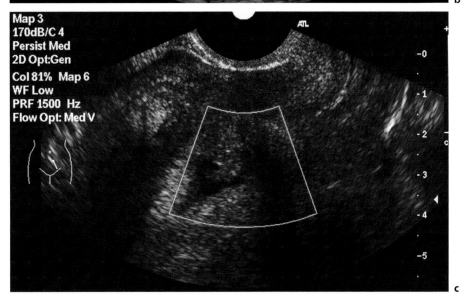

disease (uterine serosa, adnexal involvement, peritoneal cytology, intra-abdominal, and lymph nodes) has all been incorporated into the FIGO staging scheme (Table 6.3). Although the preoperative assessment of extent cannot replace the surgical staging, it enables clinicians to tailor treatment. Useful preoperative assessments include clinical examination, Pap smear, transvaginal ultrasound and CT of lungs, liver, and retroperitoneal lymph nodes. If overt metastatic disease is found, extensive surgery will not be performed. Transvaginal ultrasound is simple and readily available and has reasonable accuracy in predicting cervical and myometrial invasion from endometrial cancer [3]. A logistic regression model based on several variables was as accurate as most other proposed methods for measuring depth of myometrial invasion including frozen section of the hysterectomy specimen and CT. Contrast-enhanced MRI is currently seen as the best method for the assessment of myometrial invasion [16, 28]. Although the histological assessment of the hysterectomy specimen remains the gold standard, it is important to assess myometrial and endocervical invasion pre- or intraoperatively. Intraoperative visual estimation of the depth of myometrial invasion is accurate in 90% of cases [31]. The combination of preoperatively known tumour grade and visual estimation of the depth of myometrial invasion might guide the experienced surgeon to select candidates for lymphadenectomy. However, preoperative knowledge of deep myometrial or cervical stroma invasion allows the general gynaecologist to decide whether or not the patient requires specialised surgical expertise. Indeed, in most countries a general gynaecologist lacks the knowledge to perform lymphadenectomy (associated with a higher complication rate such as lymphedema, infection) and refers the patient to a gynaecologist specialised in surgical oncology.

Each case will be graded histologically into G1, G2, and G3. Grading is based on nuclear/cytoplasmic abnormalities rather than morphology alone.

6.5.1
MR Imaging Protocol for
Staging Endometrial Carcinoma

The MR imaging protocol at intermediate or high-field strength includes the use of a pelvic phase array coil, 3–6 h fasting prior to the examination, and an intra-muscular injection of an anti-peristaltic agent, such as 20 mg of Buscopan (butylscopalamine, Scher-

ing) at the beginning of the examination [34]. General recommendations include small section thickness of 3–4 mm and a smaller field of view than those used for bone imaging covering the pelvic content and not the hips or the entire abdomen. After the initial localizer, high resolution T2-weigthed pelvic images are acquired in a sagittal plane, oblique axial (short uterine body axis), and oblique coronal (long uterine body axis) plane to detail uterine zonal anatomy and help to choose the most appropriate imaging plane for contrast-enhanced T1-weighted sequences. At T2-weighted fast spin echo images an optimal junctional zone to external myometrium contrast is obtained with a repetition time of about 4000 ms and an echo time of about 90 ms. T1-weighted sequences should be performed at least after intra-venous bolus injection of gadolinium chelates. Contrast injection is mandatory to optimize the diagnosis of myometrial invasion [28]. On contrast-enhanced images, the tumour appears hypointense or less enhancing than the normal myometrium. At dynamic contrast-enhanced T1-weighted sequences the inner myometrial layer enhances earlier and more intensely than the outer myometrial layer [47]. Myometrial invasion can be diagnosed due to the interruption or loss of early normal subendometrial enhancement even in postmenopausal woman. These early reports demonstrated optimal myometrium to tumour contrast at 2 min (120 s) compared to delayed post-contrast images acquired at 5 min after injection [47]. A more recent study confirmed these initial results demonstrating an optimal myometrial to tumour contrast at about 2 min 30 s (150 s) compared to 30 or 90 s after intravenous contrast injection at fast dynamic 3D multiplanar spoiled gradient echo pulse sequences with chemically selected fat suppression (FSPGR). The choice of pulse sequences can be either 2D or 3D, but needs to take into consideration the optimal tumour to myometrium contrast after contrast injection and the different timing of contrast sampling in 2D versus 3D sequences. Rectilinear κ-space sampling in the y-direction takes places in most 3D sequences leading to contrast timing at the middle of the sequence acquisition time, taking place at the end of the acquisition time for 2D sequences. Therefore, a recent consensus meeting of the European Society of Urogenital Imaging (ESUR) suggested the use of high resolution 3D T1-weighted sequences with an acquisition time of about 5 min corresponding to the acquisition of gadolinium contrast at 2 min 30 s. This technical protocol might allow an increase in matrix size to 512×512 and avoid common pitfalls in staging myometrial invasion with MRI [27]. T1-weighted 2D sequences should respect an acquisition time of about 2 min 30 s due to contrast acquisition at the end of the acquisition time. If cervical invasion is suspected, additional T2-weighted sequences according to the short and long axis of the endocervical channel might be helpful.

6.5.2
MR Imaging Findings

The signal intensity of endometrial tumours is usually hyperintense to the myometrium and slightly hypointense to the normal endometrium at T2-weighted images [44]. Although MR imaging cannot differentiate benign from malignant intracavitary endometrial neoplasm, benign endometrial polyps can be suspected when a central hypointense fibrous core is identified at T2-weighted images in the enlarged uterine cavity [17]. However, hypointensity within the uterine cavity is not a specific finding and can be related to fresh blood (Fig. 6.3). Benign and malig-

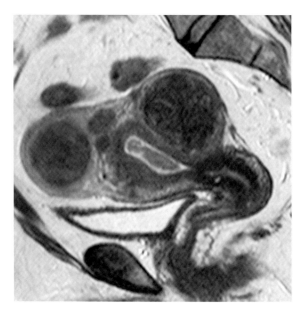

Fig. 6.3. A 52-year-old woman with metrorrhagia underwent MRI due to posterior shadowing of the myometrium at transvaginal ultrasound hiding the endometrium and failure to obtain tissue at endometrial sampling without general anesthesia. Sagittal T2-weighted fast spin echo image of the uterus shows a hypointense central part within the endometrium suggesting a polyp. Multiple subserosal leiomyoma deform the uterine contour. Tissue analysis of endometrial curettage confirmed normal endometrial glands and stroma associated with a large amount of hemorrhagic liquid mimicking a polyp at MRI

nant endometrial tumours may overstretch the cavity and cause myometrial thinning (Fig. 6.4) that should not be mistaken for myometrial invasion. Diagnostic criteria for myometrial invasion include irregular endometrium-junctional zone interface at T2-weighted and contrast-enhanced T1-weighted images or interruption of the junctional zone [41] (Figs. 6.5, 6.6). Deep myometrial invasion is defined as invasion of the external half of the myometrium (Table 6.3; Figs. 6.7, 6.8). Involvement of the endocervical glands is suspected whenever the tumour signal extends from the uterine cavity towards the endocervical channel (stage IIA) with widening of the endocervical channel and/or disruption of the normal cervical epithelium (Fig. 6.9). At contrast-enhanced sequences, endocervical glandular involvement is diagnosed when normal contrast-enhancement of the cervical epithelium is interrupted (Fig. 6.10) [35]. Stage IIB, defined as stromal invasion of the cervix requires disruption of the normal low signal intensity of the junctional zone located at the inner cervical stroma at T2-weighted images [13] (Fig. 6.10). Careful comparison between T2-weighted and T1-weighted images is helpful to avoid pitfalls in staging endometrial tumours [27] commonly due to adenomyosis or multiple leiomyoma. Stage IIIA tumours corresponding to involvement of the uterine serosa requires transmyometrial invasion without normal myometrium between the endometrial carcinoma and the peritoneal cavity (Fig. 6.11) [15]. The spread to the vagina (stage IIIB) follows the same diagnostic criteria as for cervical cancer. The diagnosis of lymph node invasion (stage IIIC) using size criteria of a small axis superior to 10 mm has poor results of sensitivity of about 50% [34]. The diagnosis of bladder or rectal mucosa invasion (stage IVA) relies on visualization of direct extension of the tumour into the normally T2-hyperintense mucosa of the bladder or the rectal wall (Fig. 6.12). At T1-weighted images the normal mucosa strongly enhances after intravenous contrast injection. Tumour invasion relies on the disruption of the normal mucosa. Before the recent change in TNM stage, diagnostic criteria relied on the disruption of the bladder or rectal wall regardless of the part of the wall. Therefore, diagnostic criteria took into consideration the hypointense bladder detrusor or rectal muscles. Due to the small numbers of patients with the newly defined stage IVA disease concerning only the bladder or rectal mucosa there are currently no published results about the performance of MRI to diagnose bladder or rectal mucosa wall invasion. In patients with cervical cancer and a pathological

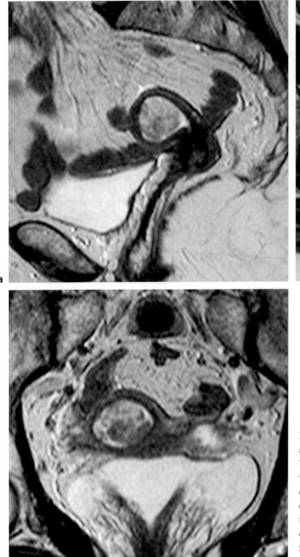

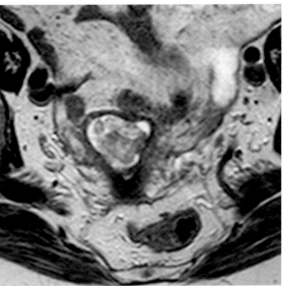

Fig. 6.4a–c. MRI of the pelvis for staging of serous papillary and endometrioid adenocarcinoma of the uterus grade 3 in a 76-year-old woman. **a** Sagittal T2-weighted image of the pelvis shows a polypoid endometrial mass distending the uterine cavity and a preserved junctional zone. Additional T2-weighted images in coronal oblique orientation (long axis view of the uterus, **b**) and axial oblique orientation (short axis view of the uterus, **c**) confirm absent interruption of the junctional zone suggesting stage 1A endometrial carcinoma. Subsequent pathology of hysterectomy specimen demonstrated no myometrial invasion (stage IA)

diagnosis of bladder or rectal wall invasion regardless of the part of the wall, accuracies of MRI varied from 75% to 94% for bladder wall invasion [4, 39] and 85% for rectal wall invasion [39]. The sensitivity of bladder wall invasion depended on the sequence used and was highest with pharmacokinetic images (94%) versus contrast-enhanced images (88%) and T2-weighted images (81%) [21]. An example of distant metastasis (stage IVB) detected at pelvic MRI is shown in Fig. 6.13.

Various approaches have been explored to increase the detection of pelvic lymph node invasion. Preliminary reports in patients with cervical cancer have used an intravenous injection of a lymph node specific contrast agent for MRI, UPSIO (Combidex/ Sinerem) that has shown lack of sensitivity (25%) to detect lymph node metastasis in this cancer. Per-operative approaches, such as sentinel lymph node ablation, are also currently under investigation. Indirect assessment of the risk of lymph node invasion is possible by the preoperative assessment of deep myometrial and cervical stroma invasion, strongly correlated to lymph node invasion and survival [6, 32]. The diagnostic performance of contrast-enhanced MRI to define myometrial invasion has been reported superior to endovaginal ultrasound or computed tomography with accuracies around 91% [28]. Bayesian analysis has shown that a positive MRI for myometrial in-

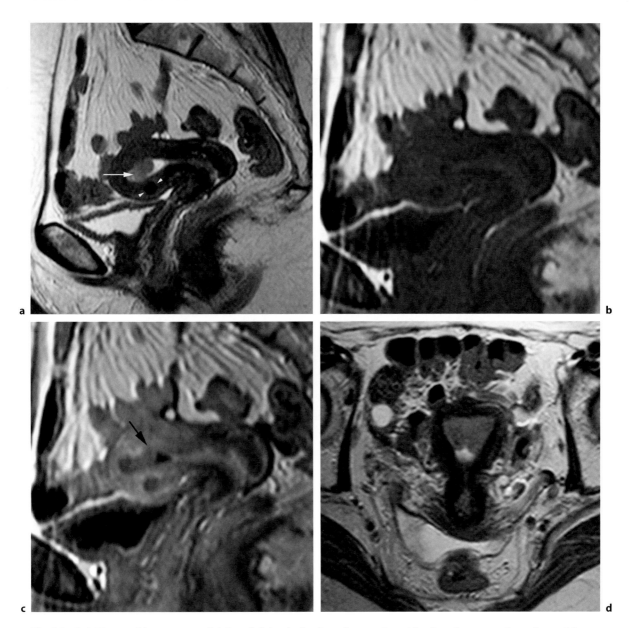

Fig. 6.5a–d. A 58-year-old woman complaining of abdominal pain and presenting with a 2-cm hypervascular endometrial mass at transvaginal ultrasound. Endometrial biopsy diagnosed endometrioid adenocarcinoma grade 1. MRI was performed for staging. **a** A sagittal T2-weighted fast spin echo image demonstrating an intermediate signal intensity of the endometrial cancer (*arrow*) associated with a hypointense anterior intramural leiomyoma (*arrowhead*). The junctional zone is not clearly identified. **b** Sagittal T1-weighted pre-contrast image fails to demonstrate the tumor. **c** Sagittal T1-weighted dynamic post-contrast image at 3 min demonstrates minimal enhancement of the endometrial tumor compared to the subendometrial enhancement of the normal myometrium. Decreased myometrial enhancement at the lower tumour-myometrial interface (*arrow*) points to superficial myometrial invasion. **d** T2-weighted long axis view of the uterus shows the fundal position of the tumor not extending to the cervix excluding stage II disease. A normal right ovary and a small amount of peritoneal fluid are also seen. Pathology of subsequent hysterectomy specimen confirmed superficial myometrial invasion (1 mm invasion of 15 mm total myometrial thickness, stage IB) with associated adenomyosis and a 7-mm leiomyoma

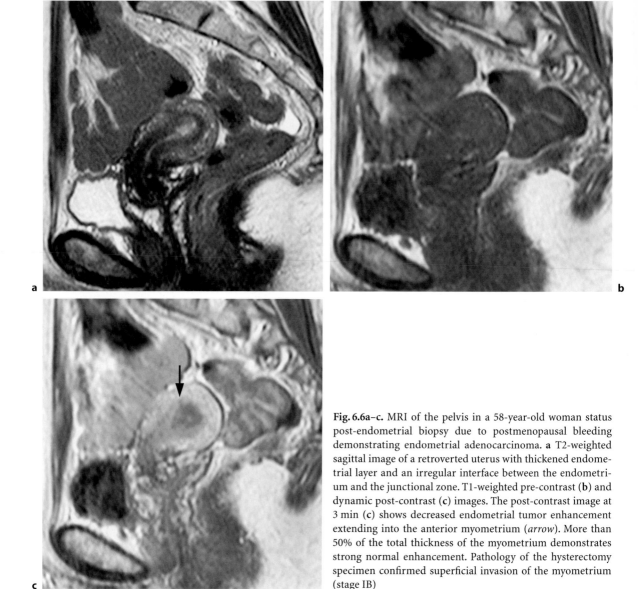

Fig. 6.6a–c. MRI of the pelvis in a 58-year-old woman status post-endometrial biopsy due to postmenopausal bleeding demonstrating endometrial adenocarcinoma. **a** T2-weighted sagittal image of a retroverted uterus with thickened endometrial layer and an irregular interface between the endometrium and the junctional zone. T1-weighted pre-contrast (**b**) and dynamic post-contrast (**c**) images. The post-contrast image at 3 min (**c**) shows decreased endometrial tumor enhancement extending into the anterior myometrium (*arrow*). More than 50% of the total thickness of the myometrium demonstrates strong normal enhancement. Pathology of the hysterectomy specimen confirmed superficial invasion of the myometrium (stage IB)

Fig. 6.7a–e. MRI of the pelvis for staging endometrioid adenocarcinoma grade 1 of the uterus in a 65-year-old woman. Sagittal (**a**) and coronal oblique (**b**) T2-weighted image of the uterus show a hypointense left-sided posterior intramural leiomyoma (*white arrow*) in a small uterus and an ill-defined or not visible junctional zone. **b** Myometrial signal intensity at the left uterine cornua (*black arrow*) cannot be differentiated from the signal intensity of the endometrium. **c** Contrast-enhanced dynamic T1-weigted image at 3 min in the long axis of the uterus clearly demonstrates two areas of decreased myometrial enhancement: the posterior leiomyoma (*white arrow*) and the anterior left-sided endometrial tumor (*black arrow*) extending into the myometrium. Residual strong enhancement of the normal myometrium (*arrowheads*) is smaller than half of the total thickness of the myometrium suggesting deep myometrial invasion. **d** Contrast between tumor and normal myometrial enhancement decreased at delayed post-contrast-enhanced image at 4 min 30 s. **e** Sagittal reconstruction of the portal phase of a contrast-enhanced helical CT also shows decreased endometrial enhancement extending into the anterior myometrium (*arrow*). Subsequent pathology of hysterectomy specimen and pelvic lymph nodes confirmed stage IC with 15 mm adenomyoma of the myometrium without lymph node invasion

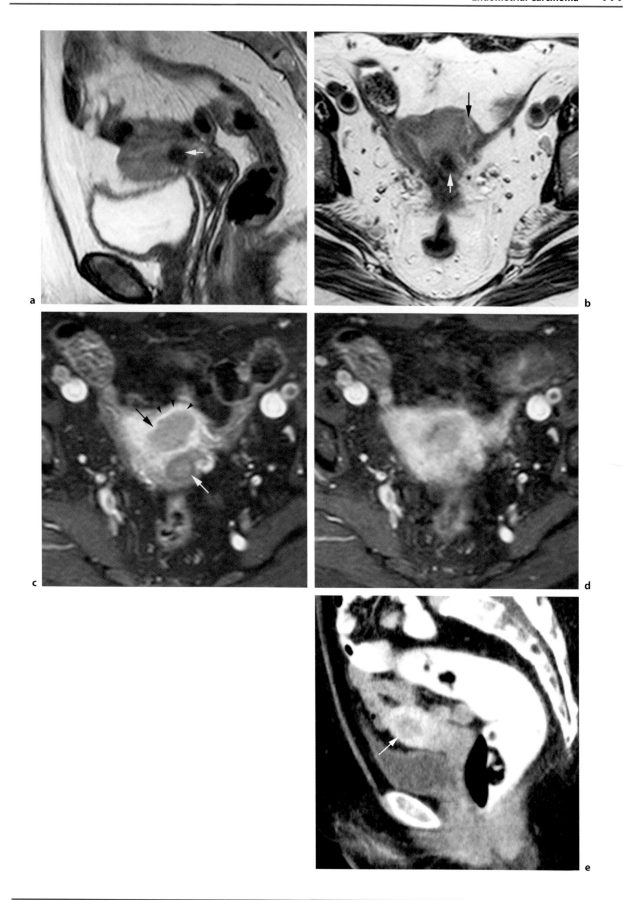

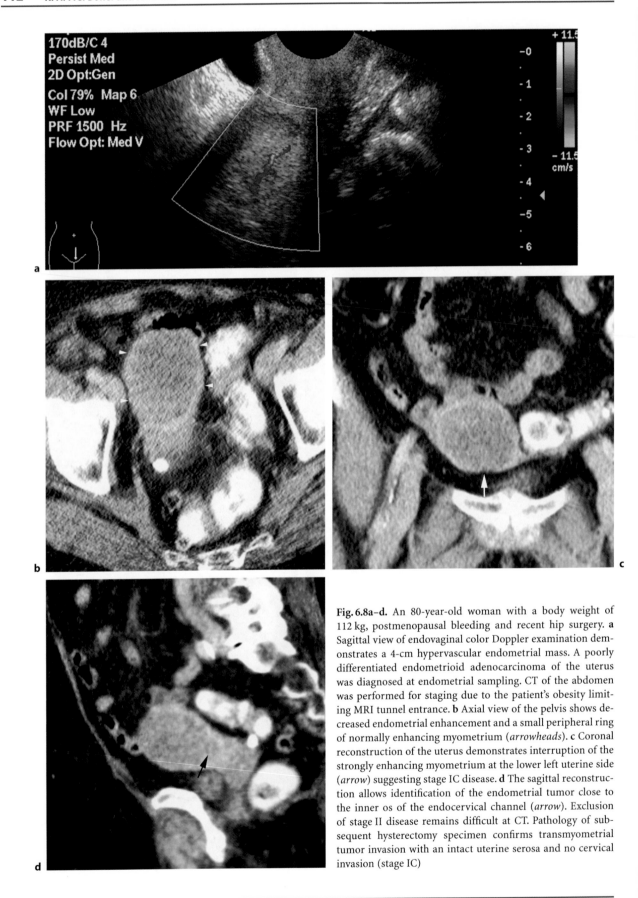

Fig. 6.8a–d. An 80-year-old woman with a body weight of 112 kg, postmenopausal bleeding and recent hip surgery. **a** Sagittal view of endovaginal color Doppler examination demonstrates a 4-cm hypervascular endometrial mass. A poorly differentiated endometrioid adenocarcinoma of the uterus was diagnosed at endometrial sampling. CT of the abdomen was performed for staging due to the patient's obesity limiting MRI tunnel entrance. **b** Axial view of the pelvis shows decreased endometrial enhancement and a small peripheral ring of normally enhancing myometrium (*arrowheads*). **c** Coronal reconstruction of the uterus demonstrates interruption of the strongly enhancing myometrium at the lower left uterine side (*arrow*) suggesting stage IC disease. **d** The sagittal reconstruction allows identification of the endometrial tumor close to the inner os of the endocervical channel (*arrow*). Exclusion of stage II disease remains difficult at CT. Pathology of subsequent hysterectomy specimen confirms transmyometrial tumor invasion with an intact uterine serosa and no cervical invasion (stage IC)

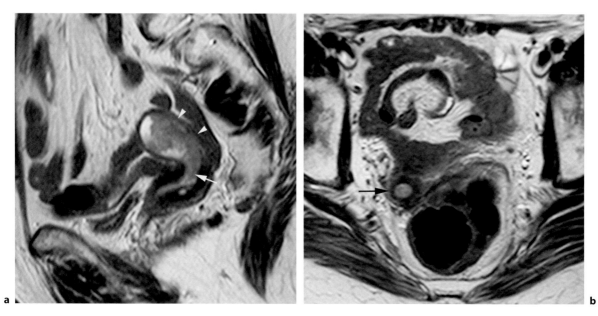

a   b

Fig. 6.9a,b. MRI of the pelvis for staging endometrioid adenocarcinoma grade 1 of the uterus diagnosed at endometrial biopsy in a 69-year-old woman with postmenopausal bleeding. **a** T2-weighted sagittal image of the uterus shows endometrial enlargement due to a mass of intermediate signal intensity extending into the inner os of the endocervical channel (*arrow*) and interrupting the posterior junctional zone (*arrowheads*). **b** Axial oblique T2-weighted image through the cervix demonstrates an intact hypointense stromal ring (*arrow*) excluding stage IIB. Prospective image interpretation concluded on stage IIA disease with at least superficial myometrial invasion. Pathology of subsequent hysterectomy specimen demonstrated 4 mm depth of myometrial invasion for a maximum thickness of 10 mm (stage IB) with associated adenomyosis and no invasion of the cervical mucosa. The false positive diagnosis of cervical mucosa invasion was explained at macroscopic examination by tumor prolapse into the cervical channel without associated cervical invasion

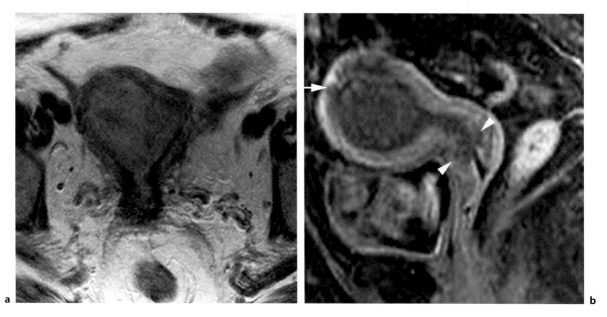

a   b

Fig. 6.10a,b. MRI of the pelvis for staging endometrial carcinoma in a 52-year-old woman. **a** T2-weighted coronal image of the uterus with a distended cavity and an ill-defined myometrial endometrial interface. **b** T1-weighted contrast-enhanced sagittal image of the uterus shows decreased enhancement of the endometrial tumor and the deeply invaded part of the myometrium (*arrow*), the cervical channel and the cervical stroma (*arrowheads*). Pathology of the hysterectomy specimen diagnosed deep myometrial and cervical stroma invasion (stage IIB disease). (Courtesy Dr. L. Oleaga, Bilbao, Spain)

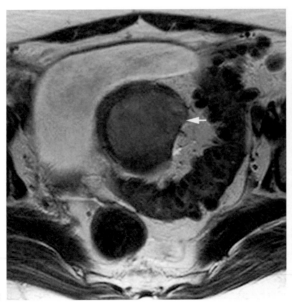
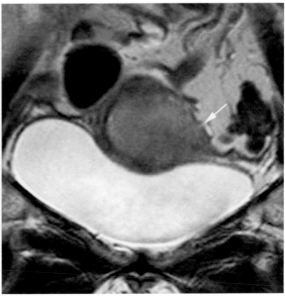

a   b

Fig. 6.11a,b. MRI of the pelvis for staging endometrial carcinoma in a 65-year-old woman. **a** T2-weighted axial image of the uterus shows a distended uterine cavity and absent myometrial signal intensity at the left part of the uterus (*arrow*). **b** The coronal orientation of the T2-weighted image suggests complete left-sided myometrial invasion (*arrow*). Pathology of the hysterectomy specimen confirmed involvement of the uterine serosa (stage IIIA disease). (Courtesy Dr. L. Oleaga, Bilbao, Spain)

vasion significantly changes post-test probabilities for myometrial invasion regardless of prior tumour grade at endometrial biopsy [16]. According to this study, a suspicious MRI for deep myometrial invasion increased the probability of this pathology to 60% for grade 1, 84% for grade 2 and 92% for grade 3. On the contrary, after a negative MRI for deep myometrial invasion, the probability of deep myometrial invasion at final pathology decreased to less than 1% for grade 1, to 5% for grade 2 and to10% for grade 3. Due to the impact of preoperative knowledge of deep myometrial invasion on patient management leading to lymphadenectomy at the time of hysterectomy, preoperative MRI has become a new standard in many European countries prior to treatment of patients with endometrial cancer. Pre-operative knowledge of adequate imaging protocols including medical supervision during image acquisition and adequate knowledge of image interpretation criteria is mandatory to ensure high quality pelvic MRI of endometrial cancer. Only at this price will gynaecologists recognize the important role of preoperative pelvic MRI and allow MRI to keep its top rang of preoperative imaging techniques for endometrial cancer staging.

Computed tomography (CT) has been used as an alternative tool for staging endometrial cancer. Its performance to diagnose myometrial and cervical invasion is not as high as magnetic resonance imaging (MRI) [28]. However, in patients with contra-indication to MRI, CT remains a diagnostic staging tool for endometrial cancer, particularly due to the possibility of multiplanar reconstruction in a sagittal and coronal plane. Optimal timing of post-contrast images, however, needs to be refined to catch the moment when greatest contrast between the strongly enhancing myometrium and the hypointense endometrial tumor is obtained. The lack of anatomical density differences between the layers of cervical stroma and the mucosa makes the diagnosis of cervical invasion quite difficult at CT.

6.6
Therapy

6.6.1
Surgery

Surgery is the treatment of choice in early-stage endometrial cancer. The surgical procedure includes total hysterectomy, bilateral salpingoooophorectomy, as well as acquisition of peritoneal fluid or washings for

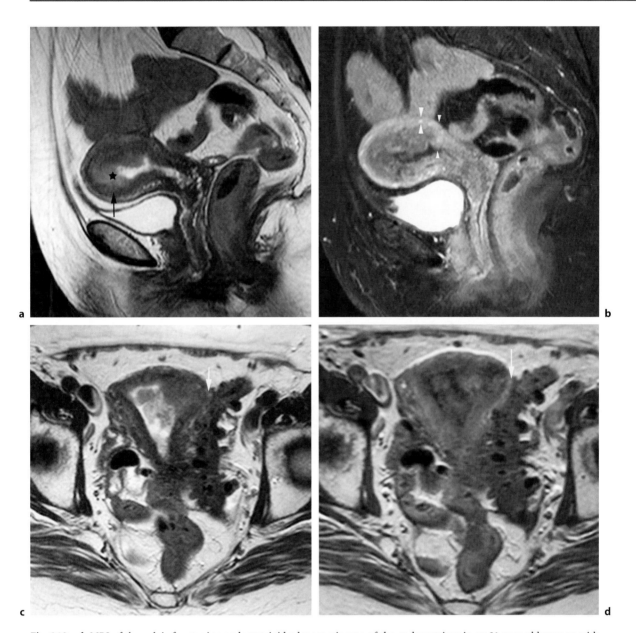

Fig. 6.12a–d. MRI of the pelvis for staging endometrioid adenocarcinoma of the endometrium in an 81-year-old woman with postmenopausal bleeding and a history of recurrent sigmoiditis. **a** T2-weighted sagittal image of the uterus shows an endometrial mass (*star*) and an irregular interface with the junctional zone (*arrow*). **b** Fat-suppressed contrast-enhanced T1-weighted sagittal image at 3 min allows easier identification of endometrial tumor limits due to decreased tumor enhancement. The remaining thickness of the hypervascular, non-invaded myometrium (*arrowheads*) measures less than 50% of the total myometrial thickness (*small arrowheads*) and suggests deep myometrial invasion. **c** T2-weighted coronal oblique image of the uterus shows absent myometrial signal intensity at the left uterine horn (*arrow*) suggesting close tumor contact with the sigmoid wall demonstrating multiple diverticula. **d** The contrast-enhanced delayed T1-weighted image in the same plane as (**c**) shows a small part of normal myometrial enhancement (*arrow*) at the left uterine horn and no abnormal invasion of the adjacent sigmoid. Surgery described adhesions between the uterus and lesions of chronic sigmoiditis. Pathology of hysterectomy specimen diagnosed stage IC disease

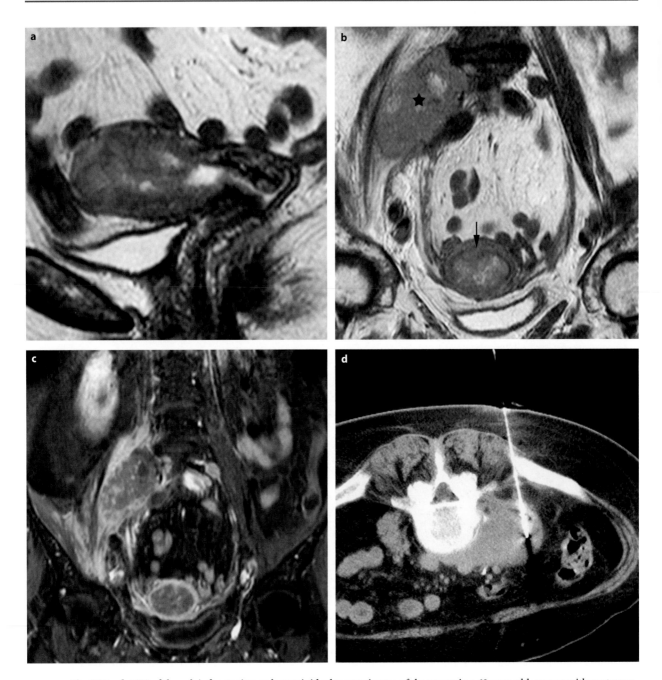

Fig. 6.13a–d. MRI of the pelvis for staging endometrioid adenocarcinoma of the uterus in a 69-year-old woman with postmeno-pausal bleeding. **a** Sagittal T2-weighted image of the uterus demonstrates a large endometrial mass of similar signal intensity as the myometrium. **b** The T2-weighted coronal image (short axis image of the uterus) shows disruption of the junctional zone (*arrow*) and a right-sided large paravertebral mass (*asterisk*). **c** Contrast-enhanced fat suppressed T1-weighted coronal image shows deep myometrial invasion by the mildly enhancing endometrial tumor coexisting with an enhancing right paraverte-bral mass. **d** CT-guided biopsy of the paravertebral mass diagnosed a metastasis of endometrioid adenocarcinoma infiltrating fibrous tissue

cytology. In selected cases such as clear-cell or serous endometrial cancer, there is a need for omentectomy and retroperitoneal lymph-node dissection. Although the results of randomised trials are still lacking, in experienced hands, laparoscopy-assisted vaginal hysterectomy is feasible in patients with endometrial cancer. Fluid for cytology, peritoneal biopsy samples, lymph nodes, and omentum can be obtained in a single laparoscopy-assisted intervention [1]. Type-1 endometrial cancer has a primarily lymphatic spread in most cases limited to pelvic nodes. If there are positive lymph nodes, those around the obturator nerve are more likely than those around the external and common iliac vessels. Isolated involvement of the para-aortic nodes is rare. Endometrial cancer presenting with grossly positive pelvic nodes, grossly positive adnexal metastasis, or serosal infiltration is associated with positive inframesenteric para-aortic lymph nodes. As the risk of lymph node metastasis depends on the stage of endometrial cancer, lymph node dissection is recommended in the following stages:

= FIGO IB, G2 and G3
= FIGO IC, G1, G2, G3
= FIGO II and FIGO III as far as the carcinoma is resectable

Lymph node dissection is also recommended in histological subtypes associated with a higher risk of lymph node metastasis (e.g., clear cell, serous papillary endometrial carcinoma). Pelvic lymph node dissection should be performed in combination with para-aortic lymph node dissection because of the high risk of metastasis at both sites [24]. Whether lymphadenectomy is curative in endometrial cancer remains controversial [38].

6.6.2
Radiotherapy

Radiation can be delivered externally to the pelvis, as vaginal brachytherapy, or as a combination. Treatment can also be directed to the whole abdomen or to an extended field that includes the pelvis and para-aortic region. Indications for radiotherapy are generally in the adjuvant setting. Radical radiotherapy with intrauterine brachytherapy is curative but should be applied only in medically inoperable patients [30]. The practice of preoperative radiotherapy has been abandoned because it interferes with adequate surgical staging and there is no proven benefit over postoperative radiotherapy. The goal of adjuvant radiotherapy is to treat the pelvic lymph node region, as well as the central pelvic region including the upper vagina as there might be microscopic disease. The purpose of radiotherapy is the risk reduction for local recurrence. Patients with surgical stage IA and grade 1 or grade 2 disease do not benefit from radiotherapy. In patients with stage IB grade 1 and grade 2 vaginal brachytherapy is indicated. For stage IA grade 3, vaginal brachytherapy associated with possible percutaneous pelvic radiotherapy should also be discussed. In higher stages a combination of brachytherapy and percutaneous pelvic radiotherapy is recommended. In stage IV disease, therapy should be planned individually [40].

6.7
Follow-Up and Prognosis

Weight loss, pain, and vaginal bleeding can suggest recurrent disease, in most cases occurring during the first 3 years after primary treatment. Although follow-up visits are organised in most settings, retrospective data suggest no difference in survival between symptomatic and asymptomatic recurrence or between women with recurrence detected during routine follow-up visits and those with recurrence detected during the interval between routine visits [2]. Furthermore, follow-up of patients treated for endometrial cancer based on routine Pap smears and systemic imaging does not permit earlier detection of recurrence. There is a psychological benefit for most patients controlled in a follow-up program. In the first 2 years a follow-up visit is recommended every 3 month, in the next 3 years every 6 months and after 5 years on an annual basis. Local recurrence occurs most often at the vagina or the vaginal cuff of hysterectomy; therefore, a vaginal exam including Pap smear and transvaginal ultrasound should be performed. As endometrial cancer is associated with a higher risk for breast cancer, breast examination and mammography are also recommended every year. The most important prognostic features in endometrial cancer are surgical FIGO stage, myometrial invasion, histological type, and differentiation grade. The FIGO stage reflects the 5-year survival, which varies according to series but is around 85% for stage I, 75% for stage II, 45% for stage III, and 25% for stage IV disease. Nonendometrioid endometrial cancers such as serous and clear-cell carcinomas account for about 10% of all endometrial cancers, but for more than 50% of all recurrences and deaths from endometrial cancer [1].

6.8
Areas of Controversy and Current Research

The following are areas of controversy and current research according to AMANT et al. [1]:

= Assessment of the role of 3D ultrasonography in the diagnosis of endometrial cancer.
= Cost–benefit analysis of tests done in women with abnormal uterine bleeding.
= Microarray analyses and proteomics are likely to further disentangle molecular pathways.
= Distillation of prognostic and predictive factors from molecular findings.
= Conservative management with anti-oestrogens or local progestogens to conserve fertility
= Long-term safety in relation to local and port-site metastases of laparoscopically assisted vaginal hysterectomy
= Accuracy of sentinel procedure for lymph-node staging
= Pelvic versus local radiotherapy to decrease local relapse
= Survival benefit of correct surgical staging (lymphadenectomy) and mode of radiotherapy
= Role of adjuvant chemotherapy in endometrial cancer of surgical stage I–II, type 2
= Role of pure anti-oestrogens (fulvestrant) and newer selective oestrogen-receptor modulators.
= Tibolone and endometrium.
= Role of ultrasonography in detection of recurrent disease.

References

1. Amant F, Moerman P, Neven P, Timmerman D, Van Limbergen E, Vergote I (2005) Endometrial cancer. Lancet 366:491–505
2. Agboola OO, Grunfeld E, Coyle D, Perry GA (1997) Costs and benefits of routine follow-up after curative treatment for endometrial cancer. CMAJ 157:879–886
3. Arko D, Takac I (2000) High frequency transvaginal ultrasonography in preoperative assessment of myometrial invasion in endometrial cancer. J Ultrasound Med 19:639–643
4. Bipat S, Glas AS, van d, V, Zwinderman AH, Bossuyt PM, Stoker J (2003) Computed tomography and magnetic resonance imaging in staging of uterine cervical carcinoma: a systematic review. Gynecol Oncol 91:59–66
5. Bokhman JV (1983) Two pathogenetic types of endometrial carcinoma. Gynecol Oncol 15:10–17
6. Boronow RC, Morrow CP, Creasman WT, DiSaia PJ, Silverberg SG, Miller A, Blessing JA (1984) Surgical staging in endometrial cancer: clinical-pathologic findings of a prospective study. Obstet Gynecol 63:825–832
7. Calle EE, Rodriguez C, Walker-Thurmond K, Thun MJ (2003) Overweight, obesity, and mortality from cancer in a prospectively studied cohort of U.S. adults. N Engl J Med 348:1625–1638
8. Clark TJ (2004) Outpatient hysteroscopy and ultrasonography in the management of endometrial disease. Curr Opin Obstet Gynecol 16:305–311
9. Clement PB, Young RH (2002) Endometrioid carcinoma of the uterine corpus: a review of its pathology with emphasis on recent advances and problematic aspects. Adv Anat Pathol 9:145–184
10. Cohen I (2004) Endometrial pathologies associated with postmenopausal tamoxifen treatment. Gynecol Oncol 94:256–266
11. Creasman WT (1990) New gynecologic cancer staging. Obstet Gynecol 75:287–288
12. Creasman WT (1995) New gynecologic cancer staging. Gynecol Oncol 58:157–158
13. Cunha TM, Felix A, Cabral I (2001) Preoperative assessment of deep myometrial and cervical invasion in endometrial carcinoma: comparison of magnetic resonance imaging and gross visual inspection. Int J Gynecol Cancer 11:130–136
14. Eifel P, Hendrickson M, Ross J, Ballon S, Martinez A, Kempson R (1982) Simultaneous presentation of carcinoma involving the ovary and the uterine corpus. Cancer 50:163–170
15. Frei KA, Kinkel K (2001) Staging endometrial cancer: role of magnetic resonance imaging. J Magn Reson Imaging 13:850–855
16. Frei KA, Kinkel K, Bonel HM, Lu Y, Zaloudek C, Hricak H (2000) Prediction of deep myometrial invasion in patients with endometrial cancer: clinical utility of contrast-enhanced MR imaging – a meta-analysis and Bayesian analysis. Radiology 216:444–449
17. Grasel RP, Outwater EK, Siegelman ES, Capuzzi D, Parker L, Hussain SM (2000) Endometrial polyps: MR imaging features and distinction from endometrial carcinoma. Radiology 214:47–52
18. Gu M, Shi W, Barakat RR, Thaler HT, Saigo PE (2001) Pap smears in women with endometrial carcinoma. Acta Cytol 45:555–560
19. Gupta JK, Chien PF, Voit D, Clark TJ, Khan KS (2002) Ultrasonographic endometrial thickness for diagnosing endometrial pathology in women with postmenopausal bleeding: a meta-analysis. Acta Obstet Gynecol Scand 81:799–816
20. Harvey EB, Brinton LA (1985) Second cancer following cancer of the breast in Connecticut, 1935–82. Natl Cancer Inst Monogr 68:99–112
21. Hawighorst H, Knapstein PG, Weikel W, Knopp MV, Schaeffer U, Brix G, Essig M, Hoffmann U, Zuna I, Schonberg S, van Kaick G (1996) Cervical carcinoma: comparison of standard and pharmacokinetic MR imaging. Radiology 201:531–539
22. Hill HA, Eley JW, Harlan LC, Greenberg RS, Barrett RJ, Chen VW (1996) Racial differences in endometrial cancer survival: the black/white cancer survival study. Obstet Gynecol 88:919–926
23. Hinkula M, Pukkala E, Kyyronen P, Kauppila A (2002) Grand multiparity and incidence of endometrial cancer: a population-based study in Finland. Int J Cancer 98:912–915

24. Hirahatake K, Hareyama H, Sakuragi N, Nishiya M, Makinoda S, Fujimoto S (1997) A clinical and pathologic study on para-aortic lymph node metastasis in endometrial carcinoma. J Surg Oncol 65:82–87

25. Hubacher D, Grimes DA (2002) Noncontraceptive health benefits of intrauterine devices: a systematic review. Obstet Gynecol Surv 57:120–128

26. Kaaks R, Lukanova A, Kurzer MS (2002) Obesity, endogenous hormones, and endometrial cancer risk: a synthetic review. Cancer Epidemiol Biomarkers Prev 11:1531–43

27. Kinkel K (2005) Pitfalls in staging uterine neoplasm with imaging: a review. Abdominal Imaging 2005 Dec 5; [Epub ahead of print]

28. Kinkel K, Kaji Y, Yu KK, Segal MR, Lu Y, Powell CB, Hricak H (1999) Radiologic staging in patients with endometrial cancer: a meta-analysis. Radiology 212:711–718

29. Kjaer SK, Mellemkjaer L, Brinton LA, Johansen C, Gridley G, Olsen JH (2004) Tubal sterilization and risk of ovarian, endometrial and cervical cancer. A Danish population-based follow-up study of more than 65 000 sterilized women. Int J Epidemiol 33:596–602

30. Kucera H, Vavra N, Weghaupt K (1990) [Value of irradiation alone of generally inoperable endometrial cancer with high dose rate iridium 192] Zum Wert der alleinigen Bestrahlung des allgemein inoperablen Endometriumkarzinoms mittels High-Dose-Rate-Iridium-192. Geburtshilfe Frauenheilkd 50:610–613

31. Kucera E, Kainz C, Reinthaller A, Sliutz G, Leodolter S, Kucera H, Breitenecker G (2000) Accuracy of intraoperative frozen-section diagnosis in stage I endometrial adenocarcinoma. Gynecol Obstet Invest 49:62–66

32. Larson DM, Connor GP, Broste SK, Krawisz BR, Johnson KK (1996) Prognostic significance of gross myometrial invasion with endometrial cancer. Obstet Gynecol 88:394–398

33. Madison T, Schottenfeld D, James SA, Schwartz AG, Gruber SB (2004) Endometrial cancer: socioeconomic status and racial/ethnic differences in stage at diagnosis, treatment, and survival. Am J Public Health 94:2104–211

34. Manfredi R, Mirk P, Maresca G, Margariti PA, Testa A, Zannoni GF, Giordano D, Scambia G, Marano P (2004) Local-regional staging of endometrial carcinoma: role of MR imaging in surgical planning. Radiology 231:372–378

35. Murakami T, Kurachi H, Nakamura H, Tsuda K, Miyake A, Tomoda K, Hori S, Kozuka T (1995) Cervical invasion of endometrial carcinoma – evaluation by parasagittal MR imaging. Acta Radiol 36:248–253

36. Obermair A, Geramou M, Gucer F, Denison U, Graf AH, Kapshammer E, Medl M, Rosen A, Wierrani F, Neunteufel W, Frech I, Preyer O, Speiser P, Kainz C (2000) Impact of hysteroscopy on disease-free survival in clinically stage I endometrial cancer patients. Int J Gynecol Cancer 10:275–279

37. Parkin DM, Pisani P, Ferlay J (1999) Global cancer statistics. CA Cancer J Clin 49:33–64, 1

38. Podratz KC, Mariani A, Webb MJ (1998) Staging and therapeutic value of lymphadenectomy in endometrial cancer. Gynecol Oncol 70:163–164

39. Popovich MJ, Hricak H, Sugimura K, Stern JL (1993) The role of MR imaging in determining surgical eligibility for pelvic exenteration. AJR Am J Roentgenol 160:525–531

40. Santin AD, Bellone S, O›Brien TJ, Pecorelli S, Cannon MJ, Roman JJ (2004) Current treatment options for endometrial cancer. Expert Rev Anticancer Ther 4:679–689

41. Sironi S, Colombo E, Villa G, Taccagni G, Belloni C, Garancini P, DelMaschio A (1992) Myometrial invasion by endometrial carcinoma: assessment with plain and gadolinium-enhanced MR imaging. Radiology 185:207–212

42. Smith-Bindman R, Kerlikowske K, Feldstein VA, Subak L, Scheidler J, Segal M, Brand R, Grady D (1998) Endovaginal ultrasound to exclude endometrial cancer and other endometrial abnormalities. JAMA 280:1510–1517

43. Tabor A, Watt HC, Wald NJ (2002) Endometrial thickness as a test for endometrial cancer in women with postmenopausal vaginal bleeding. Obstet Gynecol 99:663–670

44. Takeuchi M, Matsuzaki K, Uehara H, Yoshida S, Nishitani H, Shimazu H (2005) Pathologies of the uterine endometrial cavity: usual and unusual manifestations and pitfalls on magnetic resonance imaging. Eur Radiol 15:2244–2255

45. Ulbright TM, Roth LM (1985) Metastatic and independent cancers of the endometrium and ovary: a clinicopathologic study of 34 cases. Hum Pathol 16:28–34

46. Umar A, Risinger JI, Hawk ET, Barrett JC (2004) Testing guidelines for hereditary non-polyposis colorectal cancer. Nat Rev Cancer 4:153–158

47. Yamashita Y, Harada M, Sawada T, Takahashi M, Miyazaki K, Okamura H (1993) Normal uterus and FIGO stage I endometrial carcinoma: dynamic gadolinium-enhanced MR imaging. Radiology 186:495–501

48. Zaino RJ, Kurman RJ, Diana KL, Morrow CP (1995) The utility of the revised International Federation of Gynecology and Obstetrics histologic grading of endometrial adenocarcinoma using a defined nuclear grading system. A Gynecologic Oncology Group study. Cancer 75:81–86

Cervical Cancer

Uta Zaspel **and** Bernd Hamm

CONTENTS

U. Zaspel, MD
Institut für Radiologie (Campus Mitte), Charité – Universitäts-medizin Berlin, Charitéplatz 1, 10117 Berlin, Germany
B. Hamm, MD
Professor and Chairman, Institut für Radiologie (Campus Mitte), Klinik für Strahlenheilkunde (Campus Virchow-Klinikum und Campus Buch), Charité – Universitätsmedizin Berlin, Charitéplatz 1, 10117 Berlin, Germany

7.1
Background

7.1.1
Epidemiology

The annual incidence rate of cervical cancer is about 12 per 100,000 women in Germany and 7.9 in the United States, with the worldwide rate ranging between 5 (Spain) and 45 (Colombia) per 100,000 women. Cervical cancer accounts for about 4% of all malignant diseases and is the eighth most common malignancy in women in the more developed countries. It is the most frequent gynecologic carcinoma in women under 50 years of age and the third most common gynecologic malignancy in postmenopausal women following endometrial and ovarian cancer. About 500,000 women worldwide are diagnosed with invasive cervical carcinoma per year and about 350,000 women die from the disease. It is the second most common cause of cancer-related death in women, with the majority of affected women living in third world countries. In Germany, approximately 7,000 new cases are diagnosed per year and approximately 2,000 women die from cervical cancer every year [1–3]. The age distribution of invasive cervical cancer shows a first peak between 35 and 45 years of age and a second peak between 60 and 64 years. The mean age of onset used to be 52 years, but there is a tendency toward earlier onset. One reason for this tendency is the fact that screening programs have reduced the risk of cervical cancer, especially in women aged 50 and older (see Sect. 7.1.3). On the other hand, the baby boom generation aged 35–45 results in a larger cervical cancer population in this age range. The overall incidence of invasive cervical cancer has declined by about 75% in Europe and other industrialized countries since the 1970s. The annual incidence rate per 100,000 women in Germany was 35 in 1971 as opposed to 12 in 2001.

This decline is attributable to the availability of cytologic screening, which has led to the identification and therapy of precursor lesions of cervical cancer in younger women. Progression to invasive cervical cancer is thus prevented [4, 5]. Precursor conditions are much more common than invasive cervical cancer and typically already occur in women aged 30–40. Precancerous lesions gradually progress to invasive disease over a period of about 10 years [6]. Invasive cervical cancer occurring before the age of 35 is typically of a more malignant type.

The overall mortality from cervical cancer has declined by 55% since 1970 and the figures continue to decrease slightly. The annual mortality rate today is 3.2 per 100,000 women in the United States and ranges between 2.0 (Denmark) and 4.4 (Germany) in Europe. Death from cervical cancer thus accounts for just barely 2% of all cancer-related deaths and is no longer among the eight most common causes of cancer death. This development is primarily attributable to the installation of screening programs as a result of which more cancers are detected at a more favorable earlier stage (FIGO stages IA and IB) as compared with more advanced disease. In addition, there has been a change in therapeutic strategies as it has been shown, for instance, that certain subgroups of patients benefit from the combination of surgery and radiochemotherapy. Altogether, more patients are now treated by surgery alone than by radiotherapy alone. Novel and minimally invasive operative techniques primarily aim to improve the patient's postoperative quality of life. Despite these advances, there has been only slight change in the stage-related prognosis of invasive cervical cancer over the last decades. The average relative 5-year survival rate continues to be about 65% in Germany and 70% in the USA with a relative 10-year survival rate of 59% and 65%, respectively [7, 8].

7.1.2
Pathogenesis

The main cause of cervical cancer is infection of the cervical epithelium by one of the oncogenic human papilloma virus (HPV) types. The high-risk types of HPV are 16 and 18, which have been shown to have a high oncogenic potential [9–13]. The overall prevalence of cervical HPV infections is 5%–20%, with a peak between 20 and 25 years of age. Spontaneous regression and clearance of HPV infection with complete eradication of the virus is common. Persistence of the virus is only associated with the risk of epithelial changes of the cervical mucosa. Especially women with cofactors are at risk. These include sex at an early age, having many sexual partners, poor genital hygiene, frequent other genital infections, multiple pregnancies, immunosuppression as in women with AIDS, and long-term use of oral contraceptives [14–16]. Other cofactors are smoking and vitamin deficiencies. A genetic predisposition also appears to be involved.

Cervical cancer of the squamous cell type (see Sect. 7.1.5) develops in several stages from local epithelial proliferation, through definitive epithelial changes and dysplasia, to a truly precancerous lesion. The precancerous stages are referred to as cervical intraepithelial neoplasia (CIN) [17] or squamous intraepithelial lesion (SIL) and first progress to carcinoma in situ before they become invasive cancers. Initial changes typically have their origin in the unstable transformation zone of the uterine cervix at the junction between the squamous epithelium of the portio and the columnar epithelium of the cervical canal. About 3%–5% of sexually mature women have CIN. The incidence of advanced precancerous conditions (CIN II, III) is about 100 times higher than the incidence of cervical cancer and has continually increased over the last two decades. The earliest forms of CIN are seen in women in their mid-twenties. CIN often resolves spontaneously but may also progress to carcinoma in situ – typically between 25 and 35 years of age – and finally to invasive cervical cancer at around age 40.

7.1.3
Screening

Early detection by means of colposcopic and cytologic screening has considerably lowered the incidence and mortality of cervical cancer since the

1970s. The long lead time from the development of preinvasive lesions to invasive cancer and the accessibility of the cervix are two important factors that contribute to the detection of precursor lesions and early stages by screening [18]. Today over 80% of cervical carcinomas are detected at stage I when the tumor is still locally confined. Most of the remaining cervical cancers are detected in women who have never had a screening test (50% of eligible women in Germany) or attended only irregularly. Moreover, the usual form of cervical smear cytology and staining according to Papanicolaou (Pap) has an overall sensitivity of only about 60% with a specificity of over 90%. The Pap smear has also been shown to be of limited value in detecting the rare histologic type of cervical adenocarcinoma [19–21]. Current studies therefore investigate the effectiveness of different screening schemes and evaluate alternative screening tests such as monolayer cytology or HPV screening [5, 19, 22, 23]. Finally, a vaccine against papillomavirus has been developed and its prophylactic potential is under clinical evaluation.

7.1.4
Clinical Presentation

Early forms of cervical cancer do not present any symptoms. Clinical symptoms occur fairly late, typically when the tumor has reached the stage of invasive ulcerating cancer. The symptoms include vaginal bleeding after intercourse, vaginal discharge, and dyspareunia. Diffuse pelvic and back pain radiating into the legs may indicate advanced cervical cancer with infiltration of adjacent structures. Large cervical cancers may cause pain or bleeding with urination or passage of stools. Tumor-induced disturbance of lymphatic drainage causes unilateral leg edema, peritoneal seeding an increase in body circumference. General symptoms of advanced cervical cancer are a reduction of physical performance and loss of weight. Late complications include respiratory disturbance and cough in patients with metastatic spread to the lungs.

7.1.5
Histopathology

Histologically, approximately 80% of all cervical cancers are of the keratinizing or nonkeratinizing squamous cell type. Adenocarcinoma is the second most common histologic type, accounting for about 15% of all cervical cancers [24]. Its incidence has slightly increased over the last 25 years. Cervical adenocarcinoma has been found to correlate with recurrent or chronic cervicitis and the intake of estrogen-containing drugs. Altogether, however, the pathogenesis is unknown. Stage II and III adenocarcinoma has a slightly more unfavorable prognosis than squamous cell carcinoma [25]. A small proportion (about 3%) of adenocarcinomas is of the histologic subtype of highly differentiated mucinous adenocarcinoma. This so-called adenoma malignum has a very poor prognosis because of early spread into the abdominal cavity and a poorer response to chemotherapy or radiotherapy [26, 27]. At the same time, its well-differentiated morphology may lead to misinterpretation of its malignancy. MRI depicts a solid tumor containing multiple cysts which arises from the endocervical glands and invades the cervical stroma [28]. This malignant tumor is difficult to differentiate from cystic cervical lesions, which have a similar appearance. The solid tumor portions provide the key to the diagnosis [29]. Adenoma malignum is often seen in patients with Peutz-Jeghers syndrome, which is characterized by pigmentation of the skin and mucous membranes, multiple hamartomas of the gastrointestinal tract, and ovarian tumors [30]. Among the rarer histologic types of cervical cancer is adenosquamous carcinoma with a proportion of 3% and a poorer prognosis than squamous cell carcinoma and adenocarcinoma [31]. Other cervical tumors are neuroendocrine tumors, small cell tumors, and rhabdomyosarcoma. Small-cell cervical cancer has a poor prognosis due to early metastatic spread. Neuroendocrine tumors account for 0.3% of cervical cancers and show aggressive growth. Accompanying carcinoid syndrome is rare and the clinical symptoms do not differ from those of squamous cell carcinoma [32–34].

7.1.6
Staging

The most widely used staging system is the FIGO (International Federation of Gynecology and Obstetrics) classification, which distinguishes four stages of cervical cancer (Table 7.1) [35]. This staging system was introduced before the advent of modern imaging modalities and hence differs from all other classifications of gynecologic tumors in that it is still based on the results of bimanual palpation. FIGO stage 0 com-

Table 7.1. FIGO staging of cervical cancer

FIGO		Drawing
0	Dysplasia or cervical invasive neoplasia (CIN)	
0	Carcinoma in situ (CIN III)	
I	Cervical carcinoma strictly confined to uterus	
IA	Invasive cancer identified only microscopically	
IA1	Stromal invasion no greater than 3 mm in depth and no wider than 7 mm in diameter	
IA2	Stromal invasion greater than 3 mm but no greater than 5 mm in depth and no wider than 7 mm in diameter	
IB	Invasion of stroma greater than 5 mm in depth or greater than 7 mm in diameter or clinically visible lesion confined to the cervix	
IB1	Clinically visible lesion no greater than 4 cm in size	
IB2	Clinically visible lesion greater than 4 cm in size	
II	Carcinoma extending beyond the cervix but not involving the pelvic sidewall or the lower third of the vagina	
IIA	Tumor involves the vagina but not its lower third	
IIB	Parametrial invasion	
III	Tumor involves the lower third of the vagina or extends to the pelvic sidewall or causes hydronephrosis	
IIIA	Tumor involves the lower third of the vagina	
IIIB	Tumor extends to the pelvic sidewall or causes hydronephrosis	
IVA	Tumor invades mucosa of the bladder or rectum or extends beyond the true pelvis	
IVB	Metastatic spread to distant organs	

prises all forms of preinvasive cervical carcinoma. In FIGO stage I, cervical carcinoma is confined to the uterus (extension to corpus should be disregarded). FIGO stage II comprises cervical carcinoma invading beyond the uterus with involvement of the upper two-thirds of the vagina or of the parametria. FIGO stage III cervical carcinoma extends to the pelvic wall, involves the lower third of the vagina, or causes hydronephrosis or a nonfunctioning kidney. FIGO stage IVA is characterized by invasion of the bladder or rectum or by tumor extension beyond the true pelvis. The presence of distant metastases establishes stage IVB disease.

The FIGO classification also defines the diagnostic procedures to be used for pretreatment evaluation. These comprise biopsy, cervical conization, hysteroscopy, and endocervical curettage as invasive measures for histologic diagnosis. The radiographic modalities include intravenous pyelography, barium enema, and X-ray examinations of the lungs and skeleton. The invasive diagnostic procedures for assessing tumor extent consist of cystoscopy and proctoscopy. Findings obtained with MRI, CT, ultrasound, scintigraphy, and laparoscopy are not taken into consideration in determining the FIGO stage, which is regarded as a drawback of this staging system. The vaginal extent of cervical cancer can be determined with a high degree of accuracy by means of rectovaginal examination and colposcopy while the clinical examination is less accurate in determining tumor size and parametrial involvement. Studies comparing FIGO stages with surgical stages found an error rate of about 30% for stage IB [36, 37] and of up to 70% for advanced tumors of stages II–IV [38]. Clinical symptoms such as fever or reactive parametrial inflammation often lead to overstaging. The nodal status is not considered, although it is crucial for the patient's prognosis and survival [36, 39]. For these reasons, more and more examiners prefer surgical and histopathologic staging according to the TNM classification from the American Joint Committee on Cancer (AJCC) and the

Table 7.2. Staging of cervical cancer according to UICC and TNM criteria

FIGO	UICC	T	N	M
0	0	Tis	N0	M0
I	I	T1	N0	M0
II	II	T2	N0	M0
IIIA	IIIA	T3a	N0	M0
IIIB	IIIB	T1	N1 all N positive	M0
		T2		M0
		T3a		
		T3b		
IVA	IVA	T4	All N positive	M0
IVB	IVB	All T	All N positive	M1

UICC (United International Cancer Congress) criteria (Tables 7.1 and 7.2). These criteria correlate much better with the prognosis. According to the FIGO and TNM classification, MRI and CT are optional modalities in perioperative staging [40, 41]. Surgical lymph node staging is often performed as a supplementary procedure to determine operability or prior to neo-adjuvant therapy, primary radiotherapy. In patients with positive para-aortic lymph nodes, additional biopsies should be obtained from scalene lymph nodes. Tumor markers have a poor sensitivity and specificity and are therefore not routinely determined as part of the diagnostic work-up and follow-up of patients with cervical cancer.

7.1.7
Growth Patterns

The vast majority of cervical carcinomas arise from the squamocolumnar junction and typically show exophytic growth in the outer cervix in younger women. With retraction of the transformation zone into the cervical canal in older women, endophytic growth patterns of cervical cancer become more common (Figs. 7.1, 7.12).

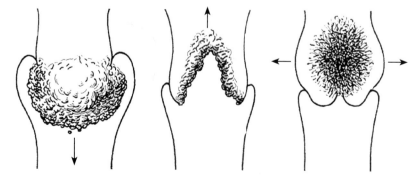

Fig. 7.1. Growth patterns of cervical cancer: exophytic, endophytic ulcerative, and endophytic expansion with barrel-shaped configuration of the cervix. (from [130])

Cervical cancer is characterized by continuous invasive growth with extension into the vagina, parametria, uterine corpus, bladder, rectum, and peritoneal cavity. In the same way, the tumor spreads to the pelvic lymph nodes. Preferred sites of nodal metastases are the obturator fossa, the nodes along the external, internal, and common iliac vessels, the presacral lymph nodes, and finally the para-aortic nodes (Fig. 7.2) [42]. The risk of lymph node metastasis correlates with the stage of cervical cancer. In stage IA1 disease (microscopic infiltration of stroma) without vascular space involvement, the probability of pelvic lymph node metastasis is less than 1% [43] vs 10%–20% in stage IB disease. When there is cancer extension beyond the cervix with involvement of the upper vagina in stage IIA, the risk of pelvic or para-aortic nodal metastases increases to 25% and to over 30% when there is parametrial invasion (stage IIB). The risk is 45% in stage III tumors with involvement of the lower third of the vagina or extension to the pelvic wall and 55% in stage IVA with infiltration of

the bladder or rectum. The probability of metastatic spread to para-aortic nodes becomes relevant for stage IIA and above, where it is 8%–17%. Para-aortic nodal metastases are regarded as distant metastases and are rare when the pelvic nodes are negative.

Hematogenous dissemination is rare and is seen only in advanced cervical cancer. The 10-year risk of distant metastases varies with the stage and ranges from 3% for IB cervical cancer and 75% for stage IVA. Preferred sites of distant metastases are the para-aortic and supraclavicular lymph nodes, the lungs, the abdominal cavity, and the skeleton [44].

The probability of tumor recurrence correlates with the disease stage and is 10%–20% for stages IB and IIA with negative lymph nodes and 50%–70% in advanced tumors of stages IIB–IVA and in patients with nodal metastases (Fig. 7.3) [45]. The incidence of pelvic recurrence and metastatic spread is highest during the first 2 years after diagnosis and primary therapy [46]. The true pelvis is the site of recurrent tumor in 60%–80% of cases [44, 47–49].

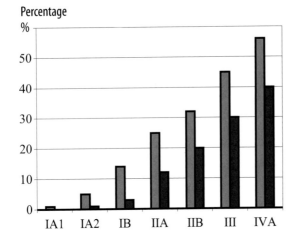

Fig. 7.2. Probability of lymph node metastasis by tumor stage

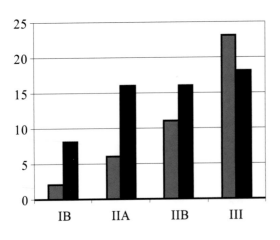

Fig. 7.3. Probability of central pelvic recurrence and distant metastasis by tumor stage

7.1.8
Treatment

Treatment of cervical cancer is individualized to the patient's disease stage, and the therapeutic scheme may also depend on the gynecologic institution. A low-grade CIN lesion (CIN I) that is confined to the transformation zone and is fully visible with the colposcope is not treated and simply followed up, as it often regresses spontaneously in healthy women. CIN I lesions in women with risk factors for the development of cervical cancer and CIN II or CIN III lesions (moderate to severe dysplasia) are treated by cervical conization. Stage I and IIA cervical cancer and some stage IIB carcinomas are treated by primary surgery. Alternatively, stage IB and IIA can be treated by primary curative radiotherapy, which has a comparable survival rate. Surgery is preferred in younger women because it has less deleterious consequences for the ovaries and vagina and less severe long-term effects on the urinary bladder and rectum as compared with radiotherapy.

Different surgical options are available to treat different tumor stages. Microinvasive cervical carcinoma of stage IA1 can be treated by simple hysterectomy or therapeutic conization to preserve fertility in younger women [50, 51]. Radical hysterectomy according to Wertheim with removal of the uterus, parametria, and upper vagina including the paracolpium (Fig. 7.4a) is considered the standard surgical approach to treat stage IB and IIA cervical cancer. The radicalness of the resection and extent of lymphadenectomy depend on the tumor stage and the result of intraoperative quick section diagnosis. Five classes of extended hysterectomy are distinguished according to Piver. Transabdominal laparoscopic and transvaginal approaches are available [52]. Alternatively, the more advanced local tumors of stages IA2 and IB1 (up to 2 cm in size) can be treated by radial trachelectomy combined with lymphadenectomy in patients who wish to preserve their fertility. This operative technique consists in transvaginal removal of the cervix and parametria with reanastomosis of the uterine corpus and vagina (Fig. 7.4b) [53–55]. This operative technique requires an experienced operator and is comparable to hysterectomy in terms of prognosis and recurrence rate. The postoperative rate of conception is 40%–70%. Pregnancies after trachelectomy have been reported to be associated with a markedly higher rate of complications [56, 57].

Lymph node dissection is performed in all cases of vascular space invasion regardless of the depth of infiltration. It includes removal of the parametrial, pelvic, and para-aortic lymph nodes. Only the parametrial and pelvic nodes may be removed in stage IA and IB1 cervical carcinoma, with a negligible risk of para-aortic lymph node metastasis [51, 58]. Surgical removal and examination of the so-called sentinel lymph node as part of surgical staging is under clinical evaluation. The results available so far suggest a high negative predictive value [59, 60]. The sentinel lymph node is the regional lymph node that is assumed to be the first lymph node affected in case of metastatic spread.

Alternatively to surgery, primary or neoadjuvant radiochemotherapy is used to treat cervical carcinomas with a large volume, with infiltration of the vagina, or with parametrial involvement. Following

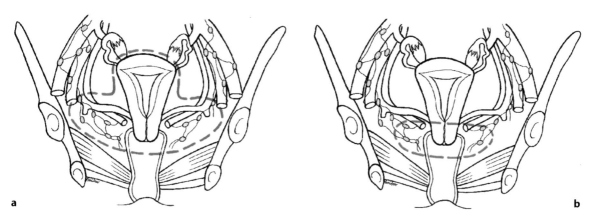

a **b**

Fig. 7.4a,b. Operative techniques. **a** Radical hysterectomy with removal of the uterus, vaginal cuff, parametria, and parailiac and para-aortic lymph nodes. Depending on the extent of parametrial removal, different types of hysterectomy are distinguished according to Piver. **b** Radical trachelectomy with removal of the uterine cervix, parametria, a vaginal cuff, and parailiac lymph nodes with subsequent uterovaginal anastomosis. (from the lecture script of the Dept. of Gynecology and Obstetrics, Jena University Hospital, Germany)

surgery, adjuvant radiochemotherapy is performed in patients with an increased risk of local pelvic recurrence. An increased risk of recurrence is assumed when there is a large tumor volume, a positive surgical margin, a very small safety margin, invasion of blood and lymphatic vessels, parametrial infiltration [7], or lymph node metastasis. A higher recurrence rate has also been identified for the histologic types of adenocarcinoma and clear cell carcinoma [61].

Advanced cervical carcinomas (FIGO stages III and IV) are not amenable to primary curative surgery due to their local extent with macroscopically visible involvement of the parametria, extension to the pelvic sidewall, or para-aortic nodal metastases. For these tumor stages, primary definitive radiochemotherapy is the treatment of first choice. Pretreatment surgical lymph node staging may be performed to exclude para-aortic lymph node metastases and may additionally serve to perform oophoropexy or to reduce the tumor bulk.

Radiotherapy consists of external beam irradiation of the uninvolved pelvic lymphatics and uninvolved parametrial tissue with a dose of up to 45 Gy and intracavitary brachytherapy with three to six fractions of 4–8 Gy each delivered to point A or the uterus [62], corresponding to a total dose equivalent of 70–80 Gy delivered to point A. The dose delivered by external beam radiotherapy is adjusted to the local tumor extent and metastatic nodal involvement (boost). A larger field of external irradiation is chosen in patients with para-aortic lymph node metastases. No brachytherapy is done in most patients with infiltration of the bladder or rectum because of the risk of fistula development. Alternatively, cervical cancer with invasion of adjacent pelvic organs can be treated by surgical pelvic exenteration. The most common therapies according to stage are summarized in Table 7.3.

The diagnosis of cervical cancer in a pregnant woman presents a therapeutic dilemma. CIN lesions or microinvasive cancer (stage IAI) can be treated by conization and cerclage with continuation of the pregnancy. Following delivery, thorough repeat evaluation is performed. In patients with more advanced cervical cancer diagnosed in early pregnancy, hysterectomy with termination of the pregnancy is recommended. Patients in advanced pregnancy have the option of premature delivery by cesarean section with subsequent definitive cancer treatment. Continuation of pregnancy with delay of cancer treatment is advocated only after the patient has been fully informed of the potential risks and counseled about the options available and undergoes close follow-up for evaluation of further tumor development.

Table 7.3. Therapy of cervical cancer

Stage	Therapy
0 (CIN I)	Cytologic follow-up
0 (CIS)	Conization
IA	Conization Simple hysterectomy Radical trachelectomy (only in patients wishing to preserve their fertility)
IB, IIA	Radical hysterectomy with lymph node dissection Radical trachelectomy with lymph node dissection (only in patients wishing to preserve their fertility) Primary, neoadjuvant radiochemotherapy Adjuvant radiochemotherapy
IIB, III, IVA	Primary, neoadjuvant radiochemotherapy Radical hysterectomy with lymph node dissection Adjuvant radiochemotherapy Exenteration
IVB	Primary radiochemotherapy

Local tumor recurrence with infiltration of the bladder or rectum but without extension to the pelvic sidewall can be treated by pelvic exenteration with curative intention. With strict patient selection, the 5-year-survival rate is 82% [63]. Various other surgical options are available for removal of recurrent tumor. In patients not having undergone radiotherapy or chemotherapy before, these therapeutic options are available for treating central pelvic recurrence. Repeat radiotherapy achieves successful local control with improvement of symptoms in cases of recurrent tumor outside the primary radiation field. Palliative chemotherapy is the final option available to all patients in whom curative surgery or radio(chemo)therapy is no longer possible.

7.1.9
Prognosis

Prognostic factors in cervical cancer are tumor volume, depth of stromal invasion, tumor stage, and lymph node status. Negative prognostic factors are invasion of blood or lymph capillaries, advanced tumor stage (Fig. 7.5), tumor diameter greater than 4 cm, lymphadenopathy, and onset at an early age. The 5-year survival rate is 95% for stage IA1 cervical carcinoma and 80% for stage IB2 tumors with a size of over 4 cm. In patients with more advanced cervical cancer, 5-year survival is 73% for those with para-

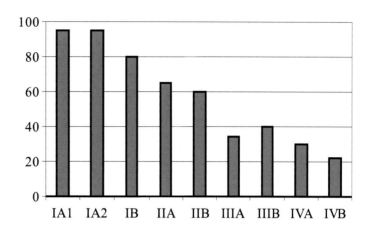

Fig. 7.5. Five-year survival rates by tumor stage

metrial invasion in stage IIB, 30% for patients with infiltration of pelvic organs, and 22% when distant metastases are present [8, 64]. Patients with negative lymph nodes have a 5-year survival rate of 90% as opposed to 60%–20% for patients with lymph node metastasis. Tumor extension to para-aortic lymph nodes reduces survival by half. For instance, the 5-year survival rate of stage IB decreases from 85% to 50%–60% in patients with pelvic lymph node metastases and to only 25% in patients with para-aortic lymph nodes.

The prognosis for patients with recurrent cervical carcinoma is reported to be less than 10% but there are subgroups of patients with a markedly better prognosis. Five-year survival rates range from 30% to 70% in patients with curative pelvic exenteration for central tumor recurrence [8, 64]. Similar survival rates of 40%–70% are reported for curative radiotherapy of recurrent cervical carcinoma in patients not having undergone primary radiation therapy. However, the prognosis strongly depends on the size of the recurrent tumor and its location. Recurrent tumor in the pelvic sidewall is associated with a disease-free 5-year survival rate of 20%–50%, which is below that of central tumor recurrence [65].

7.2
Imaging

7.2.1
Indications

Currently, MRI is recommended for pretreatment assessment of local tumor extent in patients with histologically proven FIGO stage IB or greater cervical cancer [66, 67]. It provides relevant information for deciding between primary operation and radiotherapy. It is the method of choice for local tumor staging: assessing the depth of infiltration, tumor volume, and involvement of adjacent structures. The clinical examination is inadequate to exclude parametrial invasion and infiltration of the urinary bladder and rectum while the extent of vaginal involvement can be determined more reliably by means of colposcopy. MRI is the most accurate imaging modality (90%) for distinguishing cancer confined to the cervix from cancer with parametrial infiltration (stage IB from IIB). Conventional radiologic modalities such as cystoscopy, rectosigmoidoscopy, or double-contrast barium enema as recommended in the FIGO classification have been abandoned in most cases since MRI has become firmly established as the first-line modality for evaluating the local extent of cervical cancer. MR urography has since also replaced conventional IV urography, which used to be the standard procedure in patients with advanced or recurrent cervical cancer and clinically suspected urinary obstruction. In this way, MRI evaluation of cervical cancer is even cost-effective [79]. Cervical cancer of stages 0 (carcinoma in situ) and IA (micro-invasive cervical cancer) cannot be assessed directly by MRI or CT. Nevertheless, in clinical practice, pelvic MRI could be performed for pretherapeutic evaluation of the pelvic organs and for radiologic lymph node staging at these early stages as well. Most patients already have a histologic diagnosis of cervical cancer at the time they undergo MRI. This means that MRI is performed to evaluate the extent of the cervical carcinoma and not to detect it.

MRI is considered the best method for planning radiochemotherapy and for following up tumor response to therapy. Pelvic CT scanning is the established technique for planning radiotherapy in cervical cancer.

In the aftercare of patients, MRI can distinguish postoperative scar formation or postactinic changes from recurrent tumor after about 6 months. This is why guidelines also recommend pelvic MRI in patients with suspected recurrence of cervical cancer.

With its lower soft-tissue contrast, CT is less widely used for assessing the local extent of cervical cancer. For tumor stages III and IV, German guidelines recommend a spiral CT examination to supplement MRI in the pretherapeutic staging of cervical cancer.

Positron emission tomography (PET) is currently being investigated to evaluate its usefulness in assessing primary and recurrent cervical cancer. No recommendations are available as yet.

7.2.1.1
Role of CT and MRI

The most important advantages of multislice CT over MRI are the shorter examination time and the high spatial resolution. However, direct data acquisition is restricted to the transverse plane and reformations in oblique plane from data sets causes loss of image quality. The major drawback of CT is the markedly poorer soft-tissue contrast compared with MRI (Fig. 7.6).

Hence, CT does not visualize the zonal anatomy of the pelvic organs. Therefore, the diagnostic accuracy of CT is inadequate for the detection of small cervical cancers and early parametrial infiltration and it has only a minor role in the local staging of cervical cancer [68, 69]. Unenhanced CT identifies tumors only indirectly as cervical enlargement, while tumors are depicted after contrast medium administration as contrast-enhancing lesions. Parametrial infiltration is detected indirectly by an irregular cervical demarcation or larger intraparametrial lesions. CT depicts rectal or bladder infiltration only indirectly as consumption of the fat lamella or in advanced tumor stages when there is wall thickening or a tumor mass protruding into the lumen is present [77, 78].

In cases where pelvic CT is performed, combined oral and rectal contrast medium administration is recommended. On the other hand, CT is the method of choice for excluding pulmonary metastases, which is why guidelines in Germany recommend a chest CT scan for patients with FIGO stage III or IV cervical cancer [130]. The CT of the chest is performed with IV contrast and includes the supraclavicular lymph nodes. Finally, CT can be used as an alternative modality for lymph node staging and liver imaging and is indicated for evaluating the extent of osseous damage in patients with bone metastases.

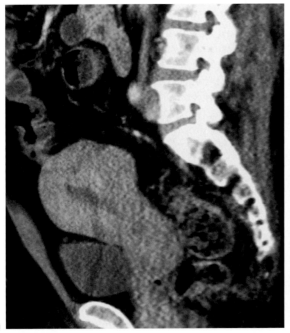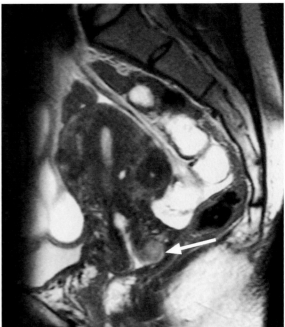

a   b

Fig. 7.6a,b. Comparison CT and MRI. **a** No cervical tumor can be delineated in the sagittal reconstruction of a CT scan. **b** A nodular cervical carcinoma is shown in the dorsal external cervix (*arrow*) in T2-weighted (T2w) sagittal MRI. Accessory finding: leiomyoma of the dorsal uterine corpus

With its excellent soft-tissue contrast on T2-weighted images, MRI is the imaging modality of pathology depiction that is ensured by the free selection of imaging planes and imaging in two planes (Table 7.4) [70, 71], which allows optimal adjustment to pelvic anatomy. MRI differentiates a tumorous lesion from surrounding tissue and allows precise determination of its size. T2-weighted images depict the organs of the true pelvis, and in part also their zonal anatomy, which is the basis for identification of intra- and extracervical tumor extension. Studies in the literature report accuracy of 90%–95% for MRI in the detection of parametrial invasion as compared to 72% for CT [72, 73]. The superior depiction of the vaginal anatomy by MRI with differentiation of the mucosal layer and muscular layer of the wall results in earlier detection of vaginal involvement, with an accuracy of 90% as opposed to 77%–82% for CT [74]. Infiltration of the bladder and rectum is demonstrated directly by MRI and is identified with an accuracy of 96%–100% [75, 76].

MRI is also the first-line modality for excluding or demonstrating local tumor recurrence. In particular, MRI enables differentiation of postoperative or radiation-induced scars from recurrent tumor. Additional contrast-enhanced dynamic T1-weighted studies are helpful to differentiate therapy-related changes from tumor tissue. In contrast, CT demonstrates most local recurrences only when they produce a mass effect or infiltrate adjacent structures or organs [80, 81].

With regard to lymph node staging, MRI and CT have similar sensitivities of only up to 70%, while specificity is high at approximately 95% [67, 70, 74]. Helical CT yields a continuous volume scan from which thin slices can be reconstructed and thus enables complete evaluation of the area of interest. However, both imaging modalities primarily rely on morphometric criteria for identifying metastatic nodes and therefore fail to detect micrometastases that do not affect lymph node size and shape. Such metastases could be identified only by surgical staging. Lymph node staging is discussed in more detail in Section 7.2.3.5.

7.2.2
Imaging Technique

7.2.2.1
MRI

A brief gynecologic history should be obtained prior to the MRI examination. As the morphologic appearance of the uterus varies with the patient's hormonal status, information on the phase of the menstrual cycle or postmenopause as well as on hormone therapy (see Chap. 3) should be gathered. Moreover, the history should comprise information on pregnancies and cesarean sections as well as on invasive diagnostic procedures such as cervical conization or curettage. In patients undergoing follow-up MRI, information on earlier pelvic surgery or radiochemotherapy is important. The radiologist needs these data to correctly interpret the morphologic MR appearance.

MRI is performed with the patient in the supine position. Fasting is not necessary prior to the examination, on the contrary, patients should have a light meal. Moderate bladder filling will straighten an anteflexed uterus. Too much bladder filling may lead to restlessness during the course of the examination or may even make it necessary to discontinue the examination.

For an optimal image quality, artifacts caused by intestinal peristalsis should be minimized, in general by administration of a spasmolytic agent at the beginning of the examination. The usual agent is butylscopolamine bromide (Buscopan) administered intravenously or intramuscularly at a dose of 40 mg. This spasmolytic agent has an elimination half-life of 2–3 h. The onset of spasmolytic activity is immediately after IV administration while it is delayed by a few minutes after IM administration. Alternatively, patients with contraindications to butylscopolamine bromide (hypersensitivity, glaucoma, driving immediately after the examination) are given an IV dose of 2 mg glucagon (GlucaGen). Technically, motion artifacts can be reduced by rapid image acquisition.

A high signal-to-noise ratio (SNR) and a high spatial resolution are important for optimal pelvic evaluation by MRI. For this reason, body phased-array surface coils are preferred. The resolution can also be improved by use

Table 7.4. Sensitivity and specificity of MRI in pretreatment staging of cervical cancer

FIGO stage	MRI Accuracy (%)	CT Accuracy (%)
IB (tumor localization)	91	
IIA (vaginal infiltration)	93	
IIB (parametrial infiltration)	94	70
IIIB (extension to pelvic sidewall)	75	
IVA (bladder infiltration)	99	
Average stage	83	63

of a small field of view (FOV), for instance 20 × 20 cm, in combination with phase oversampling to prevent wrap-around artifacts (aliasing). With surface coils being highly susceptible to artifacts caused by respiratory motion of the abdominal wall, all sequences must be acquired with presaturation of the abdominal wall.

The imaging area should comprise not only the pelvis but also the abdomen up to the renal hilum in order to include the para-aortic lymph nodes. This applies especially to patients with cervical cancer stage IIB and above.

The MRI examination begins with a localizer scan in transverse, sagittal and coronal orientation, followed by T2-weighted imaging in two planes. T2-weighted sequences have the highest soft-tissue contrast and thus provide most of the information on the localization and extent of a cervical carcinoma. They are the basis of any pelvic MRI examination. The first T2-weighted sequence should be acquired in the sagittal plane and covers the uterus and vagina to the pelvic floor. This sequence should be acquired with a high resolution

using thin slices and a small FOV, i.e., a 512 matrix, a phase resolution of a least 75%, and a slice thickness of 4–5 mm. The sagittal T2-weighted images may serve to plan the transverse angulated T2-weighted sequence. The transverse sequence should be angulated for alignment perpendicular to the axis of the cervical canal. As with the sagittal sequence, the imaging field in transverse orientation extends from the fundus uteri to the pelvic floor. Images should be acquired with a slice thickness of 4–5 mm, a 512 matrix, and a phase-resolution of at least 75% (Tables 7.5 and 7.6, Fig. 7.12).

The cervix uteri is normally anteversed and forms an angle of about 90° with the axis of the vagina. The uterine corpus is flexed forward, resulting in an angle of 70°–100° relative to the cervix. The degree of anteflexion varies with bladder filling and is also affected by the size of the uterine corpus. From puberty onwards, the cervix-to-corpus ratio is 1:2, and the corpus again becomes smaller after menopause and descends into the true pelvis. The positions of the uterus are shown in Figure 7.7.

Table 7.5. Recommended standard protocol at 1.5 Tesla

	Orientation	Area imaged	TR (ms)	TE (ms)	ST (mm)	Flip angle (degrees)	FOV (cm)/ rec FOV (%)	Matrix (pixel)	Acquisition time (min)
T2w FSE/TSE	Sagittal	Uterus and vagina	4000	100	4	150	30/75	282×512	6.09
T2w FSE/TSE	Transverse oblique	Uterus and vagina<	4000	100	4	150	30/75	282×512	4.01
T1w FSE/TSE/PD	Transverse	Pelvic floor to aortic bifurcation	500–1690	10	6	150	30/75	269×448	6.05

Table 7.6. Optional protocols at 1.5 Tesla

	Orientation	Area imaged	TR (ms)	TE (ms)	ST (mm)	Flip angle (degrees)	FOV (cm) × rec FOV(%)	Matrix (pixel)	Acquisition time (min)
T2w TSE respiratory triggering	Transverse	Renal hili to aortic bifurcation	One respiratory cycle	80	4	180	32/75	358×512	4.53
T1w FSE/TSE	Sagittal and transverse oblique	Uterus and vagina	944	8.9	5	150	29/75	256×512	3.08
T1w FSE/TSE FS post-CM	Sagittal and transverse oblique	Uterus and vagina	944	8.9	5	150	29/75	256×512	3.08
T2w Ira	Transverse	Pelvis	7770	30	6	150	50/75	384×512	3.47
T2w single-shot FSE/TSE	Coronal	Kidneys to pelvis	∞	69	5	150	40/75	256×154	0.15
T1w 3D GE post-CM	Coronal	Kidneys to pelvis	3.67	1.2	2	20	40/81.3	249×512	0.32

[a]TI = 130 ms

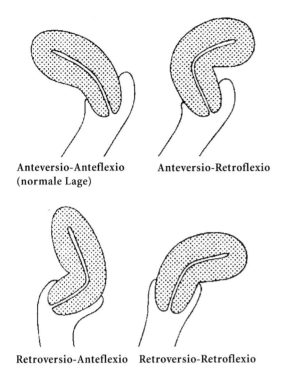

Anteversio-Anteflexio (normale Lage)   Anteversio-Retroflexio

Retroversio-Anteflexio   Retroversio-Retroflexio

Fig. 7.7. Positions of the uterus. Version is the tilting of the uterus relative to the vagina and varies with bladder filling (typically 90°). Flexion refers to the position of the uterine corpus relative to the cervix (typically 70°–100°) (from [131])

Angulated image acquisition ensures optimal depiction of the cervix and parametria and their topographic relationships (Fig. 7.8). It is important that the angulation does not exceed 45° to avoid acquisition in coronal orientation with reversal of left and right.

In cases of vaginal involvement with the risk of parametrial infiltration through the paravaginal tissue from below, additional angulation perpendicular to the vagina is useful. For optimal evaluation of vaginal infiltration, the vagina may be distended with ultrasound gel. Involvement of the pelvic floor muscles in advanced tumors is evaluated on coronal T2-weighted images, which is especially suited for evaluation of the levator ani muscle. Information on muscle involvement is important for planning the surgical procedure.

For evaluation of the pelvic sidewall and lymph node staging, an additional proton-density or a T1-weighted sequence in transverse orientation should be performed (see Fig. 7.11). The acquisition starts at the level of the aortic bifurcation and extends to below the pelvic floor. A slice thickness of 6 mm is used, with a 512 matrix and a phase resolution of at least 60%. Complete coverage of the inguinal lymph nodes should be attempted in patients with cervical cancers involving the lower third of the vagina (stage IIIA

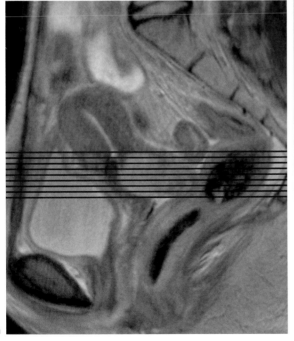

a

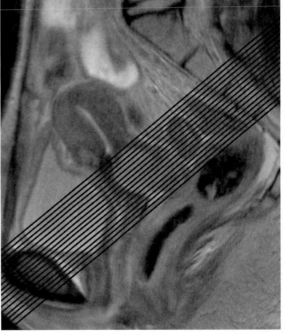

b

Fig. 7.8 a,b. Angulation. T2w TSE images in sagittal orientation of a more hyperintense cervical cancer of the posterior cervix with infiltration of the posterior vaginal fornix. The cervical cancer is shown in strictly axial orientation (**a**) and in angulated axial orientation (**b**). With angulated image acquisition, a superior anatomic view is obtained of the structures that are crucial for staging (cancer, cervical stroma, parametria) and the cancer is depicted on more slices

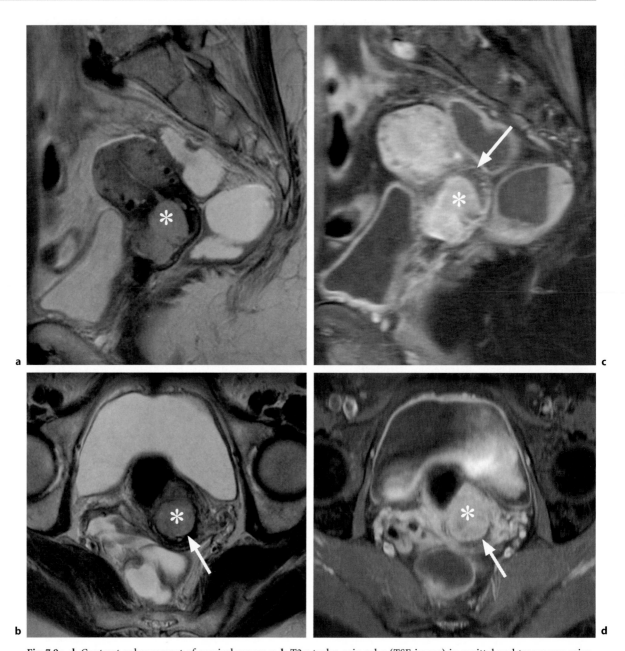

Fig. 7.9a–d. Contrast enhancement of cervical cancer. **a, b** T2w turbo-spin echo (TSE image) in sagittal and transverse orientation. The cervical cancer (*asterisks*) is seen as a hyperintense mass in the surrounding low-signal-intensity cervical stroma (*arrow*). **c, d** T1w TSE images with fat saturation (FS) in sagittal and transverse orientation with fat saturation acquired 1 min after administration of Gadopentate dimeglumine (Gd-DTPA). There is pronounced contrast medium enhancement of the hypervascularized cervical cancer (*asterisks*) with less enhancement of the hypointense cervical stroma (*arrows*)

or higher), which may be associated with inguinal lymph node metastasis.

Intravenous contrast medium administration is rarely necessary for primary staging of cervical cancer, as the contrast medium does not improve tumor delineation from surrounding tissue compared with the unenhanced T2-weighted images in most pa-

tients (Figs. 7.9, 7.10). Often, contrast enhancement even impairs differentiation of the tumor from parametrial tissue.

Contrast-enhanced images can, however, improve the diagnostic accuracy of identifying tumorous infiltration of the urinary bladder or rectum. The extent of infiltration is visualized as a disruption of

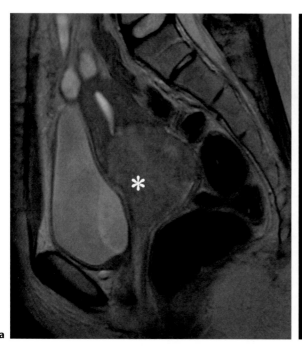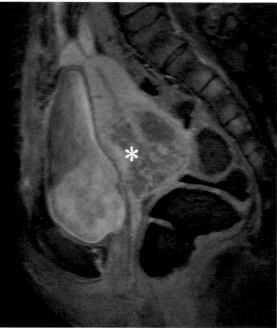

a   b

Fig. 7.10a,b. Contrast enhancement of cervical cancer. **a** T2w TSE image in sagittal orientation. The cervical cancer (*asterisk*) is seen as a large mass of intermediate to high signal intensity that is delineated against a very thin margin of low-signal-intensity cervical stroma and against the more hypointense myometrium of the uterine corpus. There is barrel-shaped expansion of the cervix. **b** T1w TSE image with FS in sagittal orientation 1 min after Gd-DTPA administration. Enhancement of the hypointense and hypovascularized cervical cancer is inhomogeneous (*asterisk*) and tumor delineation is not improved by contrast medium administration

the muscular wall of these organs, which is of lower signal intensity on T1-weighted images. It has been shown that contrast-enhanced MRI can improve the differentiation of an edematous stromal reaction (no enhancement) of the vesical or rectal wall from tumor infiltration (positive enhancement) [82]. Contrast-enhanced pelvic MRI is performed by acquiring T1-weighted sequences before and after CM administration. The contrast medium that is usually used is an unspecific gadolinium-based low-molecular agent administered at a dose of 0.5 mmol/kg body weight. The contrast-enhanced T1-weighted study can be planned by adopting the imaging area and orientation of the T2-weighted sequences.

CM administration is indicated to differentiate recurrent tumor from postoperative and postactinic changes at follow-up MRI (Fig. 7.11). A dynamic T1-weighted postcontrast study with repeated acquisitions enables temporally resolved quantification of CM enhancement.

Various other sequences are available to answer specific queries and provide specific information as required according to tumor stage. Cervical cancer extending beyond the cervix and recurrent tumors are associated with a significantly higher risk of metastatic spread to para-aortic lymph nodes. These lymph nodes are best evaluated with high-resolution respiratory triggered T2-weighted sequences for imaging of the abdomen in transverse orientation from the renal hili to the aortic bifurcation (Fig. 7.12).

In patients with locally advanced or recurrent cervical cancer, it is often necessary to exclude ureteral obstruction, which can be done on transverse T2-weighted images that also serve to assess the para-aortic lymph nodes. In addition, coronal T2-weighted turbo-spin echo (TSE) sequences enable excellent evaluation for possible urinary retention and require little extra time to acquire. In addition, contrast-enhanced MR urography can be performed to exclude tumor-induced hydronephrosis.

Rectouterine or vesicouterine fistulas may develop as a complication of radiochemotherapy. A clinically suspected fistula is an indication for contrast-enhanced MRI using an unspecific gadolinium-based low-molecular contrast medium. T1-weighted sequences in transverse and sagittal planes are acquired before and after CM administration. The postcontrast sequence is started 60 s after CM administration to image the venous phase. A fistula is typically a filiform structure of low signal intensity lumen and shows a contrast en-

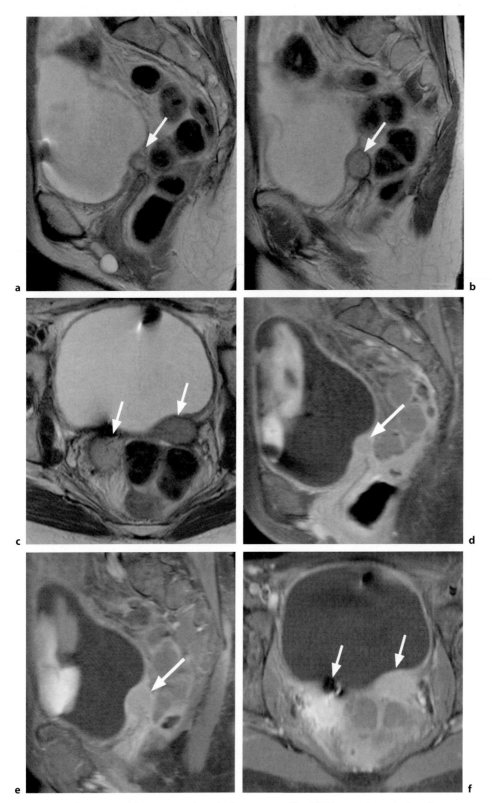

Fig. 7.11a–f. Contrast enhancement of cervical cancer. **a–c** T2w TSE images in sagittal and transverse orientation. Local recurrence of cervical cancer (*arrows*) is seen as a tumor of intermediate signal intensity above the vaginal stump. **d–f** T1w TSE images with fat saturation in sagittal and transverse orientation 1 min after Gd-DTPA administration show local recurrence as an enhancing tumor (*arrows*). Accessory finding in **a**: Bartholin cyst (*asterisk*)

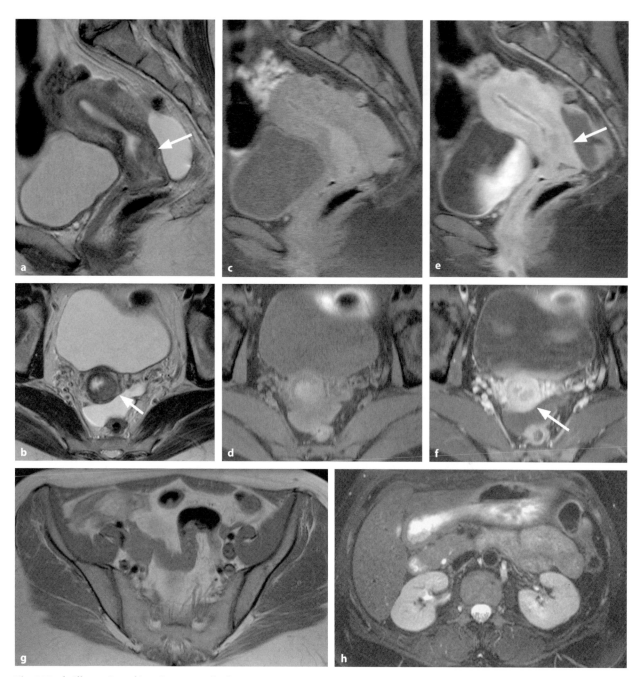

Fig. 7.12a–h. Illustration of imaging protocol. **a, b** T2w TSE images in sagittal and transverse orientation. Stage IB cervical cancer (*arrows*). The tumor is surrounded by low-signal-intensity cervical stroma. Accessory finding: small fluid collection in the pouch of Douglas, small leiomyoma in the posterior uterine corpus. **c, d** T1w TSE images with fat saturation in sagittal and transverse orientation. **e, f** T1w TSE images with FS after contrast medium administration in sagittal and transverse orientation. Cervical cancer (*arrows*). **g** PD-TSE image for lymph node assessment in the true pelvis. **h** T2w TSE image with respiratory-gating (PACE) for lymph node assessment in the abdomen

hancement of the wall. In addition, T2-weighted inversion recovery sequences that null the signal of fat have a high accuracy in detecting fistulas.

A technical overview of the recommended MR protocol is given in Tables 7.5 and 7.6.

7.2.2.2
Dynamic MRI

Dynamic contrast-enhanced MRI of the uterine cervix is performed to evaluate the course of contrast enhancement in a region-of-interest (ROI) placed in a suspicious area. First, an unenhanced sequence with an acquisition time of about 23 s is acquired, followed by the first postcontrast acquisition about 15–20 s after CM administration. Postcontrast acquisition for measurement of signal intensity in the ROI is repeated over a period of about 10 min. A dynamic MRI study is part of the routine protocol for differentiation of posttherapeutic changes from recurrent tumor but is rarely necessary in the pretreatment evaluation of patients with cervical cancer. Although vital tumor tissue typically shows earlier arterial enhancement than the surrounding cervical stroma [83], no benefit was found for differentiation of the tumor or the demonstration of parametrial infiltration in studies that evaluating color-coded dynamic MR images [84, 85]. However, the demonstration of necrosis and determination of tumor vascularization might help to estimate the radiosensitivity of a tumor prior to therapy. Moreover, a correlation was found between contrast medium time-intensity curves and angiogenic activity as an indicator of infiltration of the lymphatic system [86]. No correlation was found for other malignancy criteria such as infiltration depth and metastatic pelvic nodes.

7.2.2.3
Coil Technique

Morphologic MRI staging of cervical cancer implies high demands on SNR, signal homogenity, and spatial resolution. Therefore, body phased-array surface coils are recommended because they increase the SNR in comparison to volume coils and can also increase the spatial resolution, or, alternatively shorten the acquisition time. The surface coil is placed on the torso and must cover the entire imaging area. Local coils such as endorectal or endovaginal coils are rarely used alternatives. They improve the spatial resolution of structures in their immediate vicinity but they distort anatomy, for instance, by compressing lipid

lamellae. Moreover, an additional examination with a body phased-array coil is required in most cases to evaluate the entire pelvis including the lymph nodes. Since body phased-array coils offer a high SNR, are easy to handle, and provide better patient comfort, local coils have not become widely accepted.

7.2.2.4
Vaginal Opacification

Opacification and distention of the vagina is a controversial subject. Evaluation of vaginal involvement is not the most important goal of MRI staging, as the vagina can be adequately evaluated by clinical examination and colposcopy in most patients. On the other hand, imaging vaginal infiltration is important for planning brachytherapy. The insertion of a vaginal tampon soaked with contrast medium has been abandoned because distention of the vagina is incomplete while anatomic relationships are distorted. But intravaginal application of a contrast medium, e.g., ultrasound gel as a negative contrast medium (Fig. 7.13) was found to improve evaluation of vaginal involvement and is part of the routine protocol in some centers.

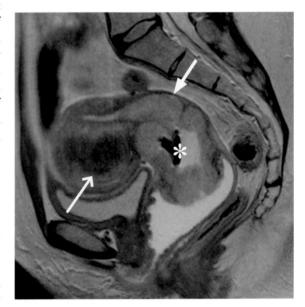

Fig. 7.13. Tumor growth and vaginal opacification. T2w TSE image in sagittal orientation. The high-signal-intensity cervical cancer has a central necrotic cavity (*asterisk*) with an air–fluid level. There is barrel-shaped expansion of the cervix and portio through the tumor. Tumor growth into the uterine cavity (*arrow*). Accessory finding: leiomyoma of the uterine corpus (*open arrow*). The vagina and fornix are distended by gel, which allows exclusion of vaginal infiltration

7.2.3
Staging

7.2.3.1.
General MR Appearance

The basis of the radiologic evaluation of cervical cancer is T2-weighted MRI sequences [87], which provide a high soft-tissue contrast for optimal differentiation of tumor from normal cervical stroma and adjacent organs. Cervical cancer is characterized by a higher signal intensity and is thus delineated against the cervical stroma, which has a lower signal intensity. Cervical cancer typically develops as a circumscribed focal lesion arising from the mucosal layer of the cervix. It may grow superficially in a circular pattern and increases in depth with invasion of the cervical stroma. Sagittal and transverse T2-weighted sequences serve to determine the localization and size of the tumor as well as the depth of cervical stroma infiltration. These sequences are also crucial for excluding extracervical extension and infiltration of the parametria, vagina, bladder, and rectum. The two critical issues – depth of infiltration and parametrial involvement – can be assessed most reliably on transverse images angulated perpendicular to the cervical axis.

Cervical cancer arises in the transitional zone that marks the junction of the squamous epithelium of the external cervix with the columnar epithelium of the cervical canal. This zone is usually located on the portio in younger women, which is where cervical cancer usually occurs with exophytic growths. In contrast, older women with retraction of the transformation zone into the cervical canal typically develop cervical cancer with an endocervical growth pattern (Fig. 7.13). This growth type usually gives rise to the typical barrel-shaped configuration of the cervix as the tumor increases in size or an endocervical ulcer develops when there is necrosis.

On T1-weighted MR images, cervical cancer is similar in signal intensity to the cervical stroma. Demarcation from the corpus uteri, vagina, and parametria is also more difficult (Fig. 7.14). Only larger cervical carcinomas can be identified on the basis of their mass effect.

However, T1-weighted images can be useful in delineation of the tumor within the lateral parametria, which have a higher fat content than the medial parametria, which results in an improved content between high-signal-intense fat vs low-signal-intense carcinoma. In the routine clinical setting, T1-weighted

sequences are primarily used for lymph node staging and for unenhanced imaging in cases where contrast medium administration is planned.

Cervical carcinomas show early enhancement 15–30 s after contrast medium administration. The increase in signal intensity can improve the contrast between the hypointense cervical stroma and the hyperintense tumor on T1-weighted images. Altogether, however, the signal intensity of cervical cancer is heterogeneous and varies with vascularization. In pretherapeutic staging where precise determination of the extent of the tumor in the cervix and its relationship to the corpus uteri, parametrial tissue, and the vagina is important, most cervical carcinomas are seen more clearly on T2-weighted images than on contrast-enhanced T1-weighted images. This does not hold true for advanced cervical carcinomas with infiltration of the bladder or rectum or extension to the pelvic sidewall and for the exclusion of recurrent tumor by posttherapeutic MRI. The indications for contrast medium administration are discussed in Sect. 7.2.2.

7.2.3.2
Rare Histologic Types

Squamous cell carcinoma is by far the most common histologic type, accounting for about 90% of all cervical carcinomas. Descriptions in this chapter and in the literature on cervical cancer in general usually refer to this histologic type, unless explicitly stated otherwise. In this section, other histologic types of cervical cancer, especially adenocarcinoma, are briefly described with regard to their clinical status and imaging features (see also Sects. 7.1.5, 7.2.6). In general, it is not possible to distinguish these less common histologic types from squamous cell carcinoma of the cervix on the basis of their MR appearance.

With a proportion of 10%–15% of all cervical cancers, adenocarcinoma is the most frequent of the rare histologic types. The histologic distinction is important. Adenocarcinomas arise from the columnar epithelium and are associated with a higher risk of infiltration of the uterine corpus, lymphatic spread, and local recurrence compared with squamous cell carcinoma. Adenocarcinoma is more difficult to demonstrate histologically, which is why the diagnosis is often delayed until the tumor has reached an advanced stage. The clinical and radiologic evaluation of tumor extent also presents a challenge, as some adenocarcinomas are characterized by subepithelial growth and diffuse infiltration. Parametrial infiltra-

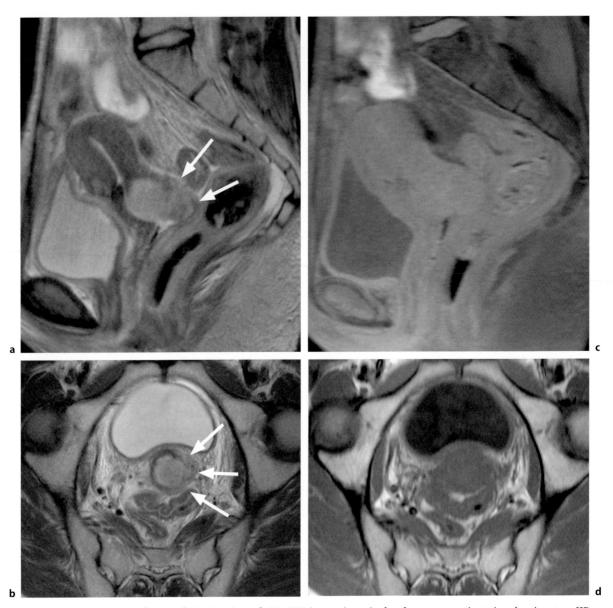

Fig. 7.14a–d. Comparison of T2w and T1w imaging. **a, b** T2w TSE images in sagittal and transverse orientation showing stage IIB cancer of the posterior cervix. There is posterior (sagittal) and left lateral (transverse) disruption of the hypointense cervical stroma (*arrows*). **c, d** T1w TSE images with FS in identical sagittal and transverse orientation. The extent of the cervical cancer in the stroma cannot be assessed due to the lower soft-tissue contrast of T1w sequences

tion is not always associated with a disruption of the cervical stroma. A focal lesion is not always apparent on MRI since small adenocarcinomas often grow diffusely and have a signal intensity similar to that of normal cervical tissue. The morphologic MR appearance varies with the histologic subtype. Mucinous adenocarcinoma is the most common subtype and may be endocervical or ectocervical in location. T2-weighted images show a tumor with an intermediate to slightly hyperintense signal intensity, depending on the mucin content. The margin is irregular and blurred. The second most common subtype is adenoma malignum, an extremely well-differentiated mucinous adenocarcinoma that is very difficult to confirm histopathologically. Adenoma malignum is composed of clusters of cystic lesions within an otherwise more or less solid tumor tissue of high signal intensity. The solid portions are the key to the differentiation from dilated cervical glands and nabothian cysts. Other histologic subtypes are endometrioid, clear cell, and serous adenocarcinoma of the cervix, which are histologically similar to carcinomas of the uterine corpus. They are of an intermediate to slightly high signal intensity on MRI and arise in the endocervix, from where they infiltrate the cervical stroma. In this type of tumor, it may be difficult to determine whether the origin is in the cervix or in the uterine corpus. In general, the part of the uterus from which the tumor arises shows deeper infiltration and more marked enlargement to the respective other part (cervix or corpus). The rare subtype of adenosquamous cervical carcinoma resembles squamous cell carcinoma with regard to its growth pattern and morphologic appearance on MR images.

Neuroendocrine cervical carcinoma is the second most frequent of the rare histologies. With its heterogeneous appearance and high signal intensity on T2-weighted images, neuroendocrine cervical carcinoma resembles squamous cell carcinoma at MRI.

7.2.3.3
Tumor Size

Cervical cancer is revealed by MRI when tumors are large enough to be macroscopically visible, which is the case when the tumor has a diameter of 1–2 cm or a volume of 2–4 cm^3 (FIGO stage IB). Tumor size is the most important prognostic factor besides lymphatic metastasis. T2-weighted MRI in at least two planes is the method of first choice for determining tumor size [88], since cervical cancer is best distinguished from surrounding tissue in these sequences. The gynecologic examination tends to underestimate tumor size, while MRI may overestimate size when the tumor is surrounded by edema (about 15%). Contrast medium administration can enable differentiation of edema and tumor since only the tumor shows enhancement.

Tumor size is usually determined by measuring the longest diameter and its perpendicular. Two-dimensional measurement is based on the WHO guidelines for evaluating the response of solid tumors to chemotherapy or radiotherapy. Since a precise description of the spatial extent of a tumor is crucial prior to surgery, the tumor should also be measured in the third dimension. However, in patients where it is important to evaluate the response to radiochemotherapy, tumor size should be measured according to the RECIST[1] (response evaluation criteria in solid tumors) guidelines

---

1 RECIST is a set of rules defining the criteria when cancer patients improve (respond), stay the same (stable), or worsen (progression) during treatments. The longest diameter of the target lesion is measured.

for one-dimensional measurement [89] (Fig. 7.15). These guidelines have superseded the two-dimensional WHO measurement as the standard.

Techniques of tumor volumetry can additionally be applied. These techniques relied on formula such as height × width × length × π/6 to calculate approximate tumor volume or determined the volume by integration of the individual slice volumes (Fig. 7.14).

7.2.3.4
Local Staging

7.2.3.4.1
Stages 0 and IA

The precursor lesions of cervical cancer, cervical intraepithelial neoplasia/CIN and carcinoma in situ (stage 0), and the earliest cancer stage, microinvasive cervical cancer (stage IA), are not amenable to clinical evaluation (see Sect. 7.1.2), nor are they detected by MRI because they do not alter the normal morphologic MR appearance of the cervix (Fig. 7.16). The normal endocervix is depicted on T2-weighted images with a hyperintense, continuous mucosal layer surrounded by hypointense cervical stroma, which consists of connective tissue and smooth muscle. The normal cervix is 3 cm long and has a diameter of 2–2.5 cm. Colposcopy and conization is the method of choice for evaluating these early forms of cervical carcinoma. The conization defect is depicted on MR images as a circumscribed lesion of the external os, quite often associated with an adjacent seroma or clot. In the further course, shrinkage of the portio can sometimes be seen.

7.2.3.4.2
Stage IB

Stage IB cervical carcinoma has a depth of more than 5 mm and a diameter of more than 7 mm or is visible clinically. The tumor is still confined to the cervix but is characterized by invasive local growth. This is the earliest stage that can be demonstrated by MRI [70, 90]. The average MRI detection rate is 95% [74]. Stage IB1 (diameter <4 cm) and stage IB2 (diameter >4 cm) are distinguished on the basis of their size. Stage IB2 cervical cancer has a poorer prognosis and may be treated by neoadjuvant radiochemotherapy prior to surgery. Transverse and sagittal T2-weighted images depict cervical carcinoma as a high-signal-intensity lesion within the low-signal-intensity oval cervical stroma (Figs. 7.12, 7.17–7.20). Cervical can-

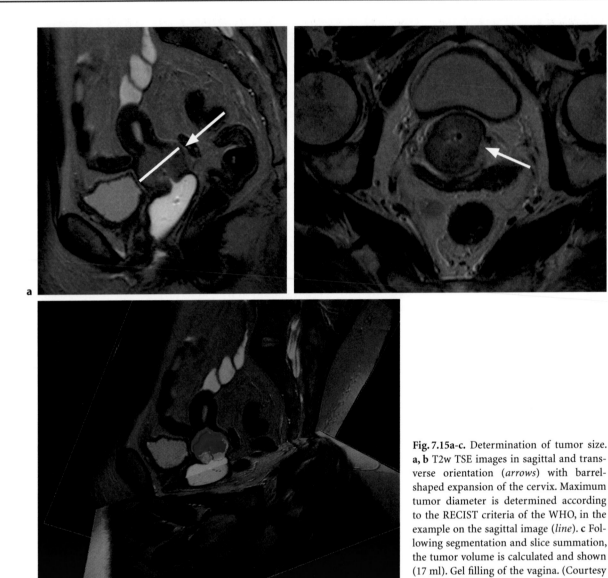

Fig. 7.15a-c. Determination of tumor size. **a, b** T2w TSE images in sagittal and transverse orientation (*arrows*) with barrel-shaped expansion of the cervix. Maximum tumor diameter is determined according to the RECIST criteria of the WHO, in the example on the sagittal image (*line*). **c** Following segmentation and slice summation, the tumor volume is calculated and shown (17 ml). Gel filling of the vagina. (Courtesy of Dr. A.J. Lemke, Berlin)

cer at this stage is fairly smoothly marginated and completely surrounded by low-signal-intensity cervical stroma. Occasional exophytic bulging of a stage IB tumor into the vagina or the parametrium may be mistaken for infiltration.

Parametrial infiltration can be reliably excluded if the tumor is surrounded by a low-signal-intensity rim on transverse T2-weighted images. A large stage IB2 cervical carcinoma can obstruct the cervical canal and lead to hydrometra or hematometra. Hydro- or serometra is suggested by a fluid collection in the uterine cavity showing hyperintensity in T2-weighted and low-signal-intensity in T1-weighted, whereas a hematometra is characterized by high-signal-intensity in T2-weighted and T1-weighted.

7.2.3.4.3
Stage IIA

In stage IIA cervical cancer, infiltration involves up to two-thirds of the proximal vagina while sparing the lower third. On T2-weighted MR images, vaginal involvement is seen as a hyperintense segmental disruption or lesion in the otherwise low-signal-intensity vaginal wall. Infiltration of the anterior and posterior fornix and of the wall is best seen in sagittal orientation (Figs. 7.21–7.24). The radiologist interpreting the images must be aware that a large exophytic cervical cancer may lead to widening of the fornix and thus mimic vaginal infiltration. In such cases, opacification and distention of the vagina can be helpful.

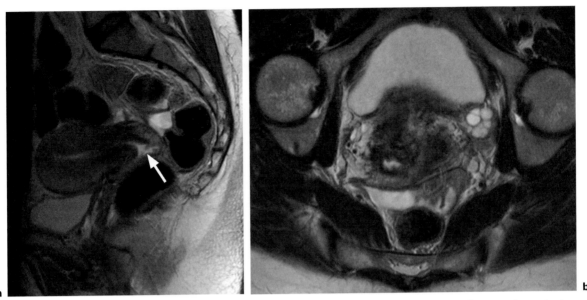

a   b

Fig. 7.16a,b. T2w TSE images in sagittal and transverse orientation showing cervical cancer histologically proven by conization. Visible conization defect of the external os (*arrow*). No tumor is seen on MRI. Microscopic tumor manifestation was demonstrated in the surgical specimen

7.2.3.4.4
Stage IIB

Stage IIB cervical cancer is characterized by parametrial infiltration but without extension to the pelvic sidewall. Parametrial infiltration has important implications for the therapeutic approach. MRI is the only noninvasive modality that allows adequate evaluation of parametrial infiltration. The accuracy of MRI in the evaluation of parametrial invasion is up to 90%. Sagittal and transverse T2-weighted images angulated perpendicular to the cervical canal are most suitable to evaluate parametrial infiltration. It is indicated by a disruption of the low-signal-intensity cervical stroma. Visualization of an uninterrupted rim of cervical stroma reliably excludes parametrial infiltration, except for the rare cases of diffusely infiltrating adenocarcinoma. Early microscopic parametrial infiltration must be suggested if high-signal-intensity tumor tissue shows irregular and unsharp margins and is disrupting the hypointense cervical stroma with no normal cervical stroma left that separates the tumor from the parametria. The most reliable MRI criterion of parametrial infiltration is the direct visualization of a tumor mass extending into the parametria (Figs. 7.25–7.28). Occasionally, the parametria may

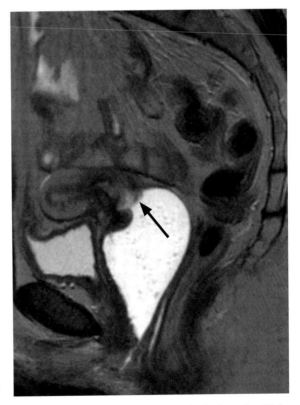

Fig. 7.17. Stage IB. T2w TSE image in sagittal orientation. High-signal-intensity cervical cancer (*arrow*) primarily involving the posterior cervix and the portio. Gel filling of the vagina

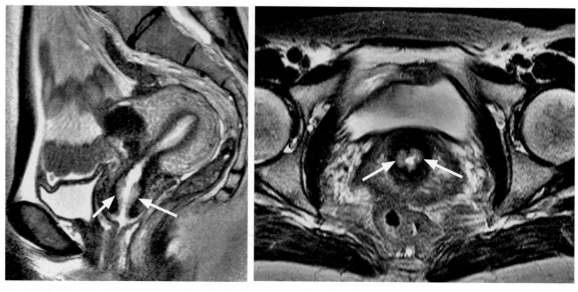

Fig. 7.18a,b. Stage IB. **a, b** T2w TSE images in sagittal and transverse orientation. The small cervical cancer is seen as a high-signal-intensity lesion primarily growing within the cervix (*arrows*). The cancer is surrounded by low-signal-intensity cervical stroma on both sagittal and transverse images. Accessory finding: uterine prolapse and leiomyomas of the anterior wall of the uterus. (from [132])

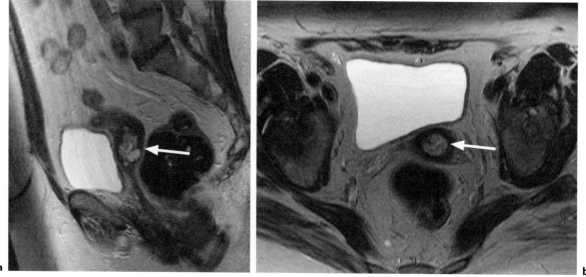

Fig. 7.19a,b. Stage IB. **a, b** T2w TSE images in sagittal and transverse orientation. The cervical cancer is seen as a high-signal-intensity lesion within the cervix (*arrows*). The cancer is surrounded by low-signal-intensity cervical stroma on both sagittal and transverse images. Accessory finding: Nabothian cysts

be invaded from below through the paravaginal space. The anatomy of the true pelvis determines the further routes of spread of cervical cancer. Infiltration of the rectouterine or vesicouterine ligaments at their cervical attachments is seen on MR images as focal thickening. In rare cases, parametrial invasion can cause retraction with displacement of the cervix to the side of infiltration.

7.2.3.4.5
Stage IIIA

Stage IIIA tumor is established when there is involvement of the lower third of the vagina. As with stage IIA tumor, sagittal and oblique transverse T2-weighted sequences are most suitable to evaluate vaginal infiltration. Tumor infiltration is indicated by

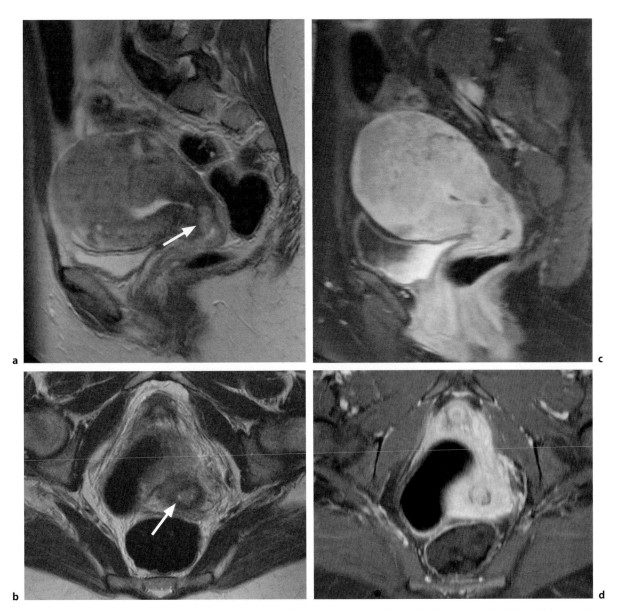

Fig. 7.20a–d. Stage IB. **a, b** T2w TSE images in sagittal and transverse orientation. High-signal-intensity lesion of the cervix (*arrows*) with preservation of low-signal-intensity stroma around the tumor. **c, d** T1w TSE images in sagittal and transverse orientation. No circumscribed cervical cancer is seen on the image obtained 1 min after Gd-DTPA administration. Accessory finding: uterine adenomyosis

a hyperintense disruption and continuous or discontinuous thickening of the vaginal wall that extends to the lower third of the vagina. This stage is also associated with an increased risk of metastatic spread to the superficial inguinal lymph nodes, which must be taken into account in the diagnostic evaluation. The lower third of the vagina corresponds to the length of the urethra (from the pelvic floor to the level of the urinary bladder).

7.2.3.4.6
Stage IIIB

Cervical cancer with invasion of the pelvic sidewall corresponds to stage IIIB. Cervical cancer can reach the pelvic sidewall by continuous lateral growth through the parametrial tissue and the sacral bone and through posterior extension along the sacrouterine ligament (Fig. 7.29). T2-weighted images depict

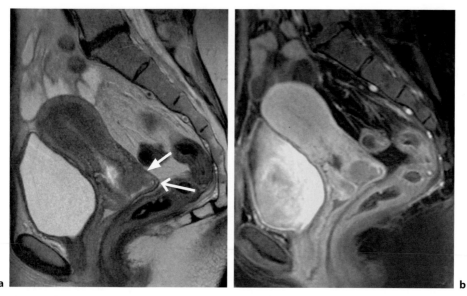

Fig. 7.21a,b. Stage IB. **a** T2w TSE image in sagittal orientation. The cervical cancer (*arrow*) is depicted as a high-signal-intensity tumor that primarily involves the posterior cervix and is surrounded by low-signal-intensity cervical stroma. There is no infiltration of the posterior vaginal fornix. (*open arrow*) **b** T1w TSE image with FS in sagittal orientation. Following administration of Gd-DTPA, a hypovascularized cervical cancer is depicted. Accessory finding: thin defect in the anterior myometrium near the isthmus 3 weeks after cesarean section

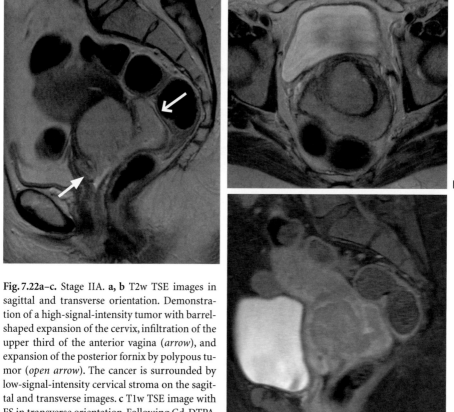

Fig. 7.22a–c. Stage IIA. **a, b** T2w TSE images in sagittal and transverse orientation. Demonstration of a high-signal-intensity tumor with barrel-shaped expansion of the cervix, infiltration of the upper third of the anterior vagina (*arrow*), and expansion of the posterior fornix by polypous tumor (*open arrow*). The cancer is surrounded by low-signal-intensity cervical stroma on the sagittal and transverse images. **c** T1w TSE image with FS in transverse orientation. Following Gd-DTPA, a moderately vascularized tumor is seen

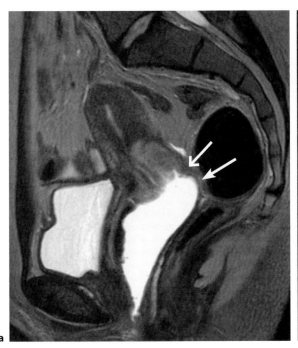 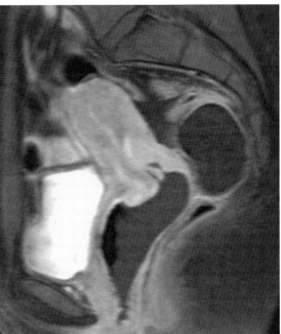

Fig. 7.23a,b. Stage IIA. **a** T2w TSE image in sagittal orientation. High-signal-intensity cervical cancer with ulceration (*open arrow*) of posterior portion and infiltration of the posterior vaginal fornix (*arrow*). **b** T1w TSE image in sagittal orientation. Following administration of Gd-DTPA, a high-signal intensity (hypervascularized) cervical cancer with ulceration and tumor infiltration of the posterior vaginal fornix is seen. Gel filling of the vagina

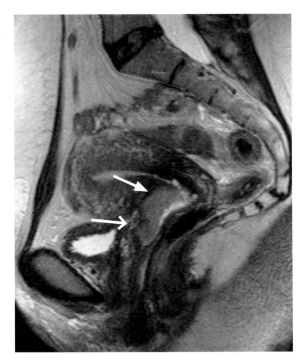

Fig. 7.24. Stage IIA. T2w TSE image in sagittal orientation. Cervical cancer seen as a high-signal-intensity mass of the anterior proximal cervix (*arrow*) with infiltration of the upper two-thirds of the vagina (*open arrow*)

tumor infiltration as hyperintense lesions in the intermediate signal intensity of the muscle, or low signal intensity of the cortical bone, or as thickening of the vascular wall. T1-weighted imaging allows evaluation of the extent of advanced parametrial infiltration and possible extension to the pelvic sidewall with good delineation of the hypointense tumor mass from the lateral parametrial tissue and the intermediate-signal-intensity muscle tissue. The tumor-related consumption of the lateral lipid lamella seen on T1-weighted images may already suggest extension to the pelvic sidewall from the surgical perspective even if direct infiltration of the sidewall is not yet apparent.

Ureteral infiltration and obstruction with hydronephrosis is also classified as stage IIIB disease (Fig. 7.30). The ureter courses over the psoas muscle from dorsolaterally before it descends into the pelvis. In the true pelvis, the ureter takes an anteromedial course from the pelvic sidewall in the inferior segment of the parametria toward the base of the bladder. At the level of the uterine isthmus, the ureter courses lateral to the uterine cervix at a distance of 1–2.5 cm and is overcrossed by the uterine artery anteriorly. The ureter is typically infiltrated by lateral tumor growth through

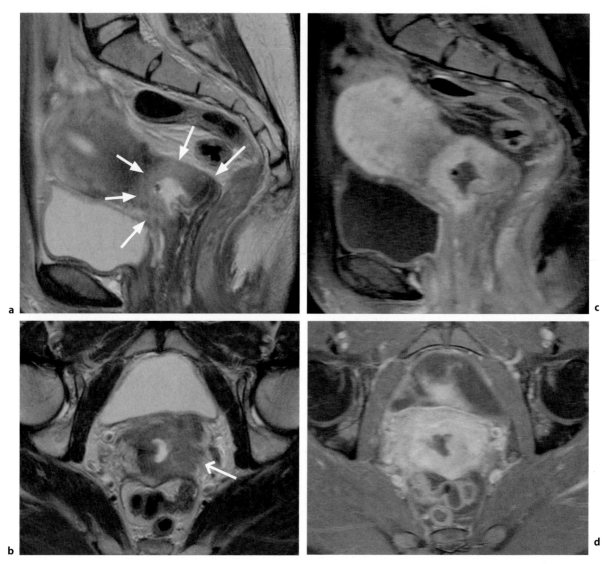

Fig. 7.25a–d. Stage IIB. **a, b** T2w TSE images in sagittal and transverse orientation. Hyperintense cervical cancer with endocervical necrotic cavity (*arrows*). Parametrium infiltration is indicated by the fact that the cervical stroma is disrupted on the left side with lateral tumor extension (*open arrow*). There is no involvement of the pelvic sidewall. **c, d** T1w TSE images with FS in sagittal and transverse orientation. Following administration of Gd-DTPA, there is pronounced enhancement indicative of a hypervascularized cervical cancer. Reliable evaluation of the extent of parametrium infiltration is no longer possible since the parametria also show contrast enhancement

the parametria. A thickening of the ureteral wall or hydronephrosis is seen. In patients with a tumor mass in the parametria, the kidneys and urinary tract should be included in the imaging volume in order to confirm or exclude ureteral obstruction and hydronephrosis.

7.2.3.4.7
Stage IVA

Stage IVA cervical cancer is characterized by infiltration of the mucosa of the rectum or urinary bladder.

The FIGO classification is based on mucosal infiltration of these organs because the outer wall layers are not amenable to evaluation by endoscopy and biopsy. MRI, on the other hand, already identifies infiltration of the outer muscular layer of the bladder and rectum. Tumor extension to the rectum is either through invasion of the sacrouterine ligament or through direct infiltration of the pouch of Douglas with subsequent extension of the tumor to the anterior rectal wall (Fig. 7.31). The peritoneal fold of the rectouterine space (pouch of Douglas), on the

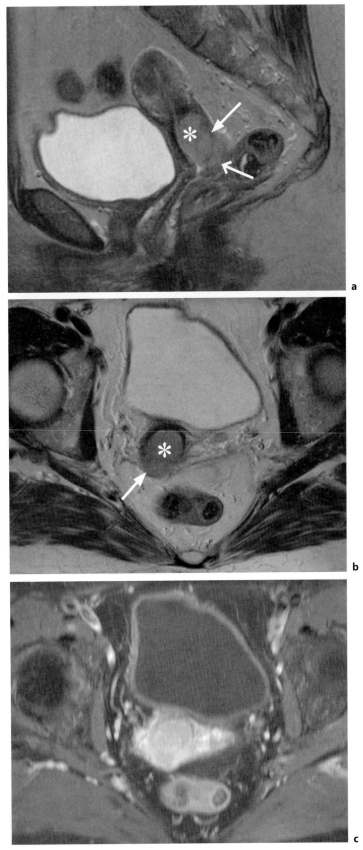

Fig. 7.26a-c. Stage IIB. **a, b** T2w TSE images in sagittal and transverse orientation. Cervical cancer (*asterisks*) with infiltration of the posterior vagina (*open arrow*). Posterior disruption of the cervical stroma and a solid tumor extending in a posterior direction (*arrows*) are seen as signs of parametrium infiltration. **c** T1w TSE image with FS in transverse orientation 1 min after administration of Gd-DTPA showing a moderately hypervascularized cervical cancer with hypovascularized cervical stroma and hypervascularized lateral parametrial tissue.

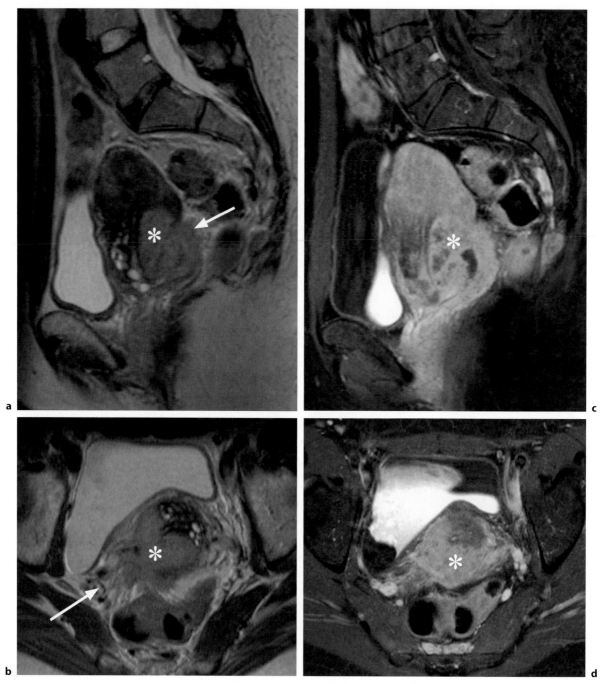

Fig. 7.27a–d. Stage IIB. **a, b** T2w TSE images in sagittal and transverse orientation. Cervical cancer (*asteriks*) with infiltration of the posterior vaginal fornix. Clearly seen are parametrium tumor extensions (*arrows*) in a posterior direction and to the right without infiltration of the pelvic sidewall or of the rectum. **c, d** T1w TSE images in sagittal and transverse orientation 1 min after administration of Gd-DTPA. Heterogeneous hypervascularized cervical cancer (*asterisks*) with hypovascularized, necrotic portions. Accessory finding: cervical cysts

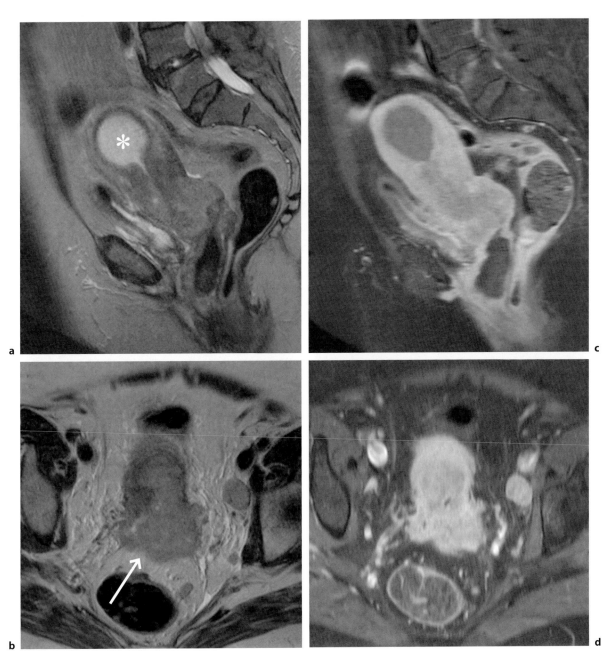

Fig. 7.28a–d. Stage IIB. **a, b** T2w TSE images in sagittal and transverse orientation. Cervical cancer with infiltration of the uterine corpus and hematometra (*asterisk*) due to tumorous stenosis of the cervical canal. Large solid tumor portions extend into the parametria posteriorly (*open arrow*) but do not infiltrate the rectum. Also seen are nodal metastases of the internal obturator group, along the internal iliac artery, and of pararectal nodes on the left. **c, d** T1w TSE images in sagittal and transverse orientation 1 min after administration of Gd-DTPA

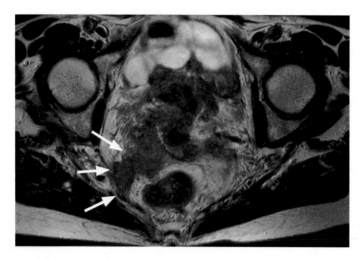

Fig. 7.29. Stage IIIB. T2w TSE image in transversal orientation. Cervical cancer with right lateral parametrial infiltration and infiltration of the right pelvic wall (*arrows*)

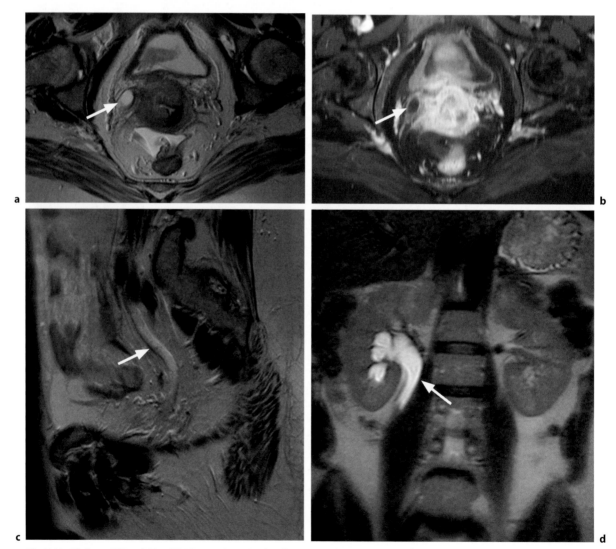

Fig. 7.30a–d. Stage IIIB. **a, b** T2w TSE images in sagittal and transverse orientation. **c** HASTE TSE image in coronal orientation. **d** T1w TSE image in transverse orientation 1 min after administration of Gd-DTPA. Cervical cancer with right lateral parametrial infiltration and infiltration of the right ureter, which is distended as a consequence (*arrows*)

other hand, acts as a natural barrier that aggravates extension to the anterior rectal wall.

The urinary bladder is infiltrated through continuous anterior growth of the cervical tumor along the peritoneal fold between the cervix and the bladder, also referred to as the vesicouterine ligament (Figs. 7.32, 7.33). Sagittal and transverse T2-weighted MR images depict infiltration as segmental disruption of the hypointense muscular layer of the wall of the bladder or rectum by hyperintense tumor. Con-trast-enhanced T1-weighted images often enable a more reliable identification of segmental disruption because of stronger enhancement of the tumor as compared with the muscular layer. Infiltration of the wall of the bladder and/or the rectum as well as contiguity of cervical cancer with either of these organs has important therapeutic implications.

Tumor infiltration of these hollow organs is quite often associated with the development of fistulas. A collection of air in the urinary bladder may indicate

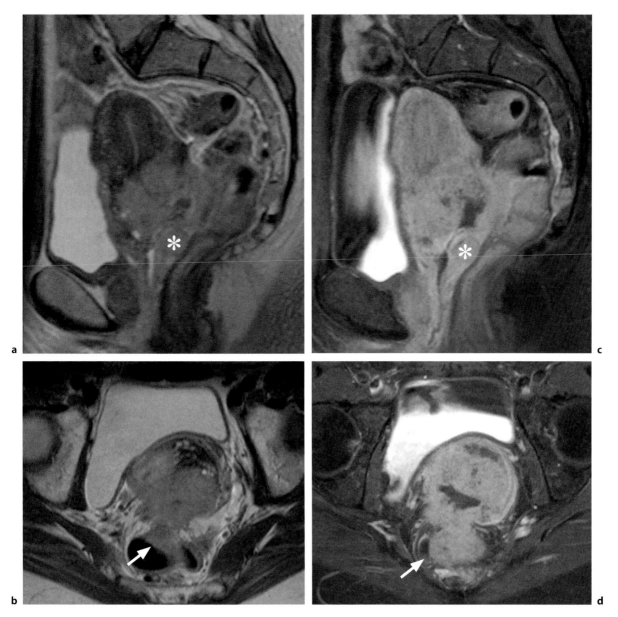

Fig. 7.31a–d. Stage IVA. **a, b** T2w TSE images in sagittal and transverse orientation. **c, d** T1w TSE images in sagittal and transverse orientation 1 min after administration of Gd-DTPA. Cervical cancer with infiltration of the posterior parametria. Rectal infiltration (*arrows*) is seen as hyperintense tumor extension disrupting the anterior rectal wall, which is of low signal intensity before and of intermediate signal intensity after CM administration. Tumor is also seen in the posterior vaginal wall (*asterisks*)

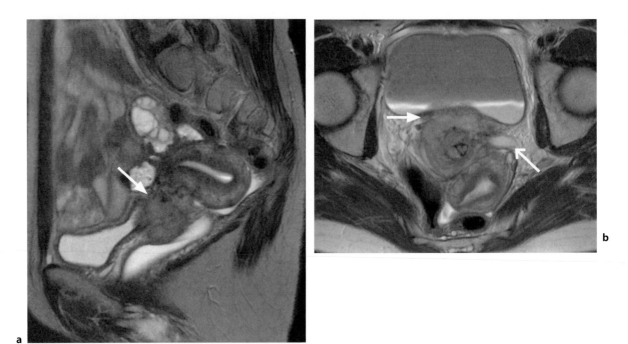

Fig. 7.32a,b. Stage IVA. **a, b** T2w TSE images in sagittal and transverse orientation showing cervical cancer with infiltration of the urinary bladder. Disruption of the hypointense bladder wall and intravesical tumor growth are seen (*arrows*). In addition, there is infiltration of the left lateral parametria and the left ureter, which is distended as a consequence (*open arrow*)

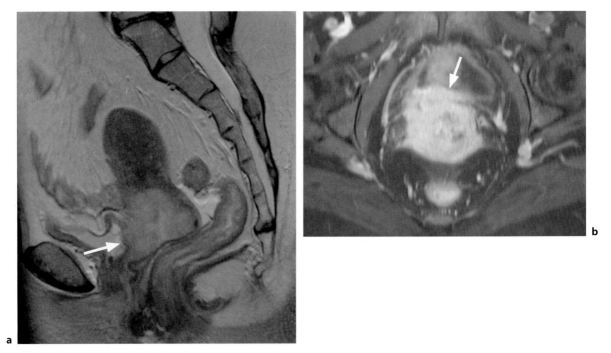

Fig. 7.33a,b. Stage IVA. **a** T2w TSE image in sagittal orientation. Cervical cancer with infiltration of the vesicouterine ligament and of the low-signal-intensity posterior bladder wall (*arrow*). T1w TSE image with FS transverse orientation 1 min after administration of Gd-DTPA. **b** After CM administration, a hypervascularized tumor (transverse image) is seen in the posterior bladder wall (*arrow*). (from [133])

a vesicouterine fistula especially under chemo- or radiotherapy (Figs. 7.47–7.49) (see Sect. 7.2.5.4). A fistula can be best demonstrated with contrast-enhanced T1-weighted sequences, which will depict the fistula as an enhancing formation with an nonenhancing filiform lumen. Alternatively, a fistula can be demonstrated as a hyperintense filiform structure with a high sensitivity by using a T2-weighted inversion recovery sequence.

7.2.3.4.8
Stage IVB

Stage IVB cervical cancer is characterized by hematogenous dissemination and is discussed in Sect. 7.2.3).

7.2.3.5
Lymph Node Staging

Following invasion of the dense network of lymphatic vessels in the parametria, cervical cancer can spread to the pelvic and para-aortic lymph nodes. Nodal metastasis is not taken into account by the FIGO classification, although it is important for therapy and is the most important prognostic factor. The earliest tumor stage associated with lymph node metastasis is IB (20%) and the risk increases with tumor size and stage (see Sects. 7.1.7, 7.1.9). The risk of metastatic lymph nodes is increased in tumor recurrence (38%) [91] and in patients with adenocarcinoma as compared with squamous cell carcinoma. Lymphatic spread usually first affects the primary lymph node stations in the parametrium, along the internal and

external iliac arteries, from where the tumor spreads to the secondary, presacral lymph nodes along the common iliac artery and to the para-aortic lymph nodes (Figs. 7.34–7.37).

Finally, there may be spread to extra-abdominal lymph nodes. These are primarily the supraclavicular lymph nodes in the venous angle (Fig. 7.37), at the termination of the azygos and hemiazygos veins into the superior vena cava, besides the less commonly affected parabronchial and axillary lymph node stations. Most metastatic lymph nodes become clinically apparent only when there is pronounced enlargement with obstruction, for instance of the ureter, or compression of nerves. The morphologic changes caused by nodal metastases range from slight increases in size of isolated nodes to large lymph node conglomerates.

Radiologic evaluation of the lymph nodes is based on size and shape. A parametrial node is considered suspicious when its short axis is 5 mm or longer. A pelvic or para-aortic lymph node with a short axis longer than 10 mm and oval in shape or with an axis longer than 8 mm and round shape is interpreted as a potentially metastatic lymph node at MRI and CT [40, 92]. Other morphologic criteria are an irregular contour, inhomogeneous contrast enhancement, and central necrosis. Intravascular contrast medium administration is especially useful to differentiate vascular structures or to identify necrotic areas [93]. Stronger contrast enhancement is not a reliable criterion as it may also indicate reactive changes.

Another modality, whole-body FDG-PET (5-fluorodesoxyglucosis-positron emission tomography), can

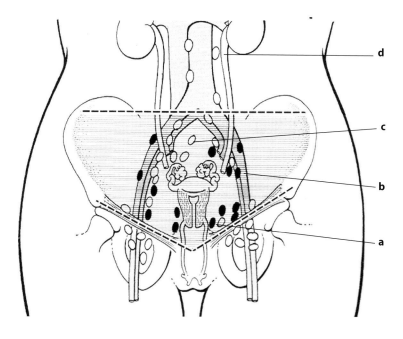

Fig. 7.34a–d. Lymph node staging. Stages of metastatic spread to the lymph nodes in cervical cancer. **a** Parametrial nodes. **b** Nodes along the external and common iliac arteries. **c** Presacral nodes. **d** Para-aortic nodes (regarded as distant metastases) (from [134])

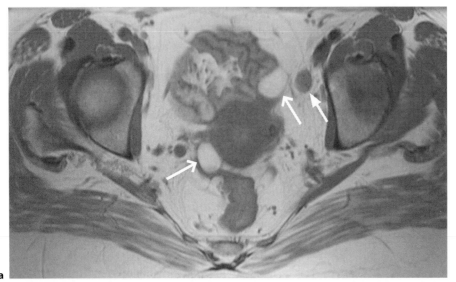

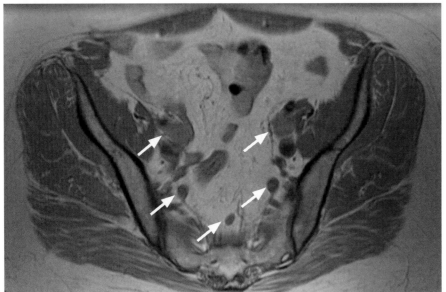

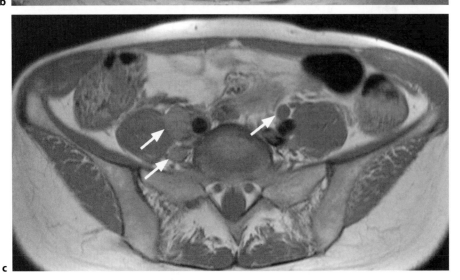

Fig. 7.35a–c. Lymph node staging in different patients. **a–c** PD-TSE images in transverse orientation. **a** Suspicious lymph node of round configuration measuring 1 cm in diameter of the external iliac artery group on the left (*arrow*) in a patient with cervical cancer with bilateral parametrial infiltration and ureteral distention (*open arrows*). **b** Suspicious round and enlarged lymph nodes along the external iliac artery on both sides and an increase in the number of presacral lymph nodes with round configuration (*arrows*). **c** Suspicious round and enlarged lymph nodes of the common iliac artery group on both sides (*arrows*). The presence of pelvic lymph node metastases is not taken into account in the FIGO staging system

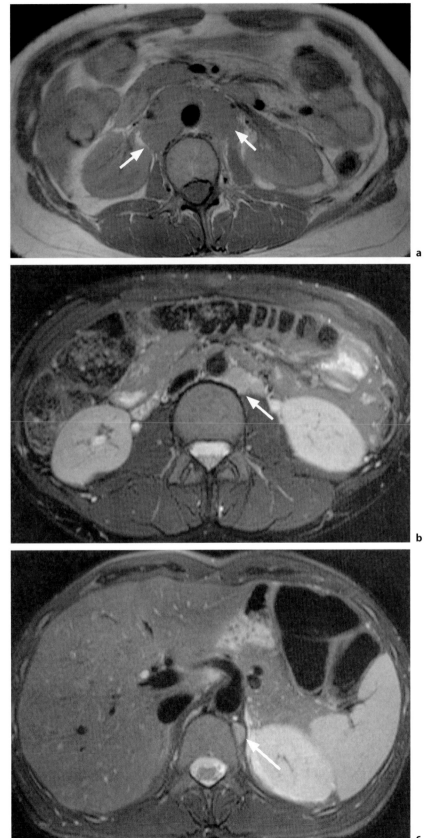

Fig. 7.36a–c. Lymph node staging in different patients. **a** PD-TSE images in transverse orientation shows para-aortic and interaortocaval lymph node metastases (*arrows*). **b, c** T1w TSE images (PACE) in transverse orientation. Suspicious round and enlarged para-aortic and retrocrural lymph nodes (*arrows*). Para-aortic lymph node metastases are regarded as distant metastases, the patient thus has FIGO stage IVB

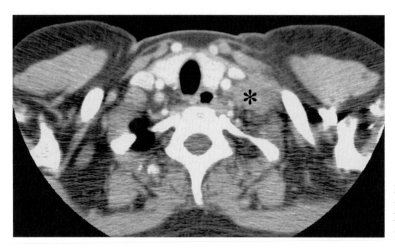

Fig. 7.37. Lymph node staging. Contrast-enhanced CT image. Supraclavicular lymph node metastasis on the left (*asterisk*). FIGO stage IVB

used as a supplementary test for lymph node staging in follow-up [94] but has similar limitations to established imaging modalities, which include identification of micrometastases and differentiation of tumor from inflammatory changes. FDG PET provides no morphologic information and has to be combined with CT or MRI, possibly using the technique of image fusion [95]. Lymphangiography has been abandoned as a modality for assessing lymph node status and is no longer recommended in the guidelines for the diagnostic management of cervical cancer [96].

7.2.3.6
Distant Metastases

Distant metastases are characteristic of stage IVB cervical cancer. In the FIGO classification, metastases of the para-aortic lymph nodes count as distant metastases. Hematogenous dissemination occurs late in cervical cancer or typically in patients with local tumor recurrence. Organ metastases most commonly affect the lungs and are less frequent in the liver, peritoneum, and skeleton. Systemic staging for the exclusion of distant metastases is indicated in stage III and IV cervical cancer. In Germany, an additional helical CT scan of the chest, abdomen, and pelvis including the supraclavicular region with oral opacification and IV bolus administration of contrast medium is recommended [130].

Autopsy studies found pulmonary metastases in about 35% of patients with recurrent cervical cancer. The probability of lung metastases is similar for squamous cell carcinoma and adenocarcinoma of the cervix. Solitary or multiple nodular pulmonary metastases may occur and are comparable to pulmonary metastases from other primaries in that clini-

cal symptoms occur late. Chest CT is recommended as the first-line modality for exclusion of pulmonary metastases. Alternatively, routine chest radiography performed before therapy for assessment of the cardiopulmonary status can likewise be used to exclude pulmonary metastases but is less sensitive than CT. Pulmonary metastases are associated with mediastinal or hilar lymphadenopathy in 30% of cases and with pleural metastases in about 27% (autopsy studies). A slightly higher risk of pleural metastases has been reported for cervical adenocarcinoma. Rare findings are pericardial metastases, bronchial spread with endobronchial obstruction (5%), and pulmonary lymphangiosis carcinomatosa (3%) [97].

Liver metastases occur in about 30% of patients with recurrent cervical carcinoma [98] (Fig. 7.38). They are identified by ultrasound as multiple focal lesions of low echogenicity and as focal lesions with heterogeneous contrast medium uptake on CT and MRI. MRI has the highest sensitivity in detecting liver metastases, especially when performed with administration of a liver-specific contrast medium [99]. Metastases of the peritoneum (Fig. 7.38), major omentum, or mesentery were identified at autopsy studies in 5%–27% of cases [98, 100]. Clinical symptoms occur late and comprise abdominal pain and an increase in abdominal circumference. Metastases in these locations are sensitively identified by MRI and CT [101, 102]. MRI is performed with contrast-enhanced fat-saturated T1-weighted sequences, optionally supplemented by oral opacification. Characteristic signs of peritoneal metastases are a wavy contour of the liver resulting from impression by the focal lesions, nodular peritoneal masses, and irregular peritoneal thickening. Ascites is unspecific but may indicate peritoneal metastases [101].

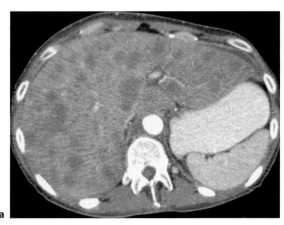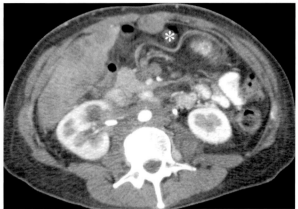

a   b

Fig. 7.38a,b. Distant metastases. **a, b** Contrast-enhanced CT images. Numerous hypovascularized metastases are seen in the liver. In addition, metastatic spread to the peritoneum (*asterisk*) and extensive para-aortic lymph node metastases. FIGO stage IVB

Recurrent cervical cancer is associated with bone metastases (Fig. 7.39) in 15%–29% of patients at autopsy [100, 103]. Typical locations are the bony pelvis as well as the lumbar and other vertebral bodies. Bone metastases in the ribs and extremities are less common. Skeletal metastases typically have an osteolytic character and originate from locally advanced or recurrent tumor in the pelvic sidewall or arise through retrograde tumor spread in patients with para-aortic lymph node metastasis [104]. Hematogenous dissemination to the skeleton occurs late. MRI with unenhanced and contrast-enhanced fat-saturated T1-weighted sequences depicts bone metastases as hyperintense lesions in the low-intensity bone marrow with a high sensitivity. CT primarily shows the extent of osseous destruction.

About 15% of patients with recurrent cervical cancer develop adrenal metastases [98]. Vary rare are splenic, pancreatic, gastrointestinal, and renal metastases.

7.2.4
Specific Diagnostic Queries

7.2.4.1
Preoperative Imaging

Pretherapeutic local tumor staging is crucial to determine resectability and to select the most suitable operative procedure (simple hysterectomy, radical hysterectomy, trachelectomy, extent of lymphadenectomy), which is primarily based on tumor size, lymph node status, and parametrial involvement. The surgical procedure chosen on the basis of the MRI findings is

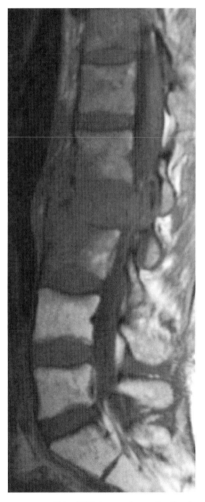

Fig. 7.39. Distant metastases. T1w TSE image in sagittal orientation. Para-aortic lymph node metastases with vertebral infiltration of L1–L3. Consecutive total collapse of vertebral body of L2. FIGO stage IVB

often specified further by surgical lymph node staging. If no primary surgery and no surgical lymph node staging are performed, the MRI findings serve to determine the target volume to be irradiated. MRI after adjuvant therapy serves to reconsider the indication for surgery. In patients with local recurrence, the MRI findings have an important role in deciding about repeat surgery and the surgical technique. Contraindications to curative exenteration are intraperitoneal implantation, nonresectable nodes, extensive involvement of the pelvic sidewall, and liver or lung metastases.

MRI also has a crucial role in establishing the indication for radical trachelectomy. Only patients in whom MRI demonstrates a tumor-free internal os of the cervical canal at the isthmus uteri are candidates for trachelectomy [105]. Therefore, it is additionally important to estimate the distance of the tumor from the uterine isthmus and from the vaginal vault. Trachelectomy is not performed if there is infiltration of the isthmus or of the myometrium of the uterine corpus. The isthmus is identified by its small diameter and the entrance of the uterine vessels.

7.2.4.2
Imaging Before and After Radiotherapy

In patients scheduled for primary radiotherapy without surgical staging, the pretreatment radiologic evaluation together with the clinical findings gains in importance. The use of two reference points, A and B, for reporting the dose of radiation stems from the times of conventional planning of radiotherapy (Fig. 7.40). Point A serves as a reference for the primary tumor and is located 2 cm lateral and superior to the level of the portio. Point B is 5 cm lateral to and 2 cm above the portio level and corresponds to the pelvic sidewall. Some investigators still report radiation doses delivered to points A and B for the sake of comparison despite individualized radiotherapy.

Although the actual radiotherapy procedure is usually planned by means of a CT scan, MRI has an increasing role in treatment planning and controlling radiation, as it is superior in visualizing the tumor volume and infiltration of surrounding tissue (Figs. 7.41, 7.42). The CT scan performed to plan radiotherapy serves to determine the physical parameters of irradiation such as number and direction of the radiation fields, collimation, and dose distribution. The use of 3D-based individual planning of radiation fields is more and more replacing the four-field box technique (Fig. 7.41). Dose-volume histograms serve to determine the respective dose corresponding to a specific organ volume such as the bladder or rectum, which are especially at risk. In planning the target volume to be irradiated (PTV, physical target volume), the primary tumor volume (GTV, gross tumor volume), the

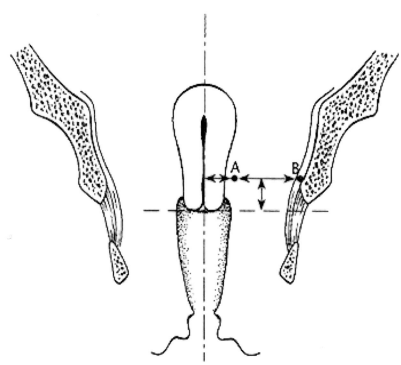

Fig. 7.40. Points *A* and *B*. The use of two reference points, *A* and *B*, for orientation stems from the times of conventional planning of radiation therapy. Point *A* is 2 cm lateral to and above the level of the portio and serves as a reference for the tumor on both sides of the cervix. Point *B* is 5 cm lateral to and 2 cm above the portio level and indicates the pelvic wall

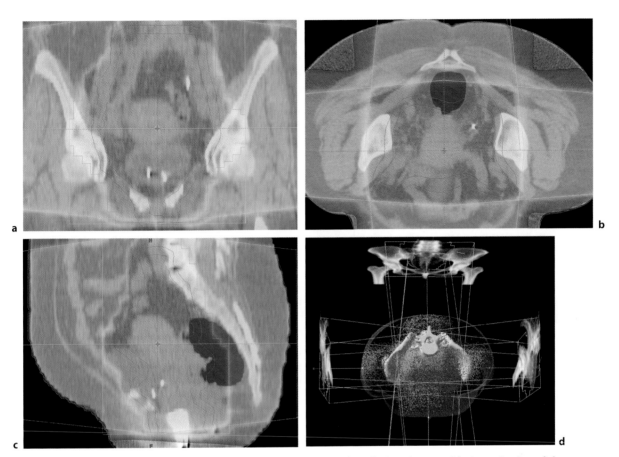

a

b

c

d

Fig. 7.41a–d. Planning CT scan prior to radiotherapy. **a–c** Planning of irradiation therapy with determination of the target volume using the transverse planes of the CT scan and transfer to the sagittal and coronal planes. **d** Dose target volume and arrangement of fields using a four-field technique. The target volume comprises the vagina, uterus, and locoregional lymphatic drainage system including a safety margin. Irradiation in the prone position to spare the small intestine. (Courtesy of Dr. L. Moser, Berlin)

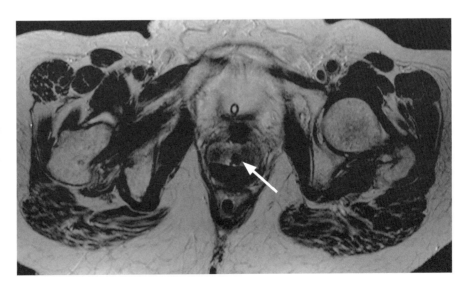

Fig. 7.42. MR-Imaging during intracavitary brachytherapy. Axial T2w image during intracavitary brachytherapy facilitates treatment planning and is useful in controlling the relationships between tumor and applicator (*arrow*). Measuring probes are placed in the rectum. (Courtesy of Dr. S. Marnitz, Berlin)

area of potential tumor extent (CTV, clinical target volume), and a safety margin that takes into account patient and organ motion are defined. The CTV comprises the uterus, at least the proximal third of the vagina, the parametrial tissue up to the pelvic wall, and the pelvic lymphatic drainage system, which is irradiated with a dose that is high enough to eliminate both micrometastases and manifest metastases. The only proven indication for para-aortic irradiation are metastatic para-aortic nodes. To spare the intestine, planning and irradiation are usually performed with the patient positioned prone on a belly board.

The results of pretherapeutic MRI and surgical tumor and nodal staging are usually available when the indication for adjuvant radiotherapy is established. Additionally, postoperative hydronephrosis should be excluded. Patients who have undergone R2 resection require follow-up MRI for evaluation of the residual tumor.

Radiation therapy is usually done with individual doses of 1.8–2 Gy per fraction with five fractions per week up to a total dose of 60–75 Gy encompassing the entire tumor volume. Treatment is continued for a maximum of 7 weeks. If external beam irradiation is supplemented by brachytherapy, the latter is performed in three to eight fractions, each with a dose of 5–8 Gy, or with delivery of one to two doses of 20–30 Gy. A cervical sheath is used in most cases to ensure identical positioning of the brachytherapy applicator.

Acute side effects of irradiation develop within 90 days and affect organs directly exposed to radiation. Typically, they include acute gastrointestinal toxicity and skin reactions. Other adverse effects such as hematologic suppression and acute toxic reactions of the genitourinary tract are rare. Chronic side effects may range from disturbed intestinal mobility to ileus, chronic diarrhea, and chronic cystitis with shrinkage of the bladder. Impaired vaginal function is typically associated with brachytherapy and can be prevented or improved by local measures. Fistulas may develop as severe complications after regression of large infiltrating tumors. Ureteral stricture is typically seen after combined surgery and radiation therapy. Loss of ovarian function may occur through scatter radiation even if the ovaries have been surgically transposed. Radio-osteonecrosis as a late complication has become rare since the introduction of 3D planning. Combination of radiotherapy with chemotherapy may occasionally require adjustment of the dose of systemic therapy since the combined approach is associated with a higher acute toxicity.

Hyperthermia is a new treatment that is currently being evaluated in phase II and III studies in combination with radiotherapy or chemotherapy for treating locally advanced cervical cancer [106,107]. Hyperthermia exerts a direct cytotoxic effect by heating the tumor tissue but primarily aims at improving the tumor's response to radiotherapy or chemotherapy through reactive hyperemia. It is performed as deep regional hyperthermia by means of electromagnetic radiation with simultaneous control of temperature in special MRI scanners.

7.2.5
Follow-up

7.2.5.1
Findings After Surgery

Scar tissue being older than 6 months has a low signal intensity similar to that of muscle on T1-weighted and T2-weighted MR images. Fresh scars are of a higher signal intensity on T2-weighted images due to inflammation and neovascularization in the first months after surgery. Signal intensity decreases with fibrosis. This is why MRI should be performed not earlier than 6 months after the end of therapy and even then the signal intensities of recurrent tumor and scar tissue may still overlap on T2-weighted images. This is why a dynamic contrast-enhanced study could be necessary, which can better distinguish recurrent tumor on the basis of its earlier and more pronounced CM enhancement.

After radical hysterectomy, the uterus and the vaginal vault are absent [108]. The vaginal stump is depicted with a smooth end and as a symmetrical, elongated, or rectangular structure that is sharply demarcated from the surrounding fatty tissue between the bladder and the rectum (Fig. 7.43). Cranial to the stump, the resection cavity is filled by parts of the urinary bladder and bowel. Images in sagittal orientation are most suitable to evaluate the vaginal wall [78]. On T2-weighted images, the vagina is characterized by a high-signal-intensity inner mucosal layer and a smooth outer muscular layer of low signal intensity. Surgical clips are depicted on MRI images as small signal voids at the vaginal stump. Some patients develop fibrotic scar tissue at the roof of the vaginal stump. It is characterized by an intermediate to low signal intensity on T2-weighted and T1-weighted images and may be difficult to differentiate from recurrence if it is of a nodular configuration.

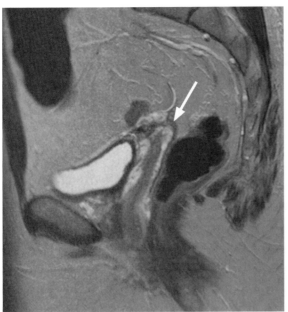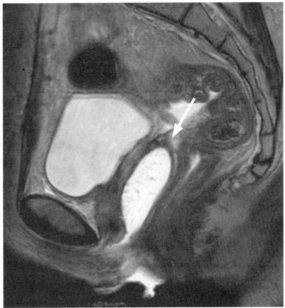

a   b

Fig. 7.43a,b. Status after hysterectomy. **a, b** T2w TSE images of different patients in sagittal orientation. Normal appearance of the vaginal stump (*arrows*) after hysterectomy without (**a**) and with (**b**) filling of the vagina. Patient is catheterized

The peri- and postoperative complications include the development of vesicovaginal fistulas, which typically occur on the basis of necrosis roughly 1–2 weeks after the operation. If they do not close spontaneously they are operated on after 8 weeks or later in patients undergoing adjuvant radiotherapy. Injury to the urinary bladder occurs in 3%–5% of patients undergoing radical hysterectomy and ureteral damage in 2%. Ureteral damage is usually treated by primary surgical repair. Ureterovaginal fistulas typically develop in the second postoperative week and have an incidence of about 1%. They close spontaneously after placement of a double-J catheter. Lymph edema of the legs has an incidence of 3% after surgery and of 5%–15% after adjuvant radiotherapy. Clinically, approximately 15% of patients develop acute bladder voiding difficulties after radical hysterectomy with lymph node dissection, caused by mechanical factors as well as damage to bladder innervation. The incidence increases with the radicalness of the operation.

In radical trachelectomy, MRI depicts the end-to-end anastomosis and the development of a posterior neofornix (Fig. 7.44). The latter may develop in the process of healing and must be carefully distinguished from a recurrent tumor. The few recurrences of cervical cancer observed after trachelectomy occurred at the site of anastomosis [109]. Occasionally, stenosis has been observed after trachelectomy. Moreover,

mobilization of the parametrial and paravaginal tissue can lead to diffuse thickening of the vaginal wall, which may mimic recurrent invasive tumor at MRI. Most of these postoperative changes recede spontaneously. In some patients, asymptomatic widening of the parametrial venous plexus has been observed. In patients becoming pregnant after trachelectomy, a cerclage is placed to keep the cervix closed.

Following lymph node dissection, metal clips are often seen at the pelvic wall as focal artifacts of low signal intensity at MRI or as metal-dense structures at CT. Lymphoceles most frequently develop after lymphadenectomy. They are usually small, cause no symptoms, and recede without therapy. If a lymphocele becomes symptomatic or infection is suspected due to contrast enhancement of the wall, therapy may be required in the form of repeat operation, puncture, drainage, or sclerotherapy.

Pelvic exenteration is the curative method of choice in patients with central pelvic tumor recurrence and comprises colpectomy and hysterectomy with removal of the bladder (anterior exenteration) or of the bladder and rectosigmoid (complete exenteration). In addition, the intervention may be performed as supralevator exenteration with partial resection of the levator plate or as translevator exenteration with vulvectomy and radical resection of the levator muscle, urogenital diaphragm, and vulvoperineal

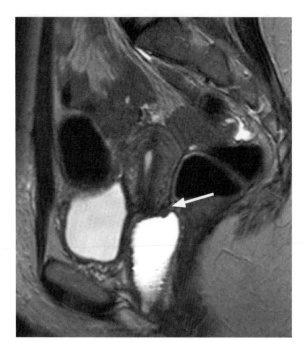

Fig. 7.44. Status after trachelectomy. A T2w TSE image in sagittal orientation. Markedly shortened uterine cervix after radical trachelectomy with fertility-sparing uterovaginal reanastomosis (*arrow*). Gel filling of the vagina

soft tissue. The patient's quality of life is improved by subsequent reconstruction of the pelvic organs with deep rectal anastomosis, creation of a urinary pouch, and possibly creation of a neovagina. The intervention-related mortality is about 5%.

7.2.5.2
Findings After Chemotherapy

The main criterion for a response to chemotherapy is a reduction of tumor size. For follow-up of tumor size under chemotherapy, the largest transverse diameter of the lesion is measured according to the RECIST criteria [89]. A size reduction of at least 30% is defined as a partial response to therapy. Tumor progression is assumed when there is an increase in size of at least 20%. Tumor regression is associated with a loss of signal already on unenhanced T2-weighted images and an inhomogeneous signal pattern resulting from regressive tumor areas with reduced perfusion. MRI is the method of choice for evaluating the response to chemotherapy in patients with cervical cancer. However, in patients on chemotherapy, both vital tumor tissue and inflammatory reactive areas are present, which are of high signal intensity on T2-weighted

images and show early contrast enhancement on T1-weighted images. This is why reliable evaluation of tumor tissue on the basis of signal intensity at T2-weighted imaging and contrast enhancement at T1-weighted imaging is not always possible at this stage. Therefore, the most important criterion for a response to therapy at this stage is the size reduction of the tumor. The concomitant reaction of the surrounding tissue and fibrosis impairs not only the radiologic diagnosis but also later surgical treatment. MR spectroscopy is being investigated experimentally as an alternative imaging modality for following up tumor response to chemotherapy [110].

7.2.5.3
Findings After Radiotherapy

MRI is the first-line radiologic modality for follow-up after radiation therapy. It may be performed 6 and 12 months after completion of irradiation and whenever tumor recurrence is suggested by the clinical or gynecologic findings. During and shortly after radiotherapy, the entire irradiated field shows a reactive signal increase on T2-weighted images and more pronounced contrast enhancement on T1-weighted images. This is why differentiation of tumor tissue from reactively inflamed tissue is impaired during and shortly after irradiation. Hence, MRI during or within the first 6 months after radiotherapy is indicated in exceptional cases as the evaluation of the tumor shrinkage or the assessment of a fistula.

Effective radiation therapy leads to a significant reduction or complete disappearance of the tumor and a decrease in signal intensity on T2-weighted images (Figs. 7.45, 7.46). A reliable sign of complete tumor remission is the return of the normal anatomy of the cervix and proximal vagina, which is suggested by the depiction of a homogeneous stroma of low signal intensity with a smooth mucosal membrane often accompanied by shrinkage of the cervix. Recurrent tumor is typically seen as a high-signal-intensity mass corresponding to the original tumor on T2-weighted images.

The signal changes seen at MRI correlate with the overall radiation dose applied. Radiation-induced edema persists in the myometrium of the uterine corpus for up to 6 months after irradiation. After completion of radiation, there is a decrease in signal intensity on T2-weighted images, the endometrium becomes narrower, and the zonal anatomy of the myometrium is eliminated. In postmenopausal women, the uterus returns to its former MRI appearance without zonal anatomy after resolution of radiation-induced edema.

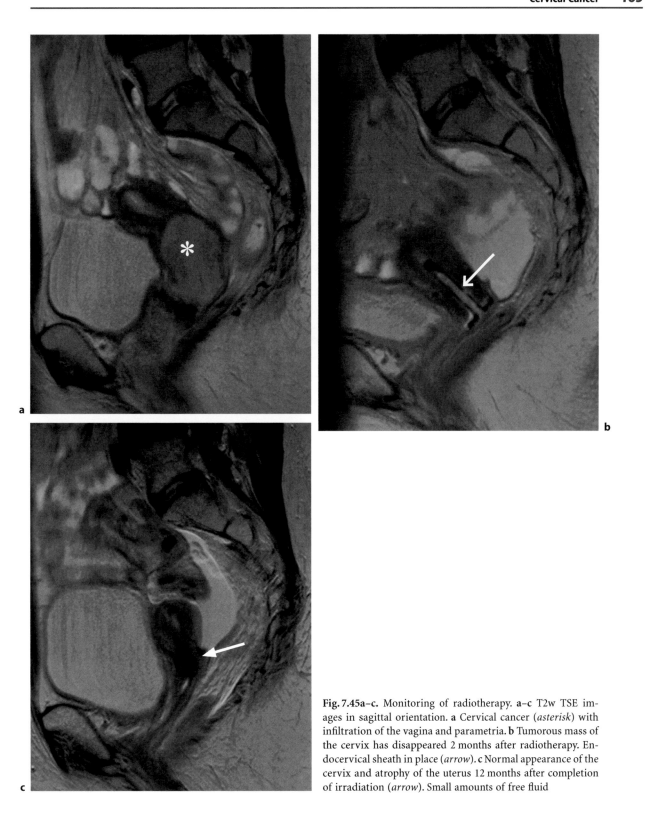

Fig. 7.45a–c. Monitoring of radiotherapy. **a–c** T2w TSE images in sagittal orientation. **a** Cervical cancer (*asterisk*) with infiltration of the vagina and parametria. **b** Tumorous mass of the cervix has disappeared 2 months after radiotherapy. Endocervical sheath in place (*arrow*). **c** Normal appearance of the cervix and atrophy of the uterus 12 months after completion of irradiation (*arrow*). Small amounts of free fluid

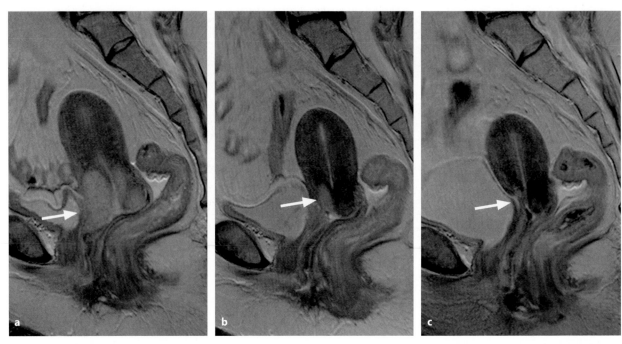

Fig. 7.46a–c. Monitoring of radiotherapy. **a–c** T2w TSE images in sagittal orientation. **a** Cervical cancer (*arrow*) with infiltration of the urinary bladder. **b** Size reduction of the tumor (*arrow*) during radiotherapy. **c** No circumscribed tumor of the cervix is depicted 3 months after completion of irradiation (*arrow*).

The vagina also has an increased signal intensity on T2-weighted images due to edematous and inflammatory changes in the acute and subacute phase after irradiation. About 6 months after the end of radiation therapy, there is a fibrosis-related signal reduction on T2-weighted images. Shrinkage of the cervix and vagina may occasionally lead to an effective stenosis (radiogenic fibrosis) with subsequent development of serometra or hematometra. This condition is associated with symmetric enlargement of the uterus with a central fluid collection, which is of high signal intensity on T2-weighted images and also on T1-weighted images if the protein or blood content is high.

A complication after irradiation is the development of fistulas due to therapy-induced regression of invasive cervical cancer (Figs. 7.47–7.49) (see Sect. 7.2.3.4.7). Contrast-enhanced T1-weighted images identify a fistula as abnormal enhancement surrounding the low-signal-intensity fistular canal. A fistula from the uterus or vagina to the bladder is suggested when there is air in the bladder [71].

Postactinic radiogenic colitis is characterized by concentric edematous thickening of the intestinal wall with preservation of the layered structure and may be associated with additional edematous thickening and infiltration of the perirectal fat. Radiation-induced stricture of the ureter or insufficiency fracture of the

sacral bone have become rare. The bone marrow of the pelvic bone in the irradiated field is regularly replaced with fat marrow, which is depicted on T1-weighted images with a high signal intensity.

7.2.5.4
Recurrent Cervical Cancer

Cervical cancer tends to recur within 2 years after the initial diagnosis. Recurrence is defined as the demonstration of renewed local tumor growth, development of nodal metastases, or hematogenous distant metastases after a tumor-free interval of at least 6 months. About 30% of patients with invasive cervical carcinoma die because of recurrent disease. Some guidelines recommend follow-up examinations at 3-month intervals during the first 3 years, every 6 months during the next 2 years, and once a year thereafter. A survival advantage from inclusion in structured follow-up has not been demonstrated. The routine follow-up tests comprise a gynecologic examination, which may be supplemented by colposcopy and cytology, and a transvaginal ultrasound examination. More extensive tests are performed in patients with suspected locoregional tumor recurrence. Recurrence is suggested by the findings of the gynecologic follow-up examination or if the patient reports difficulties passing urine or

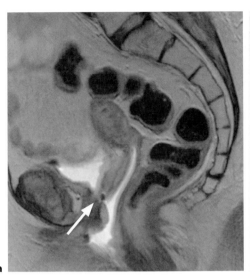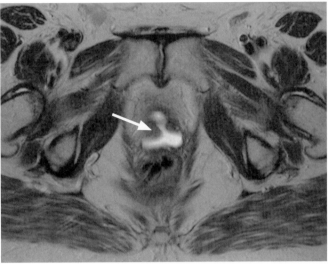

a   b

Fig. 7.47a,b. Fistula after radiochemotherapy. **a, b** T2w TSE images in sagittal and transverse orientation. Following radiochemotherapy of advanced cervical cancer, a fistula depicted as a high-signal-intensity fluid-filled connection is seen between the vagina and urinary bladder (*arrows*). There is urine in the vagina

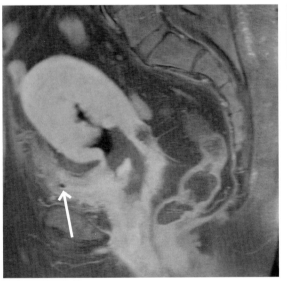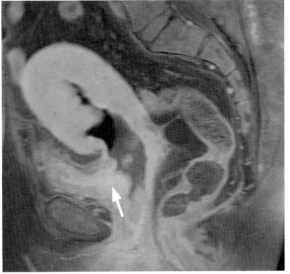

a   b

Fig. 7.48a,b. Fistula after radiochemotherapy. **a, b** T2w TSE images in sagittal and transverse orientation. Following radiochemotherapy of advanced cervical cancer, a fistula depicted as a high-signal-intensity fluid-filled connection is seen between the vagina and urinary bladder (*arrow*). There is air in the bladder (*open arrow*)

stools or other suspicious complaints. Recurrent tumor of the pelvic sidewall may manifest with pain due to nerve infiltration or leg edema due to obliteration of the lymphatics.

Usually follow-up MRI is not indicated during the first 6 months after completion of primary therapy due to limitations of MRI in differentiating recurrent tumor from acute peri- or postoperative changes [111]. As with primary staging, follow-up MRI should be performed by using sagittal and transverse T2-weighted sequences as well as a respiratory-gated T1-weighted abdominal PACE sequence and a T1-weighted pelvic sequence for lymph node staging. In contrast to pretreatment MRI, the follow-up examination should always comprise a contrast-enhanced T1-weighted sequence. These are always performed in combination with an unenhanced T1-weighted examination in identical orientations. Ideally, the con-

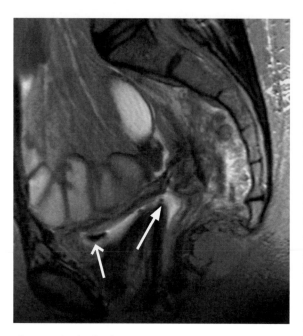

Fig. 7.49. Fistula after hysterectomy. A T2w TSE image in sagittal orientation. Following hysterectomy for cervical cancer, a fistula depicted as a high-signal-intensity fluid-filled connection is seen between the vagina and urinary bladder (*arrow*). There is air in the bladder (*open arrow*)

trast-enhanced images should allow differentiation of recurrent tumor, which shows early and pronounced enhancement, from scar tissue. If there is extension to the pelvic floor, this basic protocol can be supplemented by T2-weighted sequences in coronal orientation. If hydronephrosis is suspected, an additional coronal T2-weighted sequence or contrast-enhanced MR urography are indicated.

Recurrent cervical cancer has a variable appearance at MRI. The tumor may have a nodular appearance with a blurred contour and extensions into surrounding tissue, which may lead to fixation of bowel loops. The irregular contour is due to tumor extensions and desmoplastic reactions. Alternatively, a recurrent tumor may show diffuse growth. In this case, the absence of a circumscribed mass makes a tumor especially difficult to distinguish from a postoperative scar. In the clinical examination, both a scar and recurrent tumor may appear indurated. Problems are also posed by nodular scars and scars with adhesion to surrounding structures. T2-weighted MR images depict recurrent tumor as an inhomogeneous lesion with an irregular borders [112]. Recurrent cancer can be differentiated from scar tissue and muscle by a higher signal intensity on T2-weighted images as well as earlier and more pronounced enhancement on contrast-enhanced T1-

weighted images. Regressive tumor portions may be identified by lack of enhancement. In contrast, scar tissue resembles muscle with a low signal intensity on T1- and T2-weighted images. Moreover, scars show only little and late enhancement on condition that MRI is performed not earlier than 6 months after the end of therapy. During the first 6 months after therapy, MRI cannot differentiate vital tumor tissue from postoperative reactive changes.

Despite the short examination and the absence of artifacts caused by bowel motion, CT has little use in differentiating posttherapeutic changes and recurrent tumor in the true pelvis. However, CT of the chest, abdomen, and pelvis after oral opacification and IV contrast medium administration can be used in the follow-up of cervical cancer to exclude distant metastases and nodal involvement. The benefit of whole body FDG PET in detecting recurrent cervical cancer and distant metastasis is currently being investigated [113, 114]. As with MRI, at least 6 months should elapse after primary therapy to correctly interpret increased focal accumulation.

Recurrent tumor after surgery is most frequently seen in the operative bed, primarily the vaginal stump, and at the resection margins, in particular the pelvic sidewalls. After radical hysterectomy, most tumors show supravaginal recurrence (20%) at the roof of the vaginal stump and in the rectovaginal space, typically between the bladder and the rectum. An occasional patient may develop fibrotic scar tissue at the roof of the vaginal stump, which is characterized by moderate to low signal intensity on T2-weighted and T1-weighted images. When recurrent tumor has been identified, its relationship to the vaginal stump should be described and infiltration of the urinary bladder or rectum should be excluded (Figs. 7.11, 7.50).

Posterior tumor growth leads to infiltration of the presacral space and sacral bone or of the perirectal space and rectum. Recurrent cervical cancer is associated with rectal infiltration in about 17% of cases. The most common site is the rectosigmoid junction. Laterally, recurrent tumor may extend to the pelvic sidewall. If the recurrent local tumor grows anteriorly along the peritoneal fold, there will be infiltration of the urinary bladder. Advanced recurrent cervical cancer may involve the remaining colon or the small intestine and is typically associated with adhesion of bowel loops and may cause intestinal obstruction.

The second most common site of recurrence is the pelvic sidewall, which is the preferred site of nodal metastasis (Figs. 7.51, 7.52). An important issue is their topographic relationship to the bony pelvis

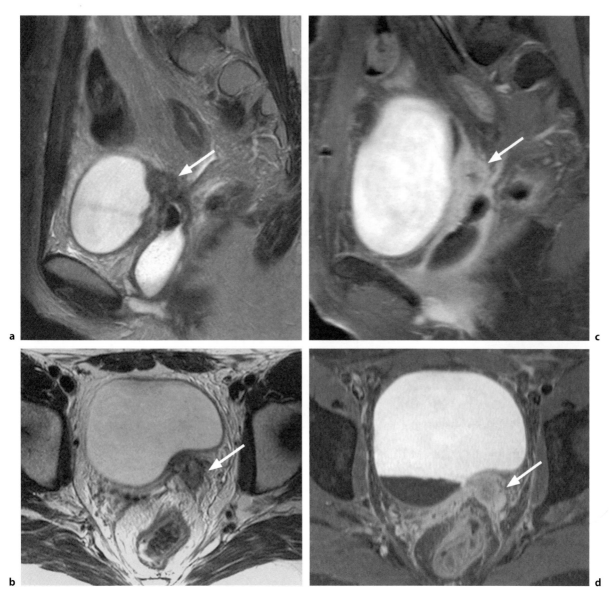

Fig. 7.50a–d. Recurrent cervical cancer after hysterectomy. **a, b** T2w TSE images in sagittal and transverse orientation. **c, d** T1w TSE images in sagittal and transverse orientation 1 min after administration of Gd-DTPA. MRI after hysterectomy depicts a nodular lesion at the roof of the vagina with enhancement on the postcontrast images (*arrows*). Note the unusually low signal intensity of the lesion (like a scar); however, tumor recurrence is indicated by the strong contrast enhancement. Gel filling of the vagina

and the iliac vessels because of its implications for the surgical technique. In relation to the iliac vessels, infra- and peri-iliac metastases are distinguished; in relation to the bones, a distinction is made between ischiopubic, acetabular, iliosacral, and sacrococcygeal metastases. Further progression may lead to destruction of the bony pelvis.

Pelvic tumor recurrence typically leads to external ureteral obstruction through encasement of the ureters and their orifices, which manifests as hydronephrosis. Follow-up MRI enables evaluation of both the etiology and the site of the obstruction.

Local recurrence after primary radiochemotherapy is characterized by the development of a new tumor in the cervix or infiltration of the vagina (Fig. 7.53). Alternatively, there may be recurrence in the parametria with lateral extension at the level of the cervix and vagina [97]. A large recurrent tumor with a mass effect within the cervix may obstruct the internal os with development of hydrometra or pyo-

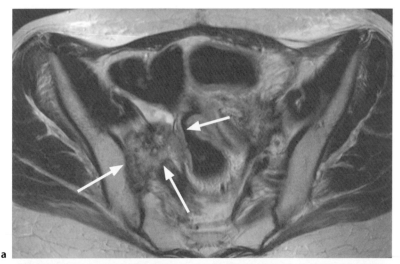

a

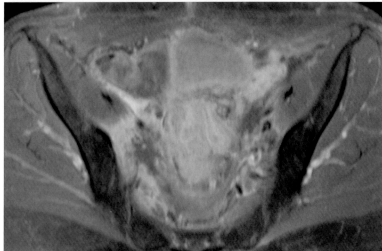

b

Fig. 7.51a,b. Recurrent tumor of the pelvic sidewall after hysterectomy. A T2w TSE image in transverse orientation. At the right pelvic sidewall, a solid, heterogeneous mass (*arrows*) is depicted that infiltrates the pelvic wall and extends to the iliac bone. Tumor adhesion to the sigmoid colon. **b** T1w TSE image with FS transverse orientation 1 min after administration of Gd-DTPA. MRI depicts an enhancement on the postcontrast image and central necrosis

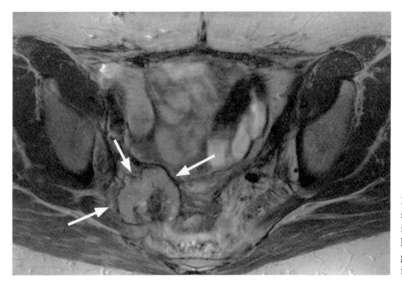

Fig. 7.52. Recurrent tumor of the pelvic sidewall after hysterectomy. T2w TSE image in sagittal orientation. A solid, heterogeneous mass with irregular margins (*arrows*) and infiltration of muscle is seen anterior to the sciatic foramen

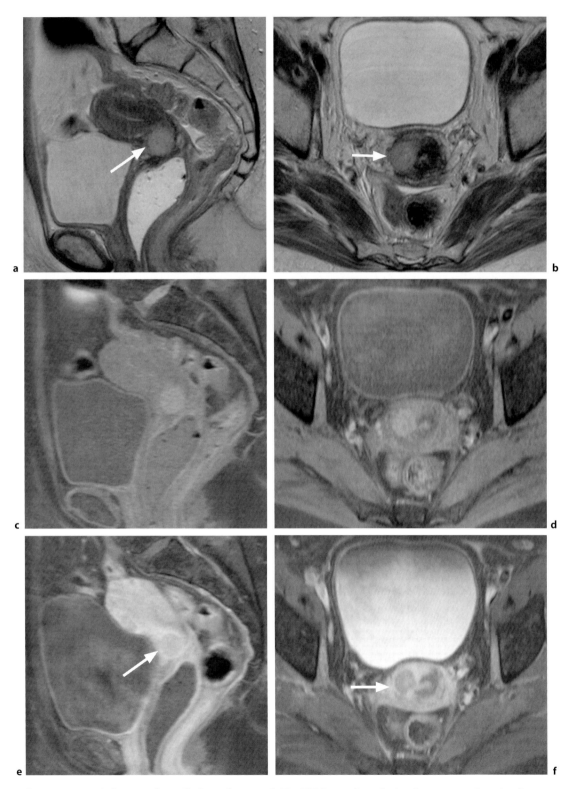

Fig. 7.53a–f. Recurrent cervical cancer after radiochemotherapy. **a, b** T2w TSE images in sagittal and transverse orientation. Recurrent cervical cancer 6 months after primary radiochemotherapy. The high-signal-intensity mass (*arrows*) is located eccentrically on the right side of the cervix. Gel filling of the vagina. **c, d** T1w TSE images with FS in sagittal and transverse orientation showing recurrent cervical cancer with slightly higher signal intensity. **e, f** T1w TSE images with FS in sagittal and transverse orientation 1 min after administration of Gd-DTPA. MRI depicts a moderate enhancement on the postcontrast image (*arrows*)

metra. Alternatively, the cervix can be obstructed by radiation-induced stenoses. This is depicted by CT and MRI as a symmetrically enlarged uterine corpus containing nonenhancing fluid.

Patients with central pelvic tumor recurrence are operated on with curative intention if possible. Curative pelvic exenteration is more difficult when the pelvic wall is infiltrated. Hence, recurrent tumor of the pelvic wall is typically treated by radiochemotherapy, which can be performed with a curative dose in patients not having undergone irradiation before. Local control of recurrence in the pelvic wall is poorer and has a more unfavorable prognosis than central pelvic recurrence. Specific surgical procedures and possibly reduced radiotherapy are available for patients having been irradiated before. However, these aggressive measures are associated with considerable side effects. Lymph node metastasis is typically treated by radiotherapy and hematogenous distant metastasis by chemotherapy.

7.2.6
Role of Other Diagnostic Modalities

7.2.6.1
Ultrasound

While ultrasonography has a role in endometrial cancer, it is of little use in detection and staging of cervical cancer. Ultrasonography does not allow reliable demonstration of parametrial infiltration. But direct imaging of cervical cancer in controlling tumor response to radiochemotherapy in 3D ultrasound is under evaluation. The sonographic evaluation of the pelvic and para-aortic lymph nodes is limited due to their location at the pelvic wall or retroperitoneally and overlying bowel gas [115]. Transrectal ultrasound is not widely used [116, 117]. Transabdominal ultrasound is routinely used in pretherapeutic staging, typically to exclude liver metastases and at follow-up, above all to exclude ureteral obstruction. Ultrasonography is limited by its dependence on the examiner and the equipment used and lacks adequate documentation and reproducibility of the findings.

7.2.6.2
PET

There exist no guidelines for the use of FDG PET in patients with cervical cancer. Studies investigating the use of whole-body FDG PET in cervical cancer demonstrated its diagnostic usefulness in lymph node staging

[94], and in demonstrating recurrent tumor [114, 118]. Results of FDG-PET in evaluating tumor extent before and after therapy show limited usefulness. Nevertheless, PET also has diagnostic limitations that include the detection of small lesions or the differentiation of tumor from reactive changes. Moreover, the FDG PET findings usually have to be combined with the morphologic information provided by MRI or CT. The cost-benefit analysis must take into account the still limited availability of FDG PET, the duration of the examination (20–60 min), and the high cost. Studies in larger patient populations aim at identifying suitable indications for this modality, as it is not universally applicable.

7.2.7
Other Malignant Tumors of the Cervix

7.2.7.1
Metastasis

Most metastases to the cervix are from endometrial cancer (Fig. 7.54) (or by tumor infiltration per continuitatem), less commonly from other primary tumors of the ovaries, breast, or stomach.

7.2.7.2
Malignant Melanoma

Between 1% and 3% of malignant melanomas in women occur in the genital tract, where they typically arise in the vaginal mucosa and infiltrate the uterine cervix. Primary cervical melanoma is rare. Melanomas of the female genital tract are characterized by a high signal intensity on T1-weighted images and a low signal on T2-weighted images. The degree of signal shortening on T1-weighted images varies with the melanin content. The signal is further altered by intralesional hemorrhages, which are quite common [119–121].

7.2.7.3
Lymphoma

Malignant lymphoma of the uterus is typically due to secondary infiltration by advanced lymphoma from other sites. Primary manifestations in the uterus account for only 2% of all primary extranodal malignant lymphomas and typically affect the cervix. Cervical lymphoma is of low signal intensity on T1-weighted images and of high signal intensity on T2-weighted images and thus resembles cervical squamous cell carcinoma. In most cases, lymphoma can be distinguished by its typically large size and the absence of infiltration of surrounding structures. In a similar manner, the uterine corpus will show diffuse infiltration and enlargement when there is lymphoma in this part of the uterus [122–124].

7.2.8
Benign Lesions of the Cervix

7.2.8.1
Nabothian Cyst

Nabothian cysts are retention cysts of the cervical glands that develop secondary to chronic cervicitis and are often discovered incidentally (Fig. 7.55). Cervicitis is associated with epithelial proliferation and may lead to localized overgrowth and obstruction of glands. Nabothian cysts usually measure only a few millimeters but may grow in size to over 4 cm and then produce a mass effect. They have an intermediate to higher signal intensity on T1-weighted images that reflects the protein content of the cyst content. On T2-weighted images, they have a high signal intensity and are depicted as round to oval lesions with

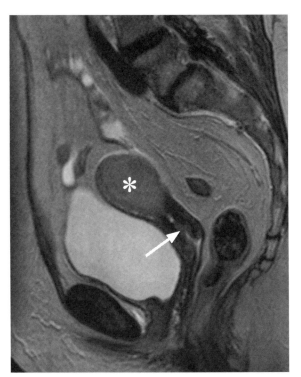

Fig. 7.54. Other tumors of the cervix. T2w TSE image in sagittal orientation. Cervical manifestation (*asterik*) of endometrial cancer (*arrow*)

a smooth margin [29]. Their differentiation from the rare adenoma malignum (well differentiated cervical adenocarcinoma with cystic portions) may be difficult by MRI. The depiction of solid portions surrounding or separating the cysts suggests malignancy [28].

7.2.8.2
Leiomyoma

Fewer than 10% of leiomyomas of the uterus affect the cervix [125, 126]. The typical clinical symptoms of cervical leiomyoma are infertility and complications during pregnancy. The lesions are characterized on T2-weighted images by a low signal intensity, a smooth contour, and a roundish shape (see Sect. 7.2.7.2).

7.2.8.3
Polyps

Cervical polyps are the most common benign lesions of the cervix. They typically occur in perimenopausal women and often cause bleeding between periods. They are usually pedicled and range in size from a few millimeters to 3 cm. Their pathogenesis is multifactorial and includes metaplastic processes and inflammatory changes of the cervical glands. Cervical polyps are diagnosed by hysteroscopy. Imaging modalities typically depict them as masses of the endocervix [127].

7.2.8.4
Rare Benign Tumors

The rare benign tumors of the cervix comprise capillary or cavernous hemangioma, lymphangioma, papillary adenofibroma, adenomyoma, fibroadenoma, and mesonephric papilloma.

7.2.8.5
Cervicitis

Cervicitis is caused by the same pathogens as vaginitis. These include *Trichomonas vaginalis*, *Candida albicans*, and Herpes simplex virus. They invade the epithelium of the portio and cause inflammation of the ectocervix. In contrast, bacteria such as *Neisseria gonorrhoeae* and *Chlamydia trachomatis* affect the cervical glands and cause mucopurulent endocervicitis. Bacterial infection may manifest with vaginal discharge or dull pelvic pain. Occasionally, retention cysts may develop in the cervix and can be demonstrated by MRI but may be difficult to differentiated

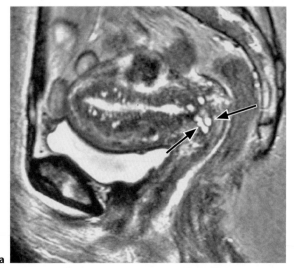

a

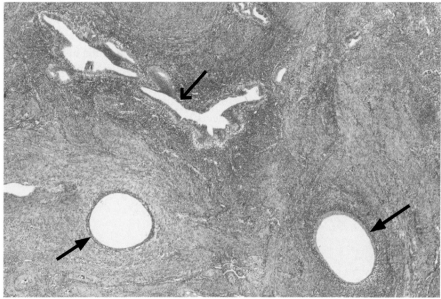

b

Fig. 7.55a,b. Nabothian cysts. **a** T2w TSE image in sagittal orientation. Cystic lesions in the cervical stroma (*arrows*). **b** H&E-stained specimen of the cervix with intrastromal cystic lesions (*arrows*). Also seen are cervical glands (*open arrow*)

from glandular hyperplasia or adenoma malignum on the basis of their MRI appearance alone when clinical symptoms are absent [128].

7.2.8.6
Endometriosis

Cervical endometriosis is rare and, when present, typically affects the portio or the endocervical canal. The solid tissue portions of an endometriosis lesion are of low signal intensity on T1-weighted and T2-weighted images and exhibit pronounced contrast enhancement. The lesions usually contain blood that often gives rise to the development of cystic portions with a high signal intensity on T1-weighted images. Alternatively, en-

dometriosis of the uterine corpus may protrude into the cervical canal as a polypoid mass that is covered by endometrial mucosa as the lesion arises from the junctional zone of the myometrium.

7.2.8.7
Ectopic Cervical Pregnancy

The number of cervical pregnancies is increasing as more women have abortions. Its rate is 1 per 1,000–24,000 pregnancies. MRI depicts a cervical pregnancy as a cervical mass of heterogeneous signal intensity with a low-signal-intensity margin that may not surround the lesion on all sides [129]. It is usually an exclusion diagnosis.

References

1. Schuz J, Schon D, Batzler W, Baumgardt-Elms C, Eisinger B, Lehnert M, Stegmaier C (2000) Cancer registration in Germany: current status, perspectives and trends in cancer incidence 1973–93. J Epidemiol Biostat 5:99–107

2. Bray F, Sankila R, Ferlay J, Parkin DM (2002) Estimates of cancer incidence and mortality in Europe in 1995. Eur J Cancer 38:99–166

3. Nagel G, Zoller D, Wiedmann T, Bussas U, El Idrissi-Lamghari C, Kneisel J, Batzler WU, Becker N (2004) [The use of the epidemiology cancer registry Baden-Wurttemberg in the follow-up of the EPIC cohort]. Gesundheitswesen 66:469–474

4. Gustafsson L, Ponten J, Bergstrom R, Adami HO (1997) International incidence rates of invasive cervical cancer before cytological screening. Int J Cancer 71:159–165

5. Womack C, Warren AY (1998) The cervical screening muddle. Lancet 351:1129

6. Plaxe SC, Saltzstein SL (1999) Estimation of the duration of the preclinical phase of cervical adenocarcinoma suggests that there is ample opportunity for screening. Gynecol Oncol 75:55–61

7. Green JA, Kirwan JM, Tierney JF, Symonds P, Fresco L, Collingwood M, Williams CJ (2001) Survival and recurrence after concomitant chemotherapy and radiotherapy for cancer of the uterine cervix: a systematic review and meta-analysis. Lancet 358:781–786

8. Brenner H (2002) Long-term survival rates of cancer patients achieved by the end of the 20th century: a period analysis. Lancet 360:1131–1135

9. Castle PE, Wacholder S, Lorincz AT, Scott DR, Sherman ME, Glass AG, Rush BB, Schussler JE, Schiffman M (2002) A prospective study of high-grade cervical neoplasia risk among human papillomavirus-infected women. J Natl Cancer Inst 94:1406–1414

10. Lorincz AT, Castle PE, Sherman ME, Scott DR, Glass AG, Wacholder S, Rush BB, Gravitt PE, Schussler JE, Schiffman M (2002) Viral load of human papillomavirus and risk of CIN3 or cervical cancer. Lancet 360:228–229

11. Walboomers JM, Jacobs MV, Manos MM, Bosch FX, Kummer JA, Shah KV, Snijders PJ, Peto J, Meijer CJ, Munoz N (1999) Human papillomavirus is a necessary cause of invasive cervical cancer worldwide. J Pathol 189:12–19

12. Yamada T, Manos MM, Peto J, Greer CE, Munoz N, Bosch FX, Wheeler CM (1997) Human papillomavirus type 16 sequence variation in cervical cancers: a worldwide perspective. J Virol 71:2463–2472

13. Bosch FX, Manos MM, Munoz N, Sherman M, Jansen AM, Peto J, Schiffman MH, Moreno V, Kurman R, Shah KV (1995) Prevalence of human papillomavirus in cervical cancer: a worldwide perspective. International biological study on cervical cancer (IBSCC) Study Group. J Natl Cancer Inst 87:796–802

14. Munoz N, Franceschi S, Bosetti C, Moreno V, Herrero R, Smith JS, Shah KV, Meijer CJ, Bosch FX (2002) Role of parity and human papillomavirus in cervical cancer: the IARC multicentric case–control study. Lancet 359:1093–1101

15. Smith JS, Herrero R, Bosetti C, Munoz N, Bosch FX, Eluf-Neto J, Castellsague X, Meijer CJ, Van den Brule AJ, Franceschi S, Ashley R (2002) Herpes simplex virus-2 as a human papillomavirus cofactor in the etiology of invasive cervical cancer. J Natl Cancer Inst 94:1604–1613

16. Smith JS, Munoz N, Herrero R, Eluf-Neto J, Ngelangel C, Franceschi S, Bosch FX, Walboomers JM, Peeling RW (2002) Evidence for Chlamydia trachomatis as a human papillomavirus cofactor in the etiology of invasive cervical cancer in Brazil and the Philippines. J Infect Dis 185:324–331

17. Richart RM (1973) Cervical intraepithelial neoplasia. Pathol Annu 8:301–328

18. Mitchell MF, Schottenfeld D, Tortolero-Luna G, Cantor SB, Richards-Kortum R (1998) Colposcopy for the diagnosis of squamous intraepithelial lesions: a meta-analysis. Obstet Gynecol 91:626–631

19. Sung HY, Kearney KA, Miller M, Kinney W, Sawaya GF, Hiatt RA (2000) Papanicolaou smear history and diagnosis of invasive cervical carcinoma among members of a large prepaid health plan. Cancer 88:2283–2289

20. McCrory DC, Matchar DB, Bastian L, Datta S, Hasselblad V, Hickey J, Myers E, Nanda K (1999) Evaluation of cervical cytology. Evid Rep Technol Assess (Summ) Jan:1–6

21. Nanda K, McCrory DC, Myers ER, Bastian LA, Hasselblad V, Hickey JD, Matchar DB (2000) Accuracy of the Papanicolaou test in screening for and follow-up of cervical cytologic abnormalities: a systematic review. Ann Intern Med 132:810–819

22. Womack C, Warren AY (1998) Achievable laboratory standards; a review of cytology of 99 women with cervical cancer. Cytopathology 9:171–177

23. Miller MG, Sung HY, Sawaya GF, Kearney KA, Kinney W, Hiatt RA (2003) Screening interval and risk of invasive squamous cell cervical cancer. Obstet Gynecol 101:29–37

24. Vizcaino AP, Moreno V, Bosch FX, Munoz N, Barros-Dios XM, Borras J, Parkin DM (2000) International trends in incidence of cervical cancer: II. Squamous-cell carcinoma. Int J Cancer 86:429–435

25. Davidson SE, Symonds RP, Lamont D, Watson ER (1989) Does adenocarcinoma of uterine cervix have a worse prognosis than squamous carcinoma when treated by radiotherapy? Gynecol Oncol 33:23–26

26. Kaminski PF, Norris HJ (1983) Minimal deviation carcinoma (adenoma malignum) of the cervix. Int J Gynecol Pathol 2:141–152

27. Fu YS, Reagan JW, Fu AS, Janiga KE (1982) Adenocarcinoma and mixed carcinoma of the uterine cervix. II. Prognostic value of nuclear DNA analysis. Cancer 49:2571–2577

28. Doi T, Yamashita Y, Yasunaga T, Fujiyoshi K, Tsunawaki A, Takahashi M, Katabuchi H, Tanaka N, Okamura H (1997) Adenoma malignum: MR imaging and pathologic study. Radiology 204:39–42

29. Li H, Sugimura K, Okizuka H, Yoshida M, Maruyama R, Takahashi K, Miyazaki K (1999) Markedly high signal intensity lesions in the uterine cervix on T2-weighted imaging: differentiation between mucin-producing carcinomas and nabothian cysts. Radiat Med 17:137–143

30. Chen KT (1986) Female genital tract tumors in Peutz-Jeghers syndrome. Hum Pathol 17:858–861

31. Lea JS, Sheets EE, Wenham RM, Duska LR, Coleman RL, Miller DS, Schorge JO (2002) Stage IIB–IVB cervical adenocarcinoma: prognostic factors and survival. Gynecol Oncol 84:115–119

32. Koch CA, Azumi N, Furlong MA, Jha RC, Kehoe TE, Trowbridge CH, O'Dorisio TM, Chrousos GP, Clement SC (1999) Carcinoid syndrome caused by an atypical

carcinoid of the uterine cervix. J Clin Endocrinol Metab 84:4209–4213

33. Ueda G, Yamasaki M (1992) Neuroendocrine carcinoma of the uterus. Curr Top Pathol 85:309–335

34. Sheridan E, Lorigan PC, Goepel J, Radstone DJ, Coleman RE (1996) Small cell carcinoma of the cervix. Clin Oncol (R Coll Radiol) 8:102–105

35. Benedet JL, Bender H, Jones H 3rd, Ngan HY, Pecorelli S (2000) FIGO staging classifications and clinical practice guidelines in the management of gynecologic cancers. FIGO Committee on Gynecologic Oncology. Int J Gynaecol Obstet 70:209–262

36. Lagasse LD, Creasman WT, Shingleton HM, Ford JH, Blessing JA (1980) Results and complications of operative staging in cervical cancer: experience of the Gynecologic Oncology Group. Gynecol Oncol 9:90–98

37. Dargent D, Frobert JL, Beau G (1985) V factor (tumor volume) and T factor (FIGO classification) in the assessment of cervix cancer prognosis: the risk of lymph node spread. Gynecol Oncol 22:15–22

38. Ho CM, Chien TY, Jeng CM, Tsang YM, Shih BY, Chang SC (1992) Staging of cervical cancer: comparison between magnetic resonance imaging, computed tomography and pelvic examination under anesthesia. J Formos Med Assoc 91:982–990

39. LaPolla JP, Schlaerth JB, Gaddis O, Morrow CP (1986) The influence of surgical staging on the evaluation and treatment of patients with cervical carcinoma. Gynecol Oncol 24:194–206

40. Scheidler J, Hricak H, Yu KK, Subak L, Segal MR (1997) Radiological evaluation of lymph node metastases in patients with cervical cancer. A meta-analysis. JAMA 278:1096–1101

41. Grigsby PW, Dehdashti F, Siegel BA (1999) FDG-PET evaluation of carcinoma of the cervix. Clin Positron Imaging 2:105–109

42. Metcalf KS, Johnson N, Calvert S, Peel KR (2000) Site specific lymph node metastasis in carcinoma of the cervix: is there a sentinel node? Int J Gynecol Cancer 10:411–416

43. Sevin BU, Nadji M, Lampe B, Lu Y, Hilsenbeck S, Koechli OR, Averette HE (1995) Prognostic factors of early stage cervical cancer treated by radical hysterectomy. Cancer 76:1978–1986

44. Fagundes H, Perez CA, Grigsby PW, Lockett MA (1992) Distant metastases after irradiation alone in carcinoma of the uterine cervix. Int J Radiat Oncol Biol Phys 24:197–204

45. Perez CA, Grigsby PW, Camel HM, Galakatos AE, Mutch D, Lockett MA (1995) Irradiation alone or combined with surgery in stage IB, IIA, and IIB carcinoma of uterine cervix: update of a nonrandomized comparison. Int J Radiat Oncol Biol Phys 31:703–716

46. Friedlander M, Grogan M (2002) Guidelines for the treatment of recurrent and metastatic cervical cancer. Oncologist 7:342–347

47. Stehman FB, Bundy BN, DiSaia PJ, Keys HM, Larson JE, Fowler WC (1991) Carcinoma of the cervix treated with radiation therapy. I. A multi-variate analysis of prognostic variables in the Gynecologic Oncology Group. Cancer 67:2776–2785

48. Burghardt E, Baltzer J, Tulusan AH, Haas J (1992) Results of surgical treatment of 1028 cervical cancers studied with volumetry. Cancer 70:648–655

49. Perez CA, Camel HM, Kuske RR, Kao MS, Galakatos A, Hederman MA, Powers WE (1986) Radiation therapy alone in the treatment of carcinoma of the uterine cervix: a 20-year experience. Gynecol Oncol 23:127–140

50. Schorge JO, Lee KR, Sheets EE (2000) Prospective management of stage IA(1) cervical adenocarcinoma by conization alone to preserve fertility: a preliminary report. Gynecol Oncol 78:217–220

51. Benedet JL, Anderson GH (1996) Stage IA carcinoma of the cervix revisited. Obstet Gynecol 87:1052–1059

52. Piver MS, Rutledge F, Smith JP (1974) Five classes of extended hysterectomy for women with cervical cancer. Obstet Gynecol 44:265–272

53. Dargent D, Martin X, Sacchetoni A, Mathevet P (2000) Laparoscopic vaginal radical trachelectomy: a treatment to preserve the fertility of cervical carcinoma patients. Cancer 88:1877–1882

54. Shepherd JH, Mould T, Oram DH (2001) Radical trachelectomy in early stage carcinoma of the cervix: outcome as judged by recurrence and fertility rates. BJOG 108:882–885

55. Covens A, Shaw P, Murphy J, DePetrillo D, Lickrish G, Laframboise S, Rosen B (1999) Is radical trachelectomy a safe alternative to radical hysterectomy for patients with stage IA–B carcinoma of the cervix? Cancer 86:2273–2279

56. Bernardini M, Barrett J, Seaward G, Covens A (2003) Pregnancy outcomes in patients after radical trachelectomy. Am J Obstet Gynecol 189:1378–1382

57. Morice P, Dargent D, Haie-Meder C, Duvillard P, Castaigne D (2004) First case of a centropelvic recurrence after radical trachelectomy: literature review and implications for the preoperative selection of patients. Gynecol Oncol 92:1002–1005

58. Committee on Practice B-G (2002) ACOG practice bulletin. Diagnosis and treatment of cervical carcinomas, number 35, May 2002.   Obstet Gynecol 99:855–867

59. Martinez-Palones JM, Gil-Moreno A, Perez-Benavente MA, Roca I, Xercavins J (2004) Intraoperative sentinel node identification in early stage cervical cancer using a combination of radiolabeled albumin injection and iso-sulfan blue dye injection. Gynecol Oncol 92:845–850

60. Marchiole P, Buenerd A, Scoazec JY, Dargent D, Mathevet P (2004) Sentinel lymph node biopsy is not accurate in predicting lymph node status for patients with cervical carcinoma. Cancer 100:2154–2159

61. Sedlis A, Bundy BN, Rotman MZ, Lentz SS, Muderspach LI, Zaino RJ (1999) A randomized trial of pelvic radiation therapy versus no further therapy in selected patients with stage IB carcinoma of the cervix after radical hysterectomy and pelvic lymphadenectomy: a Gynecologic Oncology Group Study. Gynecol Oncol 73:177–183

62. Grigsby PW, Perez CA (1991) Radiotherapy alone for medically inoperable carcinoma of the cervix: stage IA and carcinoma in situ. Int J Radiat Oncol Biol Phys 21:375–378

63. Holtz DO, Dunton C (2002) Traditional management of invasive cervical cancer. Obstet Gynecol Clin North Am 29:645–657

64. Sant M, Capocaccia R, Coleman MP, Berrino F, Gatta G, Micheli A, Verdecchia A, Faivre J, Hakulinen T, Coebergh JW, Martinez-Garcia C, Forman D, Zappone A (2001) Cancer survival increases in Europe, but international differences remain wide. Eur J Cancer 37:1659–1667

65. Hille A, Weiss E, Hess CF (2003) Therapeutic outcome and prognostic factors in the radiotherapy of recurrences of cervical carcinoma following surgery. Strahlenther Onkol 179:742–747

66. Mezrich R (1994) Magnetic resonance imaging applications in uterine cervical cancer. Magn Reson Imaging Clin N Am 2:211–243

67. Boss EA, Barentsz JO, Massuger LF, Boonstra H (2000) The role of MR imaging in invasive cervical carcinoma. Eur Radiol 10:256–270

68. Brenner DE, Whitley NO, Prempree T, Villasanta U (1982) An evaluation of the computed tomographic scanner for the staging of carcinoma of the cervix. Cancer 50:2323–2328

69. Villasanta U, Whitley NO, Haney PJ, Brenner D (1983) Computed tomography in invasive carcinoma of the cervix: an appraisal. Obstet Gynecol 62:218–224

70. Hricak H, Lacey CG, Sandles LG, Chang YC, Winkler ML, Stern JL (1988) Invasive cervical carcinoma: comparison of MR imaging and surgical findings. Radiology 166:623–631

71. Kim SH, Han MC (1997) Invasion of the urinary bladder by uterine cervical carcinoma: evaluation with MR imaging. AJR Am J Roentgenol 168:393–397

72. Kim SH, Choi BI, Han JK, Kim HD, Lee HP, Kang SB, Lee JY, Han MC (1993) Preoperative staging of uterine cervical carcinoma: comparison of CT and MRI in 99 patients. J Comput Assist Tomogr 17:633–640

73. Brodman M, Friedman F Jr, Dottino P, Janus C, Plaxe S, Cohen C (1990) A comparative study of computerized tomography, magnetic resonance imaging, and clinical staging for the detection of early cervix cancer. Gynecol Oncol 36:409–412

74. Togashi K, Nishimura K, Sagoh T, Minami S, Noma S, Fujisawa I, Nakano Y, Konishi J, Ozasa H, Konishi I et al (1989) Carcinoma of the cervix: staging with MR imaging. Radiology 171:245–251

75. Preidler KW, Tamussino K, Szolar DM, Ranner G, Ebner F (1996) Staging of cervical carcinomas. Comparison of body-coil magnetic resonance imaging and endorectal surface coil magnetic resonance imaging with histopathologic correlation. Invest Radiol 31:458–462

76. Ebner F, Tamussino K, Kressel HY (1994) Magnetic resonance imaging in cervical carcinoma: diagnosis, staging, and follow-up. Magn Reson Q 10:22–42

77. Yamashita Y, Harada M, Torashima M, Takahashi M, Miyazaki K, Tanaka N, Okamura H (1996) Dynamic MR imaging of recurrent postoperative cervical cancer. J Magn Reson Imaging 6:167–171

78. Brown JJ, Gutierrez ED, Lee JK (1992) MR appearance of the normal and abnormal vagina after hysterectomy. AJR Am J Roentgenol 158:95–99

79. Hricak H, Powell CB, Yu KK, Washington E, Subak LL, Stern JL, Cisternas MG, Arenson RL (1996) Invasive cervical carcinoma: role of MR imaging in pretreatment work-up-cost minimization and diagnostic efficacy analysis. Radiology 198:403–409

80. Heron CW, Husband JE, Williams MP, Dobbs HJ, Cosgrove DO (1988) The value of CT in the diagnosis of recurrent carcinoma of the cervix. Clin Radiol 39:496–501

81. Walsh JW, Amendola MA, Hall DJ, Tisnado J, Goplerud DR (1981) Recurrent carcinoma of the cervix: CT diagnosis. AJR Am J Roentgenol 136:117–122

82. Hawighorst H, Knapstein PG, Weikel W, Knopp MV, Schaeffer U, Essig M, Brix G, Zuna I, Schonberg S, van Kaick G (1997) [Invasive cervix carcinoma (pT2b–pT4a). Value of conventional and pharmacokinetic magnetic resonance tomography (MRI) in comparison with extensive cross sections and histopathologic findings]. Radiologe 37:130–138

83. Hricak H, Hamm B, Semelka RC, Cann CE, Nauert T, Secaf E, Stern JL, Wolf KJ (1991) Carcinoma of the uterus: use of gadopentetate dimeglumine in MR imaging. Radiology 181:95–106

84. Postema S, Pattynama PM, van Rijswijk CS, Trimbos JB (1999) Cervical carcinoma: can dynamic contrast-enhanced MR imaging help predict tumor aggressiveness? Radiology 1999; 210:217–220

85. Postema S, Pattynama PM, Broker S, van der Geest RJ, van Rijswijk CS, Baptist Trimbos J (1998) Fast dynamic contrast-enhanced colour-coded MRI in uterine cervix carcinoma: useful for tumour staging? Clin Radiol 53:729–734

86. Hawighorst H, Knapstein PG, Knopp MV, Weikel W, Schaeffer U, Zuna I, Schonberg SO, Essig M, Hoffmann U, Brix G, van Kaick G (1998) [Angiogenesis of cervix carcinoma. Contrast-enhanced dynamic MRI, histologic quantification of capillary density and lymphatic system infiltration]. Radiologe 38:50–57

87. Shiraiwa M, Joja I, Asakawa T, Okuno K, Shibutani O, Akamatsu N, Kudo T, Hiraki Y (1999) Cervical carcinoma: efficacy of thin-section oblique axial T2-weighted images for evaluating parametrial invasion. Abdom Imaging 24:514–519

88. Hawnaur JM, Johnson RJ, Buckley CH, Tindall V, Isherwood I (1994) Staging, volume estimation and assessment of nodal status in carcinoma of the cervix: comparison of magnetic resonance imaging with surgical findings. Clin Radiol 49:443–452

89. Duffaud F, Therasse P (2000) [New guidelines to evaluate the response to treatment in solid tumors]. Bull Cancer 87:881–886

90. Rubens D, Thornbury JR, Angel C, Stoler MH, Weiss SL, Lerner RM, Beecham J (1988) Stage IB cervical carcinoma: comparison of clinical, MR, and pathologic staging. AJR Am J Roentgenol 150:135–138

91. Walsh JW, Amendola MA, Konerding KF, Tisnado J, Hazra TA (1980) Computed tomographic detection of pelvic and inguinal lymph-node metastases from primary and recurrent pelvic malignant disease. Radiology 137:157–166

92. Kim SH, Kim SC, Choi BI, Han MC (1994) Uterine cervical carcinoma: evaluation of pelvic lymph node metastasis with MR imaging. Radiology 190:807–811

93. Delgado G, Bundy B, Zaino R, Sevin BU, Creasman WT, Major F (1990) Prospective surgical-pathological study of disease-free interval in patients with stage IB squamous cell carcinoma of the cervix: a Gynecologic Oncology Group study. Gynecol Oncol 38:352–357

94. Reinhardt MJ, Ehritt-Braun C, Vogelgesang D, Ihling C, Hogerle S, Mix M, Moser E, Krause TM (2001) Metastatic lymph nodes in patients with cervical cancer: detection with MR imaging and FDG PET. Radiology 218:776–782

95. Lemke AJ, Niehues SM, Amthauer H, Rohlfing T, Hosten N, Felix R (2004) [Clinical use of digital retrospective image fusion of CT, MRI, FDG-PET and SPECT – fields of indications and results]. ROFO 176:1811–1818

96. De Muylder X, Belanger R, Vauclair R, Audet-Lapointe P, Cormier A, Methot Y (1984) Value of lymphography in Stage IB cancer of the uterine cervix. Am J Obstet Gynecol 148:610–613

97. Choi JI, Kim SH, Seong CK, Sim JS, Lee HJ, Do KH (2000) Recurrent uterine cervical carcinoma: spectrum of imaging findings. Korean J Radiol 1:198–207

98. Drescher CW, Hopkins MP, Roberts JA (1989) Comparison of the pattern of metastatic spread of squamous cell cancer and adenocarcinoma of the uterine cervix. Gynecol Oncol 33:340–343

99. Hamm B, Mahfouz AE, Taupitz M, Mitchell DG, Nelson R, Halpern E, Speidel A, Wolf KJ, Saini S (1997) Liver metastases: improved detection with dynamic gadolinium-enhanced MR imaging? Radiology 202:677–682

100. Badib AO, Kurohara SS, Webster JH, Pickren JW (1968) Metastasis to organs in carcinoma of the uterine cervix. Influence of treatment on incidence and distribution. Cancer 21:434–439

101. Outwater EK, Siegelman ES, Wilson KM, Mitchell DG (1996) Benign and malignant gynecologic disease: clinical importance of fluid and peritoneal enhancement in the pelvis at MR imaging. Radiology 200:483–488

102. Low RN, Barone RM, Lacey C, Sigeti JS, Alzate GD, Sebrechts CP (1997) Peritoneal tumor: MR imaging with dilute oral barium and intravenous gadolinium-containing contrast agents compared with unenhanced MR imaging and CT. Radiology 204:513–520

103. Carlson V, Delclos L, Fletcher GH (1967) Distant metastases in squamous-cell carcinoma of the uterine cervix. Radiology 88:961–966

104. Blythe JG, Cohen MH, Buchsbaum HJ, Latourette HB (1975) Bony metastases from carcinoma of cervix. Occurrence, diagnosis, and treatment. Cancer 36:475–484

105. Peppercorn PD, Jeyarajah AR, Woolas R, Shepherd JH, Oram DH, Jacobs IJ, Armstrong P, Lowe D, Reznek RH (1999) Role of MR imaging in the selection of patients with early cervical carcinoma for fertility-preserving surgery: initial experience. Radiology 212:395–399

106. Rietbroek RC, Schilthuis MS, Bakker PJ, van Dijk JD, Postma AJ, Gonzalez Gonzalez D, Bakker AJ, van der Velden J, Helmerhorst TJ, Veenhof CH (1997) Phase II trial of weekly locoregional hyperthermia and cisplatin in patients with a previously irradiated recurrent carcinoma of the uterine cervix. Cancer 79:935–943

107. Rietbroek RC, Schilthuis MS, van der Zee J, Gonzalez Gonzalez D (1999) [Hyperthermia in combination with chemotherapy in gynecological cancers]. Ned Tijdschr Geneeskd 143:85–88

108. Kasales CJ, Langer JE, Arger PH (1995) Pelvic pathology after hysterectomy. A pictorial essay. Clin Imaging 19:210–217

109. Sahdev A, Jones J, Shepherd JH, Reznek RH (2005) MR imaging appearances of the female pelvis after trachelectomy. Radiographics 25:41–52

110. DeSouza NM, Soutter WP, Rustin G, Mahon MM, Jones B, Dina R, McIndoe GA (2004) Use of neoadjuvant chemotherapy prior to radical hysterectomy in cervical cancer: monitoring tumour shrinkage and molecular profile on magnetic resonance and assessment of 3-year outcome. Br J Cancer 90:2326–2331

111. Hricak H, Swift PS, Campos Z, Quivey JM, Gildengorin V, Goranson H (1993) Irradiation of the cervix uteri: value of unenhanced and contrast-enhanced MR imaging. Radiology 189:381–388

112. Fulcher AS, O'Sullivan SG, Segreti EM, Kavanagh BD (1999) Recurrent cervical carcinoma: typical and atypical manifestations. Radiographics 19 (Spec No.):S103–116; quiz S264–105

113. Unger JB, Ivy JJ, Connor P, Charrier A, Ramaswamy MR, Ampil FL, Monsour RP (2004) Detection of recurrent cervical cancer by whole-body FDG PET scan in asymptomatic and symptomatic women. Gynecol Oncol 94:212–216

114. Yen TC, See LC, Chang TC, Huang KG, Ng KK, Tang SG, Chang YC, Hsueh S, Tsai CS, Hong JH, Lin CT, Chao A, Ma SY, Lin WJ, Fu YK, Fan CC, Lai CH (2004) Defining the priority of using 18F-FDG PET for recurrent cervical cancer. J Nucl Med 45:1632–1639

115. Mamsen A, Ledertoug S, Horlyck A, Knudsen HJ, Rasmussen KL, Nyland MH, Jakobsen A (1995) The possible role of ultrasound in early cervical cancer. Gynecol Oncol 56:187–190

116. Innocenti P, Pulli F, Savino L, Nicolucci A, Pandimiglio A, Menchi I, Massi G (1992) Staging of cervical cancer: reliability of transrectal US. Radiology 185:201–205

117. Magee BJ, Logue JP, Swindell R, McHugh D (1991) Tumour size as a prognostic factor in carcinoma of the cervix: assessment by transrectal ultrasound. Br J Radiol 64:812–815

118. Ryu SY, Kim MH, Choi SC, Choi CW, Lee KH (2003) Detection of early recurrence with 18F-FDG PET in patients with cervical cancer. J Nucl Med 44:347–352

119. Moon WK, Kim SH, Han MC (1993) MR findings of malignant melanoma of the vagina. Clin Radiol 48:326–328

120. Miyagi Y, Yamada S, Yamamoto J, Kawanishi K, Yoshinouchi M, Kodama J, Kamimura S, Takamoto N, Kudo T, Taguchi K (1997) Malignant melanoma of the uterine cervix: a case report. J Obstet Gynaecol Res 23:511–519

121. Kristiansen SB, Anderson R, Cohen DM (1992) Primary malignant melanoma of the cervix and review of the literature. Gynecol Oncol 47:398–403

122. Dang HT, Terk MR, Colletti PM, Schlaerth JB, Curtin JP (1991) Primary lymphoma of the cervix: MRI findings with gadolinium. Magn Reson Imaging 9:941–944

123. Kim YS, Koh BH, Cho OK, Rhim HC (1997) MR imaging of primary uterine lymphoma. Abdom Imaging 22:441–444

124. Yamada I, Suzuki S (1993) Primary uterine lymphoma: MR imaging. AJR Am J Roentgenol 160:662–663

125. Ueda H, Togashi K, Konishi I, Kataoka ML, Koyama T, Fujiwara T, Kobayashi H, Fujii S, Konishi J (1999) Unusual appearances of uterine leiomyomas: MR imaging findings and their histopathologic backgrounds. Radiographics 19 (Spec No.): S131–145

126. Hricak H, Tscholakoff D, Heinrichs L, Fisher MR, Dooms GC, Reinhold C, Jaffe RB (1986) Uterine leiomyomas: correlation of MR, histopathologic findings, and symptoms. Radiology 158:385–391

127. Golan A, Ber A, Wolman I, David MP (1994) Cervical polyp: evaluation of current treatment. Gynecol Obstet Invest 37:56–58

128. Mikami Y, Hata S, Fujiwara K, Imajo Y, Kohno I, Manabe T (1999) Florid endocervical glandular hyperplasia with intestinal and pyloric gland metaplasia: worrisome benign mimic of „adenoma malignum". Gynecol Oncol 74:504–511

129. Werber J, Prasadarao PR, Harris VJ (1983) Cervical pregnancy diagnosed by ultrasound. Radiology 149:279–280

130. Schmidt-Matthiesen H, Wallwiener D (2005) Gynäkologie und Geburtshilfe. Schattauer, Stuttgart

131. Rohen JW (1999) Topographische Anatomie. Schattauer, Stuttgart

132. Hamm B et al (1999) MRT von Abdomen und Becken Thieme, Berlin

133. Nicolas CG et al (2005) Radiologic-Pathologic Correlations Springer, Berlin Heidelberg New York

134. Wittekind C, Klimpfinger M, Sobin LH (2005) TNM-Atlas, Springer, Berlin Heidelberg New York

Ovaries and Fallopian Tubes: Normal Findings and Anomalies

Rosemarie Forstner

CONTENTS

8.1
Ovaries and Fallopian Tubes: Normal Findings

8.1.1
Anatomical Relationships

The female adnexal structures are located in the lesser pelvis and include the fallopian tubes, the ovaries, and ligamentous attachments.

The fallopian tubes are 8- to 15-cm long paired tubular structures at the superior aspect of the broad ligament. They extend from the uterus to the ovaries and are composed of the intramural portion, the isthmus, the ampullary part, and the infundibulum with the abdominal ostium. The latter is trumpet shaped, opens at the ovarian end into the peritoneal cavity and is composed of irregular fingerlike extensions, the fimbriae, which overhang the ovary [1]. The infundibulum narrows gradually from about 15 mm to about 4 mm in diameter and merges medially with the serpiginous ampullary portion of the tube, which comprises more than half of the length of the fallopian tube. A thickening of the muscular wall, the isthmic portion extends for 2 cm towards the uterus. Within the uterus the 1- to 2-cm long intramural segment joins the extension of the endometrial cavity, the uterotubal junction. At its extrauterine course the fallopian tube lies within the two folds of the broad ligament [2]. The ovaries are typically located in the ovarian fossa close to the lateral pelvic side walls. In most women the ovaries can be identified laterally and superiorly of the uterine cornua near the bifurcation of the common iliac artery between internal and external iliac arteries (Fig. 8.1) [3]. Occasionally, the ovaries may be found at atypical sites (Fig. 8.2), e.g., adjacent to the uterine corpus, superior and posterior to the uterine fundus, or in the posterior cul-de-sac. Due to its anchoring to the posterior border of the broad ligament the ovary is typically located in the posterior pelvic compartment and above the uterine fundus, but not in the anterior cul-de-sac [4]. When the uterus, however, is retroverted one or both ovaries may be found anterior or posterior to the uterus (Fig. 8.3) [5]. Furthermore, pregnancy, diseases associated with uterine enlargement such as fibroids, or pelvic masses can displace the ovaries outside the lesser pelvis [4].

8.1.2
Normal Ovaries in the Reproductive Age

Adult ovaries measure approximately 3–5 cm in length, 1.5–3 cm in width, and 0.5–1.5 cm in thickness. Their size, however, varies considerably, depend-

R. FORSTNER, MD
PD, Department of Radiology, Landeskliniken Salzburg, Paracelsus Private Medical University, Müllner Hauptstrasse 48, 5020 Salzburg, Austria

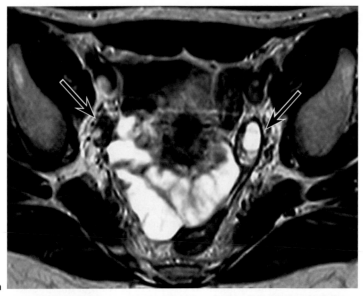

a

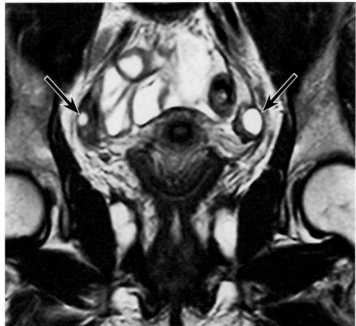

b

Fig. 8.1a,b. Ovarian fossa. Transaxial (**a**) and coronal T2-weighted (**b**) images in a 28-year-old female. Normal ovaries (*arrows*) are demonstrated in the ovarian fossa, which is a shallow peritoneal groove between external and internal iliac vessels. The ovaries are of ovoid shape and can be well identified due to follicles which display very high signal on the T2-weighting

ing on age, hormonal status, menstrual cycle, and the contents of follicular derivatives [6]. The ovaries are of ovoid, almond shape with a smooth surface in early reproductive age, that becomes more irregular thereafter. The ovary is encapsulated by a thin fibrous layer, the tunica albuginea. Within the capsule lies the ovarian stroma, which consists of fibroblasts, smooth muscle cells, arteries, veins, lymphatics, nerves, and follicles. Histologically, the ovaries contain three ill defined zones: the outer cortex, the highly vascular inner medulla, and the hilum [6]. The cortex is predominantly composed of follicles, corpora lutea, fibroblasts, and smooth muscle cells.

In childbearing age during each menstrual cycle a number of follicles are stimulated to begin to mature, but usually only a single follicle completes the process. At mid-cycle the preovulatory dominant follicle can be identified as a thin-walled cyst attaining a size of approximately 15–25 mm [7]. After formation of the corpus luteum the wall may involute and become irregular. Corpus lutea may be cystic or involuted and noncystic [3]. Furthermore,

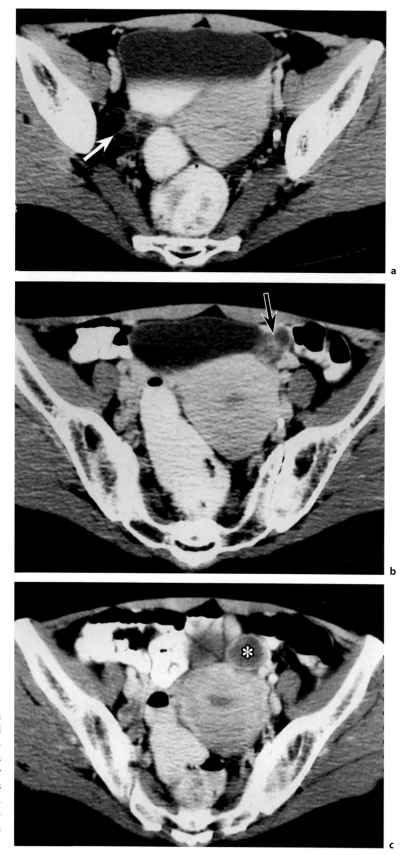

Fig. 8.2a–c. Ovarian location in a woman of childbearing age. CT scans at the level of the uterine corpus (**a–c**) The right ovary (*arrow*) is located in the ovarian fossa (**a**). Atypical location of the left ovary (*arrow*) anterior to the uterine corpus near the anterior abdominal wall (**b**). A corpus luteum cyst (*asterisk*) displays attenuation values higher than water and a distinct enhancing wall (**c**)

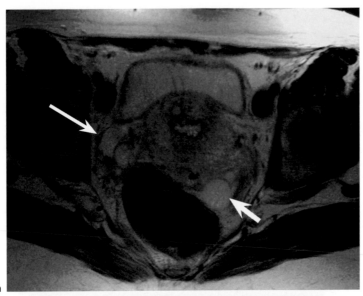

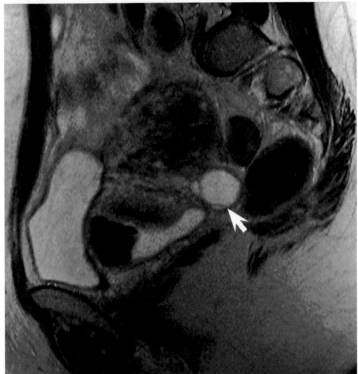

Fig. 8.3a,b. Ovarian location in cul-de-sac. Transaxial (**a**) and parasagittal T2-weighted (**b**) images demonstrate the left ovary (*arrow*) located above the posterior vaginal fornix in the left cul-de-sac. The uterus is retroflexed, distension of the vagina is due to vaginal contrast opacification. Right ovary (*long arrow*)

abundant vascularization may give rise to hemorrhage [6].

The normal fallopian tube contains a small amount of intraluminal fluid that is dispersed within multiple infoldings of the fallopian tube mucosa [3]. These infoldings usually prevent visualization of the tube as a fluid-filled structure on MRI or CT. In tubal ligation clips allow identification of the fallopian tube. (Fig. 8.4).

8.1.2.1
Imaging Findings

Ovaries can be identified on CT and MRI due to their location and soft tissue characteristics. The landmark of the ovaries are follicular structures which can be best identified on T2-weighted MRI [8]. On CT, normal ovaries can be best identified after bowel contrast opacification. They are ovoid soft tissue structures with low attenuation areas which represent normal follicles (Fig. 8.2). Presence of a dominant follicle ranging more than 1 cm in size assists in ovarian identification. Hemorrhagic corpus luteum cysts may be identified by high attenuation values or a fluid-fluid level [9].

On MRI in the majority of premenopausal women (95%) ovaries can be identified by the presence of follicles within the ovary (see Fig. 8.1) [3]. The ovaries are of low to intermediate SI on T1. In premenopausal women most ovaries (70%) display a zonal differentiation with a higher signal intensity of the medulla compared to the low signal intensity cortex on T2-weighted (Fig. 8.5) [8]. As the ovarian stroma remains of relatively low signal

intensity, follicular structures can be well discriminated on T2-weighted images. Follicular cysts are of very high signal intensity with a discrete thin walled low-signal-intensity rim and are predominantly located in the cortex. The average size of functional ovarian cysts was 1 cm (range 0.2–4.7 cm) in normal ovaries [8]. In a menstruating woman not using birth control pills a unilocular cyst of 2–3 cm in either ovary and other smaller cysts is a normal finding.

Corpus luteum cysts have thicker enhancing walls than follicle cysts following intravenous contrast application (Fig. 8.6). Corpus luteum cysts may contain blood with bright signal on T1 and T2 as a sign of subacute hemorrhage [8]. Resolution is expected in on follow-up after two to three menstrual cycles and proves the diagnosis of a functional cyst.

8.1.3
Normal Peri- and Postmenopausal Ovaries

After menopause the ovaries typically shrink to a size of half that in reproductive age [6].

Most ovaries display a shrunken gyriform external appearance, some may also have a smooth contour (Fig. 8.7). The ovarian stroma increases variably in volume, and unresolved corpora lutea may be found [6]. Follicles may persist for several years after cessation of menses. They may account for sporadic ovulation, and follicle cyst formation. Follicular activity is typically not found after 4–5 years after menopause [5]. Mild hyperplasia of the medullary and corti-

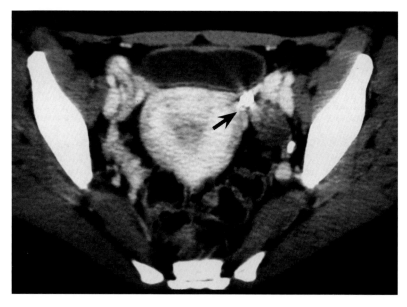

Fig. 8.4. Tubal ligation. The left fallopian tube is located at the superior margin of the broad ligament and can be identified by the clip in CT (*arrow*). Dilated tortuous vascular structures along the parametria and the right pelvic side wall present pelvic varices. Normal left ovary (*asterisk*)

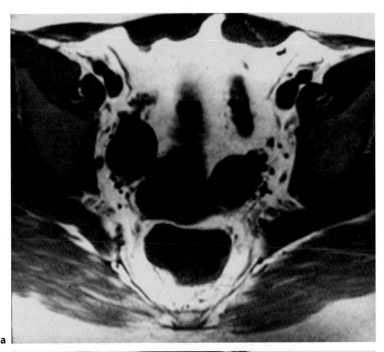

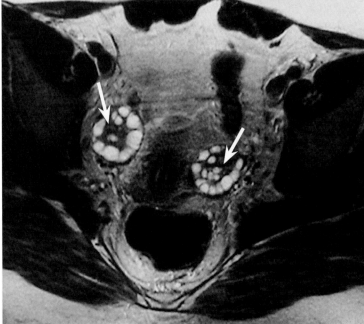

Fig. 8.5a,b. Normal zonal anatomy in a premenopausal woman. Transaxial T1-weighted (**a**) and transaxial T2-weighted (**b**) images. Both ovaries display multiple small follicles in subcortical location which show intermediate signal on T1-weighted images and very bright signal on the T2-weighted images. The low signal intensity cortex can be differentiated from the central medulla, the signal intensity of which resembles the myometrium. There seems to be an overlap between polycystic ovaries with multiple small peripheral cysts and normal ovaries as seen in this case. (Courtesy of Dr. R.N Troiano, New York)

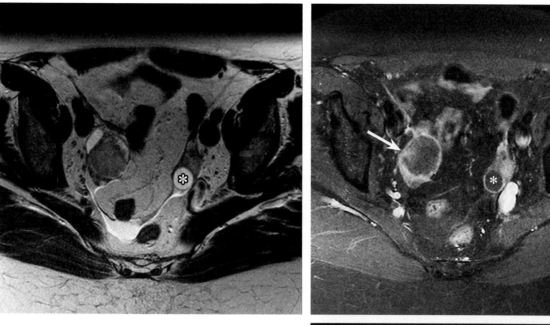

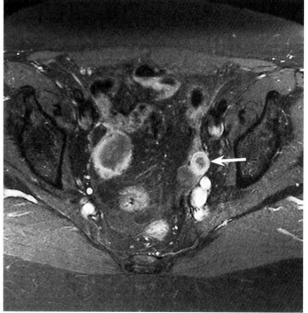

Fig. 8.6a–c. Functional ovarian cysts. Transaxial T2-weighted (**a**) and contrast enhanced T1-weighted images with fat suppression (**b,c**) at the level of the acetabulum. The normal sized left ovary contains two physiologic cysts. The follicle cyst (*asterisk*) displays a thin wall (**a**) with contrast enhancement (**b**). The corpus luteum cysts shows a thicker wall with distinct peripheral contrast enhancement (*arrow*) (**c**). The hemorrhagic cyst of the right ovary (*long arrow*) displays low signal intensity on the T2-weighted image (**a**) which is a typical finding of an endometrioma. The findings were laparoscopically proven

cal stroma is commonly found in postmenopausal women. The clinical findings are secondary to excess androgen production of the stroma, and can be associated with diabetes, obesity, and hypertension [9]. Other factors that may increase the ovarian size in postmenopausal women include multiparity or hormonal replacement therapy [6]. Ovaries may also display stromal atrophy and become extremely fibrotic [6]. Surface epithelium inclusion cysts are a common finding in postmenopausal ovaries [10] With increas-

ing age ovarian vessels within the stroma may be calcified or become hyaline [6].

8.1.3.1
Imaging Findings

Postmenopausal ovaries are more difficult to recognize than premenopausal ovaries, and especially with suboptimal bowel contrast they may be not visible on CT [11]. However, tracking down the ovarian vessels

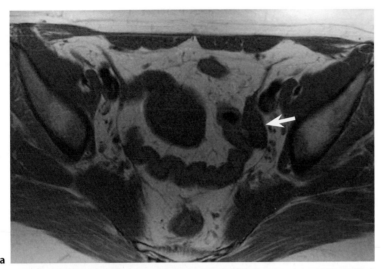

a

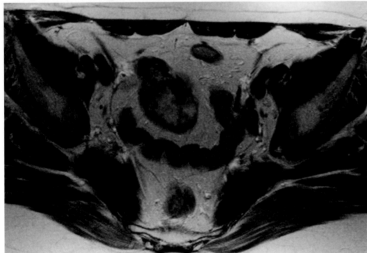

b

Fig. 8.7a,b. Normal postmenopausal ovary with a gyriform contour. T1-weighted (**a**) and T2-weighted (**b**) images show a small left ovary (*arrow*) with lobulated margins which is found in the ovarian fossa. Zonal anatomy with higher signal intensity within the central medulla is demonstrated on the T2-weighted image (**b**)

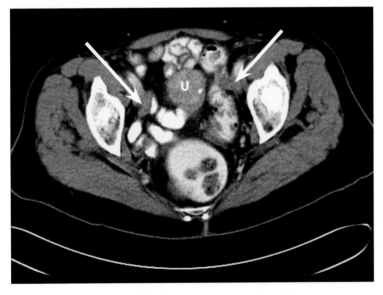

Fig. 8.8. Postmenopausal ovaries on CT. The ovaries (*arrows*) appear as bandlike soft tissue structures and are located between the iliac vessels and bowel loops. Without bowel opacification identification of normal postmenopausal ovaries is usually not possible. Uterus (*U*) with a calcified fibroid of the fundus

along the psoas muscle makes it possible to localize the ovaries, particularly in postmenopausal women with small ovaries [11]. Postmenopausal ovaries appear on CT as triangular or bandlike soft tissue structures with low or moderate contrast enhancement (Fig. 8.8). Identification of small cysts, most commonly inclusion cysts, or follicular cysts at the beginning of menopause aids in the detection of the ovaries.

On MRI, postmenopausal ovaries can be visualized as oval structures most commonly of uniformly intermediate to low signal intensity on T1-weighted and T2-weighted images [8]. They can be identified in most postmenopausal women despite their small size and nonspecific characteristics by their location in relationship to the uterus. Due to its superior soft tissue contrast, small ovarian cysts are more commonly identified than on CT in postmenopausal women.

8.1.4
Pelvic Fluid

Small amounts of pelvic fluid are best identified in the cul-de-sac or with increasing volume as tiny fluid pockets outlining bowel loops throughout the pelvis. Pelvic free fluid is a common finding throughout the menstrual cycle and peaks in the secretory phase [12]. Although some fluid may be related to ovarian cyst rupture, it seems that most of the fluid is not related to cyst rupture. Only larger amounts of pelvic fluid may be an important ancillary finding to support the diagnosis of peritoneal spread in malignancy [13]. Normal peritoneum does not enhance after the application of iv contrast media. Peritoneal enhancement, however, is not specific and is found in benign, mostly inflammatory and in malignant diseases [14].

8.1.5
Ovarian Attachments and Vascular Supply

The broad ligament is formed by two layers of peritoneum which drape over the uterus and extend laterally to the pelvic side walls [15]. Its caudal margin is defined by the cardinal ligament. The superior free margin is formed by the fallopian tube medially and the suspensory ligament of the ovary laterally. Between these peritoneal folds lies the parametrium which contains the fallopian tube, round ligament, ovarian ligament, uterine and ovarian blood vessels, nerves, lymphatics, mesonephric remnants, and in parts of the ureter [15].

Each ovary is suspended in the peritoneal cavity by three supporting structures: the mesovarium which anchors the ovary to the posterior aspect of the broad ligament; the ovarian ligament which attaches the ovary to the uterine cornu; and the suspensory ligament or infundibulopelvic which anchors the ovary to the pelvic side wall [6].

The ovarian ligament and suspensory ligament are not tight supporting structures but more comparable to a mesentery [4]. The ovarian blood vessels and lymphatics course within the peritoneal folds of the mesovarium and enter and exit the ovary through the ovarian hilum. Anastomosing branches of the ovarian and uterine vessels in close relationship with lymphatics are located within the mesovarium [6].

The suspensory ligament of the ovary is located at the superior lateral aspect of the broad ligament [6]. It extends from the ovary anterolaterally over the external and common iliac vessels and blends with connective tissue over the psoas muscle [15]. Ovarian blood vessels and lymphatics traverse the suspensory ligament to reach the ovarian hilum along the mesovarium.

The ovarian ligament is a rounded fibromuscular band extending from the ovary to the uterine cornu [6]. Its position varies with that of the ovary. It is located immediately posterior and inferior to the fallopian tube and round ligament [15]. The ovarian branches of the uterine artery pass through the ovarian ligament and anastomose with branches of ovarian artery in the mesovarium.

The ovarian artery originates from the lumbar aorta near the renal hilum. It is accompanied along its retroperitoneal course by the ovarian vein and the ureter on the anterior surface of the psoas muscle. It then crosses the ureter and common iliac vessels near the pelvic brim to enter the suspensory ligament of the ovary. The ovarian artery courses inferiorly and medially between the two layers of the broad ligament near the mesovarian border [4]. It forms multiple branches that reach the ovarian hilum via the mesovarium. It has a tortuous course that is most pronounced near the ovary.

The ovarian vein is typically single, but may also be multiple and accompanies the ovarian artery. The venous drainage is into the left ovarian vein, and the inferior vena cava on the right side.

The ovarian lymphatics ascend with the ovarian vessels along the psoas muscle and drain almost exclusively into the para-aortic lymph nodes at the level of the lower pole of the kidneys. In some patients, accessory channels pass the broad ligament and drain into the internal and common iliac and interaortic lymph nodes, or course along the round ligament to the external iliac and inguinal lymph nodes [6]. In the fallopian tube, additional lymphatic channels to presacral nodes, and occasionally from the ampulla, to gluteal nodes may exist [6].

8.1.5.1
Identifying the Ligaments on Imaging

The broad ligament and mesovarium are usually not discernible on cross-sectional imaging unless they are surrounded by large amounts of ascites. Its position, however, can be identified by the structures it contains [15]. In ascites, the ovaries can be seen suspended from the posterior surface of the broad ligament (Fig. 8.9) [4]. The ovarian ligament may occasionally be visualized as a short and narrow soft tissue band extending between the uterus and ovary (Fig. 8.10).

In the retroperitoneum at the level of the inferior renal pole the ovarian artery and vein can be identified along the psoas muscle medial to the ureter. The artery is the smaller vessel and is located medial to the vein. The ovarian artery is smaller and less constantly conspicuous on CT or MRI. They cross obliquely anterior to the ureter at the middle to the lower lumbar region and are located laterally to the ureter in the lower abdomen and pelvis (Fig. 8.11).

Tracking these vessels continuously downwards from the retroperitoneum to the pelvis, leads to the suspensory ovarian ligament [11]. The latter is an excellent landmark for localizing the ovary (Fig. 8.11). It is a short, narrow fan-shaped soft tissue band that widens as it approaches the ovary. Sometimes it can also be identified as a linear band that is thicker than the ovarian vein. Due to its vascular landmarks it is more commonly identifiable than the other ovarian ligaments [4].

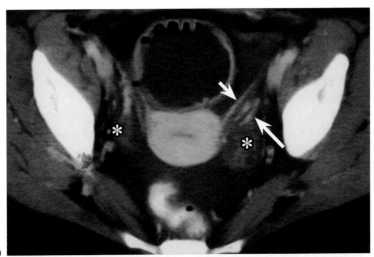

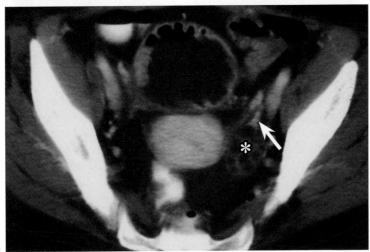

Fig. 8.9a,b. Broad ligament and ovary on CT. In a patient with free fluid the ovaries (*asterisk*) can be visualized posterolaterally of the broad ligament. The left round ligament (*arrowhead*) is visualized at the anterior aspect of the broad ligament and courses anterolaterally towards the internal inguinal canal (**a**). At the lateral free margin of the broad ligament the suspensory ligament attaches to the anterior margin of the left ovary. It transmits the ovarian artery and vein (*long arrow*) and is contiguous to the mesovarium (**a,b**)

8.2
Developmental Anomalies

Developmental anomalies of the ovaries are very rare. Although ovaries have a different developmental origin from uterus and fallopian tubes, ovarian anomalies are significantly more often associated with congenital uterine anomalies (22%), particularly with unicornuate uterus [16]. Uterus and fallopian tubes develop from the paramesonephric ducts. Defects of the paramesonephric tubes result not only in abnormalities of the uterus but also of the fallopian tubes, kidneys, and ureters.

In utero the primordial ovaries are located on the medial surface of the urogenital ridge on each side of the lower thoracic and upper lumbar spine, inside the Wolffian body. The ovaries descend during the 3rd month of fetal life with the ovaries located at the level of the iliac crest by the third month of life. They take their place in the ovarian fossa at the end of the first year of life [1]. Ovarian migration is guided by the gubernaculum which connects the lower pole of the gonad and attaches to the uterus, forming the ovarian and round ligaments of the uterus [17].

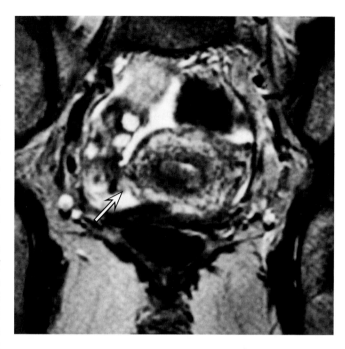

Fig. 8.10. Ovarian ligament on MRI. The right ovarian ligament is identified as a short band extending between uterus and ovary (*arrow*). The thickening of the endometrium is caused by endometrial cancer. A small amount of physiologic pelvic fluid is noted

8.2.1
Congenital Abnormalities

In phenotypic females, absence of both ovaries is usually associated with abnormal karyotypes and a syndrome of gonadal dysgenesis. These patients may have underdeveloped gonads, or uni- or bilateral streak gonads which carry a risk of malignancy (Fig. 8.12) [6]. Congenital unilateral agenesis of an ovary in a normal female is extremely rare and usually asymptomatic. It presents more likely as the result of torsion with atrophy, particularly in the prenatal period. It may be accompanied by ipsilateral renal or ureteric agenesis and/or malformation of the ipsilateral fallopian tube [18].

Accessory or supernumerary ovaries are extremely rare, and may also be associated with other congenital genitourinary abnormalities. An accessory ovary contains ovarian tissue, and is usually located in the vicinity of a normal ovary [6]. Supernumerary ovaries are not attached to the ovary, but may be found at various sites within and outside the pelvis. In most cases, they are smaller than 1 cm in size [19]. The ectopic ovarian tissue possesses the functional as well as the pathological potential of normal ovaries and may give rise to primary carcinoma of the peritoneum [20].

Adrenal cortical rests may be observed within the wall of the fallopian tubes and broad ligament.

Congenital abnormalities of the fallopian tubes are also extremely rare. As in the ovaries, they present more likely a sequelae of torsion or an inflammatory process. Tubes may be partially atretic or hypoplastic and associated with uterine abnormalities such as rudimentary uterine horn or bicornuate uterus. In infertility patients exposed to diethylstilbestrol, short sacculated or dilated fallopian tubes have been reported [21].

8.2.2
Ovarian Maldescent

Ovarian maldescent has an incidence of 0.2%–0.5% [22]. It may occur uni- or bilaterally and can be associated with Müllerian malformations [6]. In ovarian maldescent, ovaries may be found in an ectopic position along its migration pathway from the lumbar region to the ovarian fossa (Fig. 8.13). Rarely, ovaries

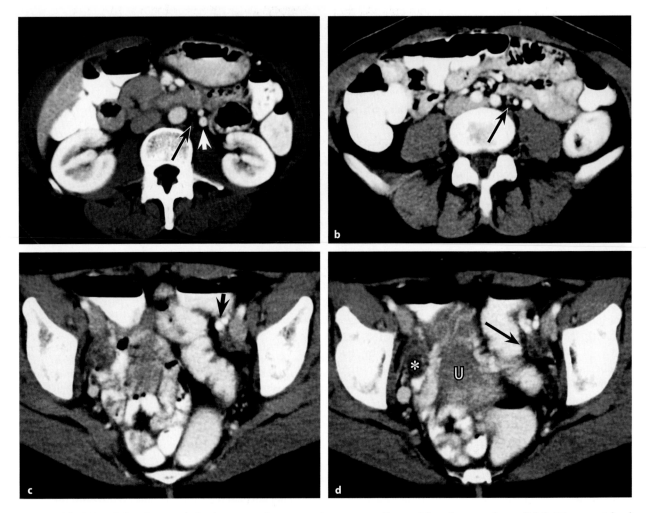

Fig. 8.11a–d. Ovarian vessels in the retroperitoneum and suspensory ligament "ovarian vascular pedicle". CT scans at level below the renal hilum (**a**), aortic bifurcation (**b**), upper pelvis (**c**), and mid pelvis (**d**). Ovarian artery and vein (***arrow***) course along the psoas muscle parallel to the ureter (***long arrow***) (**a**). At the lower lumbar region they cross obliquely (***arrow***) and are visualized lateral to the ureter (***long arrow***). The ovarian vessels (***arrow***) are continuous with the suspensory ligament, which is identified near the external iliac vessels (**c**). It demonstrates a wedging as it approaches the ovary. The latter can be identified by multiple small cystic follicles (**d**). Follicle cyst in the right ovary (***asterisk***). *U*, uterus

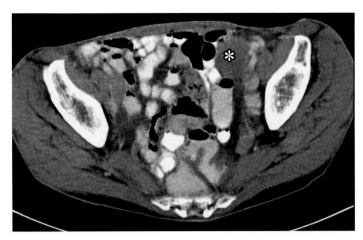

Fig. 8.12. Ovarian dysgenesis in testicular feminization. In a phenotypical 55-year-old woman no uterus can be identified. A soft tissue attenuation mass (***asterisk***) near the internal inguinal ring presents a left streak gonad. Histologically proven

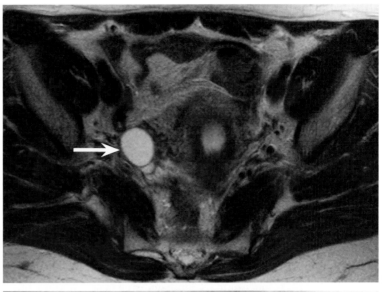

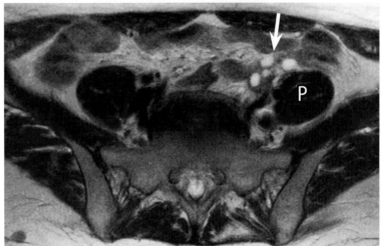

Fig. 8.13a,b. High position of the left ovary. Transaxial T2-weighted image in the mid pelvis (**a**) and upper pelvis (**b**). In a patient without history of previous surgeries or birth, normal position of the right ovary (***arrow***) (**a**) and atypical high position of the left ovary (***arrow***) at the level of S1 at the medial contour of the psoas muscle (***P***) is demonstrated (**b**)

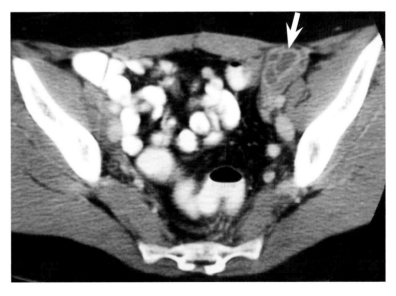

Fig. 8.14. Atypical anterior location of the left ovary. CT shows atypical anterior position of the left ovary (***arrow***) in a patient who had undergone a series of previous surgeries and suffered from chronic pelvic pain. The ovary can be identified due to the follicles which changed in size during follow-up. At surgery extensive adhesions of the ovary and anterior abdominal wall and pelvic side wall were found

may descend too far down as far as the inguinal canal [1].

The paracolic gutters present a common location of ovarian maldescent above the pelvic brim. After pregnancy the ovaries may be hindered from returning to their original position due to adhesions. Furthermore, an ectopic ovarian position may be associated with adhesions, inflammation, and surgery, or result from abnormal ovarian mobility due to elongation of the broad ligaments [4] (Fig. 8.14).

8.2.2.1
Imaging Findings

In women of childbearing age, ovaries in atypical positions can be identified on CT and MRI in the majority of patients due to the typical morphology of follicles. MRI is superior to CT for diagnosing maldescended or ectopic ovaries due to their excellent visualization on T2-weighted images. Bowel contrast opacification will facilitate identification of ovaries in atypical positions. An ovary not visualized in the ovarian fossa should be sought in other locations in proximity to the uterus and above the pelvic brim, rarely may it be located near the inguinal canal.

Differential diagnosis: differential diagnosis of an unilateral missing ovary includes ectopic ovary and atrophy resulting from adnexal torsion.

8.3
Surgically Transposed Ovaries

In young women, surgical transposition of the ovaries is performed before therapeutic irradiation of the pelvis. The ovaries are surgically removed out of the radiation field with the purpose of preserving their function.

The procedure includes mobilization of the ovaries together with the suspensory ligaments and their vascular pedicles [23]. They are most commonly repositioned laterally to the lower paracolic gutters close to the iliac fossa. Another site of transposition is the posterior intraperitoneal space in the upper pelvis lateral or anterolateral to the psoas muscle [24]. Lateral transposition is performed in patients with cervical cancer, vaginal cancer, pelvic sarcoma, and Hodgkin disease. Midline transposition can be performed in Hodgkin disease and the ovaries may be attached to the surface of the uterus [23]. Surgical clips are typically affixed to each ovary to mark its location.

8.3.1
Imaging Findings

Transposed ovaries can be identified by their characteristic morphologic features of follicles. Metallic

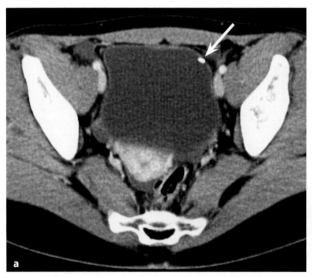
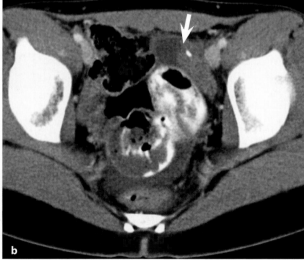

Fig. 8.15a,b. Surgical transposition. Transaxial CT after transposition of the ovary (**a**) and after radiation therapy (**b**). During endoscopic transposition the left ovary was marked by a clip (*arrow*). In the follow-up the cystic and solid lesion presents the normal transposed ovary which undergoes cyclic changes. Without the clip (*arrow*) it may easily be misdiagnosed as a tumor. Ascites is a sequelae of radiation

clips help to identify the ovaries on CT (Fig. 8.15) [24]. Furthermore, following the ovarian vessels downwards from the mid lumbar region aids in identifying the ovaries [11]. Ovarian vessels in lateral transposition deviate laterally near the iliac fossa instead of coursing inferiorly [4]. Transposed ovaries undergo the typical features of follicular maturation and may be followed in equivocal cases. Identification of featureless and small postmenopausal ovaries is possible due to the surgical clips, but it may be difficult or impossible on MRI.

Differential diagnosis: Familiarity with history of ovarian transposition is crucial to establish the correct diagnosis. The differential diagnosis includes mucocele of appendix, peritoneal implants, colonic masses, lymphoceles, and lymph node metastases.

References

1. Stevens SK (1992) The adnexa. In: Higgins CB, Hricak H, Helms CA (eds) MRI of the body. Raven Press, New York, pp 865–889
2. Wheeler JE (2002) Diseases of the fallopian tube. In: Kurman RJ (ed) Blaustein´s pathology of the female genital tract. Springer, Berlin Heidelberg New York, pp 617–648
3. Outwater EK, Talerman A, Dunton C (1996) Normal adnexa uteri specimens: anatomic basis of MR imaging features. Radiology 201:751–755
4. Saksouk FA, Johnson SC (2004) Recognition of the ovaries and ovarian origin of pelvic masses with CT. Radiographics 24:133–146
5. Hall DA (1983) Sonographic appearance of normal ovary, of polycystic disease, and of functional ovarian cysts. Semin Ultrasound CT MR 4:149–165
6. Clement PB (2002) Anatomy and histology of the ovary. In: Kurman RJ (ed) Blaustein´s pathology of the female genital tract. Springer, Berlin Heidelberg New York, pp 649–674
7. Fleischer A, Daniell J, Rodier J et al (1981) Sonographic monitoring of ovarian follicular development. J Clin Ultrasound 9:275–279
8. Outwater EK, Mitchell DG (1996) Normal ovaries and functional cysts: MR appearance. Radiology 198:397–402
9. Occhipinti KA (1999) CT and MRI of the ovary. In: Anderson JC (ed) Gynecologic imaging. Churchill Livingstone, London, pp 345–349
10. Kim JS, Lee HJ, Woo SK et al (1997) Peritoneal inclusion cysts and their relationship to the ovaries. Evaluation with sonography. Radiology 204:481–484
11. Lee JH, Jeong YK, Park JK et al (2003) Ovarian vascular pedicle sign revealing organ origin of mass lesion on helical CT. AJR Am J Roentgenol 181:131–137
12. Davis JA, Gosink BB (1986) Fluid in the female pelvis: cyclic patterns. J Ultrasound Med 5:75
13. Stevens SK, Hricak H, Stern JL (1991) Ovarian lesions: detection and characterization with gadolinium-enhanced MRI at 1.5 T. Radiology 181:481–488
14. Outwater EK, Wilson KM, Siegelman ES, Mitchell DG (1996) MRI of benign and malignant gynecologic disease: significance of fluid and peritoneal enhancement in the pelvis at MR imaging. Radiology 200:483–488
15. Foshager MC, Walsh JW (1994) CT anatomy of the female pelvis: a second look. RadioGraphics 14:51–66
16. Dabirash H, Mohammad K, Moghadami-Tabrizi N (1994) Ovarian malposition in women with uterine anomalies. Obstet Gynecol 83:293–294
17. Trinidad C, Tardaguila F, Fernandez GC (2004) Ovarian maldescent. Eur Radiol 14:805–808
18. Dueck A, Poenaru D, Jamieson MA (2001) Unilateral ovarian agenesis and fallopian tube maldescent. Pediatr Surg Int 17:228–229
19. Hahn-Pedersen J, Larsen PM (1984) Supernumerary ovary. Acta obstet Gynecol Scand 63:365–366
20. Seidman JD, Russell P, Kurman RJ (2002) Surface epithelial tumors of the ovary. In: Kurman RJ (ed) Blaustein´s pathology of the female genital tract. Springer, Berlin Heidelberg New York, pp 791–904
21. Nunley WC, Pope TL, Bateman BG (1984) Upper reproductive tract radiographic findings in DES-exposed female offspring. AJR Am J Roentgenol 142:337–339
22. Van Voohis BJ, Dokras A, Syrop CH (2000) Undescended ovaries: association with infertility and treatment with IVF. Fertil Steril 74:1041–43
23. Kier R, Chambers SK (1989) Surgical transposition of the ovaries: imaging findings in 14 patients. AJR Am J Roentgenol 153:1003–1006
24. Bashist B Freidman WN, Killackey MA (1989) Surgical transposition of the ovary: radiological appearance. Radiology 173:857–860

Adnexal Masses: Characterization of Benign Ovarian Lesions

Rosemarie Forstner and Karen Kinkel

CONTENTS

R. Forstner, MD
PD, Department of Radiology, Landeskliniken Salzburg, Paracelsus Private Medical University, Müllner Hauptstrasse 48, 5020 Salzburg, Austria
K. Kinkel, MD, PD
Institut de Radiologie, Clinique des Grangettes, chemin des Grangettes 7, 1224 Chêne-Bougeries, Switzerland

9.1 Introduction

Thorough pretreatment assessment by cross-sectional imaging plays a pivotal role in the management of suspected adnexal masses. It guides the surgeon to anticipate malignancy before starting surgery and aids in planning the adequate therapeutic approach. In this context, in benign ovarian lesions laparoscopy has been widely replacing open surgery. This is why pretreatment knowledge of imaging findings in various ovarian lesions is of utmost importance. Although a definite histopathologic diagnosis is not possible in the majority of cases, predicting the likelihood of malignancy is crucial for proper patient management [1].

In the assessment of adnexal masses the following parameters should be addressed by imaging: (a) defining the exact origin of the mass, (b) if the lesion is ovarian to define if it is a physiologic or neoplastic finding, and (c) when surgery is warranted for a neoplastic lesion, imaging findings concerning the risk of malignancy may assist the surgeon in deciding between laparoscopy or laparotomy [2].

9.2 Technical Recommendations for Ovarian Lesion Characterization

MRI of the female pelvis is performed after 5 h of fasting and with prior intramuscular injection of peristaltic inhibitors to minimize artifacts due to bowel movement. The patient lies on her back in a supine position with a pelvic, torso, or cardiac coil attached around her pelvis. The coil ideally covers the region from the symphysis pubis up to the renal hilum. Depending on the woman's height, upper coverage may be lower and require secondary adjustment of the coil if hydronephrosis or retroperitoneal lymphadenopathy is suspected.

Ovarian cyst characterization requires good anatomical coverage of the entire ovarian cyst and the uterus to be able to confirm the ovarian vs uterine origin of the mass.

The imaging protocol implies the use of both T2- and T1-weighted sequences. High-resolution fast spin echo T2-weighted images are mandatory to confirm the anatomical origin and clearly identify the ovarian nature of the mass. Further tissue characterization takes into account signal intensity at three subsequent T1-weighted sequences in the following order: native, fat-suppressed, and after intravenous injection of gadolinium. The latter contrast-enhanced sequence is mandatory to exclude malignancy. Identical slice orientation allows exact comparison of all T1-weighted sequences. Table 9.1 demonstrates differences in signal intensity according to the histological type of the most frequent ovarian neoplasm.

Table 9.1. Signal intensity of benign ovarian masses on MRI of the pelvis according to sequences and histological lesion type

Signal intensity			
Histology of ovarian neoplasm	T2	Native T1	Fat-suppressed T1
Serous cystadenoma	High	Low	Low
Mucinous cystadenoma	High	Intermediate	Intermediate
Mature cystic teratoma	Intermediate	High	Low
Endometrioma	High	High	High
Fibroma	Low-intermediate	Intermediate	Intermediate

Turbo spin echo (TSE) sequences are the sequences of choice due to their excellent image resolution. Imaging parameters include a field of view of 200–300 mm with a matrix of 512×256, slice thickness between 4 and 5 mm, and a number of signal acquisitions between two and four. T2-weighted fast spin echo (FSE) sequences use a TR/TE around 4,000/90 ms, whereas The TR for T1-weighted sequences is around 500 ms with a minimum TE. Due to time restrictions, faster T2-weighted sequences such as ultrafast half-Fourier single-shot turbo spin-echo sequences (HASTE, 3 s per slice) have been tested in 60 female pelvis examinations and compared to conventional and high-resolution turbo spin echo sequences [3]. A HASTE sequence is applied with a TR/effective TE/echotrain of infinity/90/64 and a 128×256 matrix. HASTE provided clearer visualization of large leiomyomas and ovarian tumors but slightly poorer visualization of uterine cancer compared to high-resolution turbo spin echo sequences. One of the advantages was greater time efficacy without motion and chemical shift artifacts. Lesion conspicuity was better with HASTE than with conventional TSE imaging (matrix, 128×256) but lower than with high-resolution TSE (matrix, 300×512). Because of limited image resolution, the HASTE sequence should be used when the high-resolution TSE imaging is suboptimal or to provide additional imaging planes as a complement to high-resolution TSE. T2-weighted echo planar sequences (EPI) were not successful in the female pelvis compared to fast spin echo sequences. The study showed inferior uterine zonal anatomy and ovarian visualization in 44 (56%) of 78 and 18 (33%) of 54 cases, respectively [4]. Ovarian cystic lesions were revealed more precisely by the fast spin-echo sequence than by the EPI sequence. When T1-weighted sequences were compared in a pelvic and abdominal MRI study including 70 patients, the EPI T1 sequence allowed a 40% reduction in acquisition time without difference in the diagnostic performance of three reviewers [5].

To allow the distinction of an ovarian vs uterine origin of a mass, dynamic contrast injection might be helpful to better delineate the early enhancing normal myometrium [6]. This type of sequence is acquired once before and three times after IV contrast injection and corresponds to a 2D TSE sequence with 18 slices of 4 mm at a FOV of 300 mm, a matrix of 202×512, a TSE factor of 5, a TR/TE of 550/14 with two numbers of signal acquisition and a total acquisition time of 6 min.

For ovarian lesion characterization, intravenous contrast injection has been shown to be mandatory because of its ability to identify solid intracystic portions such as papillary projections, necrosis within a solid mass, septation or wall thickening Fig. 9.1 [7]. The multivariate logistic regression analysis also demonstrated different predictive values to identify malignancy according to the MRI signs. The highest odds ratio for malignancy was found for "necrosis in a solid lesion," with an odds ration of 107, followed by the sign "vegetation in a cyst" with an odds ratio of 40. Identification of enhancement within a T1-hyperintense cyst might require a subtraction technique (contrast-enhanced fat-suppressed T1-weighted sequence minus native fat-suppressed T1-weighted sequence) to demonstrate the enhancing solid portion within a hyperintense endometrioma. This sign has recently been reported to be highly suggestive of associated ovarian carcinoma [8]. Careful inspection and comparison of T2- and T1-weighted images help identify this possibility. The number of T2-weighted acquisitions depends on imaging time but should cover at least two orthogonal imaging planes and ideally represent all three imaging planes to allow the choice of the best anatomical slice orientation for the three T1-weighted sequences.

Because of its inferior soft tissue contrast compared to MRI, CT is not the imaging modality of choice for further characterization of adnexal lesions detected at sonography. In contrast, for staging of suspected ovarian cancer it remains the primary imaging modality. Other indications for CT include contraindications for MRI, assessment of acute pelvic pain and to rule out complications of pelvic inflammatory disease. Due to its wide clinical use, however, many adnexal lesions are encountered by CT examinations. The use of bowel opacification is generally recommended in the assessment of adnexal lesions. It is crucial in the differentiation of fluid filled-bowel and cystic adnexal lesions and improves the identification of peritoneal seeding. Furthermore, especially in thin patients and in postmenopausal age, detection of normal ovaries is often only possible with bowel opacification. For this purpose, 1,000 ml of diluted contrast media or alternatively water are administered 1 h prior to the CT study. Rectal opacification is also helpful, especially if the oral contrast was not given early enough. Intravenous contrast opacification is pivotal for assessing adnexal lesions. It allows better characterization of the internal architecture and differentiation of pelvic vascular structures, including depiction of the ovarian vascular pedicle. In most cases, a venous phase enables best depiction of intralesional structures, as solid enhancing components and papillary projections may be missed in an early phase. A dual phase protocol, however, consisting of an arterial and venous phase may aid in improved assessment of the local extent or the anatomical relationships of an adnexal lesion. If a dermoid is suspected sonographically, a study without i.v. contrast media may be sufficient. However, torsion can only be assessed after contrast media application. In cases of large endometriomas a noncontrast study may also be helpful to differentiate hemorrhage from enhancing solid areas.

9.3
Defining the Origin of a Pelvic Mass: Adnexal Versus Extra-adnexal Versus Extraperitoneal

Defining the correct origin is the first diagnostic step in defining treatment of a suspected adnexal mass. Depending on the site of origin the differential diagnoses and treatment options often differ completely. Size, architecture, and location may appear similar in adnexal, extra-adnexal peritoneal masses, and even extraperitoneal lesions. However, special features determining the anatomical relationship of the mass and the surrounding pelvic anatomical structures can assist in their differentiation [9]. These parameters include visualization of ovarian structures, the type of contour deformity at the interface between the ovary and the pelvic mass, and the displacement pattern of the vessels, ureters, and other pelvic organs.

Identifying a mass separate from the ipsilateral ovary indicates its nonovarian origin (Fig. 9.2). However, especially in large pelvic lesions, the ovary may often be obscured or totally invaded by the mass [10]. Especially in smaller lesions when the ovary is not completely obscured, identifying ovarian structures, usually ovarian follicles, indicate its ovarian origin (Fig. 9.3). Furthermore, for this purpose analyzing specific signs such as the beak sign, and the embedded organ sign can aid in better defining its relationship with the ovary. When a mass deforms the edge of the ovary into a beak shape it is likely that it arises from the ovary (Fig. 9.3). In contrast, dull edges at the interface with the adjacent ovary suggest that the tumor compresses the ovary but does not arise from it [9].

Large ovarian masses typically displace the ureter posteriorly or posterolaterally. The same displacement pattern, however, can be caused by other intraperitoneal lesions, such as the bladder, and masses arising form the uterus or bowel [11]. The iliac vessels are typically displaced laterally by an adnexal lesion. In contrast, medial displacement of the iliac vessels is typical for extraovarian masses, originating from the pelvic wall or in lymphadenopathy (Fig. 9.4). The origin of a mass may be further elucidated by tracking the vascular pedicle or the ovarian suspensory ligament [9]. The presence of ovarian vessels leading to or emerging from an adnexal mass was identified in 92% of ovarian lesions on helical CT [12]. Defining the ovarian vascular pedicle allows the differentiation from lesions mim-

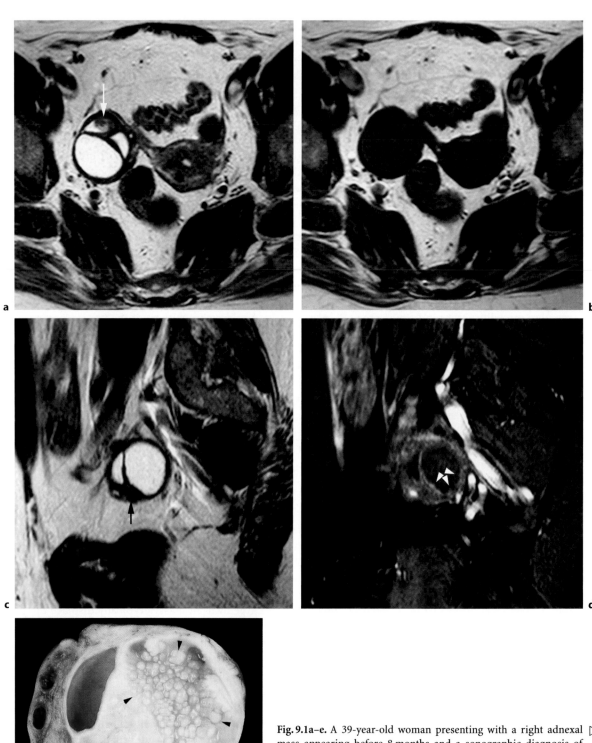

Fig. 9.1a–e. A 39-year-old woman presenting with a right adnexal ▷
mass appearing before 8 months and a sonographic diagnosis of
atypical endometriosis. MRI is performed at day 10 of the menstrual cycle for additional lesion characterization. Axial oblique T2
(**a**) and T1-weighted images (**b**), sagittal T2-weighted images (**c**),
contrast-enhanced T1-weighted images with fat saturation (FS) (**d**),
gross specimen photography (**e**). A multilocular cystic mass of the
right ovary (**a**) with a heterogeneous content in the most anterior
loculation (*arrow*). The corresponding T1-weighted image (**b**) shows
a hypointense content without any hemorrhagic portion excluding

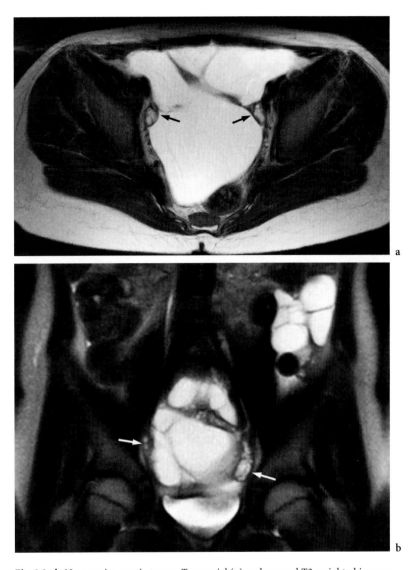

Fig. 9.2a,b. Nonovarian cystic tumor. Transaxial (**a**) and coronal T2-weighted images (**b**) in a 14-year-old girl in whom sonography, to rule out an abscess after appendectomy, found a multicystic ovarian lesion. A large bilateral multiseptate lesion extending above the umbilical level is demonstrated in both planes. Identification of normal ovaries (*arrows*) allows exclusion of an ovarian origin of the lesion. Histopathology of the surgical specimen diagnosed a chyloma

the diagnosis of endometrioma. Sagittal T2-weighted image through the heterogeneous part of the cyst shows a hypointense solid portion (*arrow*) with converging thin septa of the cyst, possibly suggesting normal ovarian parenchyma (**c**). Contrast enhancement of the ovarian parenchyma and a slightly irregular interface between the cystic content and the wall of the cyst (*arrowheads*) is demonstrated in **d**. MRI diagnosed prospectively a benign multilocular tumor of the ovary without arguments for endometriosis. Gross specimen photography (**e**) of the right ovary shows a multilocular cyst with tiny papillary projections within the wall of the posterior loculation (*arrowheads*) and a white fibrous portion. Microscopic analysis diagnosed a benign serous cystadenofibroma of the ovary

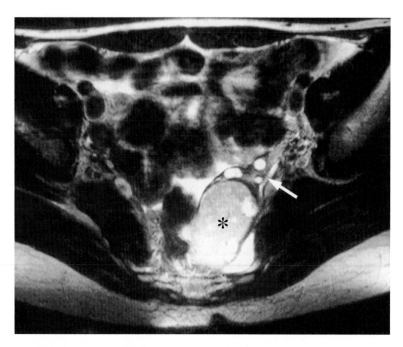

Fig. 9.3. Beak sign. Transaxial T2-weighted images shows a mass in the left cul-de-sac (*asterisk*). Its ovarian origin can be clearly identified due to multiple follicles (*arrow*). The interface to the ovarian tissue is characterized by a sharp angulation, which is typical for the beak sign. A small amount of free fluid in the cul-de-sac as seen in this patient is a physiological finding in premenopausal age and peaks in the secretory phase

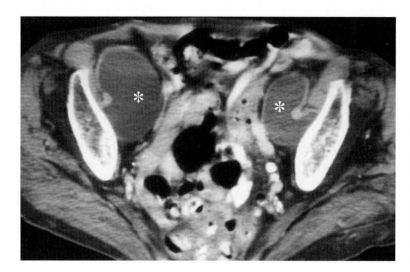

Fig. 9.4. Medial displacement of the iliac vessels. Transaxial CT in a patient with sonographically suspected bilateral ovarian cancer. Bilateral cystic lesions (*asterisks*) with mural thickening are simulating ovarian lesions. The displacement pattern of the iliac vessels, however, is typical for an origin from the pelvic sidewalls. The lesions present bilateral bursitis iliopectinea in a patient with rheumatoid arthritis

icking ovarian tumors, such as subserosal uterine leiomyoma. Furthermore, in the majority of leiomyoma cases, a vascular bridging sign at the interface between uterus and leiomyoma can be observed, which is not the case in ovarian lesions (Fig. 9.5) [13]. Because of their close anatomic relationship, masses arising from the fallopian tubes cannot be distinguished from ovarian lesions by identifying the ovarian vessels or the ovarian suspensory ligament [8]. However, incomplete septa emerging from the wall of a cystic adnexal mass indicate the fallopian origin of the mass (Fig. 9.6) [14].

9.4
Characterizing Ovarian Lesions

9.4.1
Differentiation Between Benign and Malignant Ovarian Lesions

Discrimination between benign and malignant ovarian tumors in patients who present with an adnexal mass is important for several reasons. It may directly affect the surgical decisions, including the adequate therapeutic

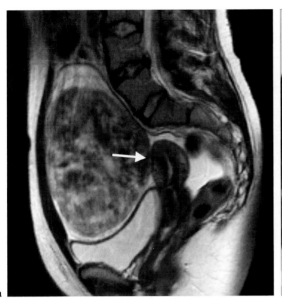
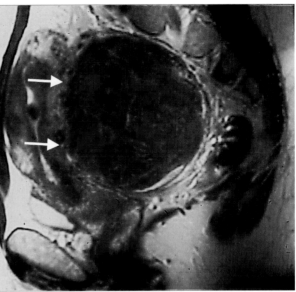

a   b

Fig. 9.5a,b. Ovarian vs extraovarian mass. Sagittal T2-weighted images images demonstrate solid lesions adjacent to the uterus in two women of reproductive age. In ovarian fibroid (**a**), the uterus can be separated from the ovarian mass (*arrowhead*). Ascites is found in the cul-de sac and surrounding the ovarian fibroid (**a**). A subserosal uterine fibroid (**b**) can be differentiated from an ovarian mass by demonstration of multiple bridging vessels. The latter (*arrows*) are found at the interface between the lesion and the myometrium

approach, surgical technique, and need of subspeciality cooperation. Furthermore, in times where endoscopic surgery has become very popular, thorough pretreatment evaluation should diminish the possibility of encountering an unexpected ovarian cancer [15].

The most commonly used criteria for differentiation between benign and malignant adnexal lesions do not differ between US, CT, and MRI. They include size, internal architecture of the mass, and assessment of additional signs suggestive of an invasive nature of the lesion, such as presence of lymphadenopathy and peritoneal implants, or ascites. Especially in sonography, more complex tests with multiparameter scoring systems, the combination of ultrasonographic characterization and Doppler findings and/or tumor markers have been suggested to improve performance [16, 17]. A multivariate analysis reported optimal lesion characterization when a combination of morphologic sonographic and color Doppler information is used (Fig. 9.7) [18]. Tumor size, wall thickness, and internal architecture, including the presence of septations, calcifications, papillary projections, and cystic and solid internal structures, have been established as diagnostic criteria for tumor characterization in all imaging modalities. At ultrasound, the presence of solid internal structures usually implies the use of

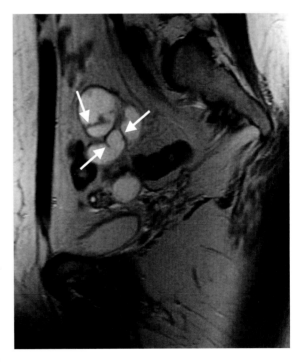

Fig. 9.6. Incomplete septations. Parasagittal T2-weighted images of a left adnexal mass. Incomplete interdigitating septa (*arrows*) are typical findings of a hydrosalpinx arising from the uterus. Widening of the fallopian tube to a diameter of 4 cm at the fimbriated end is seen

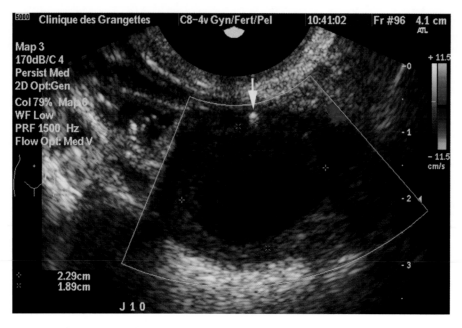

Fig. 9.7. Endometrioma with absent flow. A 34-year-old patient with chronic perimenstrual left pelvic pain. Sagittal transvaginal color Doppler sonographic image of the left ovary at day 10 of the menstrual cycle demonstrates a heterogeneous mass (between calipers) with two layers of internal low level echos, a wall calcification (*arrow*) and absent intracystic color Doppler flow. Pathology of the ovarian cyst diagnosed endometrioma

color Doppler ultrasound to identify the presence of intratumoral vessels indicative of solid tissue [19]. False-positive findings at ultrasound are possible using this specific diagnostic criteria because of the presence of vessels in solid structures in a wall thickening of a dermoid cyst, also called dermoid plug, which may contain tissue components of all three embryonic layers such as bone, lung, and skin tissue components [20]. Recognition of associated fat within the adnexal mass eases diagnosis of mature cystic teratoma. A second benign ovarian mass with solid tissue corresponds to ovarian fibromas and fibrothecomas characterized by mainly homogeneous solid tissue with a few small vessels and no or few associated cystic components (Fig. 9.8) [21].

At ultrasound, teratomas typically present as echogenic masses with acoustic shadowing due to hairballs or calcifications such as teeth or bone in the Rokitansky protuberance (Fig. 9.9) [22]. Layered lines and dots, the fat–fluid level, and isolated bright echogenic foci with acoustic shadowing are characteristic sonographic findings of dermoid cysts [23]. The majority of dermoid cysts can be reliably diagnosed by CT and MRI by the presence of intralesional fat. Endometriomas at ultrasound demonstrate diffuse low-level internal echos with hyperechoic foci

in the wall of a multilocular cyst [24]. The positive predictive value of sonography to predict endometriosis was evaluated at 75% when criteria such as diffuse low-level internal echos and absent neoplastic features were used. The use of color Doppler images helps to show absent flow within the sometimes heterogeneous cystic content. The presence of hyperechoic foci alone at the surface of the ovary is not a sign for endometriosis [25].

When CT and MRI are used, characteristics of malignancy can be best assessed in combination with contrast-enhanced studies [7, 26].

For all other ovarian lesions, features suggesting that a lesion is benign include lesion size less than 4 cm, entirely cystic architecture, wall thickness less than 3 mm, lack of internal structures, lack of ascites, and lack of peritoneal disease or lymphadenopathy. Using these criteria, MRI has been shown to have a 91%–95% accuracy for differentiating benign from malignant adnexal tumors [7, 27, 28]. Particularly the presence of papillary projections within an ovarian lesion should raise the suspicion of malignancy [19]. The presence of necrosis within a solid portion of an ovarian mass was most predictive of malignancy in a multivariate logistic regression analysis in a population of patients with complex sonographic adnexal

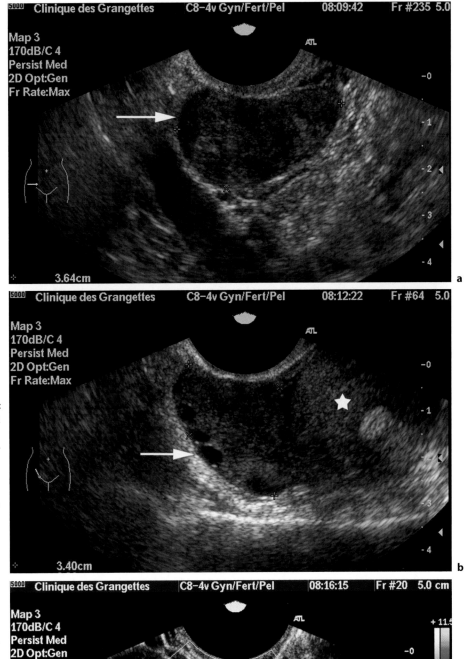

Fig. 9.8a–c. Fibroid on US: a 40-year-old patient with a right adnexal mass at physical routine examination by the gynecologist. Transvaginal US in axial, axial oblique (**a**), and sagittal oblique (**b**) plane. A 36-mm circumscribed heterogeneous oval mass (*arrow*) is demonstrated close to the right external iliac vessels (**a**) A more oblique orientation identifies a separate normal-appearing right ovary (*arrow*) close to the uterus (*star*, **b**). Color Doppler image (**c**) shows both the right ovary with parenchymal ovarian vessels (*arrow*) and the adjacent solid mass with tiny vessels (*arrowheads*). No vascular communication is seen between the ovary and the right-sided solid mass. Subsequent surgery and pathology confirmed leiomatoma of the right large ligament

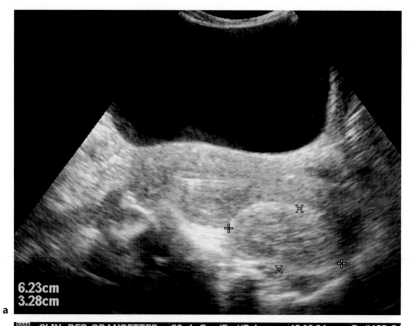

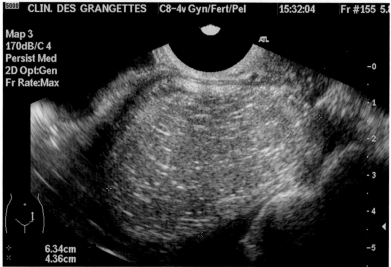

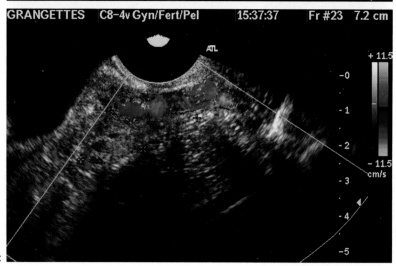

Fig. 9.9a–c. Dermoid on transvaginal sonography. Axial transabdominal US (**a**), transvaginal sagittal US (**b**), color Doppler US (**c**) in a 40-year-old woman with incidental left adnexal mass during ultrasound for intrauterine device change. Axial transabdominal ultrasound (**a**) of the pelvis demonstrates a left adnexal mass posterior to the uterus containing an intrauterine device. The left adnexal mass is isoechoic to the myometrium and contains a hyperechoic peripheral portion with posterior attenuation, suggesting calcification. The transvaginal sagittal image of the mass (**b**) shows an ovally shaped, well-circumscribed mass with hyperechoic content and wall-simulating bowel. The color Doppler transvaginal image (**c**) demonstrates utero-ovarian vessels providing blood flow to the compressed triangular ovarian parenchyma indicated by calipers at one pole of the mass. The cystic content of the heterogeneous hyperechoic ovarian mass is confirmed by absent intracystic color flow. Subsequent laparoscopy confirmed mature cystic teratoma

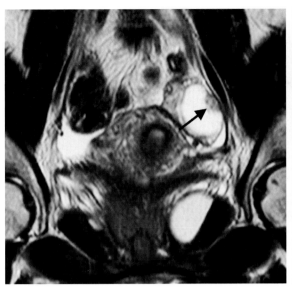
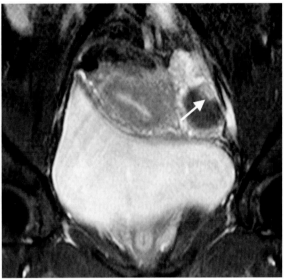

a
b

Fig. 9.10a,b. Vegetation within a cyst. Coronal T2-weighted images (**a**) and contrast-enhanced T1-weighted images with FS (**b**). In a 3.5-cm ovarian cyst, a mural nodule of 10 mm with low signal intensity on T2-weighted images (**a**) and contrast enhancement (**b**) is demonstrated. This finding should warrant the suspicion of malignancy, especially a borderline tumor as in this patient. Papillary projections in cystadenomas tend to be smaller

masses undergoing MRI for lesion characterization. "Necrosis in a solid lesion" (odds ratio, 107) was followed by "vegetations in a cystic lesion" (odds ratio, 40) identified after intravenous injection of gadolinium-based contrast material (Fig. 9.10). Interobserver (K, 0.79–0.85) and intraobserver (K, 0.84–0.86) agreement were excellent [7].

Calcifications can be easily detected in CT, whereas they are difficult to appreciate on MRI. Calcifications within the wall or the dermoid plug are a typical finding in dermoid cysts. Dense calcifications are often found in benign stromal tumors in middle-aged women. Psammoma bodies found at histologic examination in up to 30% of malignant serous tumors present a subtle finding on CT with tiny amorphic calcifications [29].

The malignancy rate in completely cystic masses in postmenopausal women is extremely low (less than 1%–2%) (Fig. 9.11) [30]. The probability of malignancy is related to lesion size. GOLDSTEIN et al. did not find cancers in cystic lesions less than 5 cm in size in postmenopausal women, and RULIN and PRESTON found in 150 ovarian masses in the same age group to be cancers in only 3%, when the size was less than 5 cm, and they were cancers in 11% of lesions with a diameter between 5 and 10 cm; however, 63% of lesions larger than 10 cm were malignant [31, 32].

Ascites alone is nonspecific with small amounts of pelvic fluid typically detected in the cul-de-sac (Fig. 9.3). Only larger amounts of pelvic fluid may be

an important ancillary finding to support the diagnosis of peritoneal spread in malignancy. Peritoneal enhancement is a pathologic finding, but is not specific and is associated with benign and malignant diseases [33]. Absence of ascites in the cul-de-sac in cases of ascites throughout the pelvis or abdomen has been described as a sign of malignancy [34].

The probability of malignancy is also related to the patient's age. In girls less than 9 years of age, 80% of ovarian masses are malignant, with the majority consisting of germ cell tumors. In women of reproductive age, the overall chance that an ovarian tumor will be malignant is 1 in 15 compared to 1 in 3 by 45 years of age [35].

9.4.2
Functioning Ovarian Tumors

Clinical and imaging findings may lead to the diagnosis of a functioning ovarian tumor.

The imaging findings comprise an ovarian mass, but also indirect findings as abnormalities of the uterus with uterine enlargement, a thickened endometrium in pre- and postmenopausal women, abnormal bleeding, features of virilization or endocrinologic symptoms [36].

Sex cord stromal tumors account for the majority of functioning ovarian tumors. These benign masses

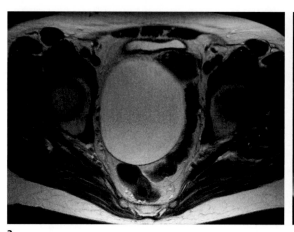
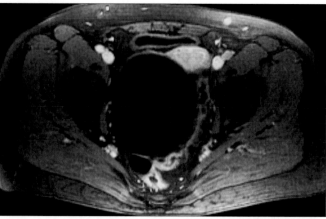

a

b

Fig. 9.11a,b. Large cystic adnexal lesion in a 55-year-old woman. Transaxial T2-weighted images (**a**) and T1-weighted images with fat saturation (**b**) show a unilocular right adnexal cyst. It displaces the uterus and the adjacent sigmoid colon. Imaging criteria include no evidence of malignancy. Due to postmenopausal age and the increase in size, surgery was performed. The histopathological diagnosis was serous cystadenoma

as well as neoplasms of low malignant potential account for the majority of estrogen-producing tumors. Granulosa cell tumors and the benign thecomas are the most common estrogen-producing tumors (Fig. 9.12). Some mucinous cystadenomas, and rarely ovarian cancer and metastases may also produce estrogens [37]. In the majority of women of reproductive age, virilization is associated with the benign disorder polycystic ovaries disease (PCOS). Virilizing ovarian tumors are rare, typically solid ovarian tumors [38]. Sertoli Leydig cell tumors are typically found in young women and account for two-thirds of these tumors causing hirsutism or virilization. In middle-aged women, steroid cell tumors can cause virilization and/or Cushing's syndrome. Further-

more, rarely granulosa cell tumors, Brenner tumors, and fibrothecomas may also have virilizing effects.

In addition to the sex-cord stromal tumors, a variety of other benign and primary and metastatic malignant ovarian tumors may have a functioning stroma with estrogenic or androgenic production. However, these elevations will remain commonly subclinical. These tumors include mucinous tumors, rarely endometrioid carcinoma, malignant germ cell tumors, and mucinous metastatic carcinomas [37].

Thyroid hormones are typically produced in struma ovarii and struma carcinoids of the ovary in subclinical levels. Hyperthyreosis seems to be present in only 25%, and thyrotoxicosis occurs in only 5% of patients with struma ovarii (Fig. 9.13) [37]. Primary

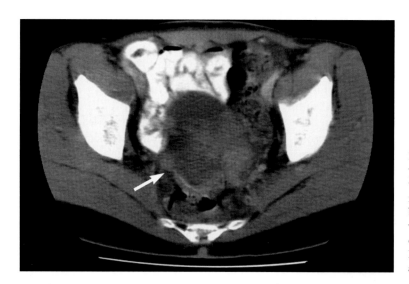

Fig. 9.12. Granulosa cell tumor. A 52-year-old female with a history of hysterectomy and unilateral oophorectomy for granulosa cell tumors several years before. A solid and cystic pelvic tumor with irregular margins displacing bowel loops is seen at the acetabular level. From imaging, it cannot be differentiated from an ovarian cancer

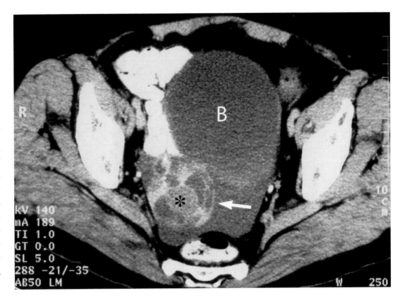

Fig. 9.13. Struma ovarii. Transaxial CT in a young woman who presented with a complex adnexal mass at sonography and no evidence of hyperthyreosis. A left adnexal (*arrow*) surrounded by ascites is demonstrated in the cul-de-sac. It is well defined, shows a thin wall, and demonstrates a solid and cystic architecture. Within the lesion a locule (*asterisk*) of high density presents hemorrhage. *B*, bladder. Courtesy of Dr. T.M. Cunha, Lisbon

carcinoids of the ovary are rarely associated with carcinoid syndrome. Metastatic carcinoids involving the ovary, however, are associated with carcinoid syndrome in 50% of cases. Benign and malignant mucinous ovarian tumors may produce gastrin within the cyst wall and present clinically with Zollinger-Ellison syndrome [39].

9.4.2.1
Value of Imaging

The value of imaging in patients with clinically suspected functioning ovarian tumors is to rule out an adnexal mass. In case of virilization, it may also confirm the diagnosis of polycystic ovaries, and rule out an adrenal mass by thorough assessment of the adrenal glands.

9.4.3
Ovarian Tumors in Children, Adolescents, and Young Women

Imaging findings, age, and clinical presentation of ovarian masses in infants and young women are the basis of treatment strategy. In this age group – unless there is histologically proven malignancy – conservative ovarian surgery and preservation of fertility is a special concern.

The type of ovarian tumor depends on the morphology and patient's age. The majority of ovarian masses in children older than 9 years and young women are benign and include follicular cysts and dermoid cysts, with fewer than 5% of ovarian malignancies occurring in this age group. However, lesions with complex architecture should be carefully assessed, as 35% of all malignant ovarian neoplasms occur during childhood and adolescence. This is especially true for children younger than 9 years, where approximately 80% of ovarian neoplasms are malignant [40]. A solid ovarian mass in childhood should also be considered malignant until proven otherwise by histology [41]. Differential diagnosis includes dysgerminoma, neuroblastoma (Fig. 9.14) rhabdomyosarcoma, lymphoma, and nongenital tumors in the pelvis. Some ovarian neoplasms occurring in this age group excrete protein tumor markers, which may aid in diagnosis and follow-up. They include alpha-fetoprotein, which is produced by endodermal sinus tumors, mixed germ cell tumors, and immature teratomas, lactate dehydrogenase, which is secreted by dysgerminomas, and human chorionic gonadotropin, which is elevated in pregnancy and pregnancy-related tumors and in embryonal ovarian carcinomas [41]. Torsion is a special problem in children and young adults presenting with an ovarian mass. Usually ovarian masses associated with torsion are benign cystic lesions (Fig. 9.15); particularly lesions presenting with a size greater than 5 cm seem to be under a special risk for torsion [42]. Acute pelvic pain is the mainstay in the differential diagnosis of a torsed ovary; however, imaging findings may be misleading and simulate a malignant ovarian tumor.

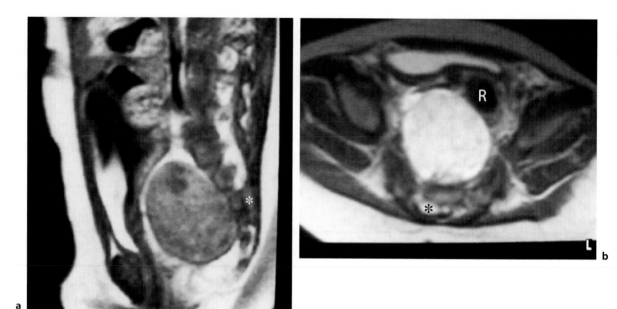

Fig. 9.14a,b. Pelvic neuroblastoma. Sagittal contrast-enhanced T1-weighted images (**a**) and transaxial T2-weighted images (**b**) of a 5-month-old girl with a sonographically detected right pelvic mass. A well-delineated solid tumor with moderate inhomogenous contrast enhancement (**a**) and bright signal on T2-weighted images (**b**) is seen in the posterior aspect of the pelvis. It compresses the bladder and displaces the rectum (*R*) anteriorly and to the left side. Furthermore, a small lesion (*asterisk*) with the same signal intensity as the tumor is seen in the sacral canal at the level of S3. At surgery, a neuroblastoma was resected, which was composed of a small intraspinal and a large pelvic tumor component

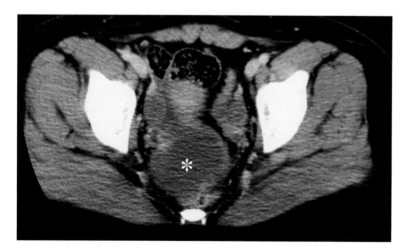

Fig. 9.15. Torsion of a paraovarian cyst. In a 14-year-old girl with severe acute pelvic pain a cystic lesion was found on sonography. CT shows normal ovaries in the ovarian fossa and a 7-cm cystic lesion (*asterisk*) in the cul-de-sac. The latter shows mild wall thickening at its left contour. Exploratory laparotomy found torsion of a right paraovarian cyst with involvement of the right fallopian tube. The ovaries were unremarkable

Ovarian cysts are uncommon before puberty. Most of these are physiologic follicular cysts that will resolve spontaneously. Some ovarian cysts may be hormonally active and result in precocious pseudopuberty, e.g., in McCune-Albright syndrome [43]. Development of cysts is extremely common between puberty and 18 years of age. Most of these cysts are functional ovarian cysts and may attain a size of up to 8–10 cm. In this age group, paraovarian or mesothelial cysts, hydrosalpinx, tubular pregnancy, and obstructive genital lesions may also simulate cystic ovarian lesions. Germ cell tumors account for half to two-thirds of the tumors in girls up to 18 years; they present 70% of ovarian tumors in the age between 10 and 30 years [44]. The vast majority are unilateral and present dermoid cysts. Only 3% of ovarian germ cell tumors are malignant. Dysgerminomas account for approximately 50% of the malignant germ cell malignancies in adolescents and young adults and are followed by endodermal sinus tumors (20%) and immature teratomas (19%). As in many ovarian malignancies, rapid growth is a typical finding; however, bilateral manifestation is more common in dysgerminomas than in other malignant germ cell tumors.

Endodermal sinus tumors are found in women at a median age of 18 years, often diffuse peritoneal dissemination is already present at the time of diagnosis [45].

Juvenile granulosa cell tumors are stromal cell tumors of low malignant potential, which occur before the age of 30. Rarely, they occur before puberty and may become clinically apparent as precocious puberty. Immature teratomas are commonly associated with a mature teratoma; they comprise 1% of all teratomas and occur most commonly in the first two decades of life. Tumor markers are usually negative [46].

9.4.3.1
Value of Imaging

Sonography is the modality of choice to determine the architecture of a suspected ovarian mass in children and young adolescents. The sonomorphologic pattern in combination with age, clinical manifestation and presence of tumor markers are pivotal to establish the diagnosis. Cystic lesions are usually followed and regress in the majority of cases. In case of growth, or presence of a complex cystic or solid ovarian lesion, further characterization by CT or MRI is usually performed (Fig. 9.2). The information obtained includes complementary evaluation of the site of origin, the nature of the mass (presence of fat or calcifications), and metastases. Because of radiation issues, MRI is the preferred imaging modality in this age group.

The imaging characteristics in CT and MRI of the different tumors are discussed in detail in this and Chap. 10.

9.4.4
Adnexal Masses in Pregnancy

With the widespread use of abdominal ultrasound during pregnancy, adnexal masses are concurrently diagnosed with increasing frequency. Adnexal mass-es have been reported to occur in 0.15%–1% of pregnancies. Most patients are asymptomatic at the age of presentation, and most adnexal masses disappear during the first 16 weeks of pregnancy [47]. The incidence of ovarian cancer associated with a persistent adnexal mass varies from 3% to 5.9% (Fig. 9.16). In a retrospective analysis of 60 adnexal masses during pregnancy, 50% included mature cystic teratomas, 20% cystadenomas, 13% functional ovarian cysts, and 13% malignant tumors. Among the latter, six out of eight were tumors of low malignant potential, and all malignant lesions were FIGO stage Ia tumors [48]. The therapeutic regimen of an adnexal mass during pregnancy depends on the size, sonomorphologic criteria, and gestational age. Lesion size seems to play an important role in the management of adnexal masses during pregnancy. Many authors recommend conservative treatment in adnexal masses 6 cm or smaller [48]. The vast majority of these are cysts, which will resolve spontaneously. Furthermore,

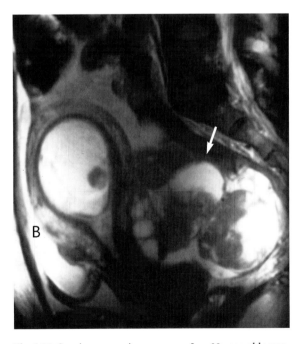

Fig. 9.16. Ovarian cancer in pregnancy. In a 38-year-old woman who underwent routine sonography during pregnancy, a suspicious adnexal lesion was found. Sagittal T2-weighted images shows dilatation of the uterine cavity and the fetus. A large solid and cystic adnexal mass is demonstrated located posterior and above the uterine cervix, compressing the rectum. Ascites is demonstrated in the upper pelvis, but not in the cul-de-sac. Surgical staging showed stage III ovarian cancer. *B*, compressed bladder

the risk of torsion of an ovarian mass of this size seems low.

SHERARD et al. reported an average size of 11.5 cm in malignant lesions, in contrast to benign lesions, which showed an average size of 7.6 cm [48]. Furthermore, papillary projections were a typical finding of borderline tumors.

Pain or an acute abdomen should alert to complications due to hemorrhage, rupture, and torsion of the adnexal mass (Fig. 9.17) or caused by nongynecological pelvic diseases.

9.4.4.1
Value of Imaging

Adnexal masses during pregnancy are often incidental findings during fetal sonography. Sonography is the modality of choice to further characterize these masses, assess their size, and plan follow-up. The aim of thorough assessment of an adnexal mass during pregnancy is to manage typical benign masses conservatively and/or to postpone surgery in the second or third trimester in order to reduce adverse fetal outcome. MRI has been used to characterize masses in pregnancy [49]. It is particularly useful to further characterize sonographically solid lesions, especially to exclude a leiomyoma and confirm the diagnosis of a dermoid. In patients with acute abdomen, MRI is also used as a complement to sonography to detect nongynecological causes, e.g., appendicitis or enteritis [50].

9.5
Benign Adnexal Lesions

9.5.1
Non-neoplastic Lesions of the Ovaries and Adnexa

9.5.1.1
Physiologic Ovarian Cysts

The ovaries change their appearance periodically during their ovarian cycle. The ovarian cycle consists of development of the ovarian follicle, rupture, discharge of the ovum, formation and regression of corpus luteum.

Ovarian cysts under 3 cm are regarded as physiologic cysts. They include follicles of various stages of development, corpus luteum cysts, and surface inclusion cysts.

Physiologic ovarian cysts constitute the vast majority of cystic adnexal lesions. They may be classified as functional, which means they are associated with hormone production, or nonfunctional.

They occur typically in women in the reproductive age; however, less commonly they may be also found in the postmenopausal age. In a series of 74 normal ovaries, the average size of the largest cyst was 1 cm (range, 0.2–4.7 cm) [51]. Functional cysts usually do not exceed 5 cm in size, but may occasionally grow as large as 8–10 cm (Fig. 9.18). In most cases, they are

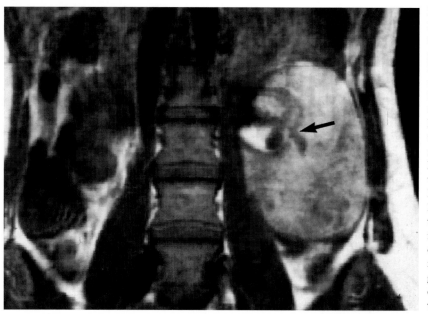

Fig. 9.17. Torsion of a dermoid. MRI was performed in a woman presenting with acute pelvic pain in the 16th week and an indeterminate mass at sonography. Coronal T1-weighted images shows a well-delineated mass 15 cm in diameter with high SI due to hemorrhage in the left mid abdomen. At its mediocranial aspect, an apple-like structure also containing very bright signal presents the Rokitansky nodule (*arrow*). Dilatation of the fallopian tube, which is a common associated finding in adnexal torsion, is demonstrated at the inferior margin of the lesion. At surgery, hemorrhagic infarction of the dermoid and left adnexa was found

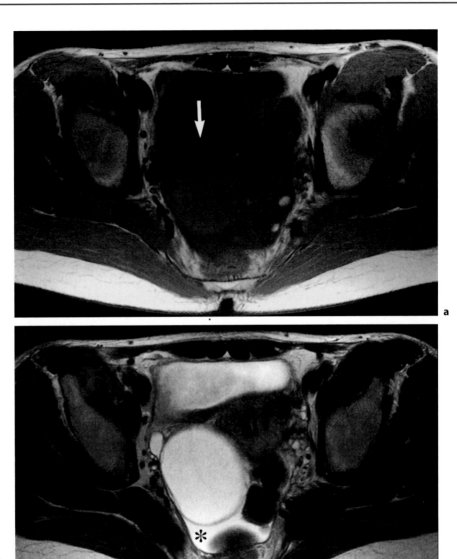

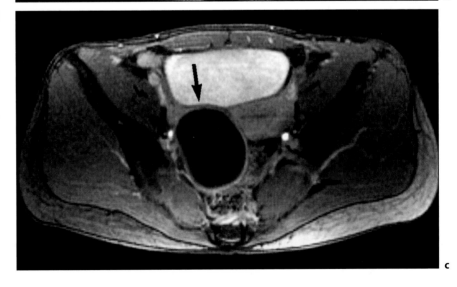

Fig. 9.18a–c. Functional cyst in a 29-year-old woman. Transaxial T1 (**a**), T2-weighted images (**b**) and contrast-enhanced T1-weighted images with FS (**c**). An 8-cm cystic ovarian lesion (*arrow*) with intermediate signal intensity on T1-weighted images similar to myometrium (**a**), and very high SI on T2-weighted images (**b**) displays a thin wall on the T2-weighted images (**b**) and after contrast administration (**c**). From imaging, a functional cyst, most likely a corpus luteum cyst, could not be differentiated from a cystadenoma. The sonographic follow-up showed a considerable decrease in size within 3 months. Small amount of ascites in the cul-de-sac

self-limiting and will regress spontaneously. In contrast to follicular cysts, corpus luteum cysts often require a period of up to 3 months to regress.

9.5.1.1.1
Follicular and Corpus Luteum Cysts

The majority of ovarian cysts are follicular cysts resulting from failure of rupture or of regression of the Graafian follicle. Under nonpregnant conditions, corpus luteum cysts derive from failure of regression or hemorrhage into the corpus luteum.

Functional cysts are asymptomatic in the majority of cases. Progesterone production may persist in corpus luteum cysts, resulting in delayed menstruation or bleeding anomalies. Large physiologic cysts may cause abdominal pressure or low back pain. Acute abdomen is caused by complications such as rupture, hemorrhage, or torsion.

9.5.1.1.2
Imaging Findings in Physiologic Ovarian Cysts

Transvaginal sonography is currently the gold standard for the diagnosis of ovarian cysts. Findings include anechoic thin walled cysts for simple follicular cysts and a fishnet like heterogeneous hypoechoic content for hemorrhagic follicular or luteal cysts also described with a fine trabecular jelly-like content (Fig. 9.19) [52]. Most of these cysts will disappear or decrease in size at short-term follow-up. In all, 65% of the cysts persisting after menstruation had resolved at the first control examination 3 months later, independently of the use of oral contraceptives [53].

Simple ovarian cysts are a common incidental finding in CT and MRI. They are unilocular and display an imperceptible or thin (<3 mm) wall. On CT they appear as round or oval water-density lesions (<20 HU). Most cysts display intermediate to low signal intensity (SI) on T1-weighted images, and very high signal intensity on T2-weighted images, due to presence of simple fluid. The thin wall is best depicted on T2-weighted images as hypointense and on contrast enhanced images as hyperintense to ovarian stroma [51]. Hemorrhagic ovarian cysts and corpus luteum cysts tend to display a high SI on T1 and intermediate to high SI on T2-weighted images [51]. Corpus luteum cysts tend to have thicker walls than follicle cysts, with distinct enhancement due to their thick luteinized cell lining. Layering by debris and internal fibrin clots in corpus luteum cysts can be differentiated from papillary projections in epithelial tumors by their lack of enhancement.

Differential Diagnosis

Functional cysts smaller than 2.5-3 cm cannot be differentiated from normal mature follicles. Unilocular cystadenomas may mimic functional cysts. Regression in a follow-up over two to three cycles, however, will allow the diagnosis of a nonneoplastic functional cyst. Unilocular cystic lesions even in postmenopausal women have an extremely low incidence of malignancy (Fig. 9.11) [32].

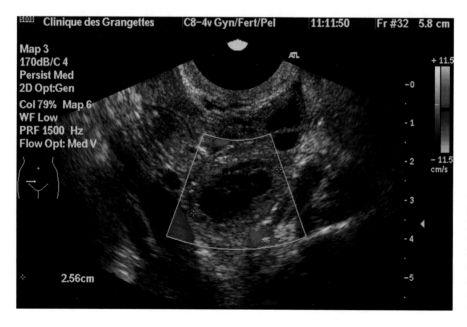

Fig. 9.19. Corpus luteum cyst in sonography. A 35-year-old woman with recent right pelvic pain. Axial transvaginal sonographic image of the right ovary shows a 25-mm ovarian cyst with hypoechoic heterogeneous content, an irregular wall, absent intracystic color Doppler flow, and increased peripheral blood flow within the ovarian parenchyma, suggesting a corpus luteum cyst. Findings where confirmed at a follow-up sonography 3 months later, demonstrating a normal right ovary

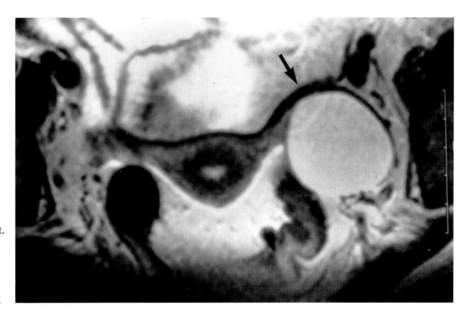

Fig. 9.20. Paraovarian cyst. Transaxial T2-weighted images shows a thin-walled cyst (*arrow*) displacing the left adnexa. Not histologically verified

Both corpus luteum cysts and endometrioma may show intracystic hemorrhage; however, only in endometrioma will a prominent T2 shortening ("shading") be observed [54]. Furthermore, in endometriosis often multiple hemorrhagic cysts may be found.

9.5.1.2
Paraovarian Cysts

Paraovarian cysts (paratubal) cysts arise from Wolffian duct remnants in the mesovarium [2]. They are often an incidental finding. Although encountered throughout life, they are most commonly found in middle-aged women. Surgical data suggest that they account for 10%–20% of adnexal masses [55]. They are round or ovoid, unilocular thin-walled cysts with a wide range of sizes between 1 and 12 cm; several have been reported as large as 28 cm [56]. Complications do not differ from those of functional ovarian cysts. Secondary transformation with foci of benign and malignant papillary neoplasms is extremely rare [57].

9.5.1.2.1
Imaging Findings

Paraovarian cysts tend to be large thin-walled unilocular cysts, located typically within the broad ligament (Fig. 9.20). Rarely they may contain internal septations. On CT and MRI, they display typical criteria of ovarian cysts, but are found separate from the ipsilateral ovary [55, 58].

9.5.1.2.2
Differential Diagnosis

A paraovarian cyst can only be distinguished from an ovarian cyst if it is clearly separate from the ovary. While paraovarian cysts are usually larger cysts, cysts of Morgagni, which arise from the fimbriated end of the tube, usually do not exceed 1 cm in diameter. The differential diagnosis of paraovarian cysts includes ovarian cystadenoma, an eccentric ovarian cyst, retroperitoneal cysts, and lymphoceles. The latter can be differentiated based on the clinical history and the pattern of vascular displacement. Hydrosalpinx may have a similar location within the broad ligament; however, it displays a tubular form and interdigitating septa. In contrast to paraovarian cysts, peritoneal inclusion cysts are often not round, but their shape is defined by the surrounding structures. Complicated paraovarian cysts cannot be differentiated from abscesses, endometriomas, and even ovarian cancer.

9.5.1.3
Peritoneal Inclusion Cysts

Peritoneal inclusion cysts (pseudocysts) are accumulations of fluid produced by the ovaries that become entrapped by peritoneal adhesions. These lesions are typically encountered in patients with previous surgery, endometriosis, or pelvic inflammatory disease (PID). They are of variable size and tend to adhere to adjacent structures. Pseudocysts have an irregular shape because the outer surface is not a true wall but defined by surrounding structures. They may become clinically apparent due to mass effect, pain, or present without symptoms [56].

9.5.1.3.1
Imaging Findings

Peritoneal inclusion cysts tend to take the shape of the space they are occupying, and may displace surrounding structures. The ovary or tubes lie typically inside or inside the cyst wall and may be mistaken as a solid nodule (Fig. 9.21). The internal architecture of peritoneal inclusion cysts depends on the contents. In most cases, they contain simple fluid with low SI on T1-weighted images and very high SI on T2-weighted images, and low density on CT. Hemorrhage and layering of hemosiderin can lead to high SI on T1 and low SI on T2 W, and higher densities on CT. In one study internal septa were found in 11/15 cases of peritoneal inclusion cysts [56].

9.5.1.3.2
Differential Diagnosis

Septations within a peritoneal inclusion cyst, the murally located ovary mimicking a solid component within a cystic mass, and distortion of pelvic anatomy may make the differentiation from a malignant ovarian tumor difficult. The coverage of adjacent organs and the history of a previous surgery or pelvic adhesions may be key arguments for the correct diagnosis [59].

9.5.1.4
Theca Lutein Cysts

Theca lutein cysts are ovarian cysts that are lined by luteinized theca cells. They develop in patients with high levels of serum human chorionic gonadotropin. They are not as common as other ovarian cysts. They are associated with multiple gestations, trophoblastic disease, and pregnancies complicated by hydrops fetalis, or in ovarian hyperstimulation syndrome.

9.5.1.4.1
Imaging Findings

Theca lutein cysts are typically large, bilateral multiseptate ovarian cysts composed of simple fluid. They may cause gross enlargement of the ovaries to 10–20 cm in diameter. T2-weighted images or contrast-enhanced MRI or CT will typically display no evidence of mural thickening (Fig. 9.22).

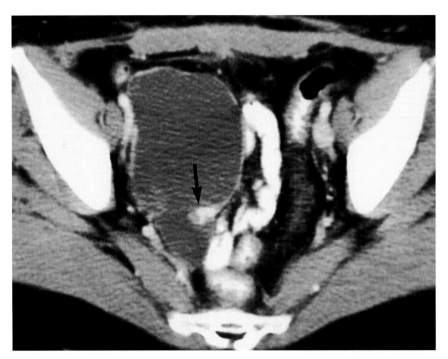

Fig. 9.21. Peritoneal inclusion cyst. In a 33-year-old woman with a history of several previous pelvic surgeries, a cystic lesion of the right adnexa was found at sonography. CT demonstrates a cystic lesion with thin enhancing walls and a solid ovoid structure (*arrow*) at its posterior wall. Surgery revealed an inclusion cyst, the solid structure presented the normal ovary

9.5.1.4.2
Differential Diagnosis

Theca lutein cysts may resemble bilateral cystadenomas; however, the clinical background is different.

9.5.1.5
Polycystic Ovary Syndrome

Polycystic ovary syndrome (PCOS) is a complex endocrinologic disorder characterized by inappropriate gonadotropin secretion that results in chronic anovulation [60]. It affects as many as 5%-10% of women of reproductive age, and is found in 50% in women with infertility problems [61].

Although most notable in Stein-Leventhal syndrome, which comprises the classical findings of amenorrhea, hirsutism, obesity, and sclerotic ovaries, a wide range of clinical presentations exist. Only one-quarter to one-half of the patients present the classical signs. Usually, infertility is the leading clinical problem of patients with PCOS. Recently, ultrasonographic studies reported a prevalence of polycystic ovaries in young women of at least 20%. However, there seems to be an overlap of polycystic ovaries and normal ovaries [62].

An increased risk of endometrial cancer in patients has been noted in patients with PCOS younger than 40 years of age due to chronic estrogen stimulation [63]. PCOS may also be associated in women with venous congestion who suffer from pelvic pain [64].

The morphologic hallmark is mild enlargement of both ovaries, which contain multiple small cysts surrounding the increased central ovarian stroma. The follicles may concurrently exist in different stages of growth, maturation, or atresia.

9.5.1.5.1
Imaging Findings

As there seems to be an overlap of normal and polycystic ovaries in imaging, the diagnosis of polycystic ovary syndrome is based on hormonal changes as well as clinical and imaging findings [65].

The imaging modality of choice is transvaginal US [55]. MRI is used as a complement to US to confirm the diagnosis of PCOS or to exclude a virilizing ovarian tumor.

The imaging findings in PCOS include bilateral moderately enlarged (up to 5 cm) spherical ovaries with an abnormally high number of follicles (Fig. 9.23) These follicles are typically found in a peripheral distribution. At least ten follicles ranging between 2 and 8 mm in size encircle the abnormally hypointense central stroma (Fig. 9.24). A dominant follicle is typically not seen [66]. Rarely, a normal contralateral ovary may be identified. The ovaries are surrounded by a thickened sclerotic capsule and typically display abundant low signal central stroma on T1- and T2-weighted images (Fig. 9.24).

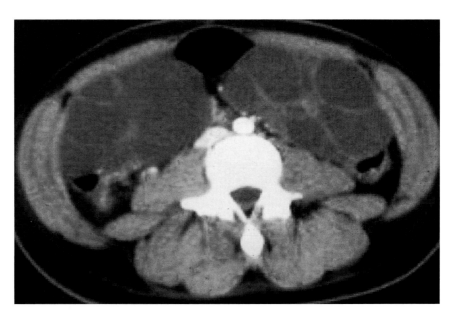

Fig. 9.22. Bilateral theca lutein cysts CT at the umbilical level in a 27-year-old patient with a hydatiform mole. Bilaterally enlarged ovaries are demonstrated displaying numerous thin-walled cysts of water-like density. No enhancing solid structures or papillary projections could be identified. Theca lutein cysts are found in up to 20% of patients with a hydatiform mole

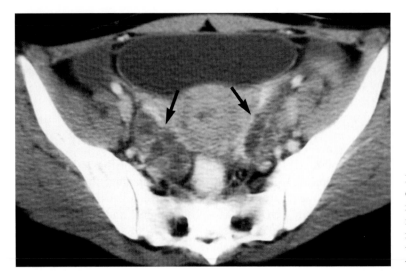

Fig. 9.23. Polycystic ovaries in CT. Bilateral spherical ovaries (*arrows*) can be identified lateral of the uterine corpus in the ovarian fossa. Numerous uniformly sized follicles are found within the ovaries in this case of PCO, which was surgically verified

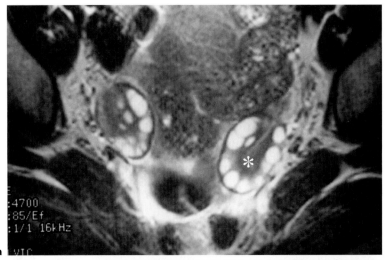

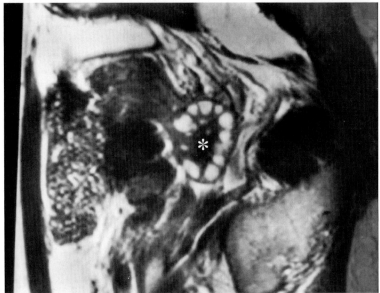

Fig. 9.24a,b. Polycystic ovaries in MRI. Transaxial T2-weighted images (**a**) and parasagittal T2 WI (**b**) in a patient with Stein-Leventhal syndrome. Bilateral spherical ovaries are demonstrated showing numerous small follicles of uniform size. The latter are located in the periphery of the ovary and surround the ovarian stroma (*asterisk*), which typically is of very low signal intensity on T2-weighted images in PCO

9.5.1.5.2
Differential Diagnosis

Multifollicular ovaries are found in mid to late puberty as a normal finding. Multifollicular ovaries may also result from hyperprolactinemia, hypothalamic anovulation, and weight-related amenorrhea. They may be differentiated from PCO by fewer cysts, the different size of follicles, lack of stromal hypertrophy, and the distribution of the often larger follicles throughout the ovary. In contrast to PCO, the ovaries resume normal appearance after treatment.

9.5.2
Benign Neoplastic Lesions of the Ovaries

Benign ovarian neoplasm account for 80% of all tumors involving the ovaries. Although there is large spectrum of benign ovarian neoplasm, the vast majority are encompassed by only a few different histologic types. It is a matter of debate whether cystadenomas or teratomas are most frequent. In a large series cystic teratomas accounted for the majority of benign lesions (58%) followed by serous cystadenomas (25%) and mucinous cystadenomas (12%), benign stromal tumors (fibromas/fibrothecomas) (4%), and Brenner tumors (1%) [67].

9.5.2.1
Cystadenoma

Cystadenomas account for 37%-50% of benign ovarian tumors in the reproductive age. Their frequency tends to increase with age, and after menopause, cystadenomas account for up to 80% of the benign ovarian tumors [1]. Cystadenomas are thin-walled unilocular or multilocular cystic lesions filled with serous mucinous, and sometimes hemorrhagic contents. Papillary projections within the cyst walls may be rarely found, but they should principally raise the suspicion of a borderline malignancy [68, 69]. The two types serous and mucinous cystadenomas differ in pathology, prognosis, and disease course.

Serous cystadenomas account for up to 40% of all benign ovarian neoplasms. They show a peak incidence in the fourth and fifth decades and are in up to 20% bilateral. Mucinous cystadenomas account for 20%-25% of all benign ovarian neoplasms, and are bilateral in only 2%-3% of cases. Both are cystic lesions filled with water-like or higher proteinaceous contents. Calcified psammoma bodies are a typical feature of serous cystadenomas. Mucinous cystadenomas tend to be filled with sticky gelatinous fluid. They tend to be larger at the time of presentation. In contrast to serous cystadenomas, mucinous cystadenomas are typically multilocular with different contents of the loculi (Fig. 9.25) [1]. These loculi are small and multiple and separated by thin septations. Rupture of a mucinous cystadenoma can result in pseudomyxoma peritonei.

9.5.2.1.1
Imaging Findings

Although an overlap exists, imaging features may aid in the differentiation of serous from mucinous cystadenomas [1]. Cystadenomas are well-circumscribed cystic tumors with enhancing thin walls and – if present – internal septations on CT and MRI (Fig. 9.25). The wall and septa are regular and thin (<3 mm) (Fig. 9.26). Papillary projections are rarely found in benign cystadenomas, and tend to be small (Fig. 9.1) [68].

The cystic loculi of serous cystadenomas display signal of simple fluid and tend to be low in signal on T1 and high on T2-weighted images (Fig. 9.11). In contrast, mucinous cystadenomas have often various signal intensities depending on the contents within the different loculi, which varies from watery to proteinaceous to hemorrhagic. The sticky gelatinous contents or mucin in mucinous cystadenomas display SI intensity higher than water on T2 and lower SI on T2-weighted images relative to serous fluid. When hemorrhage is present, blood products may be identified on MRI. The loculi of mucinous cystadenomas are often small and multiple. Multiple loculi with different contents within one lesion is a typical finding of mucinous cystadenomas. Rarely, they can manifest as a simple cyst.

Mucinous cystadenomas tend to be multilocular and larger at the time of presentation than serous cystadenomas. They present with a mean size of 10 cm, but may be as large as 30 cm [1].

9.5.2.1.2
Differential Diagnosis

Serous and mucinous cystadenomas may display similar imaging findings in CT and MRI. If papillary projections are found in cystadenomas, they tend to be fewer and smaller than in borderline

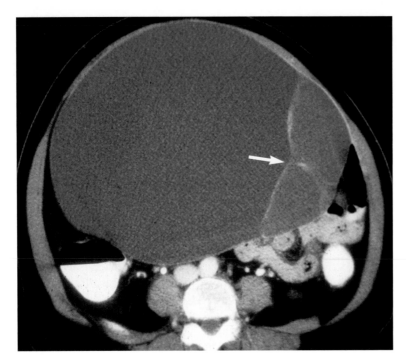

Fig. 9.25. Mucinous cystadenoma in CT. At the level of L5, a cystic ovarian lesion extending to the upper abdomen and measuring 25 cm in diameter is demonstrated. It bulges the abdominal wall and displaces bowel loops posteriorly. It displays multiple thin septations (*arrow*). Loculi in the left periphery display attenuation values which are higher than water. The large lesion size and different densities of the loculi are findings suggesting the diagnosis of a mucinous cystadenoma

tumors [68]. The presence of a mural nodule or focal wall thickening are signs highly indicative of malignancy. Microscopic foci of cystadenocarcinoma, which may arise in serous cystadenomas, will invariably be missed on imaging. Endometriomas may resemble mucinous cystadenomas, especially when they are complicated by hemorrhage. Low SI shading on the T2-weighted images is only found in endometrioma [54]. Furthermore, the walls in endometriomas tend to be thicker and irregular, and endometrioma usually are smaller than 10 cm. Hydrosalpinx can also display as a multiloculated uni- or bilateral adnexal lesion. In contrast to cystadenomas, the loculi communicate and incomplete septa are found. Furthermore, their origin from the tubal angle may enable the correct differential diagnosis.

9.5.2.2
Cystadenofibroma

Cystadenofibromas account for 1.7% of ovarian tumors. They are benign serous ovarian tumors that display as cystic tumors with variable amounts of fibrous stroma. They can also be purely cystic with small foci of stroma detected microscopically. The margin tends to be well defined and smooth. Endocrine activity is not found.

9.5.2.2.1
Imaging Features

The imaging features are nonspecific and may be similar to malignant tumors or borderline tumors. Variable amounts of fibrous stroma in ovarian cystadenofibromas produces imaging features that vary from purely cystic to a complex cystic tumor with one ore more solid components (Fig. 9.27). In one series of 32 ovarian cystadenofibromas, 50% displayed as multiloculated masses identical to cystadenomas. The other half were complex cystic tumors with one or more solid components and smooth thickened septa [70].

9.5.2.3
Benign Teratoma

Teratomas are the most common ovarian neoplasm in women under 45 years of age, and account for up to 70% of tumors in females less than 19 years of age [67]. Ovarian teratomas derive from germ cells and are classified into three main categories, among which the mature cystic teratomas account for 99%. Less common types of mature teratomas are the monodermal teratomas, which include the struma ovarii and carcinoid tumors. It is typical for monodermal teratomas not to be cystic but contain

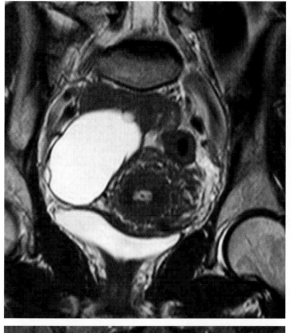

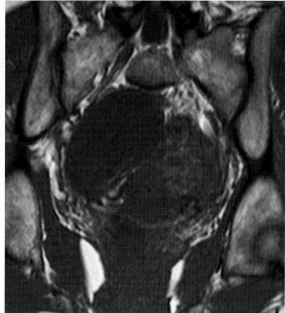

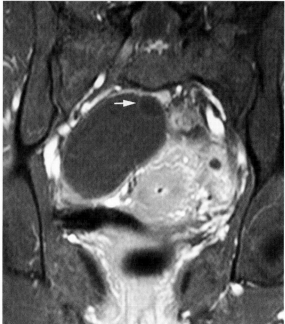

Fig. 9.26a–c. Mucinous cystadenoma. In a 48-year-old woman with a cystic mass in sonography, complementary MRI with coronal T2-weighted images (**a**), coronal T1-weighted images (**b**), and contrast-enhanced T1-weighted images (**c**) are demonstrated. Coronal T2-weighted MR image of the pelvis shows a hyperintense multilocular cystic mass with thin septation (**a**) in the right adnexal region. T1-weighted image confirms the purely cystic content of the cyst (**b**). The septations are thin and demonstrate contrast enhancement (**c**). Pathology after laparoscopic removal of the ovary showed benign mucinous cystadenoma of the ovary

primarily solid structures. Cystic teratomas typically contain lipid material consisting of sebaceous fluid within the cyst cavity or adipose tissue within the cyst wall or the dermoid plug [71].

9.5.2.3.1
Dermoid Cysts

Dermoid cysts or mature cystic teratomas are composed of mature tissue from at least two of the three germ cell layers: ectoderm, mesoderm, and endoderm. They are typically unilateral lesions, with only 10%-15% of dermoids found in both ovaries.

In the vast majority (88%), dermoid cysts are unilocular cystic lesions filled with sebaceous material. A protuberance, the Rokitansky nodule, or dermoid plug, projects into the cavity and is the hallmark of dermoids (Fig. 9.17). It contains a variety of tissues, often including fat and calcifications, which represent teeth or abortive bone. Fat is detected in over 90%,

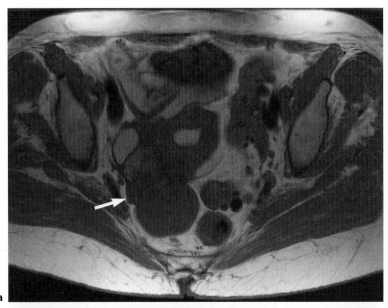

a

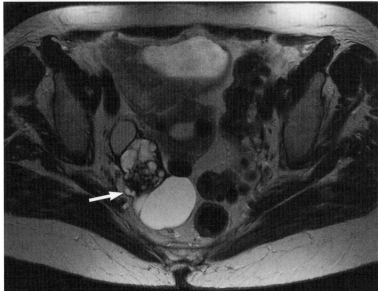

b

Fig. 9.27a,b. Cystadenofibroma. Trans-axial T1 (**a**) and T2-weighted images (**b**). In a 77-year-old female, a cystic adnexal mass showing an increase in size in a follow-up underwent preoperative MRI. A multiseptate cystic right adnexal lesion (*arrow*) with multiple hemorrhagic-proteinaceous loculi displaying high SI on the T1-weighted images (**a**) is demonstrated. It displays irregular septa of very low SI on T2-weighted images (**b**). The uterus is enlarged due to fibroids; the uterine cavity is widened by hematometra

teeth in 31% and calcifications in the wall in 56% [72].

A minority of dermoid cysts will demonstrate no fat or only small foci of fat within the wall or the Rokitansky nodule (Fig. 9.28) [73]. YAMASHITA et al. reported that 15% of mature teratomas did not show fat within the cystic cavity. Approximately half of these cases displayed small amounts of fat within the wall of the dermoid or the dermoid plug. In 8% of benign teratomas, no fat could be detected [73].

Dermoids are usually asymptomatic and tend to grow slowly. This is why some gynecologists advo-cate surgery in lesions larger than 6 cm in size [74]. Complications encountered with dermoid cysts are malignant degeneration and rupture, and with up to 16% torsion [75]. Malignant degeneration occurs in up to 2% and is usually found in the sixth to seventh decade; it is extremely rare and arises from the dermoid plug. The risk of malignancy is associated with large size (>10 cm) and postmenopausal age [76]. Rupture of a dermoid can cause acute abdomen due to granulomatous peritonitis caused by leakage of the fatty contents. Rarely, giant dermoids are found occupying the pelvis and abdomen.

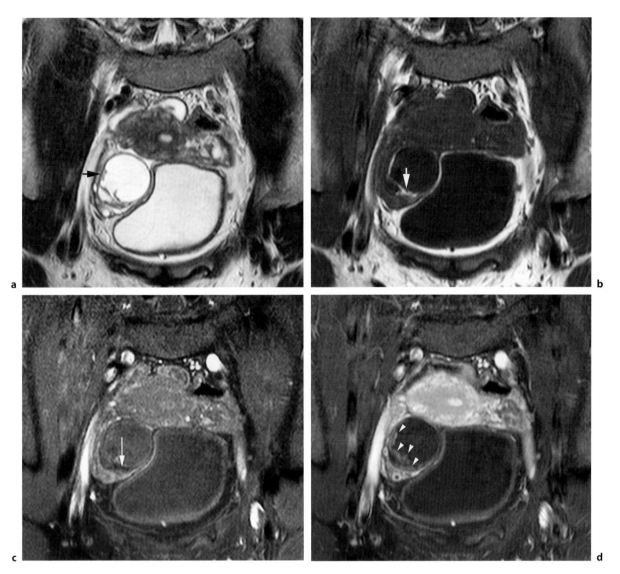

Fig. 9.28a–d. Dermoid with little fat. MRI was performed for further characterization of a sonographically suspicious cystic and solid mass in a 31-year-old woman. Coronal T2-weighted images (**a**), T1-weighted images (**b**), T1-weighted images with FS (**c**), contrast-enhanced T1-weighted images with FS (**d**). A multilocular mass with irregular wall thickening (*arrow*) (**a**) arising from the right adnexa is demonstrated. Coronal native T1-weighted image (**b**) confirms the cystic nature of the mass. A linear hyperintense portion is located at the lower part of the cyst (*white arrow*). The corresponding coronal fat-suppressed T1-weighted image (**c**) shows vanishing of the hyperintense linear part confirming the presence of a small amount of fat in the linear hypointense lower portion of the cyst (*white arrow*). The contrast-enhanced fat-suppressed T1-weighted image (**c**) shows enhancement of an irregular wall and septa (*arrowheads*) corresponding to the Rokitansky nodule of a dermoid cyst with little fat. Contrast enhancement of the mural protrusion of a mature cystic teratoma can be mistaken for ovarian cancer

Imaging Findings

Sonographic assessment of dermoid cysts is often limited by its variety of appearance.

At CT and MRI, however, the diagnosis of fat within a cystic mass is pathognomonic for a mature cystic teratoma [73]. The fatty elements display characteristic low CT attenuation (–20 to –120 HU) (Fig. 9.29). Another typical feature on CT is the presence of calcifications within the cyst wall or the dermoid plug.

The typical MRI findings include a round or oval, sharply delineated lesion with high SI on T1-weighted images, and loss of signal on the fat-saturated T1-weighted images, representing fat (Fig. 9.30). This fatty content may display a broad spectrum of

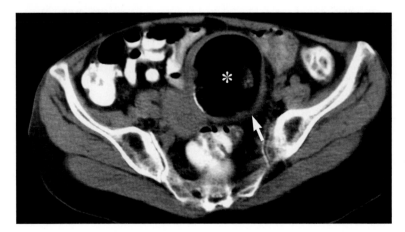

Fig. 9.29. Dermoid torsion in CT. Non-contrast transaxial CT in a 37-year-old female who presented with acute pelvic pain. A well-demarcated left adnexal lesion with fatty attenuation values (*asterisk*) is located adjacent to the uterus. Linear calcifications are found at its medial wall. An area of higher density within the fatty tissue correlated with floating hair in the macroscopic specimen. The homogenous wall thickening (*arrow*) is caused by edema due to torsion of the dermoid

appearance, including a fat-filled cavity, foci of fat within the lesion or its wall, and a fat–fluid interface often representing a floating mass of hair.

On T2-weighted images, the signal may be variable, but it tends to be similar to subcutaneous fat. Furthermore, chemical shift artifacts in the frequency-encoding direction can be observed, which confirms the presence of fat and differentiates it from hemorrhage [77]. Calcification in the wall of cystic teratomas and in the dermoid plug will often be missed on MRI due to the low SI on T1- and T2-weighted images.

In a patient with acute abdomen and a dermoid, the presence of sebaceous fluid floating in the peritoneal cavity can suggest rupture [75].

Differential Diagnosis

Although hemorrhagic lesions including endometrioma, hemorrhagic cysts, and neoplasm may appear similar on the T1-weighted images and T2-weighted images, fat-suppressed or chemical shift images are most reliable for the differentiation of fat from hemorrhage [78].

When no or only small amounts of fat are present (8%), dermoids are not distinguishable from benign cystic ovarian tumors or ovarian cancer (Fig. 9.28) [75].

Capsule perforation often arising from the dermoid plug is a sign for malignant transformation of a mature teratoma [79]. The rare liposarcoma or immature teratoma may contain fat and thus may be indiscernible from a dermoid. Immature teratomas, however, are extremely rare, and occur in the first two decades of life. They may occur in association with an ipsilateral dermoid in 26%, and a contralateral dermoid in 10%. However, at the time of presentation they are usually very large, are predominantly solid or

cystic and solid, and contain only few foci of fat [80]. Collision tumors of the ovary consisting of a mature cystic teratoma and a mucinous cystadenoma show a multiloculated cystic mass with an area of pure fat (Fig. 9.31) [81].

9.5.2.3.2
Monodermal Teratoma

Monodermal teratomas are composed predominantly or solely of one tissue type. They include struma ovarii, ovarian carcinoid tumors, and tumors with neural differentiation.

Struma ovarii is the most common type, and accounts for 3% of all mature teratomas. It consists predominantly or solely of mature thyroid tissue. A mixed morphology with acini filled with thyroid colloid, hemorrhage, fibrosis, and necrosis is found. Rarely struma ovarii may produce thyrotoxicosis.

Carcinoid tumors are frequently associated with a mature cystic teratoma or a mucinous ovarian tumor. Unlike most cystic teratomas, they are predominantly found in postmenopausal women. The course is usually benign; rarely will metastases be found. Carcinoid syndrome is uncommon.

Imaging Findings

On CT and MRI, a struma ovarii displays as a heterogenous complex mass (Fig. 9.13). They present as cystic lesions or with a multilocular appearance with loculi displaying high signal intensity on T1 and T2, some with low signal intensity on T1 and T2-weighted images on MR. Fat is not seen in struma ovarii [82].

Carcinoid tumors are solid tumors indistinguishable from solid ovarian malignancies.

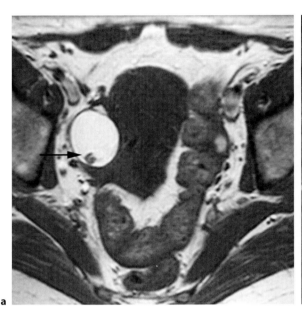
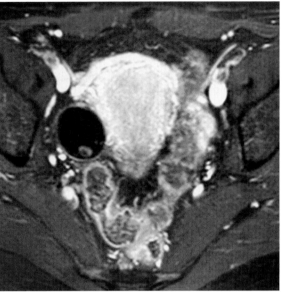

a   b

Fig. 9.30a,b. Typical findings of dermoid in MRI. A 44-year-old woman complaining about irregular menstrual cycle and a suspicious adnexal mass at transvaginal ultrasound. Axial T1-weighted images (**a**) and T1-weighted images contrast-enhanced image with fat suppression (**b**) at the acetabular level. The cystic structure of the right ovary demonstrates hyperintense contents with a round nodule in the lower part of the cyst (*arrow*) (**a**). The hypointense content after fat suppression (**b**) confirms the fatty nature of the cyst. At pathology, the round nodule corresponded to a hair ball within a mature cystic teratoma

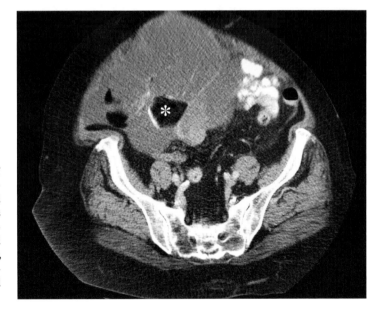

Fig. 9.31. Collision tumor of the ovary. CT at the level of the mid pelvis in a 65-year-old woman with sonographically suspected ovarian cancer. A cystic right adnexal mass is demonstrated showing multiple thin septations and a 3-cm lesion with fat density and mural calcifications (*asterisk*). Pathologically, a collision tumor composed of a benign mucinous cystadenoma and a benign dermoid was diagnosed

9.5.2.4
Benign Sex Cord Stromal Tumors

Sex cord stromal tumors include neoplasms that are composed of granulosa cells, theca cells, and their luteinized derivates, including Sertoli cells, Leydig cells, and fibroblasts of gonadal stromal origin [37].

Tumors of the thecoma-fibroma subgroup are characterized by fibrous components and include fibroma, fibrothecoma, cystadenofibroma, and Brenner tumors. They account for the vast majority of the sex cord stromal tumors and are benign, except for Brenner tumors, which may rarely be malignant.

9.5.2.4.1
Fibroma and Fibrothecoma

Fibromas and fibrothecomas are solid ovarian tumors accounting for 3%-4% of all ovarian tumors and 10% of solid adnexal masses. They are typically unilateral (90%), and occur in peri- and postmenopausal age women.

Fibromas are composed mostly of fibroblasts and spindle cells and abundant collagen contents. Fibromas are not hormonally active. Fifteen percent of fibromas are associated with ascites (Fig. 9.32), and in 1% pleural fluid is also found [83]. This triad of an ovarian fibroma, ascites and pleural effusion constitutes the benign Meigs syndrome, which can be associated with elevated Ca-125 levels [84]. In basal cell nevus syndrome, numerous basal cell carcinomas are associated with abnormalities of bones, eyes, brain, and tumors, including ovarian bilateral fibromas [85].

Thecomas are composed of thecal cells with abundant and varying amounts of fibrosis, and rarely contain calcifications. Unlike fibromas, 60% of thecomas have estrogenic activity and may present with uterine bleeding. Furthermore, in more than 20%, endometrial carcinomas may be present concomitantly [85].

Imaging Findings

Small fibromas and fibrothecomas are solid tumors with imaging features similar to nondegenerative uterine leiomyomas on CT and MRI (Fig. 9.33). They display intermediate to low SI on T1-weighted images and typically very low SI or low SI with intermediate SI on the T2-weighted images on MRI (Fig. 9.32). Large lesions may have an inhomogenous architecture with high signal intensity foci within the low signal intensity lesion, representing edema or cystic degeneration [21]. Furthermore, especially in larger lesions, dense amorphous calcifications may be seen, which are easily detected on CT. On MRI, calcifications are typically not appreciated because of their low SI on the T2-weighted images. Fibromas and fibrothecomas tend to show mild or delayed gadolinium enhancement (Fig. 9.32) [86]. Ascites may be

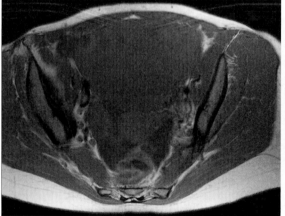
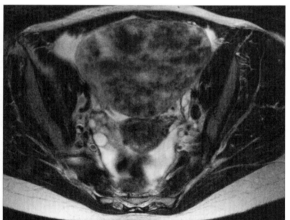

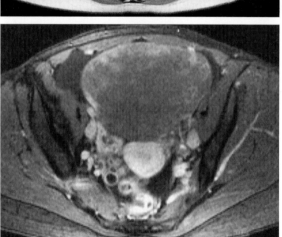

Fig. 9.32a–c. Ovarian fibroid. Transaxial T1-weighted images (a), T2-weighted images (b) and contrast-enhanced T1-weighted images with FS (c). In a 38-year-old woman with abdominal fullness, a large solid tumor was found. It is separated from the right ovary and the uterus (b and c). Signal intensity on T1-weighted images is similar to myometrium (a). The transaxial T2-weighted images shows a predominantly low-signal-intensity pattern and areas of intermediate SI (b). Contrast enhancement is less than those of the myometrium (c). In the anterior periphery, areas of higher enhancement are seen. Ascites as seen in this case is a feature of Meigs syndrome

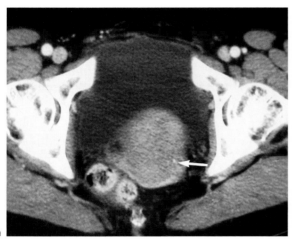
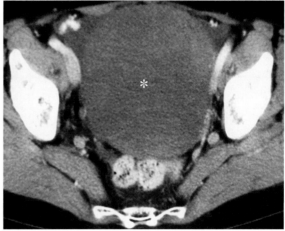

a   b

Fig. 9.33a,b. Ovarian fibroma in CT. Transaxial pelvic CT at the uterine level (**a**) and above (**b**) in a 55-year-old woman with abdominal fullness. A large lesion (*asterisk*) is found in the mid pelvis above the level of the uterus and bladder (**b**). It is well demarcated and displays a slightly inhomogeneous solid structure . Contrast enhancement is distinctly less than that of the myometrium (*arrow*). No calcifications were found throughout the lesion. Minimal ascites was seen. Histopathology revealed a 9-cm fibroid of the left ovary

present and even large amounts are no sign of malignancy.

9.5.2.4.2
Brenner Tumors

Brenner tumors present rare ovarian tumors that occur at a mean age of 50 years. Brenner tumors constitute 1%–3% of ovarian tumors. They are mostly benign, with less than 2% demonstrating borderline or malignant transformation. They are typically small, solid, unilateral ovarian tumors, with 60% of these tumors found under 2 cm in size. Extensive calcification may be observed. The vast majority is discovered incidentally in pathologic specimen of the adnexa. Brenner tumors rarely produce estrogen, and then they may be associated with endometrial thickening [87]. If cystic components are found in Brenner tumors, they may be associated with cystadenomas [88]. Up to 20% of Brenner tumors are associated with mucinous cystadenomas or other epithelial neoplasm (Fig. 9.34).

Imaging Findings

The typical finding of a Brenner tumors is a small solid tumor that displays very low SI on the T2-weighted images [87]. Dense amorphous calcifications in a small solid ovarian tumor is a typical CT finding. In one series of eight Brenner tumors, the mean size was 11.5 cm, and tumors displayed a mixed solid and cystic appearance in half of the cases, which mimicked ovarian cancer [87]. The combination of a multiseptate ovarian tumor with a solid part displaying extensive calcifications on CT or very low SI on MRI may suggest the diagnosis of a collision tumor of Brenner tumor and a cystic ovarian neoplasm, e.g., cystadenoma (Fig. 9.34).

9.5.2.4.3
Sclerosing Stromal Tumor of the Ovary

Sclerosing stromal tumor of the ovary is a rare subtype of the sex cord stromal tumor type. It is a benign tumor and affects most commonly young girls and women younger than 30 years of age, which is much earlier than in the other stromal tumor types [89]. Macroscopically, these tumors have a capsule with peripheral edematous ovarian cortical stroma surrounding nodular highly vascular cellular components [89]. These tumors may have an estrogenic effect and rarely androgenic effects, which cause prolonged menstrual irregularities. Ascites may be rarely associated.

Imaging Findings

Sclerosing stromal cell tumors tend to be well encapsulated multiloculated cystic or heterogenous ovarian lesions (Fig. 9.35). On T1 and T2-weighted images, a

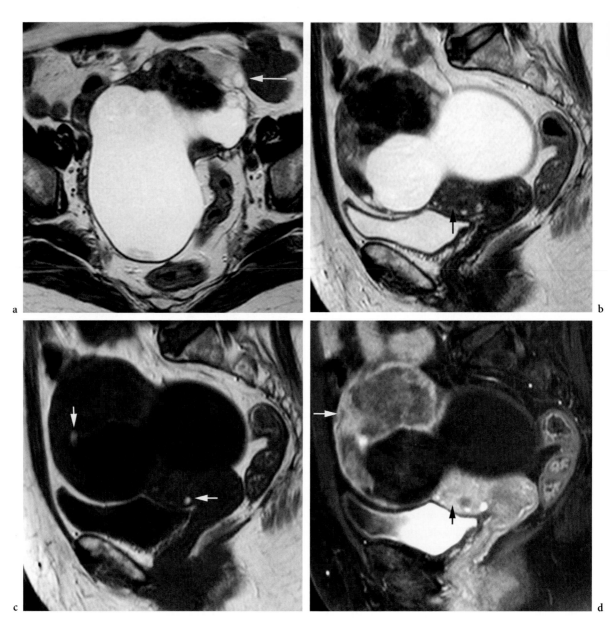

Fig. 9.34a–d. Large Brenner tumors with mucinous portion. A 75-year-old woman presenting with a large suspicious pelvic mass at ultrasound and moderate increase in Ca125 level. Axial T2-weighted images (**a**), sagittal T2-weighted images (**b**), Sagittal T1-weighted images (**c**), Sagittal T1-weighted images with FS. (**d**) A cystic mass with a solid hypointense anterior portion is demonstrated (**a**). Ovarian parenchyma with two follicles is seen at the left anterior side (*arrow*). The small uterus (*arrow*) is identified below the left ovarian mass (**b**). The interface between the cystic and solid portion of the mass is regular. Sagittal T1-weighted images (**c**) shows absent blood within the cyst except for two blood vessels seen within the solid portion of the mass and the anterior myometrium (*arrows*). At the same level as **b** and **c** contrast-enhanced T1-weighted image with fat suppression (**d**) shows heterogeneous decreased contrast enhancement of the solid portion of the cyst (*white arrow*) compared to the strongly enhancing myometrium (*black arrow*). Histology after hysterectomy and bilateral oophorectomy diagnosed a benign Brenner tumor of the left ovary with an associated benign mucinous portion

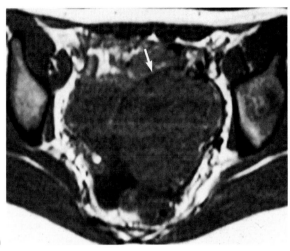

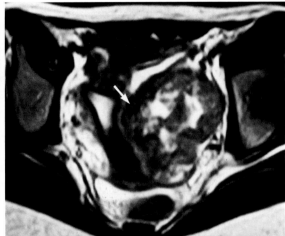

a

b

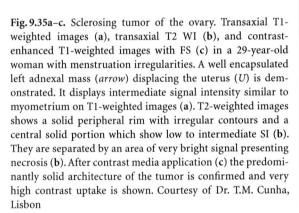

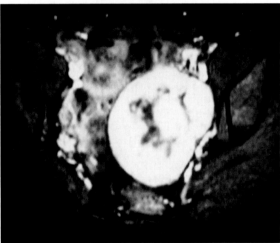

Fig. 9.35a–c. Sclerosing tumor of the ovary. Transaxial T1-weighted images (**a**), transaxial T2 WI (**b**), and contrast-enhanced T1-weighted images with FS (**c**) in a 29-year-old woman with menstruation irregularities. A well encapsulated left adnexal mass (*arrow*) displacing the uterus (*U*) is demonstrated. It displays intermediate signal intensity similar to myometrium on T1-weighted images (**a**). T2-weighted images shows a solid peripheral rim with irregular contours and a central solid portion which show low to intermediate SI (**b**). They are separated by an area of very bright signal presenting necrosis (**b**). After contrast media application (**c**) the predominantly solid architecture of the tumor is confirmed and very high contrast uptake is shown. Courtesy of Dr. T.M. Cunha, Lisbon

c

thin low-intensity rim representing a capsule is seen. On T2-weighted images, in the periphery an irregular low-signal-intensity rim is found adjacent to a very bright more central portion, which has a nodular appearance. On dynamic MRI, lack of enhancement of the outermost part and distinct early peripheral enhancement with centripetal progression on delayed images has been described [89].

Differential Diagnosis

The solid morphology and the signal characteristics of fibromas and fibrothecomas are fairly characteristic. Pedunculated uterine fibroids and fibroids of the broad ligaments can display similar imaging characteristics. The latter can only be differentiated from ovarian fibromas or fibrothecomas when they are separated from the ovary. Subserosal pedunculated fibroids can be discrimi-

nated by the bridging vascular sign. Unilateral or bilateral ovarian leiomyomas are extremely rare, and cannot be reliably differentiated by imaging. High-contrast media uptake in such a lesion might suggest ovarian leiomyoma [90]. Fibromas and fibrothecomas with large central necrotic areas cannot be reliably differentiated from malignant solid ovarian masses, especially Krukenberg tumors. In contrast to the majority of ovarian tumors, only little or delayed contrast enhancement is observed in ovarian stromal tumors. Dense calcifications in CT support also the diagnosis of stromal tumors. Small calcified solid tumors favor the diagnosis of Brenner tumors. A multicystic tumor with focal very dense calcifications, which is only reliably appreciated on CT, may suggest the diagnosis of Brenner tumor and cystadenoma. In contrast, calcifications in ovarian cancer tend to be small punctuate foci, so-called Psammoma bodies.

Sclerosing stromal cell tumors seem to have a unique distinct centripetal contrast media uptake. Morphologically, they may resemble Krukenberg tumors or dysgerminomas.

References

1. Jung SE, Lee JM, Rha SE et al (2002) CT and MRI of ovarian tumors with emphasis on the differential diagnosis. Radiographics 22:1305–1325

2. Sala EJ, Atri M (2003) MRI of benign adnexal disease. Top Magn Reson Imaging 14:305–328

3. Yamashita Y, Tang Y, Abe Y, Mitsuzaki K, Takahashi M (1998) Comparison of ultrafast half-Fourier single-shot turbo spin-echo sequence with turbo spin-echo sequences for T2-weighted imaging of the female pelvis. J Magn Reson Imaging 8:1207–1212

4. Niitsu M, Tanaka YO, Anno I, Itai Y (1997) Multishot echo-planar MR imaging of the female pelvis: comparison with fast spin-echo MR imaging in an initial clinical trial. AJR Am J Roentgenol 168:651–655

5. Maubon A, Berger V, Aubas P et al (1999) Abdominal and pelvic segmented T1-weighted echo-planar imaging and MRI. Comparison with T1-TSE and T2-UTSE sequences. J Radiol 80:291–296

6. Yamashita Y, Harada M, Sawada T, Takahashi M, Miyazaki K, Okamura H. (1993) Normal uterus and FIGO stage I endometrial carcinoma: dynamic gadolinium-enhanced MR imaging. Radiology 186:495–501

7. Hricak H, Chen M, Coakley FV et al (2000) Complex adnexal masses: detection and characterization with MRI: multivariate analysis. Radiology 214:39–46

8. Wu TT, Coakley FV, Qayyum A et al (2004) Magnetic resonance imaging of ovarian cancer arising in endometriomas. J Comput Assist Tomogr 28:836–838

9. Saksouk FA, Johnson SC (2004) Recognition of the ovarian origin of pelvic masses with CT. Radiographics 24: S133–S146

10. Levine CD, Patel UJ, Ghanekar D (1997) Benign extraovarian mimicks of ovarian cancer: distinction with imaging studies. Clin Imaging 21:350–358

11. Foshager MC, Hood LL, Walsh JW et al (1996) Masses simulating gynaecologic diseases at CT and MRI. Radiographics 16:1085–1099

12. Lee JH, Jeong YK, Park JK et al (2003) Ovarian vascular pedicle sign revealing organ origin of mass lesion on helical CT. AJR Am J Roentgenol 181:131–137

13. Kim JC, Kim SS, Park JY (2003) Bridging vascular sign in the MR diagnosis of exophytic uterine leiomyoma. J Comput Assist Tomogr 24:57–60

14. Outwater EK, Siegelman ES, Chiowanich P et al (1988) Dilated fallopian tubes: MRI characteristics. Radiology 208:463–469

15. Kobal B, Rakar S, Ribi M et al (1999) Pretreatment evaluation of adnexal tumors predicting ovarian cancer. Int J Gynecol Cancer 6:481–487

16. Brown DL, Doubilet PM, Miller FH et al (1998) Benign and malignant ovarian masses: selection of most discriminating gray scale and Doppler sonographic features. Radiology 208:103–110

17. Alcazar JL, Jurado M (1998) Using a logistic model to predict malignancy of adnexal masses based on menopausal status, ultrasound morphology, and color Doppler findings. Gynecol Oncol 69:146–150

18. Kinkel K, Hricak, H, Lu Y et al (2000) US characterization of ovarian masses: a meta-analysis. Radiology 217:803–811

19. Buy JN, Ghossain MA, Hugol D et al (1996) Characterization of adnexal masses: combination of color Doppler and conventional sonography compared with spectral Doppler analysis alone and conventional sonography alone. AJR Am J Roentgenol 166:385–393

20. Quinn SF, Erickson S, Black WC (1985) Cystic ovarian teratomas: the sonographic appearance of the dermoid plug. Radiology 155:477–478

21. Bazot M, Ghossain MA, Buy JN et al (1993) Fibrothecomas of the ovary: CT and US findings. J Comput Assist Tomogr 17:754–759

22. Atri M, Nazarnia S, Bret PM et al (1994) Endovaginal sonographic appearance of benign ovarian masses. Radiographics 14:747–760

23. Ekici E, Soysal M, Kara S, Dogan M, Gokmen O (1996) The efficiency of ultrasonography in the diagnosis of dermoid cysts. Zentralbl Gynakol 118:136–141

24. Patel MD, Feldstein VA, Chen DC et al (1999) Endometriomas: diagnostic performance of US. Radiology 210:739–745

25. Brown DL, Frates MC, Muto MG, Welch WR (2004) Small echogenic foci in the ovaries: correlation with histologic findings. J Ultrasound Med 23:307–313

26. Yamashita Y, Torashima M, Hatanaka Y et al (1995) Adnexal masses: accuracy of characterization with transvaginal US and precontrast and postcontrast MRI. Radiology 194:557–565

27. Stevens SK, Hricak H, Stern JL (1991) Ovarian lesions: detection and characterization with gadolinium-enhanced MRI at 1.5 T. Radiology 181:481–488

28. Sohaib SA, Sahdev A, Van Trappen P et al (2003) Characterization of adnexal lesions on MRI. AJR Am J Roentgenol 180:1297–1304

29. Kawamoto S, Urban BA, Fishman EK (1999) CT of epithelial ovarian tumors. Radiographics 19:85–102

30. Dorum A, Blom GP, Ekerhovd E et al (2005) Prevalence and histologic diagnosis of adnexal cysts in postmenopausal women: an autopsy study. Am J Obstet Gynecol 192:48–54

31. Goldstein SR, Subramanyam B, Synder JR et al (1989) The postmenopausal cystic adnexal mass: the potential role of ultrasound in conservative management. Obstet Gynecol 73:8–10

32. Rulin MC, Preston AI (1987) Adnexal masses in postmenopausal women. Obstet Gynecol 70:578–581

33. Outwater EK, Wilson KM, Siegelman ES, Mitchell DG (1996) MRI of benign and malignant gynecologic disease: significance of fluid and peritoneal enhancement in the pelvis. Radiology 200:483–488

34. Walkey MM, Friedman AC, Sohotra P et al (1988) CT manifestations of peritoneal carcinosis AJR Am J Roentgenol 150:1035–1041

35. Occhipinti KA (1999) CT and MRI of the ovary. In: Anderson JC (ed) Gynecologic imaging. Churchill Livingston, London pp 345–359

36. Tanaka YO, Tsunoda H, Kitagawa Y et al (2004) Functioning

ovarian tumors: direct and indirect findings at MR imaging. Radiographics 24:147–166

37. Young RH, Scully RE (2002). Sex cord stromal, steroid cell, and other ovarian tumors. In: Kurman RJ (ed) Blaustein's pathology of the female genital tract. Springer Verlag, New York, pp 903–966

38. Outwater EK, Wagner BJ, Nannion C et al (1998) Sex cord stromal and steroid cell tumors of the ovary. Radiographics 18:1523–1546

39. Garcia-Villaneuva M, Figuerola NB, del Arbol LR et al (1990) Zollinger Ellison syndrome due to a borderline mucinous cystadenoma of the ovary. Obstet Gynecol 75:549–551

40. Norris HJ, Jensen RD (1972) Relative frequency of ovarian neoplasm in children and adolescents. Cancer 30:713–719

41. Laufer MR, Goldstein DP (2005) Ovarian cysts and neoplasm in infants, children, and adolescents. www.uptodate.com

42. Cass DL, Hawkins E, Brandt ML et al (2001) Surgery for ovarian masses in infants, children, and adolescents: 102 consecutive patients treated in a 15-year period. J Pediatr Surg 36:693–699

43. Frisch LS, Copeland KC, Boepple PA (1992) Recurrent ovarian cysts in childhood: diagnosis of McCune-Albright syndrome by bone scan. Pediatrics 90:102–104

44. Van Winter JT, Simmons PS, Podratz KC (1994) Surgically treated adnexal masses in infancy, childhood, and adolescence. Am J Obstet Gynecol 170:1780–1786

45. Dorigo O, Berek JS (2005) Epidemiology, pathology, and clinical manifestations of ovarian germ cell tumors. www.Uptodate.com

46. Jabra AA, Fishman EK, Taylor GA (1993) Primary ovarian tumors in the pediatric patient: CT evaluation. Clin Imaging 17:199–203

47. Hermans RHM, Fisher DC, van der Putte HWHM et al (2003) Adnexal masses in pregnancy. Onkologie 26:167–172

48. Sherard GB, Hodson CA, Williams HJ et al (2003) Adnexal masses and pregnancy: a 12-year experience. Am J Obstet Gynecol 189:358–362

49. Nagayama M, Watanabe Y, Okumura A et al (2002) Fast MR imaging in obstetrics. Radiographics 22:363–380

50. Birchard KR, Brown MA, Hyslop WB et al (2005) MRI of acute abdominal and pelvic pain in pregnant patients. AJR Am J Roentgenol 184:452–458

51. Outwater EK, Mitchell DG (1996) Normal ovaries and functional cysts: MR appearance. Radiology 198:397–402

52. Guerriero S, Ajossa S, Lai MP et al (2003) The diagnosis of functional ovarian cysts using transvaginal ultrasound combined with clinical parameters, CA 125 determinations, and color Doppler. Eur J Obstet Gynecol Reprod Biol 110:83–88

53. Christensen JT, Boldsen JL, Westergaard JG (2002) Functional ovarian cysts in premenopausal and gynecologically healthy women. Contraception 66:153–157

54. Togashi K, Nishimura K, Kimura I (1991) Endometrial cysts: diagnosis with MRI. Radiology 180:73–78

55. Kier R (1992) Nonovarian gynaecologic cysts: MR imaging findings. AJR 158:1265–1269

56. Kim JS, Lee HJ, Woo SK et al (1997) Peritoneal inclusion cysts and their relationship to the ovaries: evaluation with sonography. Radiology 204:481–484

57. Honore LH, O'Hara KE (1980) Serous papillary neoplasms arising in paramesonephric paraovarian cysts: a report of 8 cases. Acta Obstet Gynecol Scand 59:525–528

58. Kishimoto K, Ito K, Awaya H et al (2002) Paraovarian cysts: MR imaging features. Abdom Imaging 27:685–689

59. Kurachi H, Marakami T, Nakamura H et al (1993) Imaging of peritoneal pseudocysts: value of MRI compared with sonography and CT. AJR Am J Roentgenol 161:589–591

60. Clement PB (2002) Non-neoplastic lesions of the ovary. In: Kurman RJ (ed) Blaustein's pathology of the female genital tract. Springer Verlag, New York, pp 675–728

61. Lakhani K, Seifalian AM, Atiomo WU et al (2002) Polycystic ovaries. BJR 75:9–16

62. Polson DW, Adams J, Wadsworth J et al (1988) Polycystic ovaries: a common finding in normal women. Lancet 1:870–872

63. Ginsburg J, Havard CWM (1976) Polycystic ovary syndrome. Br Med J 2:737–740

64. Park SJ, Lim JW, Ko YT et al (2004) Diagnosis of pelvic congestion syndrome using transabdominal and transvaginal sonography. AJR 182:683–688

65. Kyei-Mensah A, Zaidi J, Campbell S (1996) Ultrasound diagnosis of polycystic ovary syndrome. Baillieres Clin Endocrinol Metabol 10:249–262

66. Mitchell DG, Gefter WB, Spritzer CE et al (1986) Polycystic ovaries: MR imaging. Radiology 160:425–429

67. Koonings PP, Campbell K, Mishell DR, Grimes DA (1989) Relative frequency of primary ovarian neoplasm: a 10-year review. Obstet Gynecol 74:921–926

68. Outwater EK, Huang AB, Dunton CJ et al (1997) Papillary projections in ovarian neoplasm: appearance on MRI. J Magn Reson Imaging 7:689–695

69. Buy JN, Ghossain MA, Sciot C et al (1991) Epithelial tumors of the ovary: CT findings and correlation with US. Radiology 178:811–818

70. Cho SM, Byun JY, Rha SE et al (2004) CT and MRI findings of cystadenofibromas of the ovary. Eur Radiol 14:798–804

71. Outwater EK, Siegelman ES, Junt JL (2001) Ovarian teratomas: tumor types and imaging characteristics. Radiographics 21:475–490

72. Buy JN, Ghossain MA; Moss AA et al (1989) cystic teratoma of the ovary: CT detection. Radiology 171:697–670

73. Yamashita Y, Hatanaka Y, Torashima M et al (1994) Mature cystic teratomas of the ovary without fat in the cystic cavity: MR features in 12 cases. AJR Am J Roentgenol 163:613–616

74. Caspi B, Appelman Z, Rabinerson D et al (1997) The growth pattern of ovarian dermoid cysts: a prospective study in premenopausal and postmenopausal women. Fertil Steril 68:501–505

75. Rha SE, Byun JY, Jung SE et al (2004) Atypical CT and MRI manifestations of mature ovarian cystic teratomas. AJR Am J Roentgenol 183:743–750

76. Carrington BM (1991) The adnexae. In: Hricak H, Carrington BM (eds) MRI of the pelvis: a text atlas. Martin Dunitz, London, pp 185

77. Togashi K, Nishimura K, Itoh K et al (1987) Ovarian cystic teratomas: MR imaging. Radiology 162:669–673

78. Stevens SK, Hricak H, Campos Z (1993) Teratomas versus cystic hemorrhagic adnexal lesions; differentiation with proton-selective fat-saturation MR imaging. Radiology 186:481–488

79. Brammer HM, Buck JL, Hayes WS et al (1990) Malignant germ cell tumors of the ovary: radiologic-pathologic correlation. Radiographics 10:715–724

80. Heifetz SA, Cushing B, Giller R et al (1989) Immature tera-

tomas in children: pathologic considerations. Am J Surg Pathol 22:1115–1124

81. Kim SH, Kim YJ, Park BK et al (1999) Collision tumors of the ovary associated with teratoma: clues to the correct preoperative diagnosis. J Comput Assist Tomogr 23:929–933

82. Matsuki M, Kaji Y, Matsuo M et al (2000) Struma ovarii: MRI findings. Br J Radiol 73:87–90

83. Tailor A, Hacket E, Bourne T (1999) Ultrasonography of the ovary. In: Anderson JC (ed) Gynecologic imaging. Churchill Livingstone, London, pp 319–343

84. Timmerman D, Moerman P, Vergote I (1995) Meigs syndrome with elevated Ca-125 levels: two case reports and review of the literature. Gynecol Oncol 59:405–408

85. Outwater EK, Siegelman ES, Talerman A et al (1997) Ovarian fibromas and cystadenofibromas: MRI features of the fibrous component. J Magn Reson Imaging 7:465–71

86. Troiano RN, Lazzarini KM, Scoutt LM et al (1997) Fibroma and fibrothecoma of the ovary: MR imaging findings. Radiology 204:795–798

87. Moon WJ, Koh BH, Kim SK et al (2000) Brenner tumor of the ovary: CT and MR findings J Comput Assist Tomogr 24:72–76

88. Seidman JD, Russell P, Kurman RJ (2002) Surface epithelial tumors of the ovary. In: Kurman RJ (ed) Blaustein's pathology of the female genital tract. Springer Verlag, New York, pp 791–904

89. Matsubayashi R, Matsuo Y, Doi J, Kudo S et al (1999) Sclerosing stromal tumor of the ovary: radiologic findings. Eur Radiol 9:1335–1338

90. Yoshitake T, Asayama Y, Yoshimitsu K et al (2005) Bilateral ovarian leiomyomas: CT and MRI features. Abdom Imaging 30:117–119

CT and MRI in Ovarian Carcinoma

10

ROSEMARIE FORSTNER

10.1
General Considerations

The vast majority of ovarian carcinomas are epithelial in origin, accounting for more than 90% of the estimated 25,580 new cases of ovarian cancer diagnosed in 2004 in the United States [1]. Fallopian tube carcinomas and extraovarian peritoneal carcinomas are much less common. However, these tumors share similarities in histology, tumor growth, treatment, chemotherapy responsiveness, and overall prognosis. For this reason, most aspects of these tumors will be discussed under epithelial ovarian cancer in this chapter. For both epithelial and fallopian tube cancer, there are significant differences in the prognosis between early and advanced ovarian cancer. While early-stage cancer is often curable, advanced-stage ovarian cancer is one of the most deadly cancers in women, with an overall 5-year survival rate of 38%–53% [1].

10.2
Epidemiology and Risk Factors

Ovarian cancer accounts for 4% of cancers in women and is responsible for 5% of cancer deaths [2]. In most Western countries, ovarian cancer is the sixth most common cancer in women, and the most lethal among the gynecological cancers. The incidence of ovarian cancer has increased by 30% over the past decade, while death from ovarian cancer has increased by 18% [3]. It is estimated that one women in 70 will develop ovarian cancer, and one woman in 100 will die of the disease. Ovarian cancer is usually clinically silent and about 75% of women present with advanced stages. This is why, despite developments in diagnosis and treatment, the overall survival rate has changed only little within the last decade [4]. Although there is an

R. FORSTNER, MD
PD, Department of Radiology, Landeskliniken Salzburg, Paracelsus Private Medical University, Müllner Hauptstrasse 48, 5020 Salzburg, Austria

initial response in most patients, the majority ultimately will die from their disease [3].

The incidence of ovarian cancer is higher in North America and Northern Europe than in Japan [3]. The strongest patient related risk factor for ovarian cancer is increasing age. The vast majority of epithelial ovarian carcinomas are diagnosed in the postmenopausal period, with a mean age at diagnosis of 59 years.

In patients with a family history of breast and ovarian cancer, ovarian cancers occur up to 10 years earlier. In females younger than 20 years of age, germ cell tumors account for more than two-thirds of malignant ovarian tumors.

Genetic, reproductive, and environmental factors have been identified to play a role in the development of ovarian cancer. The vast majority of ovarian cancers are sporadic in nature. Patients with a family history are at high risk, although an identifiable genetic predisposition for hereditary ovarian cancer is found only in approximately 5% of affected women. Families with three or more first-degree relatives with ovarian and/or ovarian and breast cancer carry a substantially (16%–60%) increased risk for developing ovarian cancer.

Hereditary breast-ovarian cancer syndrome (HBOC) accounts for the vast majority (85%–90%) of all hereditary ovarian cancers [5]. The site-specific ovarian cancer syndrome with only ovarian cancer accounts for 10%–15% of hereditary ovarian cancers. In hereditary nonpolyposis colorectal cancer syndrome (HNPCC), which is also known as Lynch syndrome II, patients present with colon, endometrial, breast, ovarian and other cancers [6].

The hereditary breast/ovarian cancer syndrome, and perhaps less frequently the site-specific ovarian cancer syndrome, are linked to mutations in the *BRCA1* and *BRCA2* genes [4]. The vast majority of *BRCA1*-associated cancers are serous adenocarcinomas and present at an average age at diagnosis of 48 years. *BRCA1*-associated cancers may have a longer median survival than sporadic ovarian cancer [4].

Women with nulliparity, childbirth after 35 years, late menopause, and early onset of menses are also under an increased risk. Prolonged times of uninterrupted ovulations seem to play a role in the development of ovarian cancer [3].

Treatment with ovulation stimulation drugs may also slightly increase the risk of developing ovarian cancer [3].

Long term oral contraceptive use, however, has been associated with a protective effect.

10.3
Screening for Ovarian Cancer

10.3.1
General Population

Successful screening for ovarian cancer, by definition, is able to decrease mortality and morbidity from the disease. Clinical palpation, transvaginal sonography, and serum CA-125 have been proposed as screening tests for ovarian cancer. Unfortunately, with these tests, routine screening for ovarian cancer is currently not recommended in the general population [3, 4, 7].

Successful screening for ovarian cancer requires either detection of early invasive stage disease or of a precancerous stage [4]. Although the patterns of spread of ovarian cancer are well established, its natural course is poorly understood. It seems that the preclinical phase of ovarian cancer may last less than 2 years [7]. Furthermore, most ovarian cancers, particularly serous types, may develop without a precursor lesion, which makes early detection difficult [8].

The primary reason that screening is not recommended, however, is based upon the fact that the currently available techniques have not shown to decrease the mortality of ovarian cancer in large clinical screening trials [3]. The detection rate of ovarian cancer is low, and cost-benefit analysis of ovarian cancer screening is currently not cost-effective [9]. Most screening studies have used either serum tumor markers or ultrasonography including color Doppler imaging, or both. Although US has excellent reported sensitivity and specificity for detection of ovarian masses (90%-96% and 98%-99%, respectively), its PPV is only about 7% for ovarian cancer, mainly because of its low prevalence. Serum CA-125 levels correlate with progression or regression of established disease. This test, however, is not specific and is found in benign diseases as well. False-positive findings during screening may even lead to adverse effects with an increased morbidity due to unnecessary surgeries [10].

10.3.2
High-Risk Women

Screening may be more effective in women with a positive family history of ovarian cancer. The American College of Radiology (ACR) recommends that women with a strong family history of ovarian cancer should consult gynecologists in their early twenties and undergo a clinical follow-up in their thirties [7]. Because of the markedly increased lifetime risk of ovarian cancer, screening with annual transvaginal US and CA-125 testing is recommended for women with *BRCA1* or *BRCA2* gene mutations [11]. Prophylactic oophorectomy seems to have a protective effect in women from families with hereditary cancer. Oophorectomy may be delayed until childbearing is completed, or the age of 40. However, these patients carry a persisting risk for peritoneal carcinomatosis even after removal of normal ovaries [4].

10.4
Histologic Tumor Types and Tumor Grade

On the basis of distinct clinical and pathologic features, primary ovarian carcinomas can be separated into three major entities: epithelial carcinomas, germ cell tumors, and stromal carcinomas. Epithelial ovarian cancer accounts for 86% of tumors, the vast majority of ovarian malignancies [12]. Epithelial ovarian cancers are adenocarcinomas and comprise, depending on their histopathologic features, serous, mucinous, endometrioid, transitional cell, clear cell, undifferentiated carcinomas, and mixed carcinomas. Fallopian tube cancers show similar histologies, with serous carcinoma also identified most frequently [3]. Except for clear cell carcinomas, the histologic type has limited prognostic significance independent of clinical stage [3].

Epithelial carcinomas are characterized by histologic type and the degree of cellular differentiation (grade). Most grading systems are based upon a three-grade classification that describes the degree to which a tumor forms papillary structures or glands vs solid tumors [4]. At present, grading of ovarian carcinoma is clinically relevant only for stage I tumors, because of its direct impact on the necessity of chemotherapy and the prognosis [2].

10.5
Tumor Markers

CA-125, a glycoprotein antigen, is currently the most commonly used tumor marker for ovarian cancer. However, elevation of CA-125 of more than 35 U/ml is not specific for epithelial ovarian cancer, but can be observed as well in other malignant epithelial cancers, including pancreatic, lung, breast, and colon cancer, and in non-Hodgkin's lymphoma [13]. Furthermore, the list of benign conditions associated with an elevated CA-125 level is long and includes cirrhosis, peritonitis, pancreatitis, endometriosis, uterine fibroids, pregnancy, benign ovarian cysts, pelvic inflammatory disease, and even ascites. The level of CA-125 is associated with the menstrual cycle, and more than 90% of false-positive findings are encountered in premenopausal women [14]. This is why in premenopausal women, CA-125 is not useful as a single test, but its value is based upon the rise in serial measurements. In postmenopausal women, CA-125 is a better discriminator between benign and malignant diseases. In this age group, CA-125 levels exceeding 65 U/ml are predictive of malignancy in 75% of women with pelvic masses [7]. More than 80% of women with advanced epithelial ovarian cancer present with CA-125 elevations. It is, however, not a sensitive test for early-stage disease, where its sensitivity is only 25% [14]. In mucinous ovarian cancers, the CA-125 levels may not be markedly elevated [15].

CA-125 is pivotal in the follow-up of patients with ovarian cancer to monitor efficacy and duration of treatment and tumor recurrence [16].

Serum alpha-fetoprotein (AFP) and human chorionic gonadotropin (HCG) have been helpful in recognizing preoperatively the presence of an endodermal sinus tumor, embryonal carcinoma, choriocarcinoma, or a mixed germ cell tumor.

10.6
Imaging

10.6.1
Imaging Features of Ovarian Cancer

10.6.1.1
Characteristics of Malignant Ovarian Tumors

Most commonly used imaging features suggestive of malignancy are lesions size larger than 4 cm, thickness of wall or septa exceeding more than 3 mm, papillary projections, necrosis, partially cystic and solid internal architecture, a lobulated solid mass, and presence of tumor vessels (Fig. 10.1; Table 10.1) [17–21].

Contrast-enhanced studies in CT and MRI assist in tumor characterization, especially in the depiction of papillary projections and necrosis [17, 21]. None of

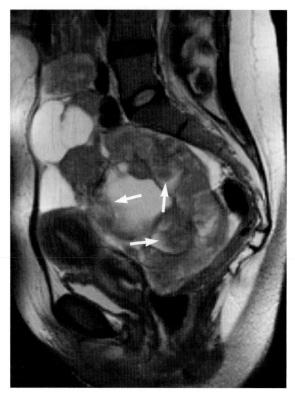

Fig. 10.1. Imaging characteristics of a malignant ovarian lesion. Sagittal T2-weighted image demonstrates a large adnexal lesion extending to above the umbilical level. It is clearly separated from the uterus and compresses the rectum. It is composed of multiple solid elements and multiple cysts. Throughout the lesion and within the cysts, papillary projections (*arrows*) can be identified. Histopathological diagnosis was a serous adenocarcinoma

Table 10.1. Imaging findings suggesting malignancy in an adnexal mass

Primary findings[a]
Lesion size >4 cm
Wall/septal thickness >3 mm
Papillary projections
Lobulated mass
Necrosis
Solid and cystic architecture
Tumor vessels
Ancillary findings
Lymph node enlargement
Peritoneal lesions
Ascites

[a]Not specific as single factors.

these imaging criteria, however, are specific enough as a single factor to reliably diagnose ovarian cancer. The likelihood of malignancy increases with solid nonfibrous elements, thickness of septa, and presence of necrosis. Ancillary findings such as presence of lymphadenopathy, peritoneal lesions, and ascites improve the diagnostic confidence to diagnose ovarian cancer. The combination of tumor size and architecture and ancillary signs improves prediction of malignancy and yields an accuracy of 89%–95% [19, 21].

Necrosis within a solid portion of an ovarian mass was most predictive sign of malignancy in a multivariate logistic regression analysis of complex adnexal masses studied by MRI (Fig. 10.2). "Necrosis in a solid lesion" (odds ratio, 107) was followed by "vegetations in a cystic lesion" (odds ratio, 40) identified after intravenous injection of gadolinium-based contrast material [21]. Solid nonfatty nonfibrous tissue with or without necrosis has also been reported as a valuable predictor of malignancy [22]. Thick walls and septations are less reliably signs of malignancy, as they may also occur in abscesses, endometriomas, and benign neoplasms such as cystadenofibromas and mucinous cystadenomas [22].

Papillary projections present folds of the proliferating neoplastic epithelium growing over a stromal core. Identification of papillary projections is impor-

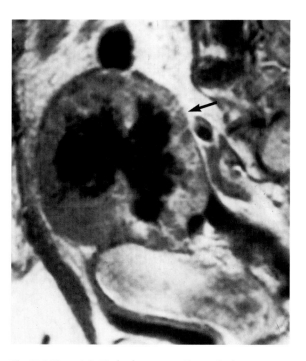

Fig. 10.2. Necrosis in Krukenberg tumor. Parasagittal contrast-enhanced T1-weighted image shows a well-delineated solid ovarian lesion (*arrow*) located cephalad of the uterus. It displays inhomogeneous contrast enhancement and a large central necrosis

tant because they are typical for an epithelial neoplasm. They are most often associated with epithelial cancers with low malignant potential, and may also be found in 38% of invasive carcinomas (Fig. 10.3). In the latter, the gross appearance is usually dominated by a solid component [17, 22].

Psammoma bodies, which are tiny calcifications, are found in CT in approximately 10% of serous epithelial ovarian cancers (Fig. 10.4). Calcifications are also found in benign ovarian stromal tumors, e.g., Brenner tumors or thecomas. These tumors are typically solid and tend to show extensive coarse calcifications.

10.6.1.2
Peritoneal Carcinomatosis

Peritoneal implants appear as solitary, or more often as multiple soft tissues lesions (Fig. 10.5), which display a wide range of size and patterns. Implants may be distributed along the peritoneal surfaces in a linear and often linear and nodular pattern (Fig. 10.6); they may also coalesce and surround the viscera or the diaphragm in a plaque- or coatlike manner. The majority of these implants enhance with contrast media; some are cystlike and may mimic loculated fluid. Implants from serous tumors may have calcifications (Fig. 10.7).

The omentum accounts for the most common sites of peritoneal metastases, with the inframesocolic omentum more often involved than the supramesocolic omentum. Most common types of omental implants include a netlike pattern, nodules of various sizes, and broad, bandlike soft-tissue lesions, an omental cake (Fig. 10.8). Nodular enhancing implants and omental cake are typically located between the abdominal wall and bowel loops.

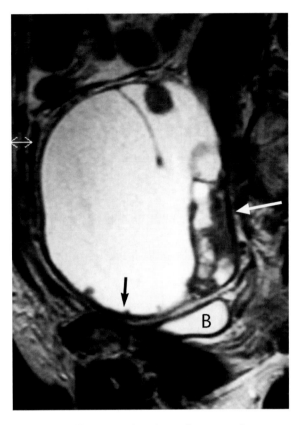

Fig. 10.3. Papillary projections in ovarian cancer. On a parasagittal T2-weighted image, a cystic ovarian lesion with septations and multiple papillary projections is demonstrated. Some small isolated papillary projections are located at the base of the lesion (*arrow*). At the top, a 1.5-cm papillary projection protrudes into the fluid-filled cavity. At the posterior aspect of the tumor, septal wall thickening and coalescence of papillary projections forming broad-based formations (*long arrow*) is demonstrated. Papillary projections typically display low signal intensity on T2-weighted image. *B*, bladder

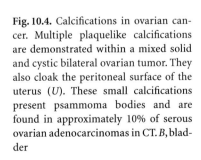

Fig. 10.4. Calcifications in ovarian cancer. Multiple plaquelike calcifications are demonstrated within a mixed solid and cystic bilateral ovarian tumor. They also cloak the peritoneal surface of the uterus (*U*). These small calcifications present psammoma bodies and are found in approximately 10% of serous ovarian adenocarcinomas in CT. *B*, bladder

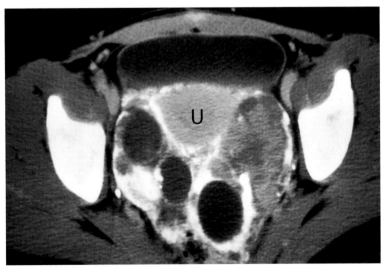

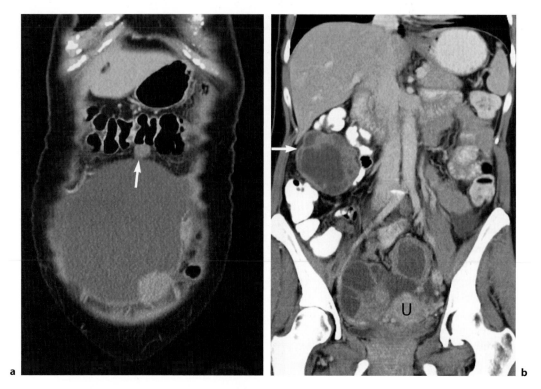

Fig. 10.5a,b. Peritoneal implants. Findings in FIGO stage IIIc ovarian cancer are shown in an anterior (**a**) and posterior (**b**) coronal CT plane. Ascites, mild peritoneal thickening and multiple solid peritoneal implants along the anterior abdominal wall and in the transverse mesocolon (*arrow*) are demonstrated in **a**. A large implant in the right paracolic gutter (*arrow*) resembles the morphology of the thick-walled cystic and solid adnexal tumors, which present bilateral ovarian cancer (**b**). (*U*), uterus

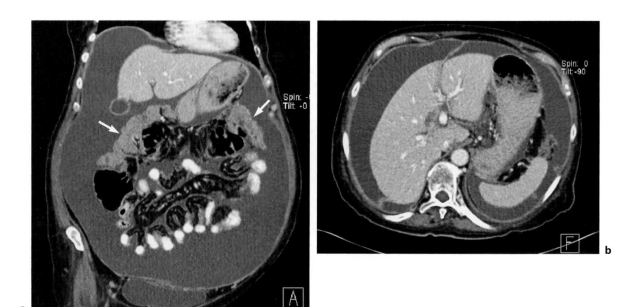

Fig. 10.6a,b. Peritoneal implants. Coronal (**a**) and transaxial CT of the upper abdomen (**b**). Linear thickening of the parietal peritoneum is seen throughout the abdomen and pelvis in a patient with large amounts of ascites (**a**). The diffuse linear thickening of the diaphragm is better appreciated on the transaxial plane (**b**). Other findings include bilateral focal diaphragmatic implants and broad bandlike tumors (*arrows*) adjacent to the transverse colon presenting omental cake

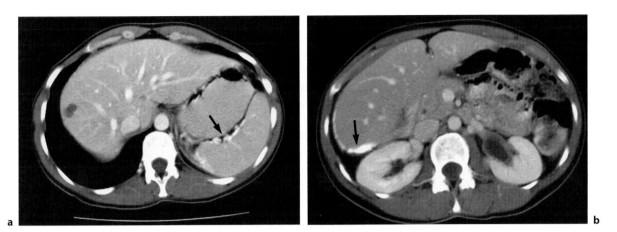

Fig. 10.7a,b. Calcified peritoneal metastases in CT. Multiple tiny calcifications (*arrows*) coat the surface of the spleen (**a**) and liver (**b**) in a patient with recurrent serous ovarian cancer. A simple cyst is found in the right lobe of the liver (**a**)

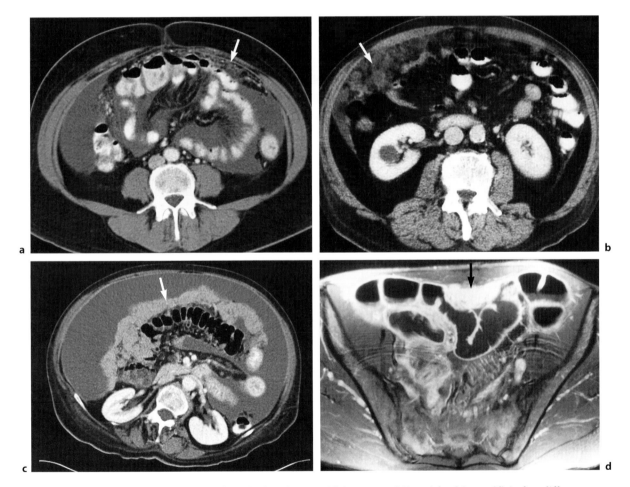

Fig. 10.8a–d. Omental implants. Transaxial CT (**a–c**) and transaxial fat-saturated T1-weighted image (**d**) in four different patients. Omental implants (*arrows*) may display a broad spectrum of findings ranging from a netlike pattern (**a**) to cottonlike (**b**) and nodular lesions (**d**). They are typically located between the abdominal wall and bowel loops. If they coalesce they are termed omental cake (**c**)

Netlike omental involvement is more difficult to evaluate. Implants of the diaphragm consist of nodular or plaquelike lesions. Peritoneal implants of liver or spleen may result in scalloping of the surface. Ligaments may appear thickened due to peritoneal metastases. Implants on bowel or mesentery can cause tethering of loops and may lead to obstruction. Bowel obstruction, however, results more commonly from intestinal wall involvement than from serous implants. Mesenteric lesions appear as thickening of the root of the mesentery, and often display a stellate radiating pattern.

Sister Mary Joseph's nodule presents metastatic cancer to the umbilicus. It usually ranges from 1 to 1.5 cm in size, but can attain a size of up to 10 cm (Fig. 10.9).

The depiction of peritoneal implants depends on the size and presence of ascites. The latter improves the conspicuity, especially of smaller lesions. However, implants less than 1 cm are detected with a sensitivity of only 25%-50% with spiral CT technique [23]. In this study, CT performance improved to a sensitivity of 85%-93% and a specificity of 91%-96% in detecting extrapelvic peritoneal disease larger than 1 cm in size [23]. Contrast-enhanced CT and MRI aid in the depiction of peritoneal implants. MRI seems similar to CT in the assessment of abdominal peritoneal implants and seems superior in the assessment of pelvic peritoneal details [24].

10.6.1.3
Ascites

Ascites alone is generally nonspecific, and small amounts of pelvic fluid are commonly detected in the cul-de-sac in normal patients. In ovarian cancer, pelvic ascites may be a sign of stage I disease; however, involvement of the diaphragmatic lymphatics, which presents stage III, should generally be a concern [25]. Large amounts of ascites in a patient with ovarian cancer usually indicate presence of peritoneal metastases. Coakley found that the presence of ascites alone had a PPV of 72%–80% for peritoneal metastases [23]. Furthermore, a direct relationship between stage of ovarian cancer and volume of ascites has been found [26]. Absence of ascites may not exclude a malignant disease, as 50% of borderline tumors and 83% of early-stage ovarian cancers are not associated with ascites [4]. Peritoneal carcinosis is characterized by various amounts of ascites and diffuse or focal peritoneal thickening. Benign forms of ascites displaying the same pattern such as postoperative inflammatory changes, bacterial peritonitis, or chronic hemodialysis cannot be differentiated from peritoneal carcinosis [27]. Absence of ascites in the cul-de sac in cases of ascites throughout the pelvis or abdomen has been described as a sign of malignancy [28].

10.6.2
Pathways of Spread in Ovarian Cancer

Knowledge of the pathways of tumor spread is pivotal for the interpretations of findings in CT and MRI, and they are the basis for staging of ovarian cancer.

Ovarian cancer spreads primarily by direct extension to neighboring organs by exfoliating cells into the peri-

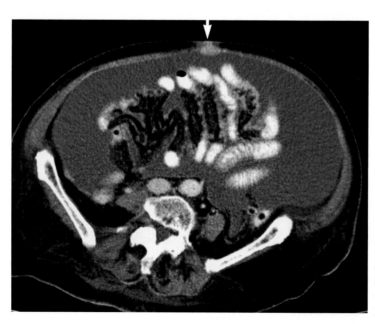

Fig. 10.9. Umbilical metastasis. Sister Mary Josef's nodule is a peritoneal implant to the umbilicus. In this patient, a solid 1.5-cm lesion (*arrow*) is demonstrated. Other signs of peritoneal tumor spread include large amounts of ascites and focal thickening of the peritoneum in the right paracolic gutter

toneal cavity that can implant on parietal and visceral peritoneum throughout the peritoneal cavity. It also disseminates by lymphatic pathways, and less commonly metastasizes hematogenously. Locoregional spread of ovarian cancer occurs by continuous growth along the surfaces of the pelvic organs and pelvic side walls. Peritoneal spread and implantation outside the pelvis is caused by tumor cells that are able to slough off the ovary and enter the peritoneal circulation. Peritoneal implants are also disseminated throughout the lymphatic vessels of the peritoneum. Due to the hemodynamics of the peritoneal fluid, the sites most often involved are the right subphrenic space, including the diaphragm, the liver surface, and Morrison's pouch. Further sites of peritoneal implants include the omentum, the surface of the left diaphragm and spleen, paracolic gutters, mesentery, and small and large bowel surfaces.

Tumor spread along the lymphatic pathways is found along three routes. The main pathway of lymphatic spread is along the broad ligament and parametria to the pelvic sidewall lymph nodes (external iliac and obturator chains), and along the ovarian vessels to the upper common iliac and para-aortic lymph nodes between the renal hilum and aortic bifurcation. Drainage to external and inguinal nodes via the round ligaments accounts for the rarest route of lymphatic tumor spread. At surgery, lymph node metastases are directly correlated with tumor stage: in stages I and II, 14% of lymph node metastases may be positive for metastases, whereas in stages III and IV, up to 64% of lymph node metastases are detected [29]. Furthermore, pelvic lymph nodes are more often involved than para-aortic nodes.

Hematogenous spread occurs later in the course of the disease. Distant metastases are most commonly found in the liver, lung, pleura, and kidneys. At the time of the initial presentation, parenchymal liver metastases are extremely rare, and patients are more likely to present with liver surface metastases [28].

10.6.3
Staging of Ovarian Cancer

Staging of ovarian cancer is based on the extent and location of disease noted at initial exploratory staging laparotomy. The most commonly used staging system of ovarian cancer is the International Federation of Gynecologists and Obstetricians (FIGO) classification system. Complete surgical staging has been established as the gold standard for assessing ovarian cancer. This procedure includes a staging laparotomy with a total abdominal hysterectomy, bilateral salpingo-oophorectomy, infracolic omentectomy, and lymphadenectomy [4, 29]. Furthermore, peritoneal cytology and multiple peritoneal biopsies are obtained throughout the pelvis and upper abdomen. More recently, laparoscopic staging procedures for ovarian cancer have also been proposed.

Understaging of ovarian cancer remains a common problem (20%–40%) in clinical routine. It occurs frequently, when the initial surgery had been performed under the presumption of a benign process, due to laparoscopy technique, and lack of oncologic specialist expertise [4].

10.6.3.1
Staging by CT and MRI

Surgical staging is regarded as the gold standard to evaluate a patient with ovarian cancer, and it is the basis to determine whether additional therapy is necessary [4]. Surgical staging can be preceded by a series of preoperative tests. Routine chest X-ray has been recommended to screen for lung metastases. Intravenous urography and contrast enema have previously been used in the preoperative evaluation of the urinary tract, and to exclude colon wall invasion or stenosis. Recently, CT and MRI have been widely accepted as adjunct imaging modalities for preoperative decision making in ovarian cancer [4, 11, 24, 30, 31].

Although definitive staging of ovarian cancer is based upon the findings at surgery, preoperative assessment of the tumor extent by imaging may influence patient management. Accurate preoperative assessment of ovarian cancer may aid the surgeon in better determining sites for biopsy, and also allow the depiction of tumor deposits that might be difficult to visualize intraoperatively, e.g., the diaphragm, splenic hilum, stomach, lesser sac, mesenteric root, and para-aortic nodes above the level of the renal hilum [4]. Furthermore, it may alert the surgeon of the need for subspecialist cooperation or for referral to an oncology center. In case of extensive cancer and signs of nonresectability on CT or MRI, candidates may be selected who may benefit from neoadjuvant therapy prior to surgery [15].

10.6.3.1.1
Imaging Findings According to Stages

A CT and MRI modified staging system of ovarian cancer is summarized in Table 10.2 [24, 25].

Table 10.2. Modified FIGO staging of ovarian cancer by CT and MRI

Stage	Imaging findings[a]
Stage I	Tumor limited to the ovaries
IA	Limited to one ovary, no ascites (intact capsule and no tumor on the external surface)
IB	Limited to both ovaries, no ascites (as in stage IA)
IC	Stage IA or IB with ascites (or with tumor on surface). Capsule ruptured, peritoneal washings positive for malignant cells
Stage II	Growth involving one or both ovaries, pelvic extension
IIA	Extension and/or metastases to the uterus and/or fallopian tubes
IIB	Extension to other pelvic tissues
IIC	Tumor either IIA or IIB with ascites
Stage III	Tumor involving one or both ovaries, peritoneal implants (including liver surface, small bowel, and omentum) outside the pelvis and/or implants of retroperitoneal or inguinal lymph nodes
IIIA	Tumor grossly limited to the true pelvis (including microscopical implants of abdominal peritoneum)
IIIB	≤2 cm implants of abdominal peritoneal surfaces
IIIC	>2 cm implants of abdominal peritoneal surface and/or retroperitoneal or inguinal lymph nodes
Stage IV	Growth involving one or both ovaries, distant metastases, parenchymal liver metastases.

[a]Additional staging criteria used in histopathological and surgical staging in parentheses.

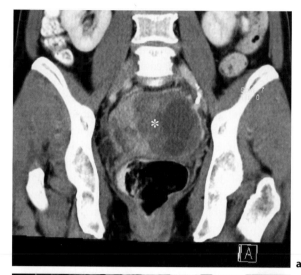

a

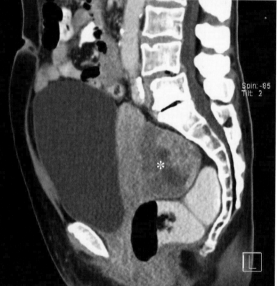

b

Fig. 10.10a,b. Stage I borderline tumor. Coronal (**a**) and parasagittal (**b**) CT. A 7-cm predominantly solid tumor (*asterisk*) with cystic areas is located in the cul-de-sac. The sagittal plane shows broad-based contact to the uterus (**b**). No evidence of ascites was found in the pelvis or abdomen. At surgery, a grayish tumor deriving from the left ovary was found. Histopathology revealed the rare endometrioid subtype of ovarian tumor of low malignant potential, which was classified as FIGO stage Ia

In stage I, tumor is confined to one (stage IA) or both ovaries (stage IB) (Fig. 10.10). The capsule of the tumor is intact and there is no evidence of spread of the tumor to the ovarian surface. In stage IC disease, tumor is detected on the ovarian surface or capsule rupture has occurred. Ascites may also be present.

Stage II is characterized by local tumor extension into the pelvic soft tissues and to organs within the true pelvis. In stage IIA, either direct tumor extension or implants on the uterus or fallopian tubes can be identified. Findings suggesting this stage include distortion or irregularity between the interface of the tumor and the myometrium. Stage IIB is characterized by involvement of pelvic tissues, such as bladder, rectum and pelvic peritoneum. Invasion of sigmoid colon or rectum is diagnosed when loss of tissue plane between the solid component of the tumor, encasement, or localized wall thickening is noted (Fig. 10.11). A distance of less than 3 mm between the lesion and the pelvic sidewall or displacement or encasement of iliac vessels is suggestive of pelvic sidewall invasion (Fig. 10.12). Stage IIC describes ovarian cancer as in stage IIA or IIB plus ascites.

Stage III consists of extrapelvic peritoneal implants and/or inguinal or retroperitoneal lymphadenopathy. Peritoneal lesions outside the pelvis, omental, or mesenteric implants are typical findings in stage III ovarian cancer. Peritoneal tumor spread is characterized by peritoneal thickening or lesions projecting from the peritoneal surfaces, or lesions that are located within the mesentery or the omentum. Stages IIIA–IIIC differ in the size of abdominal peritoneal lesions. In Stage IIIA, tumor is grossly limited to the pelvis; however, large amounts of ascites are a sign of upper abdominal tumor spread. In stage IIIB, lesion size is 2 cm or less (Fig. 10.13); in stage IIIC it exceeds 2 cm (Fig. 10.5). Retroperitoneal and inguinal lymphadenopathy also constitute stage IIIC ovarian cancer.

Ascites is a common finding in stage III disease; delayed enhancement of ascites was described as a sign of malignant ascites [32].

Stage IV ovarian cancer is characterized by distant metastases that include any location outside the pelvis, which is not spread peritoneally. Malignant pleural effusion is the most common clinical manifestation of stage IV ovarian cancer. Typical imaging findings include pleural effusion associated with pleural nodularity and focal pleural thickening (Fig. 10.14). Hematogenously spread metastases,

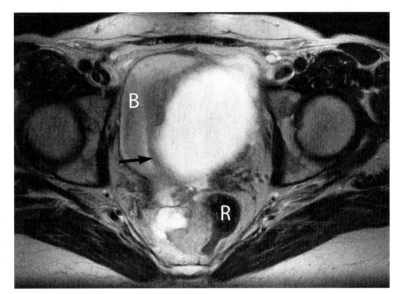

Fig. 10.11. Rectal wall invasion. Transaxial T2-weighted image. A cystic and solid left ovarian cancer (*arrow*) compresses bladder (*B*) and rectum (*R*). The latter shows broad contact with the solid tumor component located in the cul-de-sac. *B*, bladder

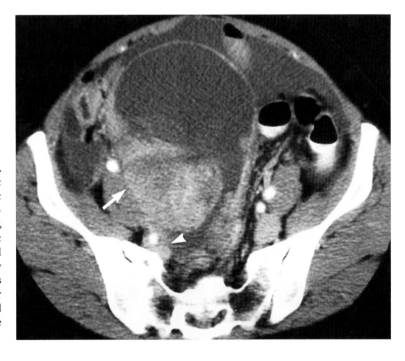

Fig. 10.12. Pelvic sidewall invasion. Transaxial CT at the level of the iliac bifurcation. A mixed solid and cystic adnexal tumor, which was nondifferentiated ovarian cancer at histopathology, is located in the pelvis. The left pelvic sidewall, including iliac vessels and psoas muscle, are clearly separated by fat. The right pelvic sidewall (*arrow*) is in direct contact with the solid tumor component. Furthermore, external and internal iliac arteries are displaced, the latter is encased by tumor (*arrowhead*)

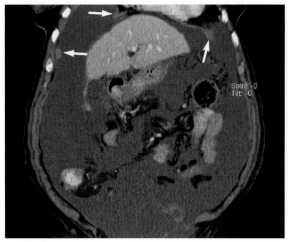 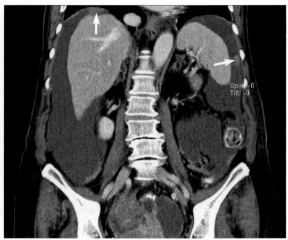

Fig. 10.13a,b. Stage IIIb ovarian cancer. Coronal CT at an anterior (**a**) and posterior level (**b**) demonstrate a pelvic ovarian mass and multiple small implants of the right and left diaphragm (*arrows*). Other findings include plaquelike and linear thickening of the peritoneum along the diaphragm, paracolic gutters, and in the pelvis (**b**). Because of large amounts of ascites, the peritoneal lesions can be well differentiated from adjacent anatomical structures

e.g., in the lung or liver parenchyma, are also typical manifestations in stage IV disease. It is particularly important to differentiate between liver surface metastases, which display smooth margins and an elliptic or biconvex shape, from liver parenchymal metastases (Fig. 10.15).

10.6.3.1.2
Value of Imaging

CT and MRI perform similarly in staging of ovarian cancer, with reported accuracy of 70%–90%, sensitivity of 63%–69% and specificity of 100% [23, 24, 25, 30, 33]. The decision to use CT or MRI is based on many factors, including cost, availability, contraindications, radiologist expertise, and clinician preference. CT is currently the primary imaging modality for staging ovarian cancer because of better availability and shorter examination times [24, 30]. Sensitivity for metastases declines with implant size less than 1 cm in diameter to 25%–50%. MRI may show advantages for detecting metastases within the pelvis. Helical CT improves the performance, with a reported sensitivity of 85%–93% and a specificity of 91%–96% for detection of peritoneal implants [23, 30]. Double-dose contrast-enhanced MR imaging including delayed images (5 min) may aid in the detection of subtle implants. In one study, this technique approximated the performance of laparotomy [16].

The diagnosis of lymphadenopathy is based on the short diameter of detectable lymph nodes. Based on

a threshold of 1 cm or less in diameter the sensitivity for lymph node metastases is only 50%, and the specificity is 95% [34].

10.6.3.2
Prediction of Resectability

Cytoreductive surgery followed by chemotherapy is the cornerstone for the treatment of advanced ovarian cancer. Tumor debulking is generally considered successful or optimal when no residual tumor larger than 1–2 cm is left after the initial staging laparotomy [4]. A significant benefit in terms of response to chemotherapy and survival has been reported only in patients with residual tumor diameters of less than 2 cm [35]. Because of local anatomical limitations despite aggressive surgery, optimal cytoreduction rates range from 50% to 60%. Neoadjuvant chemotherapy followed by surgical debulking has been suggested as an alternative treatment approach in patients with bulky nonoptimally resectable disease [36]. This treatment option, however, is a complex issue and depends on the underlying medical condition of the patient, surgical risks, and expertise of the institution. Several studies have addressed the role of imaging in predicting resectability of patients with advanced ovarian cancer [24, 31, 27]. Identifying inoperable disease may help the surgeon to select candidates in whom chemotherapy seems the appropriate therapy. Resectability, as defined by imaging, is a function of location and size of peritoneal implants. Most commonly used criteria indicating suboptimal cytoreduction include (a) retroperitoneal presacral implants, (b) lesions in the root of the mesentery, extensive disease (larger than 2 cm) along the undersurface of the diaphragm or lesser sac, liver surface implants in the gall bladder fossa, and interhepatic fissure, (c) suprarenal para-aortic lymph nodes, and d) liver parenchymal, pleural, and pulmonary metastases (Fig. 10.16) [24, 31]. Meyer et al. reported that inclusion of other factors such as ascites or CA-125 does not improve prediction and also suggested a scoring system [31]. CT and MRI performed with equal accuracy in detecting inoperable tumor and prediction of suboptimal debulking in ovarian cancer, with reported sensitivity of 76%, specificity of 99%, PPV of 99%, and NPV of 96% [37].

10.6.3.2.1
Value of Imaging

In the vast majority of patients, surgery remains the mainstay for treatment of ovarian cancer. It has been established that the maximal dimension of residual tumor remaining is an important prognostic factor. However, aggressiveness of surgery varies among the institutions and specialties. CT and MRI seem equally suitable to aid in patient management, especially to alert the surgeon to disease that may complicate the surgery or to the need of subspeciality assistance. Furthermore, imaging may aid in selecting patients with bulky unresectable disease who may benefit from neoadjuvant chemotherapy [37].

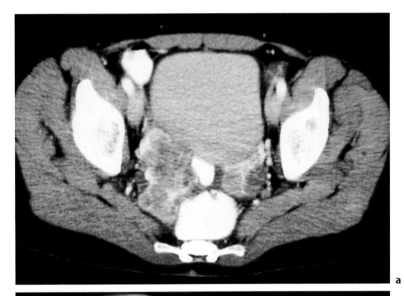

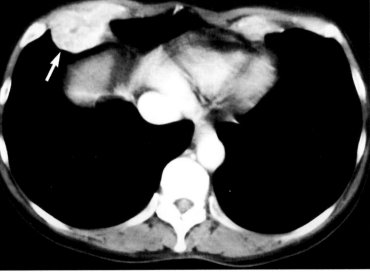

Fig. 10.14a,b. Stage IV ovarian cancer. CT in the pelvis (**a**) and lower thorax (**b**). At the time of diagnosis, the patient presented with bilateral ovarian tumors encasing the uterus (**a**). Furthermore, left cardiophrenic lymph node enlargement and a pleural mass (*arrow*) were found (**b**). Biopsy of the latter confirmed metastases from ovarian adenocarcinoma. No evidence of ascites or peritoneal dissemination was found at imaging and surgery

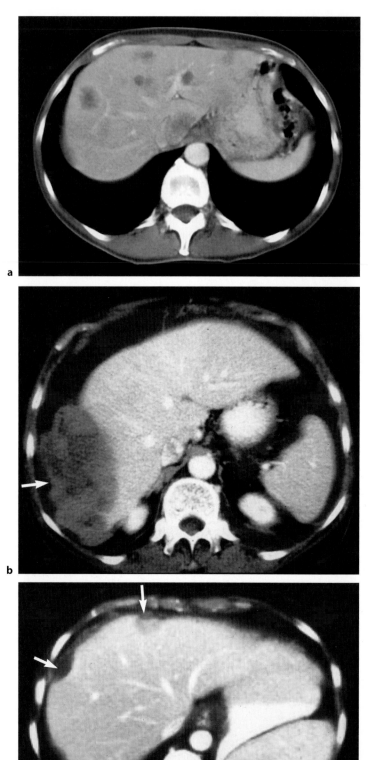

Fig. 10.15a–c. Spectrum of liver metastases in ovarian cancer. Transaxial CT shows multiple liver parenchymal metastases (**a**) and liver surface metastases (*arrows*) (**b, c**) in different patients with ovarian cancer. Liver surface metastases are typically crescent-shaped and may cause scalloping of the surface of the liver. Surface implants may be solid (**b**) or cystic (**c**). Splenic surface metastases are also found in **c**, which shows a morphology similar to the liver implants

10.6.4
Tumor Types

Patients with malignant tumors of the ovary and borderline tumors account for 21% and 4% of primary ovarian tumors, respectively [12]. Among these, epithelial cancer constitutes for the vast majority with 85%. Serous epithelial and mucinous ovarian cancer account for the majority of epithelial ovarian cancers and present approximately 49% and 36% of all ovarian epithelial tumors, respectively [3]. Endometrioid cell cancers account for 8%. The other cancers occur with equal frequency of 2% [3].

Malignant germ cell and malignant stromal neoplasm are responsible for 7% each. Germ cell tumors represent two-thirds of malignancies in females less than 20 years of age.

Unfortunately, there is a poor correlation between the gross appearance on pathology and the histologic type, and the aggressiveness cannot be determined on the basis of imaging studies.

10.6.4.1
Epithelial Ovarian Cancer

10.6.4.1.1
Serous Ovarian Carcinoma

Serous adenocarcinoma is the most common type of ovarian cancer and accounts for approximately half of the epithelial ovarian cancers [2]. Two-thirds of these tumors involve both ovaries [2].

At macroscopy, serous adenocarcinomas appear typically as multilocular cystic tumors with intracystic papillary projections. These excrescences fill the cyst cavity, or they may contain serous, hemorrhagic, or turbid fluid (Fig. 10.17) [2]. Psammoma bodies within the tumor or implants, presenting tiny calcifications, are detected in 30% at histology, but only in 12% of cases in CT [38]. In up to 12% of women with advanced serous cystadenocarcinomas, the ovaries may be small and display predominantly surface involvement, warranting the diagnosis of primary carcinoma of the peritoneum [2].

10.6.4.1.2
Mucinous Adenocarcinomas

Mucinous cystadenocarcinomas comprise 36% of ovarian carcinomas. They tend to be large at diagnosis, and contain loculi with hemorrhagic or proteinaceous contents. Macroscopically, they present

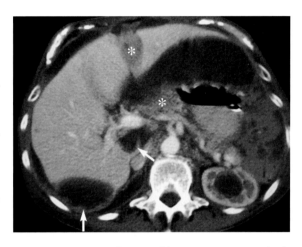

Fig. 10.16. Nonoptimally resectable ovarian cancer. Multiple peritoneal implants (*arrows*) are demonstrated on the liver surface and lesser sac. The latter is distended due to ascites. The implants located in the interlobar fissure (*asterisk*) and lesser sac (*asterisk*) are considered nonoptimally resectable

multiloculated cystic lesions with solid areas and intracystic nodules. Rarely, the tumor may be predominantly solid. Approximately 63% of mucinous adenocarcinomas are diagnosed as FIGO stage I tumors. Bilateral involvement is only found in 5%–10% [2]. Pseudomyxoma peritonei may be associated with mucinous adenocarcinomas. It consists of implants of mucinous contents on the abdominal and pelvic peritoneal surfaces.

10.6.4.1.3
Endometrioid Carcinomas

Endometrioid carcinomas represent 8% of all ovarian carcinomas. They occur with synchronous endometrial carcinomas or endometrial hyperplasia in up to 33% of cases [39]. Furthermore, an association with breast cancer has been reported [2]. Rarely, endometrioid carcinoma may arise from endometriosis [40]. Bilateral ovarian involvement is encountered in 30%–50% of cases. Macroscopically, these tumors are solid and cystic, the cysts may contain mucinous or greenish fluid. Rarely, solid tumors with extensive hemorrhage or necrosis may be found [2].

10.6.4.1.4
Clear Cell Carcinomas

Clear cell carcinomas present approximately 2%–7% of all ovarian cancers. Seventy-five percent of patients are diagnosed with stage I disease; however,

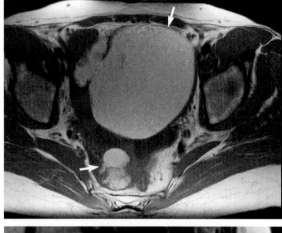

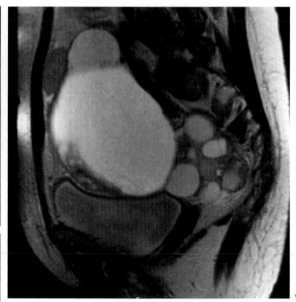

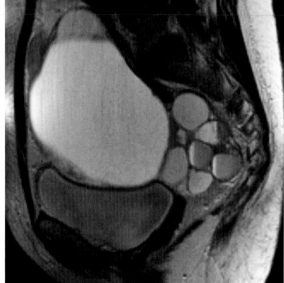

Fig. 10.17a–c. Serous adenocarcinoma. Transaxial T1-weighted image (**a**) and sagittal T2-weighted image (**b, c**). A large cystic multiloculated lesion with papillary projections and solid components is demonstrated. Most loculi show high signal on T1-weighted image (*arrow*) due to proteinaceous or hemorrhagic contents (**a**). Some locules at the posterior aspect show typical hemorrhagic fluid–fluid levels (**b**). Broad-based solid areas are identified at the anterior aspect of the lesion (**b, c**) and papillary projections are seen within some small posterior loculi (**c**)

the prognosis is worse compared to stage I of the other histologic subtypes [2]. The relationship with endometriosis is strongest (25%) among the ovarian cancers. The tumor may arise within endometriosis (Fig. 10.18), or endometriotic implants may be found commonly in relationship to the tumor or elsewhere in the pelvis [2]. Hypercalcemia as a paraneoplastic syndrome and thromboembolic complications are more common than in other ovarian cancers [41]. Most common gross appearance is a thick-walled unilocular cyst with multiple protruding nodules or a multilocular cystic mass (Fig. 10.19) [2].

Imaging Findings of Epithelial Ovarian Cancers

Epithelial ovarian cancers are typically larger than 4–5 cm at time of presentation. On CT and MRI, they present as a complex cystic or multiloculated ovarian lesion. Although differentiation between the subtypes is not reliably possible by imaging, there might be some differential diagnostic clues. Bilateral ovarian involvement is typically found in serous cystadenocarcinomas, which is the most common ovarian cancer; rarely is it encountered in endometrioid cancer. Psammoma bodies, which can only be detected on CT, are characteristic of serous ovarian cancers. Enhancement of a mural nodule within an endometrioma is highly suggestive of a malignant ovarian neoplasm. Endometriosis is associated with endometrioid, and especially with clear cell cancer. The latter appears most commonly as a large unilocular cyst with one or more solid mural nodules [42]. In endometrioid ovarian cancer, endometrial thickening or abnormal uterine bleeding can also be found.

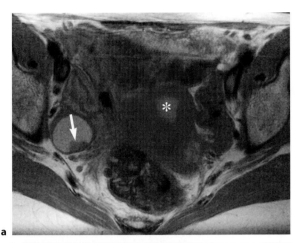

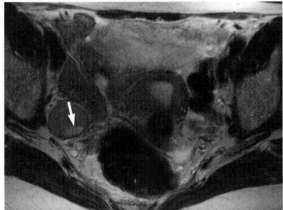

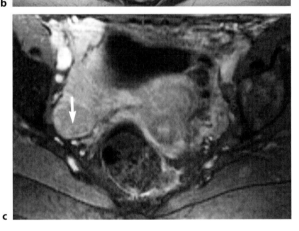

Differential Diagnosis

Benign serous and mucinous cystadenomas are usually entirely cystic and display thin walls and septa. Small papillary projections may also be present in cystadenomas. Metastases, particularly from primary cancer of the appendix or gastrointestinal tract may display similar imaging characteristics as ovarian cancer. Calcifications may also be present in metastases of mucinous adenocarcinoma of the colon and papillary thyroid cancer [39]. Malignant ovarian tumors of other origins may display similar imaging characteristics as ovarian cancer. Age and hormonal effects may help in the differential diagnosis. Other differential diagnoses include benign cystic and/or solid tumors, e.g., cystadenofibroma (Fig. 10.20) and rarely dermoids without fat. Mesothelioma and papillary serous carcinoma of the peritoneum may have an appearance similar to ovarian cancer. Normal size of the ovaries may be a diagnostic clue to exclude ovarian cancer. In case of

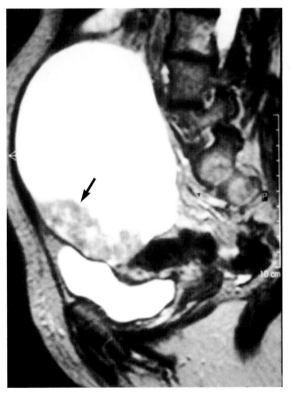

Fig. 10.18a–c. Clear cell carcinoma arising in an endometrioma. Transaxial T1-weighted image (**a**), T2-weighted image (**b**), and contrast-enhanced fat-saturated (FS) T1-weighted image (**c**). A typical endometrioma of the right ovary is demonstrated in **a** and **b**, showing high signal intensity (SI) on T1-weighted image and shading with low SI on the T2-weighted image. Within the posterior wall of the endometrioma a band-like mural lesion (*arrow*) with low SI on T1-weighted image (**a**) and high SI on T2-weighted image (**b**) is seen. Due to contrast enhancement it is obscured in **c**. Contrast enhancement is not found in a clot in endometrioma, but is indicative of a tumor within the endometrial cyst. Hematometra (*asterisk*)

Fig. 10.19. Clear cell carcinoma. Parasagittal T2-weighted image shows a large, well-delineated cystic ovarian lesion cephalad of the bladder (*B*), which extends to the midlumbar region. At its anterior wall, broad-based protruding nodules (*arrow*) with a thickness of more than 2 cm are demonstrated, a typical finding of an ovarian malignancy. Courtesy of Dr. M.T. Cunha, Lisbon

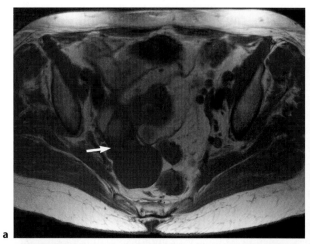

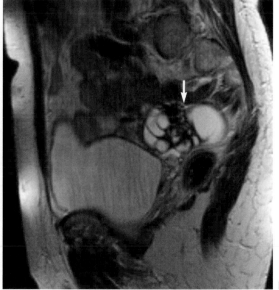

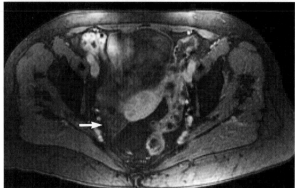

Fig. 10.20a–c. Cystadenofibroma mimicking ovarian cancer. Transaxial T1 (**a**) WI, sagittal T2-weighted image (**b**), and transaxial contrast-enhanced T1-weighted image with FS (**c**). In a 77-year-old female, a multiseptate right adnexal mass (*arrow*) is demonstrated with multiple hemorrhagic proteinaceous loculi showing high SI on the T1-weighted image (**a**) and irregular septa of very low SI on T2-weighted image (**b**). Only little discrete septal enhancement is found after contrast administration

extensive peritoneal disease, differentiation of ovarian cancer from extraovarian pelvic tumors may be difficult, especially by CT. In the majority of cases, tuboovarian abscesses can be distinguished from ovarian cancer based upon imaging and clinical findings. Endometriomas can be differentiated by MRI by typical findings such as shading, thick capsules, and lack of enhancing solid components. However, especially in CT, extensive endometriomas may be a diagnostic problem and mimic ovarian cancer (Fig. 10.21).

10.6.4.1.5
Borderline Tumors

Borderline tumors are epithelial ovarian cancers with low malignant potential. They account for approximately 4%–14% of all ovarian malignancies and present a different entity from invasive epithelial cancers. Serous and mucinous borderline tumors can be distinguished by specific histologic features including epithelial budding, multilayering of the epithelium, increased mitotic activity, nuclear atypia, and lack of stromal invasion cancer [2].

The medium age is 40 years, which is approximately 20 years earlier than for women with epithelial ovarian cancers. Compared to epithelial ovarian cancer, the survival rate stage for stage is much better. A 7-year follow-up of survival of stage I diseases was 99% and for stage II and III disease 92% [4].

Borderline tumors may be large, with diameters ranging from 7 to 20 cm; bilaterality is common. Mucinous tumors of borderline malignant potential tend to be larger, and may be associated with pseudomyxoma peritonei.

Imaging Findings

Borderline tumors tend to be large unilateral or bilateral ovarian tumors that cannot be distinguished from invasive ovarian cancers in CT or MRI. Papillary projections ranging from 10 to 15 mm in size and protrude into the cyst wall are more frequently found in borderline tumors compared to benign and malignant epithelial ovarian tumors (Fig. 10.22) [22]. Rarely, borderline tumors may present as a unilocular cyst larger than 6 cm in size [43].

10.6.4.1.6
Recurrent Ovarian Cancer

Although the initial response to treatment is good, persistence or recurrence of ovarian cancer remains a major problem. This is reflected by the 5-year survival rate for patients with advanced stages of ovarian cancer of 10%–30% [15].

Survival correlates with the disease-free interval before tumor recurrence and the residual disease following primary cytorective surgery [4, 44]. Patients who have a disease-free interval of more than 6 months or 1 year have a markedly improved prognosis. These patients have also been shown to benefit from following secondary cytoreductive surgery [4].

Pelvic recurrences develop after an average of 1.8 years, and hematogenous metastases (liver, spleen, lungs, and brain) after an average of 2.5 years [29]. The pelvis, particularly the vaginal vault and the cul-de-sac, is the most common site of tumor recurrence, and it is followed by abdominal peritoneal implants. Typical abdominal locations include the surface of the diaphragm and liver, paracolic gutters, the large-

and small-bowel surface, and mesentery. Because of the surgical technique, omental recurrence is rare. This is also true for pelvic lymph node metastases in recurrent ovarian cancer. Lymph node metastases are typically located in the para-aortal region and found in 18%–33% (Fig. 10.23) [29]. Small- and large-bowel obstruction is a common complication in patients with recurrent ovarian cancer and presents the leading cause of mortality.

Unlike in primary ovarian cancer, recurrent ovarian cancer is not strongly associated with ascites. In one study, ascites was only found in 38% of patients with ovarian cancer, and in the vast majority the amount of fluid detected was small. Furthermore, small amounts of ascites were also demonstrated in patients without evidence of tumor recurrence [45].

Serum tumor markers (CA-125) are pivotal in the follow-up of patients with a history of ovarian cancer. A rising CA-125 level in a patient in a clinically complete remission is highly predictive of recurrence. However, this may precede the median time to physical or radiographic evidence of recurrent disease by 4–6 months [4].

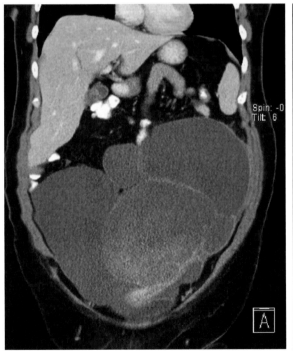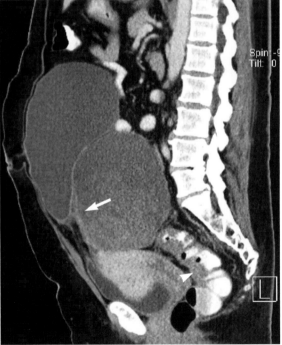

a b

Fig. 10.21a,b. Endometrioma mimicking ovarian cancer in CT. Coronal (**a**) and sagittal CT (**b**). In a 47-year-old woman with elevated tumor markers, a multicystic mass with a diameter of 25 cm occupies the pelvis and midabdomen. Focal mural and septal thickening (*arrow*) and high density within some cysts are demonstrated. There was no evidence of lymph node enlargement or ascites. At surgery, extensive endometriosis of the ovaries and peritoneum was found. Furthermore, mural wall thickening of the rectum and sigmoid colon by endometriosis (*arrowhead*) and thickening of the uterine corpus due to endometriosis was detected (**b**)

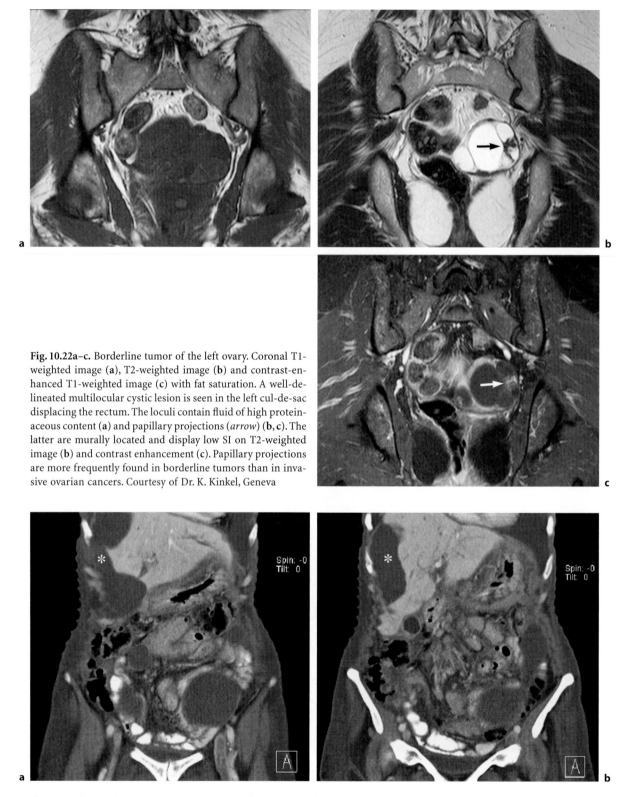

Fig. 10.22a–c. Borderline tumor of the left ovary. Coronal T1-weighted image (**a**), T2-weighted image (**b**) and contrast-enhanced T1-weighted image (**c**) with fat saturation. A well-delineated multilocular cystic lesion is seen in the left cul-de-sac displacing the rectum. The loculi contain fluid of high protein-aceous content (**a**) and papillary projections (*arrow*) (**b,c**). The latter are murally located and display low SI on T2-weighted image (**b**) and contrast enhancement (**c**). Papillary projections are more frequently found in borderline tumors than in invasive ovarian cancers. Courtesy of Dr. K. Kinkel, Geneva

Fig. 10.23a,b. Ovarian cancer recurrence. Coronal CT scans (**a, b**) in a patient with advanced recurrent clear cell cancer show multiple, predominantly cystic peritoneal implants throughout the abdomen and pelvis. The liver surface is compressed by surface implants (*asterisk*) (**a, b**). Multiple enlarged lymph nodes are seen in the right pelvis and root of the mesentery (**b**). Associated findings in this case include bilateral pleural effusion and a thrombus in the left femoral vein

Imaging Findings

Recurrent ovarian cancer most frequently presents as solid, followed by mixed solid and cystic lesions located within the pelvis (Fig. 10.23). Entirely cystic lesions are rarely found [45]. In CT, recurrent disease usually displays moderate contrast enhancement. In MRI, the imaging findings depend on the morphology of the lesions. Usually smaller lesions display low to intermediate SI on T1-weighted images and intermediate to high SI on T2-weighted images (Fig. 10.24). Contrast-enhanced images improve characterization of the architecture of the lesions and facilitate the detection of small peritoneal surface lesions, especially their differentiation from bowel loops. Diffuse or focal peritoneal enhancement presents carcinosis peritonei. The pattern of peritoneal involvement is similar to primary ovarian cancer, with diffuse thin lining of the peritoneal surfaces 2–5 mm thick to plaquelike lesions or nodules emerging from the peritoneal surfaces. Diffuse ascites is found less commonly in localized recurrent ovarian cancer and presents usually a sign of diffuse peritoneal recurrent disease. Omental caking is usually encountered only in patients who had received primary chemotherapy treatment. Small-bowel obstruction is a common complication as ovarian cancer advances and occurs in 5%–42% of ovarian cancer cases [46]. Signs of malignant bowel

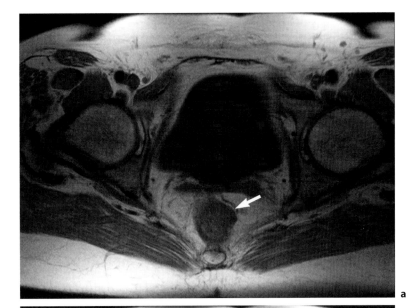

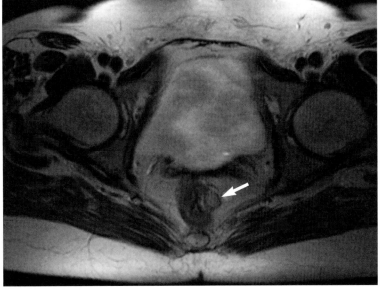

Fig. 10.24a,b. Recurrent ovarian cancer. Transaxial T1-weighted image (**a**) and T2-weighted image (**b**) at the level of the vaginal stump. In a patient with a history of surgery and chemotherapy for ovarian cancer, rising tumor markers were found. The vaginal stump is unremarkable; however, a focal nodular surface lesion of the left rectal wall (*arrow*) is demonstrated, which is protruding minimally into the mesorectal fat. This metastasis was the only manifestation of recurrent ovarian cancer

obstruction include bowel dilatation, an obstructing mass, focal mural thickening, and peritoneal carcinomatosis [46]. A pseudo-small-bowel obstruction pattern can mimic small-bowel obstruction. It is typically encountered late in the course of the disease and is caused by tumor infiltration of the myenteric plexus of the small bowel [4].

Secondary cytoreduction, which is usually performed in pelvic recurrence, is only considered successful when complete resection without a residual tumor is possible. Preoperatively, it is crucial to assess pelvic side wall invasion rather than tumor size [44]. Pelvic side-wall invasion can be excluded when the tumor shows a distance of 3 mm or more to the pelvic sidewall and no involvement of the iliac vessels is found [24].

Differential Diagnosis

Not every solid lesion in a postoperative patient means ovarian cancer recurrence. The combination of CA-125 and a baseline imaging study usually aids in the differential diagnosis. Postoperative hematomas, adhesions between bowel loops, or localized trapped fluid may mimic recurrent disease. Benign forms of diffuse peritoneal thickening such as a result of postoperative inflammatory complications or bacterial peritonitis cannot be differentiated from peritonitis carcinomatosa. Furthermore, chemical peritonitis following intraperitoneal chemotherapy also results in diffuse peritoneal thickening [32].

Value of Imaging

Second look surgery no longer plays a role as a routine procedure in the follow-up of ovarian cancer. Tumor markers, particularly CA-125, play a pivotal role in monitoring patients with ovarian cancer. Imaging in conjunction with this tumor marker is used to assess disease progression and response to therapy. Baseline examinations after surgery or before chemotherapy have been advocated to allow an objective follow-up [47]. However, in many institutions imaging is only performed when tumor markers persist or increase, or when the patients present with clinical symptoms. The exact assessment of the location and volume of recurrent ovarian cancer by imaging has a direct impact on patient management. Only patients with recurrent resectable pelvic disease may be considered as candidates for a secondary cytoreductive surgery. Furthermore, patients can be selected who will benefit from a relieving colostomy [4]. Among the imaging modalities, CT has been widely used for the assessment of recurrent ovarian cancer. MRI may assist in predicting tumor respectability, particularly in the pelvis. Recently, excellent performance has been reported for MRI in predicting the presence of residual ovarian tumors, comparable to the performance of laparotomy and superior to CA-125 values [16]. Abnormal MRI findings with a normal CA-125 value is a strong indicator of residual or recurrent tumor [16]. FDG PET or integrated PET/CT plays an increasing role in the assessment of recurrent ovarian cancer. It is particularly useful in assessing persistent ovarian cancer and serves as a complementary imaging technique when tumor markers are rising and CT or MRI findings are inconclusive or negative [48]. It seems superior to the other imaging techniques in assessing small implants within the mesentery or bowel surface [49].

10.6.4.2
Nonepithelial Ovarian Malignancies

10.6.4.2.1
Malignant Germ Cell Tumors

Malignant germ cell tumors of the ovary are much less common than epithelial ovarian neoplasms. Although germ cell ovarian malignancies account for 2%–3% of all ovarian malignancies, their clinical importance is based upon their potential for cure and the typical age distribution [4]. In women younger than 20 years of age they account for approximately two-thirds of all ovarian malignancies. They are often very large solid tumors with rapid and predominantly unilateral growth [50]. The most frequent sites of dissemination are the peritoneum and retroperitoneal lymph nodes. Compared with epithelial tumors, they have a greater tendency for hematogenous metastases, and liver and lung involvement can be observed at diagnosis. Ascites is only found in approximately 20% of cases [4]. Serum levels of HCG and AFP may assist in the diagnosis and follow-up of some germ cell tumors.

Malignant germ cell tumors comprise, in order of decreasing frequency, dysgerminomas, immature teratomas, endodermal sinus tumors, and embryonal and nongestational choriocarcinomas. The latter three are extremely rare. In these patients, tumor markers may be helpful for assessing response and tumor recurrence. Endodermal sinus tumors secrete AFP. Embryonal carcinomas can secrete both AFP and HCG, whereas pure choriocarcinomas secrete only HCG [4].

10.6.4.2.2
Dysgerminomas

Dysgerminomas present the most common type of malignant germ cell tumors and have been considered the female equivalent of seminoma of the testis. Seventy-five percent occur in early reproductive age, 10% in prepubertal girls, and 15%–20% are diagnosed during pregnancy or postpartally [51]. The vast majority of patients with dysgerminomas are diagnosed with early-stage disease. In contrast to the other germ cell tumor types, dysgerminomas may also occur bilaterally.

Imaging Findings

Dysgerminoma presents as a multilobulated, well-delineated solid lesion. In CT, speckled calcifications may be observed. Furthermore, they may contain low attenuation areas representing necrosis or hemorrhage. Contrast-enhanced CT may also demonstrate strongly enhancing fibrovascular septa. In MRI, the tumor displays low signal intensity on T1-weighted images and intermediate signal with low SI septa and high signal intensity areas of necrosis on T2-weighted images (Fig. 10.25). As in CT, intralesional septa may display strong enhancement [52].

Differential Diagnosis

Differential diagnosis includes solid ovarian tumors in younger age, e.g., granulosa cell tumors and teratomas. In MRI, uterine fibroma and fibrothecoma may display a similar appearance on T2-weighted images; however, contrast enhancement in these tumors is less and delayed. Especially in CT, differentiation of subserosal uterine fibroids from solid dysgerminomas is not possible.

10.6.4.2.3
Immature Teratomas

Immature teratomas or malignant teratomas are the second most common germ cell malignancies. They may rarely be encountered in postmenopausal women. The typical age group is the same as in dermoid cysts, typically young women between 10 and 20 years of age. However, in contrast to benign teratomas, they are extremely rare, with less than 1% consisting of immature teratomas. They are typically large at the time of diagnosis and present as solid or predominantly solid tumors with cystic elements and areas of fat and calcifications. Immature teratomas are associated with dermoid cysts, more commonly in the ipsilateral (26%) than in the contralateral ovary [53]. Immature teratomas contain embryonic tissues and can also occur in combination with other germ cell tumors (mixed germ cell tumors). Yolk sac tumors within immature teratomas give rise to alpha fetoprotein elevation and are an important prognostic factor in these patients [53]. Immature teratomas may also rarely produce steroids and cause pseudoprecosity in prepubertal girls [54].

Imaging Findings

The appearance is variable with heterogenous, predominantly solid lesions or cystic or mixed solid and cystic lesions with scattered or coarse calcifications or hemorrhage [55, 56]. In CT, punctate foci of fat and calcifications are diagnostic clues for the pres-

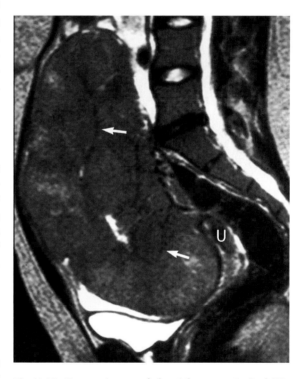

Fig. 10.25. Dysgerminoma of the right ovary. Sagittal T2-weighted image with FS. In an adolescent, a large, well-delineated solid lesion is located cranially and anterior of the uterus (*U*). It displays predominantly low to intermediate SI on the T2-weighted image. Centrally a region of high signal is seen presenting necrosis; furthermore, multiple septa (*arrows*) of low SI can be identified. The lesions showed intense homogenous contrast enhancement (not shown) and small central necrosis. Small amount of ascites is found between bladder and the tumor. Courtesy of Dr. T.M. Cunha, Lisbon

ence of a teratoma [55]. In case of cystic lesions, they are typically filled with serous fluid and may rarely contain fatty sebaceous material [56]. In MRI, small foci of fat with high SI on T1 (Fig. 10.26) and signal loss on the fat sat sequence are typically found [56]. Capsule penetration allows the differentiation from a mature teratoma [50].

Differential Diagnosis

The presence of fat is the diagnostic clue for the diagnosis of teratomas. Immature teratomas are usually large at presentation. In contrast to the majority of benign teratomas, which are cystic, malignant teratomas tend to be predominantly solid with small foci of fat and scattered calcifications. Elevation of alpha 1 fetoprotein assists in establishing the diagnosis, and is found in 33%–65% of immature teratomas [56]. Concomitant mature and immature teratomas occur in approximately 20% of cases. If no fat is identified immature teratoma cannot be differentiated from ovarian cancer.

10.6.4.2.4
Sex Cord Stromal Tumors

Sex cord stromal tumors derive from coelomic epithelium or mesenchymal cells of the embryonic gonads [54]. Eight percent of all ovarian neoplasms account for this tumor type, with granulosa cell tumors, fibrothecomas, and Sertoli-Leydig cell tumors comprising the majority of these tumors. In contrast

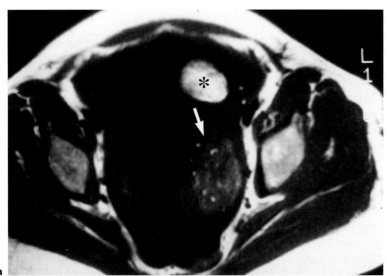

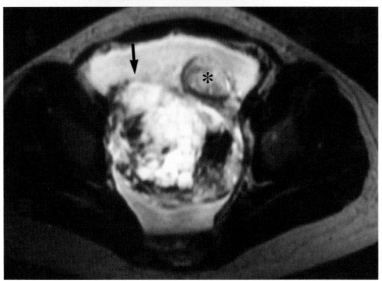

Fig. 10.26a,b. Mature and immature teratoma in a 20-year-old female. T1-weighted image (**a**) and T2-weighted image with FS (**b**) at the acetabular level. Ascites surrounds bilateral ovarian lesions. The left tumor (*asterisk*) represents a benign dermoid with predominantly fatty tissue. Posteriorly an inhomogeneous mixed solid and cystic lesion (*arrow*) with small hemorrhagic loculi is seen, which is better identified on the T2-weighted image (**b**). The tiny spots of high SI on T1-weighted image represent areas of fat (*arrow*, **a**)

to the benign fibrothecomas, granulosa cell tumors are classified as tumors of low-grade malignancy. Sertoli-Leydig cell and steroid tumors may be malignant depending on the degree of differentiation [54]. Sex cord stromal tumors affect all age groups, but are commonly encountered in peri- and postmenopausal women [57]. Their clinical and differential diagnostic importance is based upon their hormone activity. Granulosa cell tumors may typically produce estrogens; Sertoli-Leydig cell tumors and steroid cell tumors are androgen-producing tumors. The majority of sex cord stromal tumors are confined to the ovary at the time of diagnosis [58].

10.6.4.2.5
Granulosa Cell Tumors

Granulosa cell tumors are classified as neoplasm of a low-grade malignancy. Two subgroups of granulosa cell tumors, the juvenile and adult subtype, which differ in several important aspects, can be differentiated. Adult granulosa cell tumors account for 1%–2% of all ovarian tumors and for 95% of all granulosa cell tumors [54]. Granulosa cell tumors are the most common ovarian tumors with estrogen production. Juvenile granulosa cell tumors are hormonally active in 80% and occur typically before the age of 30. The vast majority are found in prepubertal girls who present with the signs of precocious pseudopuberty with development of breasts and pubic and axillary hair. An association with Ollier's disease (enchondromatosis) and Maffucci's syndrome

(enchondromatosis and hemangiomatosis) has been reported in some cases [54].

The adult granulosa cell tumors usually occur after the age of 30 years and have their peak incidence in the perimenopausal age [54]. Because of their estrogen activity, they can become clinically apparent with abnormal uterine bleeding and endometrial hyperplasia. Endometrial cancer is associated with these tumors in 5%–25% of cases [58]. Both types of granulosa cell tumors are typical unilateral ovarian tumors that vary considerably in size and show an average diameter of approximately 12 cm [54].

In adult granulosa cell tumors, late recurrence years after the initial therapy tumor manifestation may be seen. The recurrent tumor is typically confined to the pelvis and abdomen (Fig. 10.27). However, distant metastases to the bone, supraclavicular lymph nodes, liver, and lungs have been reported [29].

Imaging Findings

Granulosa cell tumors can display a broad spectrum from entirely cystic to completely solid ovarian lesions (Fig. 10.28) [22]. The latter may display homogenous contrast enhancement and high SI on T2-weighted images. They may also manifest as a solid and cystic neoplasm, and cysts may contain hemorrhagic fluid. The adult type of granulosa cell tumor manifests mostly as a predominantly sponge-like cystic multilocular tumor with blood clots and solid tissue [59].

Fig. 10.27. Late recurrence of granulosa cell tumor. Transaxial T2-weighted image in a 45-year-old patient with a history of hysterectomy and resection of a granulosa cell tumor 16 years before. Recurrent granulosa cell tumor is identified as a solid and cystic lesion above the vaginal vault. The right border is well defined, the left posterior margin shows irregular contours (*arrow*) extending to the posterior pelvic sidewall. Small amounts of ascites are demonstrated in the pelvis. At surgery, invasion of the iliac internal vessels was confirmed

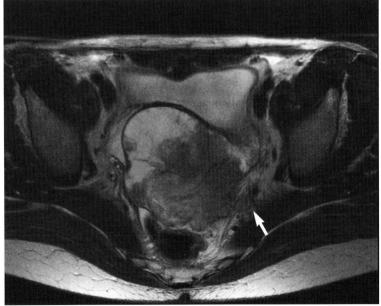

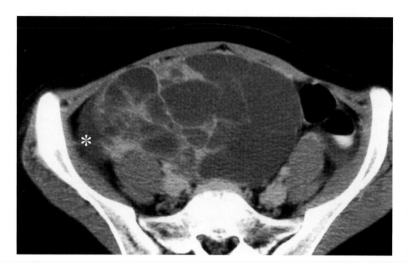

Fig. 10.28. Juvenile type of granulosa cell tumor. CT in a 17-year-old girl who presented with primary amenorrhea. A large, well-defined cystic ovarian tumor with multiple irregular septations and solid areas is demonstrated in the midpelvis. Small amounts of ascites (*asterisk*) without evidence of peritoneal seeding at surgery

10.6.4.2.6
Sertoli-Leydig Cell Tumor

Sertoli-Leydig cell tumors account for less than 0.5% of ovarian tumors. The majority (75%) of Sertoli-Leydig cell tumors occur in women younger than 30 years [57]. Less than 10% are found in women over 50 years of age [54]. Although virilization caused by androgen production is the most striking clinical feature, it occurs in only one-third of patients [54]. Other symptoms include menstrual irregularities or abnormal bleeding. Approximately 50% of women with Sertoli-Leydig tumors have no endocrine effects. Most Sertoli-Leydig cell tumors are unilateral and the majority are diagnosed as stage I disease. They vary in size between 5 and 15 cm (average, 13.5 cm). Some of these tumors, however, may be very small and difficult to detect by imaging, although they cause hormonal effects [60]. Depending upon the degree of differentiation, 1%–59% of Sertoli-Leydig cell tumors were malignant in one series [54]. In contrast to granulosa cell tumors, Leydig cell tumors tend to recur typically within the 1st year after surgery.

Imaging Findings

Sertoli-Leydig cell tumors vary greatly in gross appearance. They tend to be solid, sometimes lobulated masses. They may also appear as predominantly solid masses often with peripheral cysts or as a cystic lesion with polypoid mural structures [57]. Cysts may display a slightly high signal intensity on T1-weighted images. The solid components display intermediate to high SI on T2-weighted images and good contrast

enhancement in MRI and CT [22]. Rarely, these tumors may manifest as a cystic lesion [60]. Less differentiated types of Sertoli-Leydig cell tumors tend to display an inhomogenous architecture with areas of necrosis and hemorrhage.

10.6.4.2.7
Ovarian Lymphoma

Although the ovaries are not infrequently found to be involved by malignant lymphoma at autopsy, enlargement of the ovaries is rare. Less than 1% of patients with lymphoma initially present with unilateral or bilateral ovarian tumors [61]. Ovarian lymphoma is almost always a manifestation of a systemic disease, most commonly of B-cell lymphomas. Primary lymphoma of the ovary without lymph node or bone marrow involvement is extremely rare. It is encountered most commonly in premenopausal women.

Imaging Findings

Lymphomas appear as unilateral or more commonly as bilateral ovarian solid, often homogenous masses without ascites [62]. In CT, they appear as well defined solid masses with mild contrast enhancement. In MRI, they display intermediate signal on T1 and low to intermediate SI on T2-weighted images. Similar to CT, mild contrast enhancement is noted (Fig. 10.29).

Differential Diagnosis

Ovarian cancer may resemble ovarian lymphoma. Bilateral involvement is most commonly found in serous, undifferentiated ovarian cancers, and in borderline tumors. Ovarian cancer displays a heterogenous architecture, typically with solid and cystic elements. Furthermore, signal intensity on the T2-weighted image is often very high, and ascites is found in the majority of cases. Metastases may also present as a unilateral or bilateral solid ovarian masses. They usually display strong contrast enhancement and central necrosis or cysts. Clinical history, evidence of multiple lymph nodes, and splenomegaly support the diagnosis of lymphoma.

10.6.4.3
Ovarian Metastases

Approximately 5%–15% of malignant ovarian tumors are metastases to the ovaries. Colon, stomach, breast, and lymphoma are the most commonly encountered neoplasm to metastasize to the ovaries. Metastases from numerous other sites including melanoma, endometrial cancer, cancer of the pancreas, gallbladder, and carcinoid account for less common sources for ovarian metastases [63]. Ovarian metastases seem more common in premenopausal women because of higher vascularity of the ovaries in this age group, and they may be associated with hormonal activity [63]. Although metastases may occur unilaterally (especially in endometrial cancer), bilateral involvement is more typical and occurs in up to 75% of cases [14]. Approximately 50% of ovarian metastases consist of Krukenberg tumors, which display characteristic

features at histopathology and imaging. Krukenberg tumors originate from the stomach, gastrointestinal tumors, or the breast, and contain mucin-secreting signet ring cells surrounded by ovarian stroma. Compared to other neoplasms, Krukenberg tumors have a fourfold risk to metastasize into the ovaries. In patients with a history of Krukenberg tumors, complex ovarian tumors should be highly suspicious of metastases. In a multicenter study assessing 86 patients with primary ovarian and 24 patients with secondary cancers, only multilocularity favored the diagnosis of a primary ovarian cancer [64].

Ovarian metastases are often asymptomatic. They may rarely even precede the primary neoplasm. In general, ovarian metastases are associated with a poor prognosis and the majority of patients will die within the first year after detection [54].

10.6.4.3.1
Imaging Findings

On imaging, two types of ovarian metastases may be differentiated [14]. Krukenberg tumors display characteristic imaging features that typically include bilateral oval or kidney-shaped tumors, which tend to preserve the contour of the ovary. They are solid or predominantly solid with central necrosis or cysts and may attain a large size. On MRI, they display medium signal intensity on T1-weighted images, and an inhomogeneous low to intermediate SI on T2-weighted images (Fig. 10.30) [65, 66]. In CT and

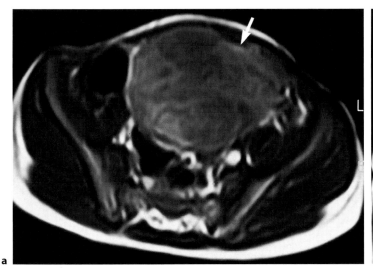
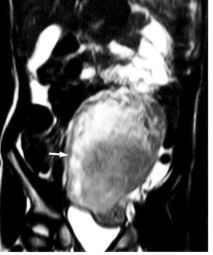

a   b

Fig. 10.29a,b. Ovarian lymphoma in a child. Contrast-enhanced T1-weighted image in the midpelvis (**a**) and coronal T2-weighted image (**b**) Non-Hodgkin lymphoma only confined to the left ovary presents as a large solid mass (*arrow*) with moderate contrast enhancement (**a**) and inhomogenous low to intermediate SI on T2-weighted image (**b**)

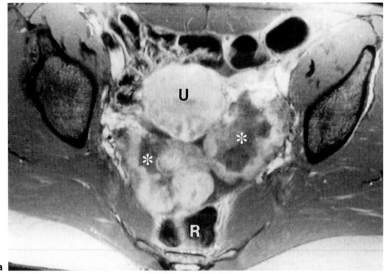

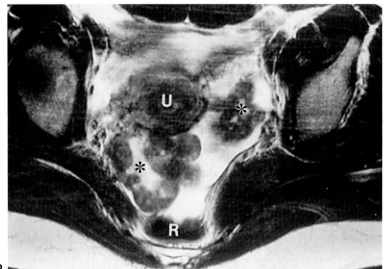

Fig. 10.30a,b. Bilateral Krukenberg tumors. Contrast-enhanced T1-weighted image (**a**) and T2-weighted image (**b**) show bilateral ovarian lesions with the typical imaging features of Krukenberg tumors. These include lobulated solid lesions with central necrosis (*asterisks*), which display strong contrast enhancement (**a**) and low SI of the solid components on T2-weighted image (**b**).The lesions are well delineated due to ascites. *R*, rectum. *U*, uterus. Courtesy of Dr. A. Heuck, Munich

contrast-enhanced MRI, they tend to show strong enhancement of solid components or septations.

Metastatic cancers different from Krukenberg tumors may have a variable appearance resembling other malignant ovarian lesions with cystic and mixed cystic and solid patterns [64, 67].

Colon cancer metastases commonly present as unilateral or bilateral, multiloculated, predominantly cystic tumors (Fig. 10.31) [63]. Presence of nodules or multinodularity at the ovarian surface may also be a sign of metastatic ovarian involvement. Ascites may be present.

The presence of another tumor outside the ovaries should warrant the diagnosis of metastases to the ovaries if the pattern of spread is atypical for ovarian cancer. In particular, the presence of pulmonary and hepatic metastases in absence of extensive peritoneal

spread is unusual for ovarian cancer and favors another primary neoplasm [54].

10.6.4.3.2
Differential Diagnosis

Confident distinction between primary and metastatic ovarian cancers is not possible because of overlapping findings in imaging. Bilateral, sharply delineated, purely solid or predominantly solid tumors with necrosis strongly favor the diagnosis of a metastatic ovarian tumor, most likely Krukenberg tumors [68]. Contrast uptake aids in the differentiation of solid ovarian metastases from stromal tumors. Stromal tumors typically display a mild and delayed contrast uptake [69]. If metastases are cystic

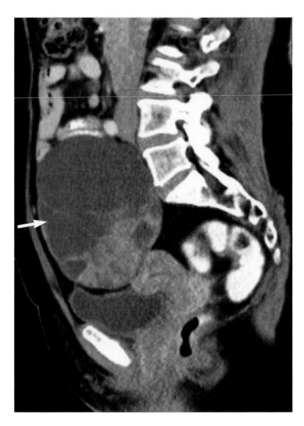

Fig. 10.31. Metastases from colon cancer. Sagittal CT shows a well-delineated mixed cystic and solid ovarian mass (*arrow*), which abuts the uterus fundus and elevates small bowel loops. No ascites was found in the pelvis or abdomen. In this patient with stage T4 colon cancer, differentiation of metastasis from ovarian cancer is not possible by imaging

and hemorrhagic, they may resemble endometriomas, which also occur in younger women. However, distinct contrast enhancement is not found in endometriomas. Abscesses usually present with different clinical features than the clinically silent metastases.

10.6.4.4
Fallopian Tube Cancer

Primary malignant neoplasms of the fallopian tube are extremely rare and account for only 0.3%–1.1% of all gynecologic cancers [4]. Most fallopian tube carcinomas present as papillary serous adenocarcinomas. The intraperitoneal spread of fallopian tube carcinomas is

similar to that of epithelial ovarian cancer. However, there seems to be a higher propensity for distant metastases [4]. In contrast to ovarian cancer, the majority of patients with tubal carcinoma are diagnosed at an early stage. Because of pain caused by tubal distension or abnormal uterine bleeding, tubal cancer often becomes clinically apparent early. Most fallopian tube cancers arise from the ampullary part of the fallopian tube and may cause tubal occlusion. In approximately 50% of all cases, fallopian tube cancer resembles hydrosalpinx and is often mistaken as such at surgery [70].

10.6.4.4.1
Imaging Findings

A unilateral adnexal complex cystic or solid mass associated with hydrosalpinx is the most common finding. CT and MR demonstrate complex solid and cystic enhancing masses similar to ovarian cancer. A cystic tubular structure with interdigitating septa adjacent to the mass represents the dilated tube. Signal intensity on T1 and T2 higher than serous fluid suggests hematosalpinx. Occasionally, focal nodularity within a hydrosalpinx may be found in fallopian cancer. Common associated findings are distension of the uterine cavity and ascites [70]. Peritoneal metastases are similar to those in ovarian cancer. Lymph node metastases may be found more often than in ovarian cancer.

10.6.4.4.2
Differential Diagnosis

Primary ovarian cancers cannot be reliably differentiated from fallopian tube cancers; however, the latter are exceedingly rare. In presence of associated hydrosalpinx, tubal cancer may mimic ovarian cancer with cystic and solid components. Especially with T2-weighted images, however, identification of the cystic areas representing the loops of the distended tube is usually possible. Metastases to the fallopian tubes, which result most commonly from direct extension of gynecologic cancers, cannot be reliably differentiated from primary fallopian tube cancers. Rarely, leiomyomas of the fallopian tube may be encountered, which resemble ovarian stromal tumors or fibroids of the broad ligament.

References

1. American Cancer society (2004) Ovarian cancer facts and figures: 2004. American Cancer Society, Atlanta
2. Seidman JD, Russell P, Kurman RJ (2002) Surface epithelial tumors of the ovary. In: Kurman RJ (ed) Blaustein's pathology of the female genital tract. Springer Verlag, Berlin Heidelberg New York pp 791–904
3. Hensley ML, Alektiar KM, Chi DS (2001) Ovarian and fallopian-tube cancer. In: Barakat RR, Bevers MW, Gershenson, HoskinsWJ (eds) Handbook of gynecologic oncology. Martin Dunitz, London, pp 243–263
4. Ozols RF, Schwartz PE, Eifel PJ (2001) Ovarian cancer, fallopian tube carcinoma, and peritoneal carcinoma. In: De Vita VT Jr, Hellman S, Rosenberg SA (eds) Cancer: principles and practice of oncology, 6th edn. Lippincott Williams & Wilkins, Philadelphia, pp 1597–1632
5. Boyd J (1998) Molecular genetics of hereditary ovarian cancer. Oncology 12:399–406
6. Chung DC, Rustgi AK (2003). The hereditary nonpolyposis colorectal cancer syndrome: genetics and clinical implications. Ann Intern Med 138:660–570
7. Bohm-Velez M, Mendelson E, Bree R et al (2000) Ovarian cancer screening. American College of Radiology. ACR Appropriateness criteria. Radiology 215:861–871
8. Scully RE (2000) Influence of origin of ovarian cancer on efficacy of screening. Lancet 355:1028–1029
9. Schwartz PE, Taylor KJ, (1995) Is early detection of ovarian cancer possible? Ann Med 27:519–528
10. Outwater EK, Dunton CJ (1995) Imaging of the ovaries and adnexa: clinical issues and applications of MR imaging. Radiology 194:1–18
11. NIH consensus conference (1995) ovarian cancer: screening, treatment and follow-up. NIH Consensus Development Panel on Ovarian Cancer. JAMA 273:491–497
12. Koonings PP, Campbell K, Mishell DR, Grimes DA (1989) Relative frequency of primary ovarian neoplasm: a 10-year review. Obstet Gynecol 74:921–926
13. Bairey O, Blickstein D, Stark P et al (2003) Serum CA 125 as a prognostic factor in non-Hodgkin's lymphoma. Leuk Lymphoma 44:1733–1738
14. Togashi K (2003) Ovarian cancer: the role of US, CT and MRI. Eur Radiol 13 [Suppl 4]:L87–L104
15. Cannistra SA (2004) Cancer of the ovary. N Engl J Med 351:2519–2529
16. Low RN, Duggan B, Barone RM et al (2005) Treated ovarian cancer: MR imaging, laparotomy assessment, and serum CA-125 values compared with clinical outcome at 1 year. Radiology 235:918–927
17. Buy JN, Ghossain MA, Sciot C et al (1991) Epithelial tumors of the ovary: CT findings and correlation with US. Radiology 178:811–818
18. Sohaib SAA, Sahdev A, Van Trappen et al (2003) Characterization of adnexal lesions on MRI. AJR Am J Roentgenol 180:1297–1304
19. Stevens SK, Hricak H, Stern JL (1991) Ovarian lesions: detection and characterization with gadolinium-enhanced MRI at 1.5 T. Radiology 181:481–488
20. Komatsu KI, Konishi I, Mandai M et al (1996) Adnexal masses: transvaginal US and gadolinium-enhanced MR imaging assessment of intratumoral structure. Radiology 198:109–115
21. Hricak H, Chen M, Coakley FV et al (2000) Complex adnexal masses: detection and characterization with MRI: multivariate analysis. Radiology 214:39–46
22. Jung SE, Lee JM, Rha SE et al (2002) CT and MR imaging of ovarian tumors with emphasis on differential diagnosis. Radiographics 22:1305–1325
23. Coakley FV, Choi PH, Gougoutas CA et al (2002) Peritoneal metastases: detection with spiral CT in patients with ovarian cancer. Radiology 223:495–499
24. Forstner R, Hricak H, Occhipinti K et al (1995) Ovarian cancer: staging with CT and MRI. Radiology 197:619–626
25. Woodward PJ, Hosseinzadeh K, Saenger JS (2004) Radiologic staging of ovarian carcinoma with pathologic correlation. Radiographics 24:225–246
26. Shen-Gunther J, Mannel RS (2002) Ascites as a predictor of ovarian malignancy .Gynecol Oncol 87:77–83
27. Outwater EK, Wilson KM, Siegelman ES, Mitchell DG (1996) MRI of benign and malignant gynecologic disease: significance of fluid and peritoneal enhancement in the pelvis at MR imaging. Radiology 200:483–488
28. Walkey MM, Friedman AC, Sohotra P et al (1988) CT manifestations of peritoneal carcinosis. AJR Am J Roentgenol 150:1035–1041
29. Burghardt E (1993) Epithelial ovarian cancer. Recurrence. In: Burghardt E (ed) Surgical gynecological oncology. Thieme, Stuttgart, p 494
30. Tempany CM, Zou KH, Silverman et al (2000) Staging of advanced ovarian cancer: comparison of imaging modalities-report from the Radiology Oncology Group. Radiology 215:761–767
31. Meyer JI, Kennedy AW, Friedman R et al (1995) Ovarian carcinoma: value of CT in predicting success of debulking surgery. AJR Am J Roentgenol 165:875–878
32. Low RN, Sigeti JS (1994) MR imaging of peritoneal disease: comparison of contrast-enhanced fast multiplanar spoiled gradient-recalled and spin echo sequences. AJR Am J Roentgenol 163:1131–1140
33. Low RN, Saleh F, Song SYT et al (1999) Treated ovarian cancer: comparison of MR imaging with serum CA-125 level and physical examination: a longitudinal study. Radiology 211:519–528
34. Low RN, Semelka RC, Worawattanakul S et al (1999) Extrahepatic abdominal imaging in patients with malignancy: comparison of MRI and helical CT with subsequential surgical correlation. Radiology 210:625–632
35. Bristow RE, Tomacruz RS, Armstrong DK et al (2002) Survival effects of maximal cytoreductive surgery for advanced ovarian carcinoma during the platinum era: a meta-analysis. J Clin Oncol 20:1248–1259
36. Huober J, Meyer A, Wagner U, Wallwiener D (2002) The role of neoadjuvant chemotherapy and interval laparotomy in advanced ovarian cancer. Cancer Res Clin Oncol 128:153–160
37. Quayyum A, Coakley FV, Westphalen AC et al (2005) Role of CT and MR imaging in predicting optimal cytoreduction of newly diagnosed primary epithelial ovarian cancer. Gynecol Oncol 96:301–305
38. Mitchell DG, Hill MC, Hill S et al (1986) Serous carcinoma of the ovary: CT identification of metastatic calcified implants. Radiology 158:649–652
39. Kawamoto S, Urban BA, Fishman EK (1999) CT of epithelial ovarian tumors. Radiographics 19:S85–S102

40. Tanaka YO, Yoshizako T, Nishida M et al (2000) Ovarian carcinoma in patients with endometriosis: MR imaging findings. AJR Am J Roentgenol 175:1423–1430
41. Hricak H, Reinhold C, Ascher SM (2004) Ovarian clear cell carcinoma. In: Hricak H, Reinhold C, Ascher SM (eds) Gynecology top 100 diagnoses. WB Saunders Company, Amirsys, Salt Lake City, pp 104–106
42. Matsuoka Y, Ohtomo K, Araki T et al (2001) MR imaging of clear cell carcinoma of the ovary. Eur Radiol 11:946–951
43. Exacoustos C, Romanini ME, Rinaldo D et al (2005) Preoperative sonographic features of borderline ovarian tumors. Ultrasound Obstet Gynecol 25:50–59
44. Funt AS, Hricak H (2003) Ovarian malignancies. TMRI 14:329–338
45. Forstner R, Hricak H, Azizi L et al (1995) Ovarian cancer recurrence: value of MR imaging. Radiology 196:715–720
46. Low RN, Chen SC, Barone R (2003) Distinguishing benign from malignant bowel obstruction in patients with malignancy: findings at MRI. Radiology 228:157–165
47. Johnson RJ (1993) Radiology in the management of ovarian cancer. Clin Radiol 48:75–82
48. Sironi S, Messa C, Mangili G et al (2004) Integrated FDG PET/CT in patients with persistent ovarian cancer: correlation with histologic findings. Radiology 233:433–440
49. Kubich-Huch RA, Dorffler W, von Schulthess GK et al (2000) Value of FDG positron emission tomography, computed tomography, and magnetic resonance imaging in diagnosing primary and recurrent ovarian cancer. Eur Radiol 10:761–767
50. Brammer HM, Buck JL, Hayes WS et al (1990) Malignant germ cell tumors of the ovary: radiologic pathologic correlation. Radiographics: 10715–10724
51. Hricak H, Reinhold C, Ascher SM (2004) Ovarian dysgerminomas. In: Hricak H, Reinhold C, Ascher SM (eds) Gynecology top 100 diagnoses. WB Saunders Company, Amirsys, Salt Lake City, pp 98–100
52. Tanaka YU, Kurosaki Y, Nishida M et al (1994) Ovarian dysgerminoma: MR and CT appearance. J Comput Assist Tomogr 18:443–448
53. Heifetz SA, Cushing B, Giller R et al (1998) Immature teratomas in children: pathologic considerations. Am J Surg Pathol 22:1115–1124
54. Young RH, Scully RE (2002) Sex-cord-stromal, steroid cell, and other ovarian tumors. In: Kurman RJ (ed) Blaustein's pathology of the female genital tract, 5th edn. Springer, Berlin Heidelberg New York, pp 905–965
55. Bazot M, Cortez A, Sananes S, Boudghene F et al (1999) Imaging of dermoid cysts with foci of immature tissue. J Comput Assist Tomogr 23:703–706
56. Yamaoka T, Togashi K, Koyama T et al (2003) Immature teratoma of the ovary: correlation of MR imaging and pathologic findings. Eur Radiol 13:313–319
57. Tanaka YO, Tsunoda H, Kitagawa et al (2004) Functioning ovarian tumors: direct and indirect findings at MRI. Radiographics 24:S147–S166
58. Outwater EK, Wagner BJ, Mannion C et al (1998) Sex cord-stromal and steroid cell tumors of the ovary. Radiographics 18:1523–1546
59. Kim SH (2002) Granulosa cell tumor of the ovary: common findings and unusual appearances on CT and MR. J Comput Assist Tomogr 26:756–761
60. Outwater EK, Marchetto B, Wagner BJ (2000) Virilizing tumors of the ovary: imaging features. Ultrasound Obstet Gynecol 15:365–371
61. Monterroso V, Jaffe ES, Merino MJ et al (1993) Malignant lymphoma involving the ovary. A clinico-pathologic analysis of 39 cases. Am J Surg Pathol 17:154–170
62. Ferrozzi F, Tognini G, Bova D et al (2000) Non-Hodgkin lymphomas of the ovaries: MR findings. J Comput Assist Tomogr 24:416–420
63. Young RH, Scully RE (2002) Metastatic tumors of the ovary. In: Kurmann RJ (ed) Blausteins's pathology of the female genital tract, 5th edn. Springer, Berlin Heidelberg New York, pp 1063–1101
64. Brown DL, Zou KH, Tempany CMC et al (2001) Primary versus secondary ovarian malignancy: imaging findings of adnexal masses in the radiology diagnostic oncology group study. 219:213–218
65. Ha HK, Baek SY, Kim SH et al (1995) Krukenberg's tumors of the ovary: MR imaging features. AJR Am J Roentgenol 164:1435–1439
66. Kim SH, Kim WH, Park KL et al (1996) CT and MR findings of Krukenberg tumors: comparison with primary ovarian tumors. J Comput Assist Tomogr 20:393–398
67. Megibow AJ, Hulnik DH, Bosniak MA et al (1985) Ovarian metastases: computed tomographic appearances. Radiology 156:161–164
68. Alcazar JL, Galan MJ, Ceamanos C et al (2003). Transvaginal gray scale and color Doppler sonography in primary ovarian cancer and metastatic tumors to the ovary. J Ultrasound Med 22:243–247
69. Troiano RN, Lazzarini KM, Scoutt LM et al (1997) Fibroma and fibrothecoma of the ovary: MR imaging findings. Radiology 204:795–798
70. Kawakami S, Togashi K, Kimura I et al (1993) Primary malignant tumor of the fallopian tube: appearance at CT and MR imaging. Radiology 186:503–508

Endometriosis

Karen Kinkel and Didier Chardonnens

11.1
Introduction

Endometriosis is among the most common disorders associated with pelvic pain (dysmenorrhea, dyspareunia, dysuria, dyschezia and/or cyclical haematochezia) and infertility, although it may be asymptomatic. The prevalence estimates of endometriosis vary by population selection, mode of diagnosis, surgeon's training and thoroughness of investigations. Among women seeking tubal ligation, endometriosis prevalence ranges from 2% to 18% [1, 2]. Within infertile populations, it ranges from 5% to 50% [3–7] and in pelvic pain clinics from 5% to 21% [3–6]. Endometriosis lesions may be active or inactive, superficial or deep infiltrating. It affects primarily the female pelvis (peritoneum, ovaries, tubes, uterus, bladder, colon, ureters and rectovaginal septum) but may be seen in uncommon sites such as diaphragm [8–9], lungs [10–13], peripheral nerves and brain [14–18]. Subtle endometriosis lesion recognition increased from 15% in 1986 to 65% in 1988 [19–20]. An increased awareness of the variations in the appearance of endometriosis lesions has resulted in almost a twofold increase in the diagnosis of endometriosis at laparoscopy [21].

K. Kinkel, MD, PD
Institut de Radiologie, Clinique des Grangettes, chemin des Grangettes 7, 1224 Chêne-Bougeries, Switzerland
D. Chardonnens, MD, PD
Hôpital de la Tour, Meyrins, Switzerland

The precise aetiology and pathogenesis of endometriosis remain largely unknown despite intense research in this field. Retrograde menstrual bleeding, subtle immunologic disturbances, hormonal and cytokine milieu imbalance, genetic predisposition, embryologic remnants, lifestyle, environmental factors and/or coelomic metaplasia may all play a role. Whatever the causes, the effects of the disease may be mentally and physically debilitating. Since lesion sites and appearance are numerous and symptoms not very specific, onset of symptoms to precise diagnosis may unfortunately average 6 years or even more [22]. So far, surgical intervention remains the gold standard to allow proper visual assessment and biopsy of lesions for histology identification of ectopic endometrial glands and stroma, thus allowing proper diagnosis, staging and treatment modalities. However, the development of noninvasive diagnostic techniques may be crucial preoperatively and postoperatively. This could lead preoperatively to a more accurate description of endometriosis lesion extension and their potential impact on adjacent anatomical structures, allowing a better surgical strategy and treatment after obtaining proper informed consent by the patient. Postoperatively, early detection of endometriosis recurrence may prove useful to medical treatment follow-up. Thus, the development of noninvasive diagnostic techniques will greatly help clinical and basic research, leading to a better understanding of the natural history and future management of endometriosis.

11.2
Imaging Techniques and Findings

11.2.1
Sonography

Ultrasound remains the most easily accessible and initial imaging technique of choice to diagnose endometriomas and other sites of endometriosis. For the diagnosis of endometrioma, transabdominal and transvaginal ultrasound of the pelvis helps to identify and confirm a persistent hypoechoic ovarian cyst, with low-level internal echos demonstrating no intracystic colour Doppler flow [23] (Fig. 11.1a). Among the nonfunctional neoplastic cysts, the differential diagnosis include dermoid cyst containing more echogenic portions with layered lines and dots and posterior shadowing [24, 25]. Mucinous cystadenoma are often hypoechoic with internal low-level echos but no menstrual cycle-related pain [26]. When endometriomas present atypical features such as mural nodules related to blood clots, contrast-enhanced MRI is useful to confirm the diagnosis of endometrioma without mural enhancement and to exclude the possibility of associated ovarian cancer [27]. Ultrasound may identify other sites of endometriosis such as abnormal nodules in the vesicouterine pouch or the bladder wall, suggesting bladder endometriosis [28, 29]. However the value of ultrasound in diagnosing posterior lesions of endometriosis, such as hypoechoic nodules of the uterosacral ligaments, rectal or vaginal wall or retrocervical lesions are more difficult due to the noncystic appearance and the more fibrous nature of these lesions [30].

11.2.2
MRI

MRI of the pelvis remains the method of choice to diagnose all lesion sites of endometriosis, particularly in patients with cycle-related dysmenorrhea, dyspareunia or pain during defecation [31]. Due to spontaneous T1 hyperintensity of blood after 8 days of bleeding, MRI should not be scheduled earlier than day 8 of the menstrual cycle. In our institution, MRI of the pelvis requires 6 h of prior fasting and an intramuscular injection of a peristaltic inhibitor and is performed with a pelvic phase array coil in a 1.5-T magnet. The patient is asked not to void the bladder during the hour preceding the examination. The MR imaging protocol for patients with suspected endometriosis uses anterior and posterior saturation bands covering subcutaneous fat and includes at least two T2-weighted sequences (repetition time 4,000 ms, echo time 90 ms, matrix 256×512, three signals acquired, 4- to 5-mm section thickness) in different slice orientations (sagittal and coronal oblique or axial oblique according to the axis of the uterine cavity), followed by three T1-weighted sequences in

an identical imaging plane that best demonstrates the pathology (TR 500 ms, TE 14 ms): native T1 without fat suppression, fat-suppressed T1 before and after intravenous injection of gadolinium contrast media [32].

The high-resolution characteristics should allow detailed visualization of small structures such as uterosacral ligaments or bowel wall layers. Sonographic gel used as an intravaginal contrast agent or rectal water enema may be useful according to the suspected location of the lesion [33]. A delayed contrast-enhanced MR urography sequence can help to demonstrate the position and dilatation of ureters. The 3D gradient echo HI-RES sequence is performed for 21 s of apnea (TR/TE = 4.9/1.38 ms, flip angle 40°, 50 sections of 1.5 mm, 400×400 matrix) and followed by postprocessing using MIP to superimpose the entire urinary system in one image [32].

Image interpretation uses a check list of possible locations of endometriosis including adnexa, vesicouterine pouch, retrouterine excavation, torus uterinus (upper portion of posterior cervix), uterosacral ligaments, anterior rectum, sigmoid, caecum and ileum. Endometriomas are easily diagnosed as ovarian cysts with a native T1- and fat-suppressed T1-hyperintense content of gradual variation of signal inten-

Fig. 11.1a–e. A 49-year-old woman with chronic left pelvic pain and an office ultrasound suspicious for bilateral ovarian cancer. **a** Oblique view of the right ovary at colour Doppler transvaginal ultrasound demonstrates a heterogeneous right ovarian mass with small calcification in the wall of the cyst (*arrowheads*). The intra- or extracystic location of peripheral colour Doppler flow (*arrow*) is difficult to diagnose. Pelvic MRI is performed to exclude ovarian cancer. **b** Axial T2-weighted FSE image of the pelvis shows two right-sided ovarian cysts of intermediate signal intensity and one left-sided ovarian cyst with shading of signal intensity (*arrow*). **c** Axial T1-weighted image shows bilateral T1-hyperintense content of all three cysts and a spiculated nodule between the two ovaries (*arrow*) with one hypointense line extending from the nodule towards the anterior rectum. **d** Axial fat-suppressed T1-weighted image at the same level as **c** confirms the haemorrhagic nature of all ovarian cysts and the interovarian peritoneal implant, suggesting endometriosis. **e** Contrast-enhanced T1-weighted image at the same level as (**c**) and (**d**) shows enhancement of the normal ovarian parenchyma and the interovarian peritoneal nodule. At surgery, bilateral endometriomas were attached to each other (kissing ovaries) and associated with severe adhesions towards the rectosigmoid. Pathology confirmed bilateral endometriomas without malignancy

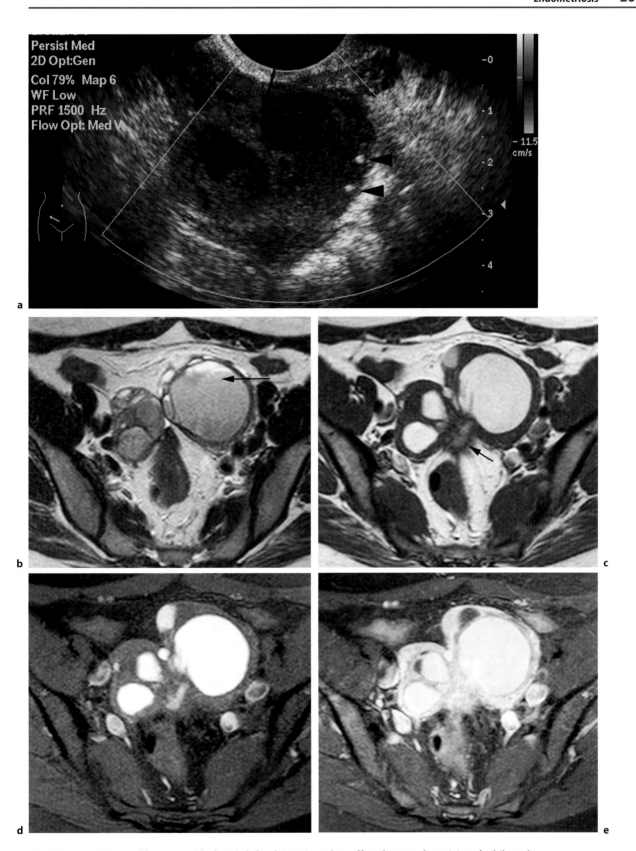

Fig. 11.1a–e. A 49-year-old woman with chronic left pelvic pain and an office ultrasound suspicious for bilateral ovarian cancer. .....(*see page 266*)

sity at T2-weighted imaging, often called shading [34] (11.1b–d). No wall thickening or intracystic portion enhances after intravenous contrast-injection. If these signs are present associated ovarian cancer has been described [27].

To diagnose bladder endometriosis at MRI, natural bladder distention by urine helps to identify small T2- and T1-hypointense nodules, most often located in the bladder dome, anterior to the vesicouterine pouch. Small T1-hyperintense portions may co-exist and correspond to haemorrhagic portions of the lesion. At contrast-enhanced imaging, the lesion enhances more than the noninvaded normal bladder detrusor [35] (Fig. 11.2).

Posterior lesions occur most often at the upper posterior cervix as a band-like T2- and T1-hypointense structure extending laterally to one or both uterosacral ligaments [33] (Fig. 11.3). Nodular thickening with regular or stellate margins at the initial uterine portion of the uterosacral ligament are easier to identify at T2-weighted images obtained in an oblique orientation perpendicular to the long axis of the cervical channel [32]. Associated T1-hyperintense portions have been described in 5%–61% of posterior lesions, corresponding to cystic haemorrhagic portions at pathology [33, 35]. When the lesion is located at the torus uterinus, uterine retroversion or angular anterior rectal attraction is often associated.

Deep endometriotic lesions of the bowel have been described in decreasing order of frequency at the rectosigmoid junction, the anterior rectum, the lower surface of the sigmoid, the appendix and the terminal ileum. At MRI these lesion appeared as fibrotic asymmetric thickening of the rectal wall forming an obtuse angle with the normal wall and enhancing less than the rectal mucosa [33] (Fig. 11.4). They are like most fibrotic lesions, T2 hypointense and T1 iso-intense to muscle. As for most posterior lesions of endometriosis, associated T1-hyperintense spots are not systematic. Locations at the anterior rectum often demonstrate a triangular shape pointing towards the uterus (Fig. 11.3). The precise extent of bowel wall invasion remains a challenge with all imaging methods and warrants further research.

Endometriosis of the vagina is usually diagnosed at physical examination and predominantly located at the upper posterior third of the vaginal wall. The extent of disease and locations at the posterior vaginal pouch are clinically difficult to assess and warrant subsequent imaging with vaginal contrast filling at transvaginal sonography [36] or at MRI. The value of standard transvaginal sonography without vaginal

contrast lacks sensitivity, with published values ranging from 29% to 44% [33, 36]. At MRI the sensitivity to detect vaginal lesions was reported at 76% [33]. Most vaginal lesions are associated with an obliteration of the pouch of Douglas. Locations of the rectovaginal septum are always associated with endometriotic lesions of the vagina or the rectosigmoid or uterosacral ligaments. Vaginal lesions present as a T2-hypointense and T1-iso-intense nodule (Fig. 11.5). Associated T2- and T1-hyperintense spots are frequently described but not reported in a systematic fashion in the published literature.

Adhesions are often not identified at any imaging modality except if fluid is present at both sides. In this circumstance, they correspond to an abnormal line or sheet within the pelvis. Indirect signs of adhesions include anterior rectal triangular attraction, angulation of bowel loops, too large changes in bowel diameter with peritoneal nodules, elevation of the posterior vaginal fornix, posterior displacement of the uterus or the ovaries, loculated fluid collections and hydrosalpinx [37]. Spiculated low signal intensity strands converging towards deep peritoneal lesions of endometriosis are also suggestive of adhesions [38].

To help the gynecologist to determine optimal treatment choices, preoperative knowledge of all lesion locations is mandatory. A complete preoperative lesion map allows scheduling of concomitant bowel, bladder or vaginal surgery and avoid intraoperative diagnoses of lesion location that postpone complete lesion removal at surgery.

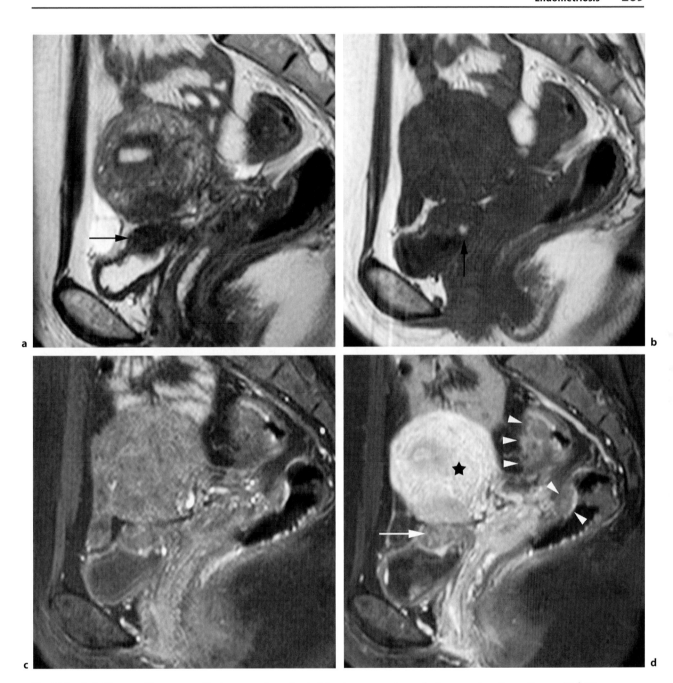

Fig. 11.2a–d. A 39-year-old woman with dyspareunia and painful urinary symptoms during menstruation. **a** Parasagittal T2-weighted image of the pelvis shows hypointense wall thickening of the upper posterior bladder wall (*arrow*). **b** Corresponding native T1-weighted image shows a hyperintense dot close to the bladder lumen (*arrow*). **c** Fat-suppressed T1-weighted image confirms the haemorrhagic nature of the dot seen in (**b**) and (**d**). Contrast-enhanced T1-weighted image at the same level as (**a**), (**b**) and (**c**) shows moderate enhancement of the bladder mass (*arrow*) compared to the strong enhancement of the myometrium (*star*). Associated thickening of the anterior rectal and lower sigmoid wall (*arrowheads*) is more easily identified after contrast enhancement than in (**a**), (**b**) or (**c**). Surgery and pathology confirmed bladder endometriosis and multiple sites of rectal and sigmoid endometriosis

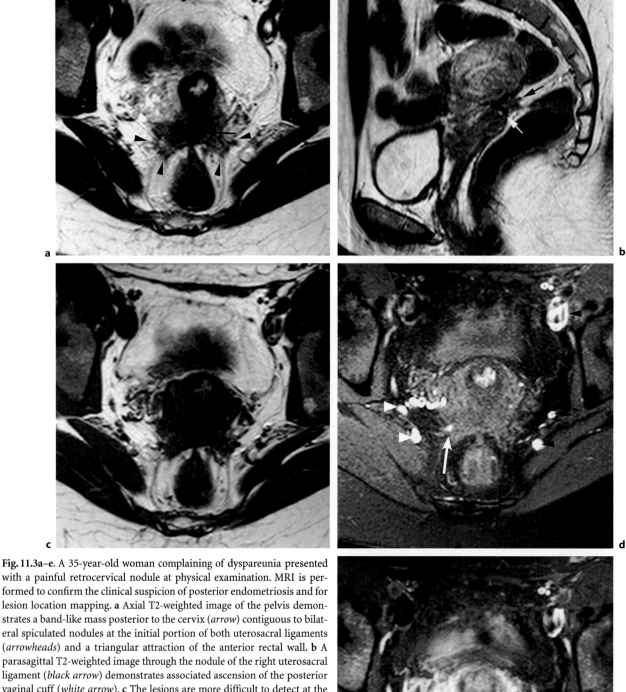

Fig. 11.3a–e. A 35-year-old woman complaining of dyspareunia presented with a painful retrocervical nodule at physical examination. MRI is performed to confirm the clinical suspicion of posterior endometriosis and for lesion location mapping. **a** Axial T2-weighted image of the pelvis demonstrates a band-like mass posterior to the cervix (*arrow*) contiguous to bilateral spiculated nodules at the initial portion of both uterosacral ligaments (*arrowheads*) and a triangular attraction of the anterior rectal wall. **b** A parasagittal T2-weighted image through the nodule of the right uterosacral ligament (*black arrow*) demonstrates associated ascension of the posterior vaginal cuff (*white arrow*). **c** The lesions are more difficult to detect at the corresponding T1-weighted image, only demonstrating an irregular contour of the initial portion of both uterosacral ligaments and the triangular attraction of the anterior rectal wall. **d** Fat-suppressed T1-weighted image at the same level as (**c**) shows several normal hyperintense vessels (*arrowheads*), blood in the endocervical channel and one small haemorrhagic cyst in the nodule of the right uterosacral ligament (*arrow*). **e** The contrast-enhanced image of the same level as (**a**), (**c**) and (**d**) confirms asymmetric thickening of the enhancing left anterior rectal wall (*arrow*) suspicious for rectal endometriosis. Pathology confirmed endometriosis of both uterosacral ligaments associated with rectal endometriosis

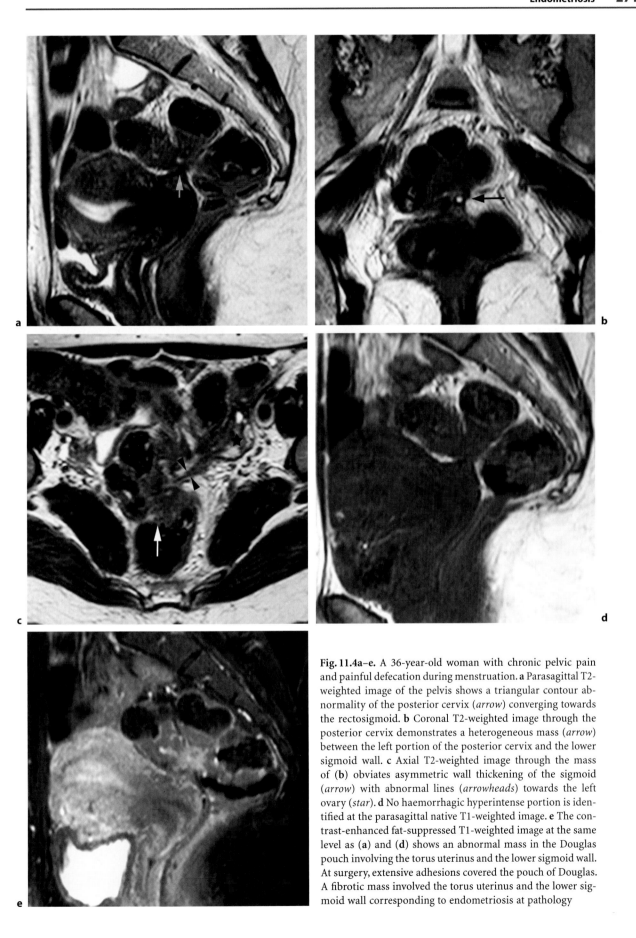

Fig. 11.4a–e. A 36-year-old woman with chronic pelvic pain and painful defecation during menstruation. **a** Parasagittal T2-weighted image of the pelvis shows a triangular contour abnormality of the posterior cervix (*arrow*) converging towards the rectosigmoid. **b** Coronal T2-weighted image through the posterior cervix demonstrates a heterogeneous mass (*arrow*) between the left portion of the posterior cervix and the lower sigmoid wall. **c** Axial T2-weighted image through the mass of (**b**) obviates asymmetric wall thickening of the sigmoid (*arrow*) with abnormal lines (*arrowheads*) towards the left ovary (*star*). **d** No haemorrhagic hyperintense portion is identified at the parasagittal native T1-weighted image. **e** The contrast-enhanced fat-suppressed T1-weighted image at the same level as (**a**) and (**d**) shows an abnormal mass in the Douglas pouch involving the torus uterinus and the lower sigmoid wall. At surgery, extensive adhesions covered the pouch of Douglas. A fibrotic mass involved the torus uterinus and the lower sigmoid wall corresponding to endometriosis at pathology

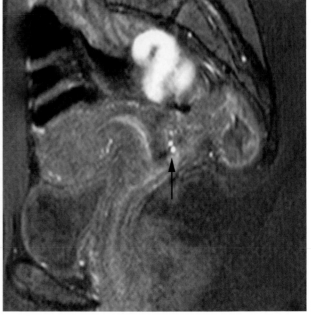

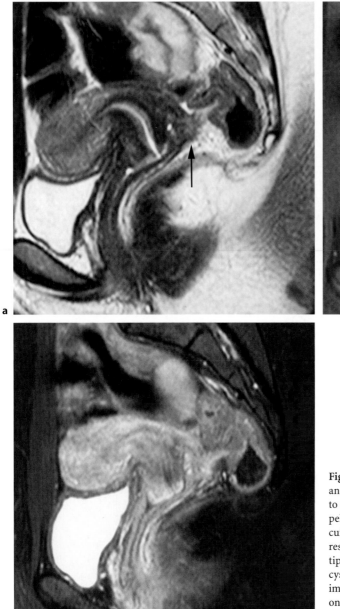

Fig. 11.5a–c. A 26-year-old woman with abnormal vaginal bleeding and clinical suspicion of vaginal endometriosis. MRI is performed to define the extent of disease. **a** Sagittal T2-weighted image of the pelvis shows an abnormal mass (*arrow*) in the posterior vaginal cuff without abnormal findings at the torus uterinus. **b** The corresponding fat-suppressed T1-weighted image clearly shows multiple hyperintense dots (*arrow*) corresponding to haemorrhagic cystic portions of the lesion. **c** Contrast-enhanced T1-weighted image shows peripheral increased contrast-enhancement with one line extending towards the anterior rectum separated from the mass by fat tissue. Lesion ablation was performed by vaginal surgery alone. Pathology confirmed vaginal endometriosis

References

1. Moen MH (1987) Endometriosis in women at interval sterilisation. Acta Obstet Scand 66:451–453
2. Strathy JH, Molgaard CA, Coulan CV et al (1982) Endometriosis and infertility: a laparoscopic survey of endometriosis among fertile and infertile women. Fertil Steril 38:667–673
3. Duignan NH, Jordan JA, Coughlan BM et al (1972) One thousand consecutive cases of diagnostic laparoscopy. J Obstet Gynecol Br Commonw 79:1016–1020
4. Hasson HM (1976) Incidence of endometriosis in diagnostic laparoscopy. J Reprod Med 16:135–140
5. Kleppinger RK (1974) One thousand laparoscopies at a community hospital. J Reprod Med 13:13–17
6. Liston WA, Bradford WP, Downie J et al (1974) Laparoscopy in a general gynaecologic unit. Am J Obstet Gynecol 43:896–900
7. Peterson EP, Behrman SJ (1970) Laparoscopy of the infertile patient. Obstet Gynecol 36:363–370
8. Cooper MJ, Russel P, Gallagher PJ (1999) Diaphragmatic endometriosis. Med J Aust 171:142–143
9. Redwine DB (2002) Diaphragmatic endometriosis, surgical management, and long-term results of treatment. Fertil Steril 77:288–296
10. Slasky BS, Siewers RD, Lecky JW, Zajko A, Burkholder JA (1982) Catamenial pneumothorax: the roles of diaphragmatic defects and endometriosis. AJR Am J Roentgenol 138:639–643
11. Velasco Oses A, Hilario Rodriguez E, Santamaria Garcia JL et al (1982) Catamenial pneumothorax with pleural endometriosis and hemoptysis. Diag Gynecol Obstet 4:295–299
12. Elliot DL, Barker AF, Dixon LM (1985) Catamenial hemoptysis. New methods of diagnosis and therapy. Chest 87:687–688
13. Rychlik DF, Bieber EJ (2001) Thoracic endometriosis syndrome resembling pulmonary embolism. J Am Assoc Gynecol Laparosc 8:445–448
14. Thibodeau LL, Prioleau GR, Manuelidis EE, Merino MJ, Heafner MD (1987) Cerebral endometriosis. Case report. J Neurosurg 66:609–610
15. Moeser P, Donofrio PD, Karstaedt N, Bechtold R, Greiss FC Jr (1990) MRI findings of sciatic endometriosis. Clin Imag 14:64–66
16. Descamps P, Cottier JP, Barre I et al (1995) Endometriosis of the sciatic nerve: case report demonstrating the value of MR imaging. Eur J Obstet Gynecol Reprod Biol 58:199–202
17. Fedele L, Bianchi S, Raffaeli R, Zanconato G, Zanette G (1999) Phantom endometriosis of the sciatic nerve. Fertil Steril 72:727–729
18. Silver MD, Jokl P (1999) Endometriosis of the pelvis presenting as a hip pain. Clin Orthop 368:207–211
19. Jansen RPS, Russel P (1986) Non-pigmented endometriosis: clinical laparoscopic and pathologic definition. Am J Obstet Gynecol 155:1154–1159
20. Stripling MC, Martin DC, Chatman DL, Zwaag RV, Poston WM (1988) Subtle appearances of pelvic endometriosis. Fertil Steril 49:427–431
21. Martin DC, Hubert GD, Vander Zwaag R, el-Zeky FA (1989) Laparoscopic appearances of peritoneal endometriosis. Fertil Steril 51:63–67
22. Hadfield R, Mardon H, Barlow DH et al (1996) Delay in the diagnosis of endometriosis: a survey of women from the USA and the UK. Hum Reprod 11:878–880
23. Patel MD, Feldstein VA, Chen DC, Lipson SD, Filly RA (1999) Endometriomas: diagnostic performance of US. Radiology 210:739–745
24. Atri M, Nazarnia S, Bret PM, Aldis AE, Kintzen G, Reinhold C (1994) Endovaginal sonographic appearance of benign ovarian masses. Radiographics 14:747–760; discussion 761–762
25. Ekici E, Soysal M, Kara S, Dogan M, Gokmen O (1996) The efficiency of ultrasonography in the diagnosis of dermoid cysts. Zentralbl Gynakol 118:136–141
26. Buy JN, Ghossain MA, Sciot C, Bazot M, Guinet C, Prevot S, Hugol D, Laromiguiere M, Truc JB, Poitout P et al (1991) Epithelial tumors of the ovary: CT findings and correlation with US. Radiology 178:811–818
27. Wu TT, Coakley FV, Qayyum A, Yeh BM, Joe BN, Chen LM (2004) Magnetic resonance imaging of ovarian cancer arising in endometriomas. J Comput Assist Tomogr 28:836–838
28. Fedele L, Bianchi S, Raffaelli R, Portuese A (1997) Pre-operative assessment of bladder endometriosis. Hum Reprod 12:2519–2522
29. Balleyguier C, Chapron C, Dubuisson JB, Kinkel K, Fauconnier A, Vieira M, Helenon O, Menu Y (2002) Comparison of magnetic resonance imaging and transvaginal ultrasonography in diagnosing bladder endometriosis. J Am Assoc Gynecol Laparosc 9:15–23
30. Bazot M, Thomassin I, Hourani R, Cortez A, Darai E (2004) Diagnostic accuracy of transvaginal sonography for deep pelvic endometriosis. Ultrasound Obstet Gynecol 24:180–185
31. Fauconnier A, Chapron C, Dubuisson JB, Vieira M, Dousset B, Breart G (2002) Relation between pain symptoms and the anatomic location of deep infiltrating endometriosis. Fertil Steril 78:719–726
32. Kinkel K, Frei KA, Balleyguier C, Chapron C (2006) Diagnosis of endometriosis with imaging: a review. Eur Radiol 16:285–298
33. Bazot M, Darai E, Hourani R, Thomassin I, Cortez A, Uzan S, Buy JN (2004) Deep pelvic endometriosis: MR imaging for diagnosis and prediction of extension of disease. Radiology 232:379–389
34. Togashi K, Nishimura K, Kimura I, Tsuda Y, Yamashita K, Shibata T, Nakano Y, Konishi J, Konishi I, Mori T (1991) Endometrial cysts: diagnosis with MR imaging. Radiology 180:73–78
35. Kinkel K, Chapron C, Balleyguier C, Fritel X, Dubuisson JB, Moreau JF (1999) Magnetic resonance imaging characteristics of deep endometriosis. Hum Reprod 14:1080–1086
36. Dessole S, Farina M, Rubattu G, Cosmi E, Ambrosini G, Nardelli GB (2003) Sonovaginography is a new technique for assessing rectovaginal endometriosis. Fertil Steril 79:1023–1027
37. Woodward PJ, Sohaey R, Mezzetti TP Jr (2001) Endometriosis: radiologic-pathologic correlation. Radiographics 21:193–216; questionnaire 288–294
38. Togashi K (2002) [MR imaging in obstetrics and gynecology]. Nippon Igaku Hoshasen Gakkai Zasshi 62:7–16

Vagina

12

UTA ZASPEL and BERND HAMM

CONTENTS

12.1
Anatomy

The vagina is a fibromuscular sheath-like structure connecting the external genitals with the uterus. It is lined with nonkeratinizing squamous epithelium and is 8–12 cm long. The vagina protects the internal genital organs against ascending infections, forms part of the birth canal, and receives the penis in copulation.

The proximal third of the vagina is at the level of the lateral vaginal fornices, the middle third at the level of the urinary bladder base, and the lower third at the level of the urethra. The anterior and posterior walls of the vagina are usually pressed together by the surrounding soft tissue, which ensures functional mechanical closure. On axial sections, this results in a shape that resembles the letter H (see Fig. 12.3a). The concertina barrier-like arrangement of the muscular layer of the vaginal wall and an abundance of elastic fibers in the subepithelial and adventitial connective tissue layer enable extreme passive extension and active contraction. The squamous epithelium of the vagina is highly susceptible to hormonal effects. The epithelium consists of up to 30 cell layers in women of reproductive age but of only a few layers in childhood and after menopause. The vagina is supplied with blood through the descending branch of the uterine artery as well as through branches from the rectal, vesical, and pudendal arteries. Lymph is drained from the vagina to the iliac, sacral, and para-aortic nodes from the upper two thirds and to inguinal and anorectal nodes from the lower third and vestibule.

U. ZASPEL, MD
Institut für Radiologie (Campus Mitte), Charité – Universitätsmedizin Berlin, Charitéplatz 1, 10117 Berlin, Germany
B. HAMM, MD
Professor and Chairman, Institut für Radiologie (Campus Mitte), Klinik für Strahlenheilkunde (Campus Virchow-Klinikum und Campus Buch), Charité – Universitätsmedizin Berlin, Charitéplatz 1, 10117 Berlin, Germany

12.2
Imaging Appearance of the Vagina

On axial CT scans, the vagina is difficult to differentiate from the urethra (Fig. 12.1) and it is not possible to distinguish the vaginal epithelium/mucus from the layers of the vaginal wall.

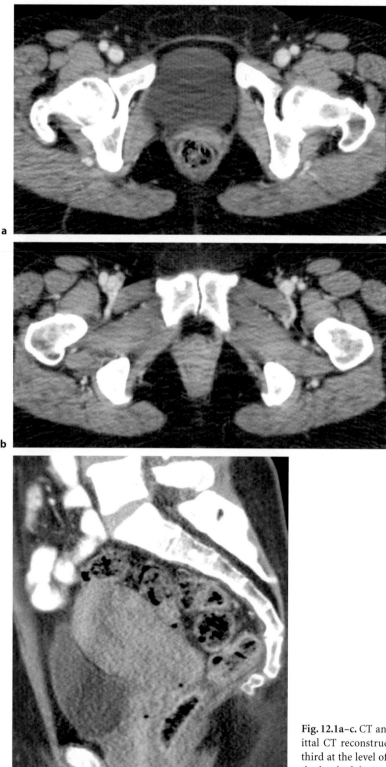

Fig. 12.1a–c. CT anatomy of the normal vagina. **a,b** CT. **c** Sagittal CT reconstruction. CT anatomy of the vagina – middle third at the level of the urinary bladder (**a**) and distal third at the level of the urethra (**b**). The vagina has the same density as the walls of the bladder, urethra, and rectum and can be distinguished from these structures on CT by the presence of a small fat layer. For differentiation of the vagina, it is also helpful if the bladder is filled with urine and the rectum is filled with air

On T1-weighted MR images with fat saturation, the vagina is of intermediate to low signal intensity and the mucosa, epithelium, and muscular layer cannot be distinguished (Fig. 12.2).

The individual layers can be appreciated much better on T2-weighted images and contrast-enhanced T1-weighted images (Figs. 12.3–12.5). T2-weighted images depict the mucosal layer and the secretions within the vaginal canal with a high signal intensity, which is thus clearly distinct from the lower-signal-intensity muscular wall and the middle layer. The paravaginal tissue or adventitia with its dense venous plexus has a high signal intensity on T2-weighted images [1].

The posterior vaginal fornix can be distinguished most readily from the cervix and the anterior rectal wall in sagittal orientation (Fig. 12.5). The smaller anterior fornix is often more difficult to differentiate from the cervix.

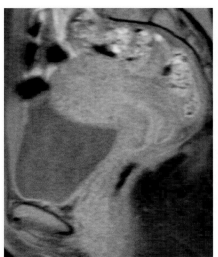
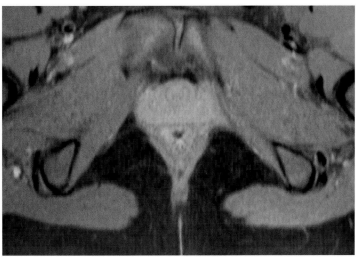

a   b

Fig. 12.2a,b. MR anatomy of the normal vagina on FS T1-weighted images. **a,b** T1-weighted images with fat sat in axial and sagittal orientation. On T1-weighted images, the vagina is of a similar signal intensity as the walls of the urinary bladder, urethra, and rectum. Thus, the vagina can only be localized indirectly between the filled bladder and the air-filled rectum

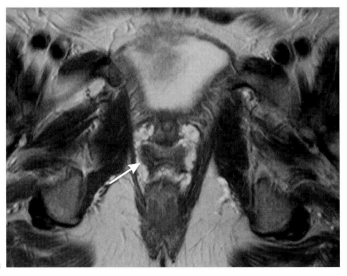
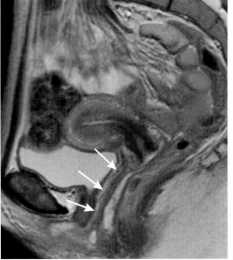

a   b

Fig. 12.3a,b. MR anatomy of the normal vagina on T2-weighted images. **a,b** T2-weighted images in axial and sagittal orientation. T2-weighted MR images allow differentiation of the three layers forming the vaginal wall (*arrows*). The innermost layer, the vaginal mucosa, is of high signal intensity; the middle layer, the muscularis, is of low signal intensity; and the outer layer, consisting of paravaginal fatty tissue and the venous plexus, is of high signal intensity. On transverse images, the vagina has an H-shaped appearance (*arrow*). The vagina is located between the urethra anteriorly and rectum posteriorly

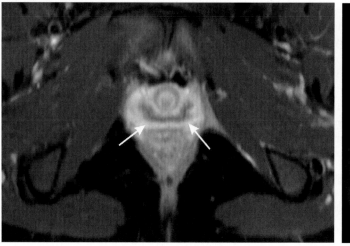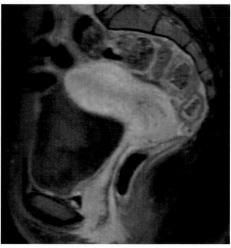

a   b

Fig. 12.4a,b. MR anatomy of the normal vagina on contrast-enhanced images. **a,b** T1-weighted images with fat sat after administration of Gd-DTPA in axial and sagittal orientation. After contrast medium administration, two layers of the vaginal wall (*arrow*) can be distinguished, a low-signal-intensity inner mucosa with intraluminal secretion and a contrast-enhancing muscularis and the outer venous plexus, which are of high signal intensity

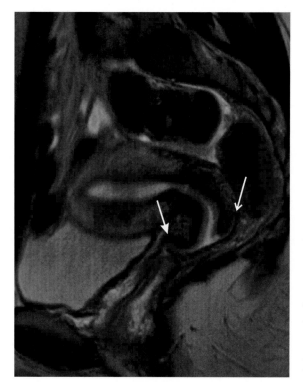

Fig. 12.5. MR anatomy of the normal vaginal fornices on T2-weighted images. T2-weighted image in sagittal orientation. The uterine cervix protrudes into the vagina, forming the posterior vaginal fornix (*open arrow*) and the somewhat smaller anterior vaginal fornix (*arrow*)

Insertion of a tampon is not necessary for adequate evaluation and may even distort vaginal anatomy (Fig. 12.6a). Instead, evaluation can be improved by filling and distending the vagina with ultrasound gel (Fig. 12.6b).

Hormone intake not only alters the thickness of the vaginal epithelium and the vaginal mucus but also affects the signal characteristics on MR images. Before the onset of menstruation, the vagina has lower signal intensity on T2-weighted images and a very thin central epithelial/fluid layer of high signal intensity. In women of reproductive age, the contrast between the vaginal mucosa and the wall is highest during the early proliferative phase. In this phase, the vaginal wall has a low signal intensity on T2-weighted images with a central stripe of high signal intensity (epithelium and mucus) (Fig. 12.7a, b). During the secretory phase, the central stripe shows moderate widening while there is a simultaneous increase in the signal of the vaginal wall, which makes it more difficult to distinguish these two layers. In postmenopausal women without hormonal replacement, the vagina has a low signal intensity on T2-weighted images and the central stripe of high signal intensity is very thin (Fig. 12.7c, d). In postmenopausal women on estrogen substitution, the vagina has the same appearance as during the proliferative phase in premenopausal women.

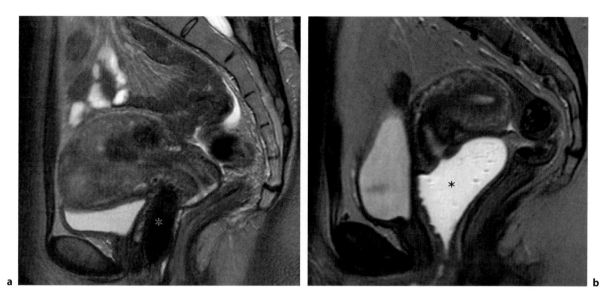

Fig. 12.6a,b. Intravaginal tampon and gel filling of the vagina. **a** T2-weighted image in sagittal orientation. Distortion of the vagina through an intravaginal tampon (*asterisk*). The tampon does not improve evaluation of vaginal morphology. **b** T2-weighted image in sagittal orientation. Gel filling unfolds the vagina and fornix (*asterisk*). The uterus is retroflexed

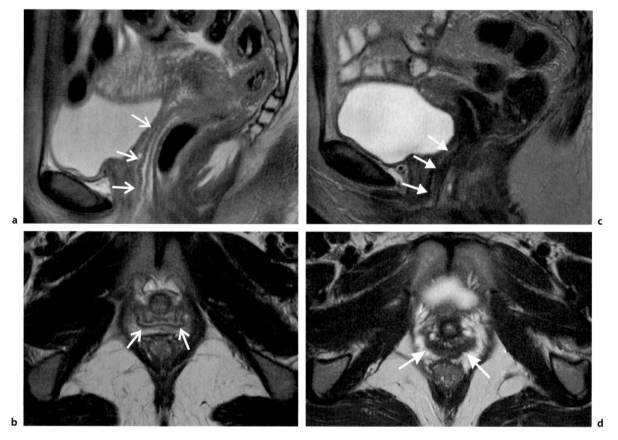

Fig. 12.7a–d. Pre- and postmenopausal vaginal anatomy. T2-weighted images in sagittal and axial orientation. A premenopausal (**a,b**) and a postmenopausal (**c,d**) woman: Two-layered appearance of the wall of the vagina (*open arrows*) is demonstrated in the postmenopausal woman. The low-signal-intensity muscularis layer and the high-signal-intensity paravaginal fatty tissue can be distinguished. Hypoplasia of the mucosa, which is just barely visible as high-signal-intensity stripe in sagittal orientation (**c,d**). Compare the thick high-signal-intensity vaginal mucosa in premenopausal age (**a,b**) (*arrows*)

12.3.
Congenital Malformations

The upper third of the vagina develops from the müllerian ducts, which descend during embryonic life and also give rise to the uterus, uterine cervix, and fallopian tubes. This is why vaginal malformations are typically associated with other developmental anomalies of the müllerian ducts. The lower and middle thirds of the vagina develop as a result of embryologic interactions between the müllerian ducts and the urogenital sinus. The close proximity to the wolffian duct (also known as the mesonephric duct) explains the association of vaginal malformations with renal anomalies. Congenital vaginal malformations are agenesis, duplication, and vaginal septa. Congenital absence (Fig. 12.8) and hypoplasia of the vagina are rare and are typically part of the Mayer-Rokitansky-Küster-Hauser (MRKH) syndrome. MRI shows a rudimentary vagina, often with concurrent hypoplasia of the uterus. Because agenesis of the vagina may be associated with renal agenesis or ectopic kidneys, the kidneys should always be included in the examination.

A longitudinal vaginal septum (Fig. 12.9) occurs as a consequence of incomplete fusion of the müllerian ducts or resorption failure of the vaginal septum. This anomaly is also typically associated with other malformations of the müllerian ducts [septate uterus, bicornuate uterus, uterus didelphys (Fig. 12.9), cervical duplication] [2].

Fibrous horizontal vaginal septa can occur anywhere in the vagina as a result of defective fusion of the descending müllerian ducts and ascending urogenital sinus. A horizontal septum causes primary amenorrhea, abdominal pain, an abdominal mass, or dyspareunia. MR imaging shows the vagina to be distended with retained secretion and allows evaluation of the location and thickness of the membrane for planning the surgical approach. Ectopic ureters inserting into the vagina are another anomaly but they are typically diagnosed by excretory urography.

In general, patients with vaginal malformations can be examined by hysterosalpingography, ultrasonography, or MRI [3]. MRI provides a good overview of pelvic anatomy in patients with suspected congenital malformations of the vagina or other structures of the urogenital tract and is very helpful in planning surgical measures for treating vaginal malformations [4].

12.4.
Benign Lesions

12.4.1
Bartholin's Gland Cysts

Bartholin's gland cysts are among the most common incidental findings in the posterolateral portion of the lower vagina (Fig. 12.10).

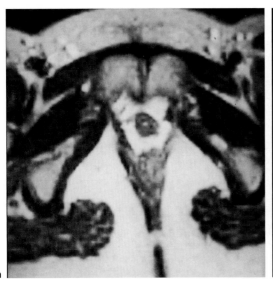
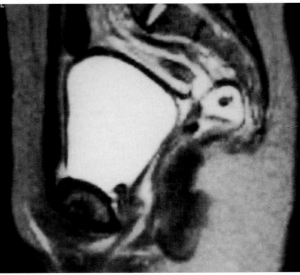

a   b

Fig. 12.8a,b. Agenesis of uterus and vagina. **a,b** T2-weighted images in axial and sagittal orientation. (Reproduced with permission from [13])

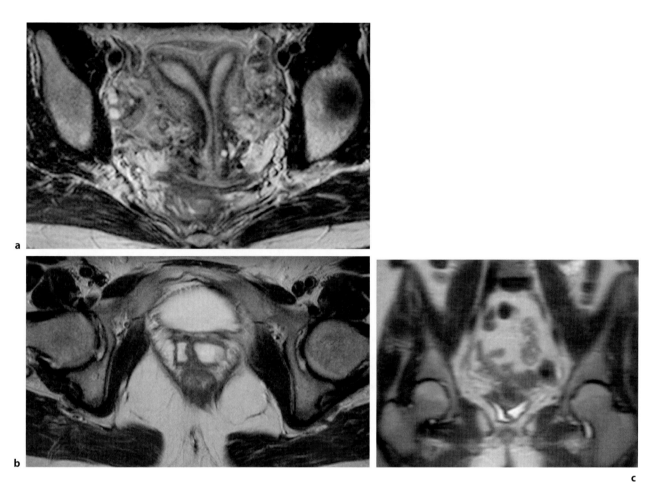

Fig. 12.9a–c. Uterus didelphys. T2-weighted images in transverse and coronal orientation. Good visualization of the duplicated uterus (**a**) and the two fluid-filled vaginas (**b,c**)

The cysts develop when secretion is retained in the ducts of the vulvovaginal glands opening in the area of the vestibule. Bartholin's cysts are characterized on T2-weighted MR images as cystic lesions of high signal intensity with a delicate and sharply delineated wall. On T1-weighted images, they are of intermediate to high signal intensity, depending on the protein content. Large cysts can cause symptoms with walking and sitting. As a complication Bartholin's cysts may develop inflammation and form an abscess. As a consequence those symptomatic cysts are treated by a wide incision of the glandular duct (marsupialization).

12.4.2
Condylomata Acuminata

Condylomata acuminata are papillomas caused by the human papilloma virus and are the most common benign tumors of the vulva but rarely occur within the vagina. They are usually diagnosed by inspection, which may be supplemented by colposcopy and biopsy as required.

12.4.3
Gartner's Duct Cysts

Gartner's duct cysts are another malformation of the vagina [3]. They develop as retention cysts from remnants of the wolffian duct system and typically occur in the anterolateral portion of the vagina and vulva (Fig. 12.11).

Gartner's duct cysts vary in size from a few millimeters to several centimeters and may occur in large numbers. Small Gartner's duct cysts are asymptomatic and may be detected incidentally while larger cysts can compress the vagina or urethra. T1- and T2-weighted MR images depict cystic lesions with a delicate wall and high signal intensity due to their high protein content.

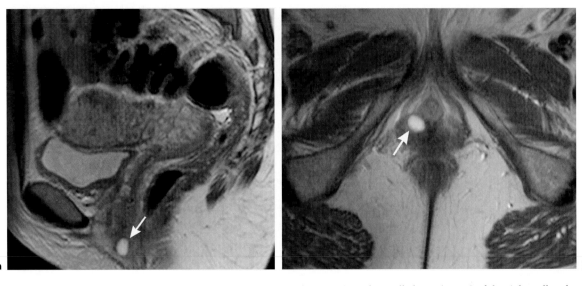

Fig. 12.10a,b. Bartholin's duct cyst. **a** T2-weighted image in sagittal orientation. Thin walled cyst (*arrow*) of the right wall at the vestibule of the vagina

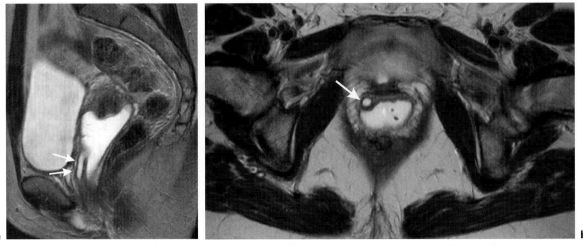

Fig. 12.11a,b. Gartner's duct cyst. T2-weighted images in sagittal and transverse orientation. Depiction of a Gartner's duct cyst (*arrows*) in the anterolateral portion of the right vagina

12.4.4
Inflammatory Conditions of the Vagina

Infections of the vagina are frequent and may be caused by a wide variety of pathogens (viruses, bacteria, fungi). MRI is rarely needed to diagnose vaginal infection. There may be thickening of the vaginal wall and vaginal secretion may be increased. Vaginal inflammation is associated with an increased signal intensity of the vaginal mucosa or of the entire vaginal wall on T2-weighted and STIR images. Contrast-enhanced T1-weighted images show more marked enhancement with a higher signal of the vaginal wall.

12.4.5
Crohn's Disease

Crohn's disease is a chronic inflammatory condition that may occur in any part of the gastrointestinal tract but commonly involves the terminal ileum or right colon frame. Gynecologic involvement with inflammation of the organs of the true pelvis or of the vulva is not uncommon. Another manifestation are fistulas between the vagina and the colon or rectum [5]. MRI is the method of choice for the diagnostic evaluation of pelvic fistulas.

12.4.6
Trauma

Traumatic injury to the vagina is usually caused by childbirth and is diagnosed clinically in the majority of cases. MRI has a diagnostic role in excluding or evaluating fistula formation after trauma.

12.4.7
Benign Tumors of the Vagina

Benign mesenchymal tumors are very rare and include lipoma, fibroma, and neurofibroma. They may be pedunculated and protrude from the vagina.

12.5
Malignant Tumors of the Vagina

12.5.1
Secondary Vaginal Malignancies

Secondary tumors account for about 80% of all vaginal malignancies. Direct tumor spread from adjacent organs such as the urinary bladder, vulva, uterine cervix (Fig. 12.12), or rectum is not uncommon. More-

over, the vagina is a common site of recurrence after surgical resection of cervical or ovarian cancer.

Vaginal metastases are typically from primary tumors of the genital tract. Other malignancies that metastasize to the vagina are melanomas (Fig. 12.13). MRI does not allow etiologic or histologic classification of secondary vaginal malignancies. Most secondary vaginal tumors have an intermediate signal intensity on T1-weighted images and a high signal on T2-weighted images.

12.5.2
Primary Vaginal Malignancies

12.5.2.1
Background

Most primary vaginal malignancies are carcinomas. Vaginal carcinoma is rare, accounting for 1%–2 % of the malignant tumors of the female genital tract. Their incidence is 0.5/100,000 women. The major histologic type is squamous epithelial carcinoma, which makes up over 90% of all primary vaginal malignancies. Vaginal cancer typically occurs in women aged 50–70 years. About 4% of vaginal cancers are adenocarcinomas. This histologic type mostly affects younger women from 17 to 32 years of age. Vaginal sarcoma in the form of leiomyosarcoma or fibrosarcoma is rare [6]. Embryonal rhabdomyosarcoma (Fig. 12.14) is the

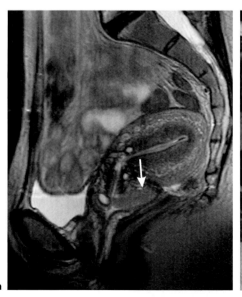
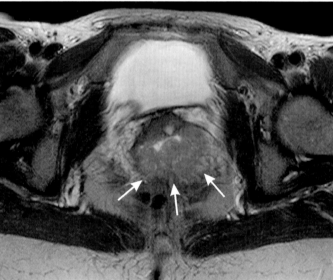

a   b

Fig. 12.12a,b. Cervical cancer invading the vagina. T2-weighted images in axial and sagittal orientation. Cervical cancer invading the proximal third of the posterior vaginal wall (*arrows*)

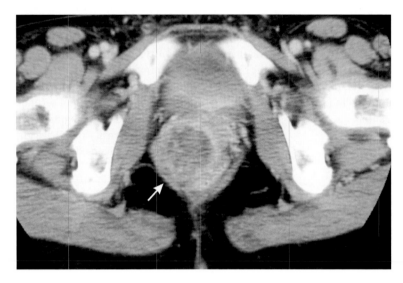

Fig. 12.13. Vaginal metastasis of malignant melanoma. Contrast enhanced CT. An unspecific mass with inhomogeneous contrast enhancement in the vagina is shown. The right levator ani muscle (*arrow*) can not be well delineated suggesting tumor involvement. (Figure courtesy of Dr. Forstner)

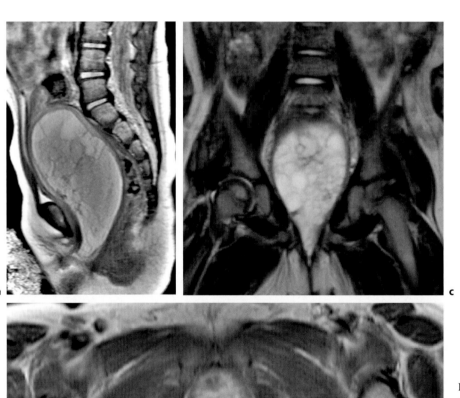

Fig. 12.14a–c. Botryoid sarcoma. Sagittal, transaxial, and coronal T2-weighted images in a 2-year-old girl. A multiseptated mass with numerous thin septations causes extensive enlargement of the vagina which extends up to the level of the promontorium

commonest type of genital rhabdomyosarcoma. It occurs in infancy and is mostly located at the vagina, vulva, and perineum. When occurring in adolescence it more often affects the cervix or corpus uteri. Due to good response to chemotherapy its prognosis has improved. Chemotherapy is usually followed by an organ preserving surgical treatment [7].

The risk factors for the occurrence of vaginal cancer are similar to those for cervical cancer and include having many sexual partners, chronic infection with high-risk types of HPV, immunosuppression, and smoking. Vaginal adenocarcinoma is associated with an increased intrauterine exposure to diethylstilbestrol. Furthermore, it has been shown that there is an association with tumors of the cervix or vulva and status post hysterectomy [8]. Vaginal cancer typically involves the proximal third and the posterior wall of the vagina [6]. Early vaginal cancer is asymptomatic. More advanced tumors may cause painless vaginal bleeding or contact bleeding, vaginal discharge, dysuria, and dyspareunia.

The growth pattern of vaginal tumors includes the whole spectrum from exophytic and papillomatous, through infiltrating, to ulcerating forms. The tumor primarily extends by direct spread to the paracolpium, parametria, vulva, uterine cervix, and rectovaginal and vesicovaginal septa. Fistulas are not infrequent when there is tumor invasion of the rectum and bladder. Lymphatic spread of tumors involving the proximal two thirds of the vagina is to the lymph nodes along the external and common iliac arteries, and the abdominal aorta. Vaginal tumors in the lower third of the vagina

drain into inguinal lymph nodes (Fig. 12.15), from where lymphatic spread continues to the lymph node stations along the external and common iliac arteries and to para-aortic lymph nodes.

Hematogenous metastatic spread from vaginal cancer is rare and occurs late in the disease. Organ metastases primarily involve the liver, lung, or bones. Vaginal cancer is staged using the FIGO and TNM classifications (Table 12.1). Treatment depends on the stage of cancer and ranges from radical hysterectomy with widening of the vaginal cuff to complete colpectomy with removal of the paracolpium. Vaginal cancer with invasion of adjacent organs is treated by exenteration with adjuvant radiotherapy. Patients in whom distant metastases outside the pelvis are present are treated by chemotherapy.

Table 12.1. Staging of vaginal cancer according to FIGO and TNM criteria

FIGO	TNM	
0	Tis	Cis
I	T1	Tumor confined to vagina
II	T2	Tumor invades paravaginal tissues but does not extend to pelvic wall
III	T3	Tumor extends to pelvic wall
IVa	T4	Tumor invades bladder and rectum, tumor extends beyond the true pelvis
IVb	M1	Distant metastasis
	N1	Pelvic lymph node metastasis
	N2	Unilateral inguinal lymph node metastasis
	N3	Bilateral inguinal lymph node metastasis

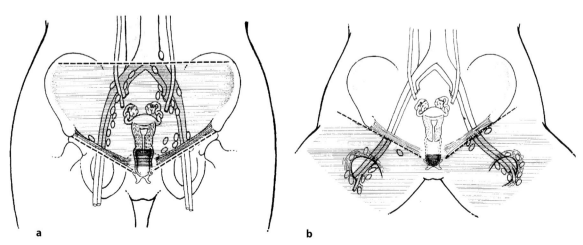

Fig. 12.15a,b. Regional lymph node stations. **a** Vaginal cancer of the proximal two thirds of the vagina drains into the pelvic lymph node stations. **b** The inguinal lymph nodes are the first lymph node stations invaded by vaginal cancer of the distal third of the vagina. (Reproduced with permission from [14])

12.5.2.2
MR Imaging

MRI has its most important diagnostic role in staging vaginal cancer that has been confirmed by colposcopy and biopsy. Staging by MRI serves to determine local tumor extent and to classify the cancer according to TNM and FIGO criteria [9]. In addition, MRI allows assessment of inguinal and pelvic lymph nodes. Because the signal intensity of vaginal tumors, except for vaginal melanoma, is unspecific, MRI does not allow differentiation of the different primary and secondary malignancies involving the vagina and thus cannot replace histologic diagnosis [10]. The protocol recommended for MR imaging of vaginal cancer is summarized in Table 12.2.

Table 12.2. MRI sequences recommended for imaging of vaginal cancer

Sequence	T2w TSE	PD TSE	T1w TSE	Contrast-enhanced T1w TSE
	Sagittal Transverse	Transverse	Sagittal Transverse	Sagittal Transverse
Area imaged	Uterus to pelvic floor	Aortic bifurcation to groin	Uterus to pelvic floor	Uterus to pelvic floor

Prior to MR imaging, patients are administered a spasmolytic agent to reduce intestinal motility, e.g. 2 ml Buscopan ^{R} (40 mg butylscopolamine). Distention of the vagina, e.g. by filling with ultrasound gel, may improve diagnostic assessment. In women with an oblique orientation of the vagina, angulation of the transverse T2-weighted sequence perpendicular to the axis of the vagina will improve evaluation of anatomy and tumor extent.

On T2-weighted images, vaginal tumors have an intermediate to high signal intensity, enabling their differentiation from the low-signal-intensity muscular vaginal wall (Fig. 12.16).

On T1-weighted images, a vaginal tumor is identified as a contour deformity of the vagina and not by a difference in signal intensity. Following administration of a contrast medium, most vaginal tumors display more marked signal enhancement than the vaginal wall (Fig. 12.14c,d). Because vaginal tumors may show a marginal inflammatory reaction, their extent may be overestimated [9]. Moreover, it may be difficult to differentiate cervical cancer and tumors of the proximal vagina when there is invasion of both organs. In such cases, the tumor often arises from the organ containing the largest tumor mass. However, only biopsy enables reliable differentiation in such cases and between primary and secondary vaginal tumors in general. An exception are vaginal melanomas which show a distinct signal behavior that depends on their composition such as presence of intralesional hemorrhage or pigments. Melanin is paramagnetic and shortens relaxation times, resulting in a higher signal on T1-weighted images and a lower signal on T2-weighted images. There is no paramagnetic effect amelanotic melanomas.

12.5.2.3
Staging

Stage T1 vaginal cancer is confined to the vagina (Fig. 12.17). T2-weighted images show a hyperintense disruption of the low-signal-intensity muscular vaginal wall. To exclude cancer growth beyond the vagina, it is important to differentiate the tumor from the fatty layer surrounding the vagina. The differentiation of tumor and fat may be easier on T1-weighted images because there is superior contrast between low-signal-intensity tumor and high-signal-intensity fat. On T2-weighted images, on the other hand, both tumor and paravaginal fat with its rich venous network have a high signal intensity. However, this is not a reliable criterion because the fatty layer surrounding the vagina is very thin.

Stage II tumors are characterized by invasion of paravaginal fatty tissue, which is seen as a blurred and irregular delineation of the vaginal wall (Figs. 12.16, 12.18, 12.19). Larger tumors extending beyond the vagina are seen as low-signal-intensity lesions surrounded by hyperintense paravaginal tissue on T1-weighted images. On T2-weighted images both the vaginal tumor and the paravaginal tissue have a high signal intensity and are difficult to distinguish.

In stage III disease with tumor extension to the pelvic sidewall (Fig. 12.20), muscular infiltration of the pelvic wall is best appreciated on T2-weighted images. Muscle is of a lower signal intensity and can thus be differentiated from the high-signal-intensity tumor. Other important muscles that need to be evaluated are the levator ani, piriform, and internal obturator muscles. Invasion of the internal anal sphincter muscle can be evaluated on coronal T2-weighted images.

Stage IV vaginal cancer is characterized by invasion of the bladder and rectum (Fig. 12.21), which is identified as a disruption of the low-signal-intensity muscular layer of these organs on T2-weighted images.

Fistulas can be identified on contrast-enhanced T1-weighted images. They are characterized by more pronounced contrast enhancement and there may be a central signal void in the fistula canal.

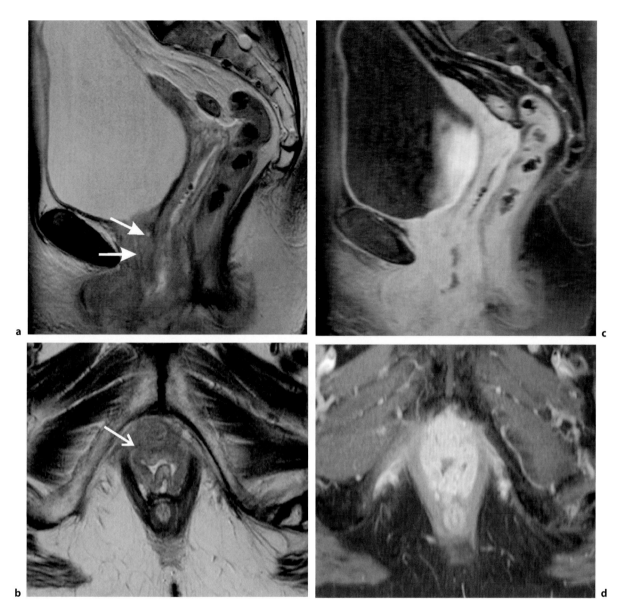

Fig. 12.16a–d. Vaginal cancer. **a,b** T2-weighted images in sagittal and axial orientation. FIGO stage II vaginal cancer of intermediate signal intensity (status post hysterectomy). There is tumor throughout the anterior wall of the distal vagina (*arrows*). Tumor extension to the urethra (*open arrow*). **c,d** T1-weighted images with fat sat after administration of Gd-DTPA in axial and sagittal orientation. Contrast medium administration does not improve delineation of the cancer

12.5.2.4
MR Appearance After Radiotherapy

Edematous and inflammatory reactions of the vagina that persist for up to about 6 months after radiotherapy are associated with an increased signal intensity of the vaginal wall on T2-weighted images. The observed increase in signal intensity is directly proportion to the total radiation dose administered and always occurs above a threshold dose of 45 Gy. The mode of admin-istration (percutaneous radiation, brachytherapy) appears not to affect the degree of signal change. Irradiated tissue also shows increased enhancement after contrast medium administration. About 6 months after completion of radiotherapy, fibrosis leads to a decreased signal intensity of the vagina on T1- and T2-weighted images and there is again less pronounced contrast medium enhancement [11]. A rare complication of radiotherapy is vaginal stenosis with subsequent development of serometra or hematometra (Fig. 12.22).

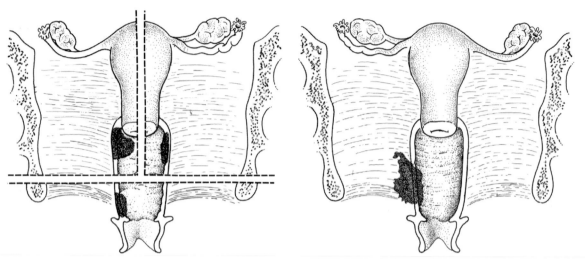

Fig. 12.17. FIGO stage I. Vaginal cancer is limited to the vagina. (Reproduced with permission from [14])

Fig. 12.18. FIGO stage II. Tumour involves the paravaginal tissue but does not extend to the pelvic wall. (Reproduced with permission from [14])

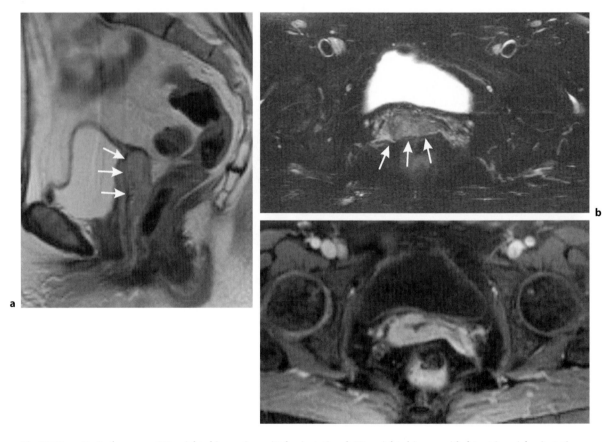

Fig. 12.19a–c. Vaginal cancer. **a** T2-weighted image in sagittal orientation. **b** T2-weighted image with fat sat in axial orientation. **c** T1-weighted image with fat sat after administration of Gd-DTPA in axial orientation. **a** Status post hysterectomy for leiomyomas of the uterus. Vaginal cancer (*arrows*) of in the proximal two thirds of the vagina with infiltration of the vaginal wall. Accessory finding: air inclusion in the urinary bladder after catheterization. **b,c** Fairly good differentiation of the solid tumor (*arrows*) from the high-signal-intensity venous plexus. There is no obvious infiltration of the paracolpal fat. (Figure courtesy of Dr. Forstner)

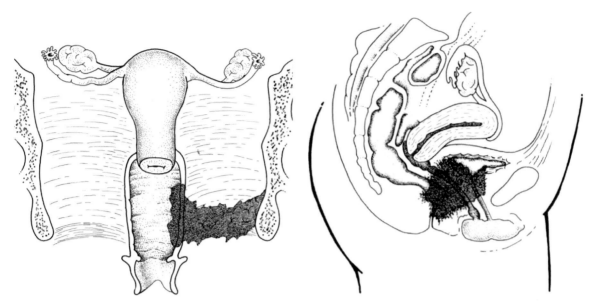

Fig. 12.20. FIGO stage III. Cancer extends to the pelvic wall. (Reproduced with permission from [14])

Fig. 12.21. FIGO stage IV. Tumour involves the mucosa of the bladder or rectum or extends beyond the true pelvis. (Reproduced with permission from [14])

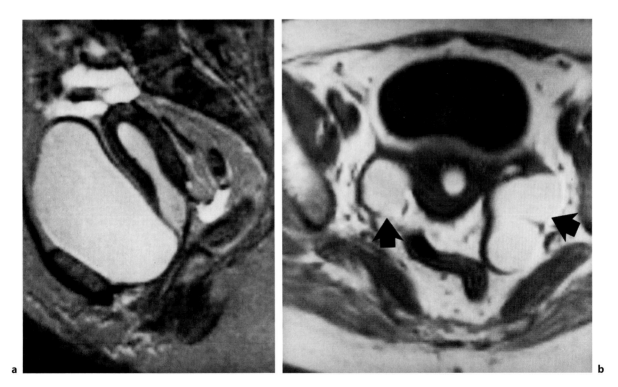

Fig. 12.22a,b. Vaginal stenosis. T2-weighted images in axial and sagittal orientation. Vaginal stenosis in the proximal third of the vagina after radiotherapy. There is hematometra (**a**) and hematosalpinx (**b**) (*short arrows*). (Reproduced with permission from [13])

12.5.2.5
MR Appearance After Surgery

The postoperative appearance varies with the type of surgery performed. Shortly after surgery, scars are characterized by a high signal intensity on T2-weighted images and there is abnormally increased contrast enhancement on T1-weighted images due to postoperative edema formation and neovascularization. These reactive changes are difficult to distinguish from residual or recurrent tumor in the early postoperative phase [12].

12.5.2.6
Residual and Recurrent Tumor

With its intrinsic high soft-tissue contrast, MRI is the method of choice for demonstrating residual tumor or tumor recurrence. Moreover, MRI allows identification of radiation-induced changes of the organs of the true pelvis. Postoperative scars or postactinic changes can be differentiated from recurrent or residual tumor on MR images on condition that the examination is performed at least 6 months after the end of therapy. This interval is necessary because acute reactive increases in signal due to edema and inflammation immediately after irradiation or surgery cannot be differentiated from vital tumor tissue. After about 6 months, the vagina has returned to its normal low signal intensity on T2-weighted images and residual or recurrent tumor can be identified as a high-signal-intensity disruption of the vaginal wall [12]. Recurrent tumor has an increased signal intensity on T2-weighted images and typically shows an inhomogeneous structure. On contrast-enhanced images, recurrent tumor is characterized by a higher signal enhancement compared with surrounding tissue. However, the examiner must be aware that even after 6 months following radiation or surgery, increased signal intensities may be due to posttherapeutic reactive changes. In such cases, a dynamic contrast-enhanced fast GRE study may be helpful. Here, recurrent or residual tumor will show significantly earlier and more pronounced contrast enhancement than scar tissue. As in pretherapeutic staging, contrast-enhanced T1-weighted images are helpful to identify possible invasion of the bladder or rectum by recurrent or residual tumor. Tumor invasion of these organs is indicated by circumscribed areas of abnormally increased contrast enhancement in the wall. As in preoperative staging, muscular infiltration is best seen on T2-weighted images.

Ultrasonography and CT have only a limited role in detecting recurrent or residual vaginal tumor because they rely on the configuration of the lesion as the only criterion. The sensitivity of both modalities is too low for differentiation of tumor from posttherapeutic changes and for the detection of small tumors. The accuracy of the clinical examination is also limited, in particular when postoperative scar tissue is present.

12.5.2.7
Lymph Nodes

Imaging of the inguinal, pelvic, and, where necessary, para-aortic lymph node stages by means of MRI/CT may provide additional information for primary therapeutic decision making. Although the inguinal lymph nodes are easily accessible to palpation, palpation has a poor sensitivity in detecting inguinal lymph node metastasis. Evaluation for lymph node metastasis is clinically relevant before surgery and before primary or adjuvant radiotherapy. Moreover, a considerable proportion of recurrent vaginal tumors arise from lymph node metastases. The criteria for lymph node imaging are described in Chapter 14.

References

1. Hricak H, Chang YC, Thurnher S (1988) Vagina: evaluation with MR imaging. Part I. Normal anatomy and congenital anomalies. Radiology 169:169–174
2. Haddad B, Louis-Sylvestre C, Poitout P, Paniel BJ (1997) Longitudinal vaginal septum: a retrospective study of 202 cases. Eur J Obstet Gynecol Reprod Biol 74:197–199
3. Carrington BM, Hricak H, Nuruddin RN, Secaf E, Laros RK, Jr., Hill EC (1990) Mullerian duct anomalies: MR imaging evaluation. Radiology 176:715–720
4. Pellerito JS, McCarthy SM, Doyle MB, Glickman MG, DeCherney AH (1992) Diagnosis of uterine anomalies: relative accuracy of MR imaging, endovaginal sonography, and hysterosalpingography. Radiology 183:795–800
5. Feller ER, Ribaudo S, Jackson ND (2001) Gynecologic aspects of Crohn's disease. Am Fam Physician 64:1725–1728
6. Creasman WT (2005) Vaginal cancers. Curr Opin Obstet Gynecol 17:71–76
7. Piura B, Rabinovich A, Yanai-Inbar I (2002) Primary malignant melanoma of the vagina: case report and review of literature. Eur J Gynaecol Oncol 23:195–198
8. Merino MJ (1991) Vaginal cancer: the role of infectious and environmental factors. Am J Obstet Gynecol 165:1255–1262
9. Lopez C, Balogun M, Ganesan R, Olliff JF (2005) MRI of vaginal conditions. Clin Radiol 60:648–662

10. Siegelman ES, Outwater EK, Banner MP, Ramchandani P, Anderson TL, Schnall MD (1997) High-resolution MR imaging of the vagina. Radiographics 17:1183–1203

11. Sugimura K, Carrington BM, Quivey JM, Hricak H (1990) Postirradiation changes in the pelvis: assessment with MR imaging. Radiology 175:805–813

12. Chang YC, Hricak H, Thurnher S, Lacey CG (1988) Vagina: evaluation with MR imaging. Part II. Neoplasms. Radiology 169:175–179

13. Hamm B et al. (2006) MRT von Abdomen und Becken. 2. Edition. Thieme, Stuttgart

14. Wittekind C, Greene FL, Hutter RVP, Klimpfinger M, Sobin LH (eds) (2005) TNM Atlas Illustrated Guide to the TNM/pTNM Classification of Malignant Tumours. Springer, Berlin Heidelberg New York

Functional MRI of the Pelvic Floor

Tanja Fischer and Andreas Lienemann

CONTENTS

T. Fischer, MD
Institut für Klinische Radiologie – Standort Innenstadt, Klinikum der Ludwig-Maximilians-Universität München, Ziemssenstraße 1, 80336 Munich, Germany
A. Lienemann, MD
HELIOS Kliniken Schwerin, Institut für Röntgendiagnostik, Wismarsche Str. 393–397, 19049 Schwerin, Germany

13.1
Introduction

Pelvic floor dysfunction is the cause of many different clinical problems such as genital descensus and prolapse, which is often associated with urinary and fecal incontinence or defecation disorders. These pelvic floor disorders are frequent problems among the whole population, but mostly afflict elderly, parous women. Since this group will continuously grow over the coming decades, there will be a great demand for new diagnostic tools including imaging modalities.

Up until some time ago, the only chance to gain knowledge about the pelvic floor anatomy had been by dissecting human cadavers. Besides artifacts due to the embalming process, this method does not provide any information about the complex functional interaction of the many pelvic floor structures and organs. Therefore, our notion of the pelvic floor anatomy and function may have been distorted and incomplete.

Imaging modalities have offered completely new perspectives. Starting with conventional fluoroscopic examinations like colpocystorectography and defecography in the 1960s, MRI has become is the method of choice for diagnosis and research of pelvic floor disorders. Besides the lack of ionizing radiation MRI is widely appreciated for its superb soft tissue contrast and multiplanar imaging capability, which allows an excellent morphological delineation of the anatomical situation. Yet for the understanding of the functional interactions of the pelvic floor system and the related pathologies such as descensus and prolapse, a dynamic examination is essential [49]. Here the new ultrafast MR sequences allow real-time visualization.

This chapter will review functional cine MRI as the main radiological method for the dynamic evaluation of the pelvic floor. Following a more general definition of the method, details of the technique are given in view of the literature. Then we focus on image analysis with a critical survey of the various different parameters that are in use and give an overview of typical and important findings within the different pelvic compartments. Finally, we discuss the clinical applications of this imaging technique with its strengths and limitations.

13.2
History

Functional cine MRI of the pelvic floor was first introduced in 1991 by YANG et al. [49] and KRUYT et al. [25]. They described the movement of the bladder, vagina and rectum in relation to the pubococcygeal and symphysiosacral reference line in patients and asymptomatic subjects. In 1993 GOODRICH et al. [13] recommended the technique for the pre- and postoperative evaluation of patients after pelvic floor surgery. In contrast, DELEMARRE et al. [6] did not find an advantage to dynamic MRI in comparison to defecography in the examination of the anorectum. But in the following years an increasing number of studies focused on different aspects of the method and continuously stressed the usefulness of functional cine MRI in the evaluation of the pelvic floor [1, 14, 19, 24, 30, 41] and proved it to be superior or at least equal to conventional colpocystorectography and defecography [15, 24, 30]. Unfortunately this ultimately led to a lack of standardization (see Table 13.1) and therefore the comparability of the different publications is limited.

13.3
Technique

Functional cine MRI of the pelvic floor can be explained as the conjunction of a static morphological imaging modality and an adequate functional examination with a freezing of motion. The term "functional" in this context should not be confused with dynamic MRI using intravenous or arterial contrast media or even functional imaging for metabolic activity.

At present the available MR sequences do not allow a sufficient depiction of motion with 3D techniques. To overcome this limitation two different approaches are used to record motion: either the acquisition of multiple single slices at the same slice position or one stack of slices covering a whole anatomical region. The first approach allows a higher temporal resolution and can analyze intrinsic (e.g. bowel motility) or extrinsic motion (e.g. straining) continuously at a given anatomical position. For this, the frequency of the single image acquisitions has to be faster than the expected frequency of the motion itself. A disadvantage is the limitation to only one single plane. To overcome this problem a stack of slices can be used alternatively. But in this case, due to the increased acquisition time, the temporal resolution is very limited and the specified load (e.g. contraction or strain) should not vary over the whole duration of the measurement. For the patient that means, for example to continuously strain for more than 10 s without producing blurring artifacts, which is quite difficult. In addition, with only one snapshot of a specific position, e.g. maximum straining, relevant findings might be concealed and further development of existing pathologies can be missed.

Considering the literature on functional cine MRI (see Table 13.1), the smallest common denominator for the procedure itself includes the following points: high field system, supine or sitting position of the patient with surface array coils and the use of a non-echo-planar imaging sequence to produce a midsagittal image with the patient at rest and straining.

13.3.1
MR System and Patient Positioning

As an MR system specially dedicated to the examination of the pelvic floor does not exist, most authors use an all-purpose high-field system of 1.5 Tesla with the possibility of sub-second scans and a 512 matrix in combination with an acceptable signal-to-noise ratio [1, 13, 24, 30, 36, 46, 49]. In all other studies a mid-field system of 0.5 Tesla with an open magnet configuration was used [7, 10, 19, 25]. The latter offers the advantage of evaluating the patient in an upright position. This more physiological position for defecation cannot be assumed in the close configuration system which is limited to horizontal positioning of the patient. In this case the supine position is preferable to the prone position [6, 25], as it is more stable and convenient for the patient. Disadvantages of the open configuration system include a restricted signal-to-noise ratio due to a sometimes unfavorable design of the surface coils, which may result, together with a limited spatial and temporal resolution, in a poorer image quality.

Table 13.1. Parameters used for functional cine MRI of the pelvic floor: survey of the literature

Reference	Tesla	Positioning	Type of sequence dynamic	Single slice or slab?	Slice orientation	Patient instruction	Reference line	Opacification
Bertschinger et al. (2002)	0.5/1.5	Sitting/supine	SSFSE; SP-GRE	Slice	sag	r,c,s	PCL3; grading	B emptied, R (potato mash +Gd)
Bo et al. (2001)	0.5	Sitting	GE	Slice	sag	c,s	PCL 1	-
Comiter et al. (1999)	1.5	Supine	HASTE; SSFSE	Slice	sag	r,s	HMO; grading	-
Delemarre et al. (1994)	1.5	Prone	GE	Slice	sag	r,s	SSL	B emptied
Dvorkin et al. (2004)	0.5	Sitting	GE	Slice	sag, cor	r,c,s,d	PCL 1	B emptied, R (potato mash +Gd)
Fielding et al. (1998)	0.5	Sitting/supine	FSE	Slice	ax, sag	r,s	PCL 3	B full; Rectal balloon for pressure measurement
Goh et al. (2000)	1.0	Supine	FFE	Slab	ax, sag, cor	r,s	PCL 3; grading	-
Goodrich et al. (1993)	1.5	Supine	GRASS	?	sag, cor	r,s	PSL; grading	-
Gufler et al.(1999)	1	Supine	RARE	Slice	sag	r,s	PCL 2	-
Healy et al. (1997a,b)	1.5	Supine	GRASS	Slab	sag	r,s	PCL 3	V+R (rubber tube)
Hilfiker et al. (1998)	0.5	Sitting	GE	Slice	sag	r,c,s,d	-	R (potato mash+Gd)
Hjartardottir et al. (1997)	1.0	Supine	GE,TSE	Slab	ax, sag, cor	r,c,s	PCL 1	B full
Hodroff et al. (2002)	1.5	Supine	?	Slab	sag	r,c,s	PCL1	B (NaCl+Gd), VR (Gel+Gd), U (5FKath)
Hoyte and Ratiu (2001)	1.5	Supine	?	Slice	sag	r,s	PCL ?	-
Kelvin et al. (2000)	1.5	Supine	TrueFISP	Slice	sag	r,c,s,d	PCL 1; grading	B emptied; V+R (Gel)
Kruyt et al. (1991)	0.5/1.5	Prone	GE	Slice; ?	sag	r,c,s	SSL	B emptied; R (normal air)
Lienemann et al. (2000b)	1.5	Supine	TrueFISP	Slice	ax, sag, cor	r,c,s,d	PCL 3; HL	B emptied; V+R (gel)
Lienemann et al. (1996)	1.5	Supine	True FISP; HASTE	Slice	sag	r,c,s	PCL 1	B (NaCl), U (Thread +NaCl), V+R (gel)
Pannu et al. (2000)	1.5	Supine	SSFSE	Slice	ax, sag, cor	r,s	?	R?
Rentsch et al. (2001)	1.5	Supine	TrueFISP	Slice	sag	r,s,d	PCL1	R (gel+Gd)
Roos et al. (2002)	0.5	Sitting	SP-GRE	Slice	sag, (cor)	r,c,s,d	PCL3; grading	B emptied, R (potato mash +Gd)
Schoenenberger et al. (1998)	0.5	Sitting	GE	Slice	sag	r,s	-	R (potato mash +Gd)
Singh et al. (2001, 2002)	1.5	Supine	FSE	Slab	ax, sag, cor	r,s	MPL; grading	-
Sprenger et al. (2000)	1.5	Supine	TrueFISP	Slice	ax, sag, (cor)	r,c,s,d	PCL 3; HL	B emptied; V+R (gel)
Unterweger et al. (2001)	1.5	Supine	SSFSE	Slice	sag	r,s	PCL 3	B emptied
Vanbeckevoort et al. (1999)	1.5	Supine	HASTE	Slab	sag	r,s	PCL 1	R (gel)
Yang et al. (1991)	1.5	Supine	GRASS	Slice	sag, (cor)	r,c,s	PCL 3	-

?, Not specified; sag, sagittal; cor, coronal; ax, axial; r, rest; c, contract; s, strain; d, defecate; PCL, pubococcygeal line; MPL, midpubic line; SSL, symphysiosacral line; PSL, pubosacral line; HL, horizontal line; B, bladder; U, urethra; V, vagina; R, rectum; Gd, Gd-DTPA; PCL1, symphysis-sacrococcygeal joint; PCL2, symphysis-levator insertion coccygis; PCL3, symphysis-last intervertebral joint.

13.3.2
Patient Instruction

In order to achieve satisfying results a detailed instruction of the patient prior to the examination is mandatory. The patient must be very cooperative and be able to understand and follow the commands during the examination. According to the literature most authors examine the patient only at rest and while straining [10, 12, 13, 18, 41, 46, 47, 49]. However, to assess the correct function of the levator ani muscle in view of a levator ani syndrome or stool outlet obstruction it is necessary to contract the pelvic floor at least once during the entire procedure. Furthermore, emptying of the rectum during the examination is essential. VANBECKEVOORT et al. [47] nicely showed the relevance of the defecation process when comparing colpocystodefecography to functional MRI without emptying of the rectum. The missing rectal evacuation results in a significantly lower sensitivity for the detection of pelvic floor defects with the MRI examination. Therefore, the following sequence of specified loads is advisable: rest – contract – relax – strain – defecate – relax [1, 19, 24, 36, 43]. Due to the preceding it is obvious that this kind of cycle should be repeated until complete defecation has been documented. In our experience between two and four cycles are usually necessary. If the patient is either too embarrassed to defecate inside the magnet or she cannot empty the rectum at all while lying supine, a triphasic approach as recommended by KELVIN et al. [24] may be suitable with an additional post-toilet phase after the patient has evacuated in the bathroom. Other specific loads like coughing or micturition are possible but not commonly used.

The overall time range for the examination is normally between 9 and 30 min [1, 30]. Diapers and waterproof pads placed beneath the patient reliably prevent soiling of the table or machine [18, 30]. In a survey of 60 patients who underwent both colpocystorectography and functional cine MRI, 90.7 % of the women would prefer MRI to fluoroscopy, thus yielding a high rate of acceptance [43]. Reasons for this might be the more private atmosphere within the magnet during the entire examination, as well as the possibility to repeat the cycle in case of insufficient straining and defecation.

13.3.3
Organ Opacification

On the T2-weighted sequences usually used for functional cine MRI, fluid-filled structures like the bladder or small bowel loops exhibit a high signal intensity. But other organs like the vagina, rectum, anal canal or muscles show an intermediate to low signal intensity, thus making their evaluation difficult. This is especially true for T1-weighted sequences. To avoid difficulties in the differentiation of these organs we introduced a stringent opacification of the bladder, urethra, vagina and rectum [30, 43].

In more detail, the bladder was filled with 60 ml of sterile isotone saline solution using a 26-F Foley catheter and the urethra was delineated using a twisted cotton thread soaked with isotone saline solution and gadopentetate dimeglumine (Magnevist, Schering, Berlin, Germany) [30]. Due to the increased effort, the limitation in time and the potential risk of a cystitis or even of loosing the thread into the bladder we omitted this kind of contrast in later studies with no disadvantage in diagnosis [28, 43]. Similar to us, KELVIN et al. [24] and HODROFF et al. [21] used thin catheters to outline the urethra and to fill the bladder with saline solution and gadopentetate dimeglumine. But it is important to keep in mind that the catheter might impede the movement of the urethra itself because it is splinting the organ.

The above-mentioned procedures to contrast urethra and bladder are not consistent within the literature, where most authors do not administer any contrast medium at all but instead instruct the patient to empty the bladder prior to the examination [1, 38, 46]. The latter is necessary to prevent masking of a rectocele or enterocele by the combination of a full bladder and a cystocele that blocks the entire genital hiatus.

There is also no agreement on opacification of the vagina in the literature. Usually ultrasound gel is instilled, which is an easy to handle and well tolerated contrast medium. Delineation of the entire vagina and especially of the posterior fornix and posterior wall is always achieved [24, 30]. In addition, during Valsalva's maneuver the gel in the vagina is emptied passively and thus the movement of the organ itself is not impeded [21]. In this regard rubber tubes are not a recommended alternative [18].

Looking at the rectum, again a variety of contrast media have been used. In those studies where defecation has been attempted either gel [21, 24, 43], potato mash [1, 7, 19, 38] or rubber tubes [18] have been proposed.

For our own studies today we use only ultrasound gel as contrast medium with a special rectal olive applicator, with which we first install 20–30 ml gel into the vagina and subsequently 200–300 ml into the rectum. This proved to be a fast, easy to perform and cheap method with an excellent organ opacification. As mentioned above, we do not opacify the bladder or urethra anymore, but encourage the patient to void prior to the examination.

Understandable concern exists that defecation onto the MR imaging table may contaminate the MR imaging unit. In our own experience the evacuated contents were always confined to the diaper and the MR unit was never polluted. In addition, a lavatory should be on site to minimize any discomfort for the patient associated with the evacuated gel.

13.3.4
Sequence Protocols

MR imaging of the pelvic floor usually includes a static and a dynamic part of the examination.

For the first, the sequence protocol preferred by most authors includes a set of either T1- or T2-weighted turbo spin-echo sequences with acquisition of a stack of images in two or all three orientations covering the entire pelvis. These types of sequences have been approved in various settings of diseases of the pelvis. They provide a high spatial resolution of the selected anatomic region [44, 45] and therefore allow an exact morphological assessment of the pelvic structures. The depiction of the urethral or anal sphincter complex or the perivaginal space are thus facilitated [9, 23]. In addition, the course of an organ over several slices (e.g. sigmoid) can be traced or accidental findings (e.g. Gärtner's or ovarian cysts) may be seen [28].

In the dynamic part, a variety of fast non-echo-planar sequence techniques for image acquisition has been described according to the used scanner type and manufacturer. To realize the freezing of motion the selected ultrafast sequence is repeated 15–25 times at the same slice position while the patient is simultaneously asked to relax the pelvic floor muscles, then contract them, relax again and then increase the intraabdominal pressure by straining and eventually defecate. Therefore, our group first introduced a gradient echo technique with fully refocused transverse magnetization (true fast imaging with steady precession, trueFISP). This gradient echo sequence combines both speed (high bandwidth and very short TR) and contrast (mixed T1/T2* contrast), but is very sensitive to susceptibility gradients. With this sequence we achieved an in-plane resolution of 1 mm with a temporal resolution of 1.3 images/s using a 256 matrix and a field of view of 270 mm [30]. It proved superior to gradient echo techniques with

partially refocused transverse magnetization (fast field echo, FFE [6, 12, 25] or gradient recalled acquisition in the steady state, GRASS [18, 49]), multi-echo spin-echo techniques (rapid acquisition with relaxation enhancement, RARE [10, 14, 38]) and single-shot techniques (snapshot GRASS [13] or half Fourier single-shot turbo spin-echo, HASTE [5, 47]). Recent advances in faster imaging with new methods of k-space acquisition [46], which are not sequence related ("parallel imaging"), allow for ultrafast achievement of images, but exhibit a lower signal-to-noise ratio.

In the case of an open configuration system the described ultrafast single-shot fast spin-echo sequences or gradient-echo sequences of the closed systems are not available. Instead, T1-weighted spoiled gradient-recalled echo sequences are used with a maximum time resolution of one image every 2 s [1, 2].

13.3.5
Slice Orientation

For the dynamic studies the midsagittal cut through the pelvis is the most preferred slice orientation throughout the entire literature. It was first introduced by YANG et al. [49] and KRUYT et al. [25] and provides an excellent overview of all relevant organs within the different compartments of the pelvis and the bony frame. In addition, we are familiar with this kind of view since the days of conventional cystography or evacuation proctography. But in our opinion, for a sufficient depiction of the complexity of the pelvic floor, at least two different slice orientations perpendicular to each other are required. Opposed to this, in the literature coronal and axial slices are only occasionally used to achieve additional information [12, 13, 41, 43].

Therefore our own protocol routinely includes, besides the midsagittal plane, a single axial slice as well as a stack of coronal slices. The axial slice at the level of the inferior border of the symphysis bone or the ischiatic tubera nicely depicts the urogenital hiatus with its content and the puborectal portion of the levator ani muscle. Changes in the signal intensity of the femoral vein allow for the estimation of the straining effort by the patient. Unfortunately this slice orientation is prone to changes in the tilting of the pelvis.

Due to the lack of whole coverage of the pelvic floor coronal images are necessary to evaluate the entire anatomic region [12, 34, 42, 43]. We perform a coronal stack of slices while the patient is continuously straining. Those images depict the levator ani muscle in more detail and facilitate the detection of lateral rectoceles, levator ani hernias or a rectal intussusception. In addition, the sacrouterine ligaments are best visualized using this slice orientation.

If, after all, some findings on the images remain unclear, an oblique or double-oblique slice orientation adjoining the structure of interest is highly recommended. This requires an online survey of the images during the examination (e.g. asymmetric ballooning of the urogenital hiatus) and anticipation of possible findings (e.g. hernia or lateral rectocele).

13.4
Image Analysis

Once image acquisition is complete the single slices have to be rearranged according to their anatomical position and timely succession and then can be viewed in a cine loop. Although the visual impression of organ movements is decisive, certain aids have been developed to quantify the extent of the observed pathologies. Unfortunately, to date no general agreement on what and how to measure has been achieved (see Table 13.1).

A guideline for image analysis should include the following points: bony pelvis, muscles and ligaments of the pelvic floor, and the degree of movement of organs and reference structures under specified loads.

13.4.1
Bony Pelvis

Functional cine MRI should not be confused with MR pelvimetry and cannot replace it, but to have a look at bony structures can sometimes be helpful. The lower pelvis is part of the intraabdominal cavity and the pelvic floor as the inferior closure is exposed to the changing forces within this compartment. The pelvic bones as a surrounding superstructure protect and support the soft tissues and pelvic viscera. RETZKY et al. [37] describe a perpendicular relationship of the abdominal and pelvic cavity in a properly orientated bony pelvis. In their opinion this directs the pressure towards the pubic symphysis and away from the pelvic floor. LAZAREVSKI [27] compared 340 women with pelvic organ prolapse to a control group of 136 female without any evidence of organ descent. Pelvimetry on conventional X-ray pictures revealed significant differences of bony parameters between both groups. Among the patient group he noticed a more horizontal orientation or tilting of the pelvis with an upward movement of the pubic bone while straining. In addition, a significant increase in the distance between the inferior-posterior border of the pubic symphysis and either the S5-level or the tip of the coccygeal bone was measured. He concluded that this ultimately might result in an increased pressure load on the pelvic floor and thus may weaken the pelvic floor structures and lead to descensus and prolapse. Similar results were observed by HANDA et al. [16] with MR pelvimetry, who found a wider transverse inlet and a shorter obstetrical conjugate to be associated with pelvic floor disorders.

In our own experience more than half of the female patients tend to tilt the pelvis as previously described in order to promote the defecation process. In addition, most female patients demonstrate an outward bulging of the ventral abdominal wall due to relaxation of weakened abdominal muscles. Moreover, the shape of the sacral and coccygeal bones varies considerably, as can be seen on midsagittal MR images. A simple computer model of the abdominopelvic cavity can make these interrelations apparent. An increase in relaxation of the abdominal wall and/or a deep sacrococcygeal cavity diminishes the force transmission to the pelvic floor. This might alter the voluntary triggering of the defecation or voiding process.

Furthermore, Tarlov (perineural) cysts can frequently be seen at the lumbosacral transition or sacral segments of the spine. The normal prevalence of these cysts is reported to be 4.6%, but we noticed them in up to 12% of our patients. Tarlov cysts can be symptomatic by putting pressure on the nerve root [35, 48], but yet it is not proven that this can cause secondary muscular pelvic floor weakness.

Other incidental pathologies include occult stress fractures of the sacral bone or coccygodynia. In the latter, a bone edema as well as a surrounding small rim of fluid can be seen. Configuration and mobility of the coccygeal bone should be noted. Bo et al. [2] found a ventrocranial movement of 8.1 mm during contraction and a caudodorsal movement of 3.7 mm during straining, but there were no statistical differences between continent and incontinent women.

13.4.2
Pelvic Floor Muscles and Ligaments

The pelvic floor muscles on the whole do not represent a simple linear plate or hammock which is interconnected between the bony structures, but a complex 3D structure [20]. Therefore, linear measurements on 2D MR images can vary considerably. In their study Hoyte et al. [22] measured the anterior-posterior dimension of the levator hiatus using slightly rotated images. Calculated and measured values differed and showed up to 15% variation.

There are several reasons for this: (1) Most cuts through the muscles on MR images are not completely perpendicular to the muscle itself, and therefore cutting the muscle oblique the measurements of the thickness are falsified and are more or less too large. (2) The position of the subject within the MR scanner can vary. It is highly recommended to position the patient properly. On the coronal localizer both acetabular bones should be at the same level. Tilting of the pelvis in the vertical axis during contraction and straining should be eliminated. In our experience changes of more than 5 mm or 10° already account for visual asymmetry of muscular structures [3]. Interobserver accuracy has to be considered, especially in thin structures of only a few millimeters in size [4]. The accuracy of measurements is limited to about 1 mm on most workstations.

Nevertheless, in the literature a variety of parameters concerning pelvic floor muscles have been analysed on functional images: width of the levator hiatus on axial [8, 10, 12, 22, 24, 32, 43], coronal [13, 20] and sagittal images [5, 42], thickness of the iliococcygeal portion of the levator ani muscle on coronal and axial images [42], range of movement of the levator ani muscle (iliococcygeal part) on coronal images [20], cross-sectional area of the urogenital hiatus on axial images [12, 17, 32, 41], as well as the surface of the levator ani calculated on coronal images [17]. In addition, three different angles have been proposed: the levator-plate [12, 13, 17, 21], the levator-vaginal [13, 21] and the iliococcygeal angle [42].

The levator plate angle (LPA) is the angle between the posterior part of the levator ani muscle (iliococcygeal portion) as seen on the midsagittal image and the pubococcygeal reference line (PC line; see Sect. 13.4.3). In a similar way, the levator-vaginal angle is calculated by measuring the angle between the posterior portion of the levator ani plate and a line drawn through the horizontal axis of the upper third of the vagina [41]. Yet another parameter to access the orientation and slope of the iliococcygeal muscle is the angle between this muscle and the transverse plane of the pelvis on coronal images [42]. However, especially in measuring angles, there is a great inter- and even intraobserver variability because of the often not completely even, but slightly curved shape of the anatomical structures,

e.g. the levator plate or the vaginal wall. The same applies to more or less all other measurements involving muscular structures of the pelvic floor and makes all these highly questionable.

Nevertheless, looking at the shape of the various parts of the levator ani muscle reveals additional information. Muscle defects with or without hernias are best seen on coronal images. A steep orientation of the coccygeal portion of the levator ani muscle on midsagittal images together with a ballooning of the puborectal portion on axial images is indicative of pelvic floor weakness (Fig. 13.1c,d). Asymmetry or even complete loss of the right puborectal portion of the levator ani is a frequent finding in parous women after episiotomy. Intramuscular hematomas due to excessive straining or a thickened coccygeal portion in patients with levator ani syndrome or extensive scars due to previous surgery are other possible diagnoses.

Ligaments play an important role in supporting the organs of the pelvic floor and tears within these ligaments have been reported to be the cause of rectoceles or uterine/vaginal descent. Yet their anatomic existence and thus their influence on the pelvic floor remain controversial [11]. On functional MRI, with the exception of three ligamentous structures, no other corresponding structures are discernible. The three structures mentioned are: the rectovaginal interface, the anococcygeal ligaments and the sacrouterine ligaments. The first two structures are best seen on midsagittal images, whereas the sacrouterine ligaments can be nicely delineated on coronal images. On functional MRI the rectovaginal interface is seen between the posterior wall of the vagina and the anterior wall of the rectum, which are both of intermediate to low signal intensity. Separation of these two structures by a small rim of high signal intensity on T2-weighted images may just indicate a deep pouch of Douglas.

13.4.3
Assessment of
Pelvic Organ Mobility – Reference Lines

To evaluate the range of movement of the organs of the pelvic floor under load a variety of reference lines have been established. On general agreement, the ideal reference line system should accomplish certain criteria: (1) Mark the level of the levator ani muscle as the main supporting structure of the entire pelvic floor; (2) be independent of tilting of the pelvis by using two or more well defined bony landmarks; (3) describe the range of organ movement in at least two different imaging planes. (4) provide the possibility to compare findings on MR images with the results of the clinical examination and clinical classification systems. To date no single reference line or grading system meets all the above-mentioned criteria.

The most commonly used reference line is the so called pubococcygeal line (PC line) (Figs. 13.1–13.3). This line was originally used for many years for the evaluation of organ descent on cystography and evacuation proctography. It was first introduced in functional MRI by YANG et al. [49] and is the reference line most commonly used.

Unfortunately, there are three different kinds of PC lines mentioned in the literature with an additional two different types of measuring the distance between the reference organ and the PC line itself. All PC lines are drawn on midsagittal images and start at the inferior-posterior rim of the pubic symphysis. The second bony landmark is either the first sacrococcygeal joint [2, 17, 20, 21, 24, 36], the last visible coccygeal intervertebral space [1, 10, 12, 30, 49] or the point of insertion of the coccygeal portion of the levator ani [14]. While most authors measure the distance of the organ in respect to the PC line by drawing a perpendicular line, some prefer to use a vertical line instead [46, 49]. The PC line certainly fulfills criteria 1 and 2 and is suitable for comparison of clinical and MR findings [43].

The HMO system proposed by COMITER et al. [5] is also based on the PC line. In addition they used the posterior anorectal junction as a third landmark on midsagittal images and measured the width of the urogenital hiatus (H line) from here to the posterior rim of the symphysis. The M line describes the perpendicular distance of the anorectal junction to the PC line. Finally with the O classification the degree of visceral prolapse is graded qualitatively according to the descent beyond the H line. In their study of 164 consecutive patients with either pelvic pain or organ prolapse this system proved to be a straightforward and reproducible method for staging and quantification of pelvic floor relaxation and organ prolapse. However, there are several drawbacks in this study. The anorectal junction represents a muscular landmark hard to define on sagittal images especially if no opacification of the rectum has been used. No intra-/interobserver evaluation was performed and the staging of the grade of organ prolapse with the O classification is only subjective. Comparison with clinical findings was not achieved. Therefore, in view of criteria 2, 3 and 4 it remains questionable if this extension to the PC line will have any impact on image analysis in daily routine.

Other proposed reference lines are: the horizontal line at the level of the inferior border of the pubic symphysis on midsagittal images [28, 43], the symphysiosacral line on midsagittal images between the superior border of the pubic bone and the distal sacral bone [6] and the midpubic line through the longitudinal axis of the pubic bone [41]. The horizontal line is lacking the first three criteria while representing the level of the ischiatic tubera. The slope of the symphysiosacral line is too steep to reflect the levator plate. The midpubic line is of some value for comparison of clinical and MR findings [41] as it represents approximately the level of the vaginal introitus. In conclusion, the diversity of all reference lines makes it completely impossible to compare the different published results.

13.4.4
Definition of Pathological Findings

In order to establish a diagnosis several reference structures have been introduced together with the reference lines. Within the anterior compartment the bladder base or the most caudal part (mostly the dorsal wall) of the bladder are mentioned. The cervix or the posterior fornix of the vagina are reference structures within the middle compartment. The anorectal junction is the only reference structure of the posterior compartment.

By definition an organ descent is diagnosed if one or all of the previously mentioned reference structures descend below the suitable reference line. Throughout the literature the reference line commonly used for evaluating the position of the bladder and the cervix or vaginal vault is the PC line. Therefore a cystocele or a uterine descensus is diagnosed if these structures descend below the PC line. Several authors propose a grading system of organ prolapse using steps of 2 or 3 cm [1, 5, 12, 13, 41].

The diagnosis of an enterocele is more difficult and intimately related to the pouch of Douglas. The normal depth of the rectouterine space is about 5 cm as shown by KUHN et al. [26]. Depending on the depth and/or the content of the pouch a variety of definitions of an enterocele are used. In evacuation proctography most authors define an enterocele either as a widening of the distance between the vagina and rectum or a deepening of the rectovaginal space beyond the upper third of the vagina. According to this, in functional cine MRI a descent or widening of the pouch of Douglas below the PC line is considered to be pathological [30, 43]. Visible small bowel loops

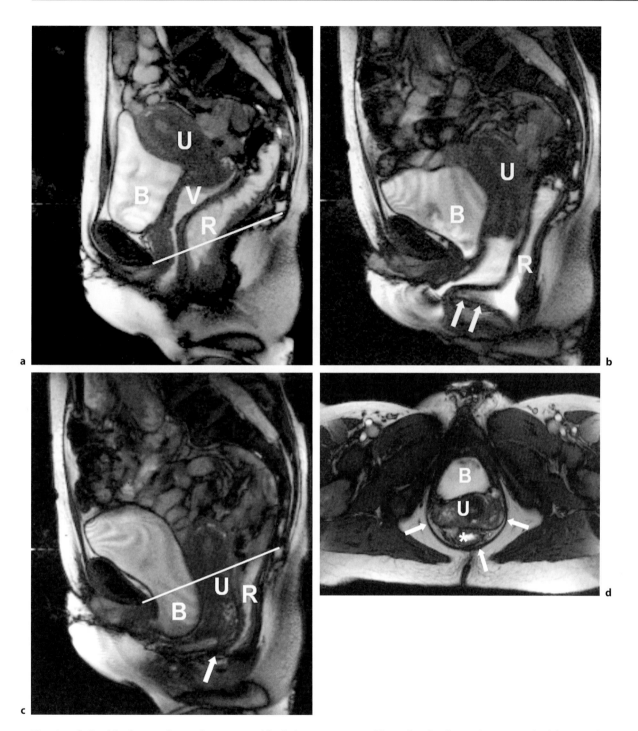

Fig. 13.1a-d. Combined organ descent in a 40-year-old primiparous woman with stool outlet obstruction. T2-weighted functional MR images of the pelvis (**a-c** midsagittal; **d** transversal) obtained with the patient at rest (**a**) and during straining (**b-d**). **a** Normal position of the bladder (*B*), vagina (*V*) and uterus (*U*) above the pubococcygeal reference line (*white line*). The rectum (*R*) shows no anterior bulging. Vagina and rectum are filled with sonography gel. **b** During the first period of straining the anterior rectal wall is protruding in an anterior direction forming a deep rectocele (*arrows*). The bladder (*B*) and the uterus (*U*) descend only slightly. **c** After repeated straining and defecation now the rectum (*R*) and the rectocele (*arrow*) are emptied. Therefore, given more space to slide into the genital hiatus, a large cystocele (*B*) and a descensus of the uterus (*U*) far below the PC line occur causing a compression of the rectal lumen. Note the relaxed levator ani muscle with a nearly vertical orientation. **d** In the axial plane (level of the pubic symphysis) a ballooning of the levator ani muscle (*arrows*) resulting from muscular weakness can be seen. The descending bladder (*B*), lower parts of the uterus (*U*) and the rectum (*asterisk*) are located between the two sides of the puborectal muscle

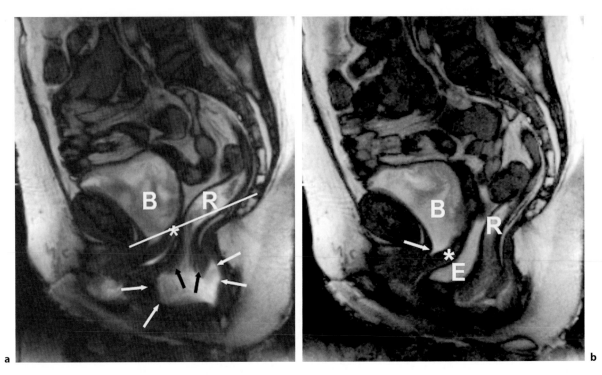

Fig. 13.2a,b. Multiparous 71-year-old woman with defecation disorder. Midsagittal T2-weighted MR images of the pelvis obtained with the patient straining repeatedly. **a** During the first straining episode the well gel-filled rectum (*R*) shows an extensive bulging of the rectal wall in the anterior-perineal as well as in the posterior direction (*white arrows*). This anterior and posterior rectocele stabilizes the position of both the bladder (*B*) and the vaginal vault (*asterisk*), which stay at the level of the PC line. Additionally, a thickening of the rectal mucosa (*black arrows*) is depicted marking a beginning intussusception. **b** After incomplete emptying of the rectocele and rectum (*R*) a large enterocele (*E*) has developed with mesenterial fatty tissue sliding down into the rectovaginal space. The sonography gel in the vagina has been evacuated passively. These findings are accompanied by a small cystocele with funneling of the urethra (*arrow*) and a vaginal vault descent (*asterisk*)

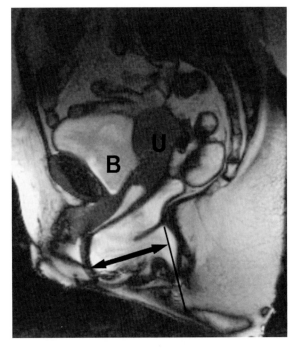

Fig. 13.3. A 69-year-old female with a partial prolapse of the posterior vaginal wall during clinical examination. Midsagittal T2-weighted MR images obtained with the patient straining. A huge bulging of the anterior rectal wall in an anterior direction occurs. The depth of the rectocele can be measured as the distance between the tip of the rectocele (*double arrow*) and a parallel line along the anal canal (*black line*). The bladder (*B*) and the uterus (*U*) descend only slightly

or sigmoid colon sliding down into the pouch during straining confirm the diagnosis of an enterocele.

The most widely accepted definition of a rectocele was proposed by YOSHIOKA et al. [50]. The depth of the rectocele is calculated by measuring the distance between a line drawn parallel to the anal canal and the most ventrocaudal part of the bulging of the anterior rectal wall (Fig. 13.4). If the depth exceeds 3 cm the rectocele is believed to be pathological [6, 12, 18]. Nevertheless, a considerable overlap between findings in normal volunteers and patients has been reported [40].

13.5
Typical Findings

13.5.1
Anterior Compartment

The bladder as a fluid-filled structure is hyperintense on T2-weighted images. Depending on the degree of filling the shape of the bladder can vary considerably, ranging from a more triangular to a round profile (Figs. 13.1b vs 13.3a). At rest it is situated superior-posterior to the pubic symphysis (Fig. 13.1a). On mid-

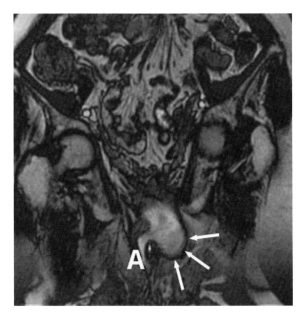

Fig. 13.4. A 74-year-old female with a history of aggravated and incomplete defecation. Coronal T2-weighted MR image during maximal straining. Large lateral rectocele (*arrows*) to the left side, detectable only in the coronal images, missed in the midsagittal and axial images. *A*, anal canal

sagittal images an area of fat-equivalent signal intensity is seen between the pubic bone and the bladder (retropubic space; space of Retzius) which adds to the displacement of the bladder (Fig. 13.1a). This area can be enlarged in patients with incontinence [45]. The urethra is normally not well delineated on the mid-sagittal images, but its typical target-like appearance can be easily noted on axial images. The supporting muscular and connective structures of the urethra are still debated and not discerned on functional MRI. Surrounding structures like small bowel loops are only partly depicted in the midsagittal plane, but adhesions between the dome of the bladder and bowel loops occur quite often. They can easily be noted as the bowel loops stick in a fixed position to the upper bladder wall and do not glide freely as they are supposed to while the patient is straining.

Both the urethra and the bladder are exposed to the increasing intraabdominal pressure during Valsalva´s maneuver. A cystocele is present if the bladder neck or any part of the posterior wall of the bladder moves below the PC line (Fig. 13.1c, 13.3b). Both the proximal urethra and the bladder neck descend and rotate around the pubic bone, initially moving posterior-inferior. A non-specific finding in patients with involuntary loss of urine is funneling of the proximal urethra (Fig. 13.2b). An additional kinking of the urethra at the urethrovesical junction can occur in large cystoceles. Furthermore, due to the limited space provided by the urogenital hiatus a large cystocele can block the prolapse of other pelvic structures and thus mask a rectocele or enterocele (Fig. 13.2a,b). Recurrence of a cystocele after retropubic or vaginal operations for stress incontinence can be nicely revealed by functional MRI. In these patients the proximal urethra and the bladder neck maintain their normal position superior to the symphysis, but the posterior wall of the bladder bulges into the anterior vaginal wall (Fig. 13.3a,b). Finally in case of previous procedures for urinary incontinence one should look for sling material or injections of bulk-enhancing agents such as collagen, all of which are normally hypointense on MR images [4].

13.5.2
Middle Compartment

In a normal anatomical setting the vagina, the rectum and the posterior components of the levator ani muscle lie one upon the other (Fig. 13.1a). Therefore, the position of the vagina and uterus is dependent on the amount of filling of the rectal ampulla.

If a vaginal or uterine descent is present, only after the rectum has been emptied both structures move ventro-caudally beyond the PC line (Fig. 13.1b,c). This is why the PC line itself might underestimate an organ descent in the middle compartment [24]. The point of reference is either the posterior fornix of the vagina or the cervix. In cases of repeated, long-standing prolapse the vagina is often shortened and the vaginal wall may be thickened or even everted. In addition the pouch of Douglas is widened, thus facilitating the development of a peritoneocele or enterocele (Fig. 13.2b). Elongated sacrouterine ligaments may be discerned on coronal images. Fascial defects, e.g. paravaginal defects or tears within the rectovaginal septum can not be appreciated on functional cine MRI alone, for this high spatial resolution static images are necessary.

The pouch of Douglas normally represents the deepest point within the intraabdominal cavity and is predisposed for an internal hernia. This posterior herniation of peritoneum may contain fat (peritoneocele), small bowel loops (enterocele) or sigmoid colon (sigmoidocele). The criterion for making the diagnosis of an enterocele is the descent of bowel loops below the PC line [24, 31]. The hernial sack follows the course of the vagina along the rectovaginal septum. A simple widening of the rectovaginal space or deepening of the pouch of Douglas below the PC line without bowel loops is defined as a peritoneocele. If the mesenteric root is too short an enterocele is unlikely to occur. Occasionally the herniation can be lateral or anterior, in this case coronal images may be helpful for a correct assessment. Again a large enterocele can mask either a cystocele or a rectocele [31, 43]. After sacrocolpopexy or uteropexy functional MRI is able to depict the foreign material and to demonstrate its intact function [33] (Fig. 13.3a,b).

13.5.3
Posterior Compartment

The rectum behaves like a flexible and expansible tube. It can fold on itself with a lateral or anterior displacement and kinking. Most often a bulging of the anterior rectal wall is noted [34]. These anterior rectoceles are normal findings and even large rectoceles may be clinically asymptomatic. In the literature a rectocele with a depth of more than 3 cm is regarded as to be a pathological finding [50]. Nevertheless it should be stressed that there is a considerable overlap between healthy volunteers and women with pelvic prolapse [40]. The

direction of a rectocele is either anteriorly (to the distal segment of the posterior vaginal wall) (Figs. 13.1b, 13.4), laterally (Fig. 13.5) or dorsally (Fig. 13.2a). It is important to notice if the rectocele empties completely with the defecation or if contrast medium is trapped in the rectocele. Lateral rectoceles are missed in the midsagittal images but clearly become apparent in the coronal images (Fig. 13.5).

Intussusceptions are mucosal or mural rectal wall invaginations which can be located anteriorly or posteriorly or can affect the whole circumference. They present as a circumscribed thickening of the rectal mucosa and the wall (Fig. 13.2a). A caudal movement of this rectal segment into the anal canal marks the beginning of an internal rectal prolapse. But note that the differentiation between an intussusception and an internal rectal prolapse is not clearly determined and the two terms are often overlapping. A more prominent internal rectal prolapse is often seen as a V-shaped or double rectal wall on the midsagittal image (Fig. 13.6). The internal rectal prolapse may eventually protrude through the anal canal and then becomes an external rectal prolapse.

Often an organ descent in/of the anterior or middle compartment typically leads to a compression of the ventral rectal wall. This finding can promote an internal rectal prolapse and might account for a stool entrapment and a stool outlet obstruction (Fig. 13.1c).

13.5.4
Levator Ani Muscle

On the midsagittal images the posterior aspects of the levator ani muscle can be delineated. An adequate relaxation of the puborectal sling during defecation with a resulting vertical orientation of the posterior levator ani should be noted. If the levator ani muscle is still contracting during straining and even defecation, this paradoxical finding is called anismus, which can cause incomplete evacuation and stool outlet obstruction symptoms. Displacement of the anorectal junction in relation to the PC line is used as a parameter to define a rectal descent [12, 18, 25, 41]. A ballooning of the levator muscle on axial images is obvious in patients with weakness of the pelvic floor muscles (Fig. 13.1d). By contrast in asymptomatic volunteers the genital hiatus and the puborectalis sling keep the typical V-like shape under load [43]. The width of the urogenital hiatus should not exceed 5 cm [32]. Again on axial images an asymmetric appearance of the puborectal part of the levator muscle can be seen in cases after episiotomy.

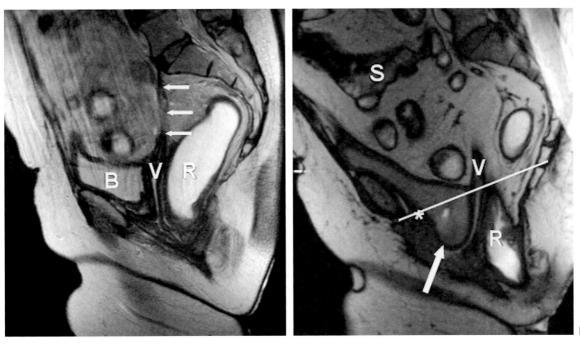

a   b

Fig. 13.5a,b. A 67-year-old female patient after sacrocolpopexy with recurrence of a cystocele. Midsagittal static (**a**) and functional (**b**) T2-weighted MR images at rest (**a**) and during straining (**b**). **a** Static MR images demonstrate the synthetic material fixing the vaginal apex (*V*) to the promontory (*arrows*). *B*, bladder; *R*, rectum. **b** Typical findings after sacrocolpopexy are the normal position of the bladder neck (*asterisk*) in contrast to the descent of the posterior wall of the bladder (*arrow*) below the PC line (*white line*). The vagina (*V*) is kept in place by the intact foreign material. *R*, rectum; *S*, small bowel

13.6
Rating of Functional Cine MRI

Most published studies focused on different technical aspects of the method and confirmed the usefulness of the method by depicting significant differences between two study groups, which differed in clinical means [5, 10, 13, 17, 19, 25, 28, 42, 46, 49].

13.6.1
Functional Cine MRI Versus Fluoroscopy/Colpocystorectography

Approximately ten studies compare functional cine MRI with conventional X-ray examinations. The majority of these studies come to the conclusion that functional cine MRI is at least equal to conventional fluoroscopic methods and in some aspects can be superior. DELEMARRE et al. [6] examined 14 patients with radiographic defecography and additionally with functional cine MRI and evaluated qualitative grading and quantitative measurements of anterior rectoceles. They stated that the potential of MRI with regard to

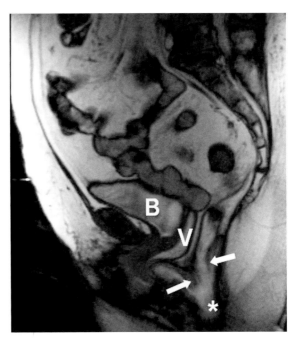

Fig. 13.6. A 66-year-old female with fecal incontinence. Midsagittal T2-weighted MR images obtained during defecation. The *arrows* mark an internal rectal prolapse with folding of the rectal mucosa and rectal wall in the direction of the opened anal canal (*asterisk*). Moderate descensus of the bladder (*B*) and vagina (*V*)

anterior rectoceles seems absent. Drawbacks of the study are the prone position of the patient and the missing opacification of the rectum. Our own results on two occasions are more in favour of functional cine MRI [30]. We examined five asymptomatic volunteers and 44 female patients with both imaging modalities. In terms of diagnosis MRI was either identical (21 cases) or superior (18 cases) to dynamic fluoroscopy. As a result sensitivity and specificity rated higher for MRI than for dynamic fluoroscopy. Functional MRI was especially helpful in the depiction of pathologies within the middle compartment (descent of uterus, enteroceles) and in revealing changes in the dominant type of prolapse. HEALY et al. [18] found a significant correlation of standard measurements of the anorectal configuration using functional MRI and evacuation proctography in ten women with constipation. In addition, functional MRI was able to show significant changes of muscular parameters in 11 women with otherwise normal proctograms [17]. SCHOENENBERGER et al. [39] examined 15 patients with defecation disorders using an open-configuration MR system. MR images showed all pathologic findings except for one case of intussusception in a patient with spastic pelvic floor syndrome, whereas defecography missed four pathologic conditions. Thus MR defecography was rated superior to fluoroscopic defecography. In the study performed by GUFLER et al. [14] 32 women with urinary incontinence or organ prolapse were examined using bead-chain cystourethrography or colpocystorectography and functional MRI. MRI correctly diagnosed the degree of bladder descent with a coefficient of determination of 0.81 and 0.85. Cystourethrography alone missed all rectoceles, whereas MRI as well as colpocystorectography correctly depicted this pathologic finding. Enteroceles could only be diagnosed by MRI. In an additional study in 2004 GUFLER et al. compared colpocystorectography in the upright and supine position with functional MRI [15]. They did not find a significant difference between MRI and colpocystorectography either in the supine or in the upright position. Another study comparing conventional X-ray methods with functional MRI was published by VANBECKEVOORT et al. [47]. Functional MRI was compared to colpocystodefecography with maximum straining and during voiding and defecation in 35 women with pelvic floor descent. When compared to the X-ray method MRI exhibited a specificity of 100% in all compartments. But the sensitivity of MRI proved to be inferior, being as low as 13% for the detection of vaginal vault descent and 56% for the diagnosis of a rectocele. The authors state that MRI is unreliable especially in the anterior and middle compartment. This study nicely demonstrates the impact of the defecation process on diagnosis: here functional MRI without defecation was compared to colpocystodefecography with defecation.

In their study KELVIN et al. (24) compared cystocolpoproctography with opacification of all relevant organs to functional MRI in the supine position with opacification of the bladder, vagina and rectum. In addition to our own protocol they added a post-toilet phase. They conclude that MR imaging and cystocolpoproctography showed similar detection rates for prolapse of pelvic organs but with the advantage of MRI that it reveals all pelvic organs and pelvic floor musculature.

13.6.2
Functional Cine MRI in Asymptomatic Subjects

Although most studies include asymptomatic volunteers as a control study group there are only two reports in the literature which exclusively define the normal range of findings in asymptomatic individuals.

GOH et al. [12] examined 25 men and 25 women on a 1.0-Tesla system in the supine position with the volunteers being at rest and during straining. All volunteers had to pass a detailed questionnaire. They measured the descent of the bladder base, cervix and anorectal junction in relation to the PC line and calculated the pelvic floor hiatus area and perimeter as well as the anorectal and levator plate angle.

Our own study included 20 female volunteers who showed no pathologic findings on clinical examination and urodynamics [32]. Functional MRI was performed in the supine position using a 1.5-Tesla system. Vagina and rectum were opacified with ultrasound gel. Among others we calculated the position of the bladder base, posterior vaginal fornix and the anorectal junction in relation to the PC line and the horizontal reference line. The width and area of the levator hiatus, as well as several bony parameters, were calculated. Unfortunately due to the lack of standardization these two studies stand by themselves.

13.6.3
Functional Cine MRI Versus Clinical Pelvic Organ Prolapse Quantification Staging System

In 1996 the International Continence Society (ICS) introduced the ICS score to standardize the measurement of pelvic organ descent and prolapse at the gynaecological examination [3]. To date such a widely accepted pelvic organ prolapse quantification staging system (POPQ) has not been developed for imaging of the pelvic floor. Two questions are of considerable interest: (1) Is functional MRI able to detect relevant morphological changes in patients with only minor or no clinical findings (POPQ stages I or O)? (2) Does the reference line system adopted by the radiologists correlate with the POP-Q system?

So far there are only two studies mentioned in the literature which address the above problems. HODROFF et al. [21] showed in their study that functional MRI was able to detect significant anatomic changes in POP stage O patients. In addition SINGH et al. [41] tried to define a grading system by functional MRI using the same landmarks as the clinical grading system. They introduced the midpubic reference line as an approximation to the plane of the hymen. By using it they found a good correlation between the radiological and the clinical reference systems.

13.7
Conclusion

Taking all the above-mentioned into account, indications for functional cine MRI still remain controversial. The method itself is not yet standardized, and so far only a 2D approach for functional imaging of the pelvic floor exists. With the advance of fast "parallel imaging" a stack of two to three slices within the same acquisition time seems possible.

In patients with disorders of pelvic support functional MRI is an alternative to conventional X-ray procedures like urethrocystography, colpocystorectography or evacuation proctography. Functional MRI proved to be equal or superior to these methods. Due to its multiplanar capability, superb soft tissue contrast and lack of superimposition additional findings, e.g. muscular or even ligamentous defects, may be well outlined. No other radiological modalities can provide such comprehensive information to the operating physician. Functional cine MRI proved to be especially helpful in patients with equivocal clinical findings, e.g. to determine a dominant hernial orifice, to outline an enterocele or for postoperative follow-up examinations. But further studies will be needed to determine, among others, the cost effectiveness of this method. In summary, functional cine MRI will be the modality of choice in patients with pelvic floor dysfunction.

References

1. Bertschinger KM, Hetzer FH, Roos JE, et al. (2002) Dynamic MR imaging of the pelvic floor performed with patient sitting in an open-magnet unit versus with patient supine in a closed-magnet unit. Radiology 223:501–508
2. Bo K, Lilleas F, Talseth T, et al. (2001) Dynamic MRI of the pelvic floor muscles in an upright sitting position. Neurourol Urodyn 20:167–174
3. Bump RC, Mattiasson A, Bo K, et al. (1996) The standardization of terminology of female pelvic organ prolapse and pelvic floor dysfunction. Am J Obstet Gynecol 175:10–17
4. Carr LK, Herschorn S and Leonhardt C (1996) Magnetic resonance imaging after intraurethral collagen injected for stress urinary incontinence. J Urol 155:1253–1255
5. Comiter CV, Vasavada SP, Barbaric ZL, et al. (1999) Grading pelvic prolapse and pelvic floor relaxation using dynamic magnetic resonance imaging. Urology 54:454–457
6. Delemarre JB, Kruyt RH, Doornbos J, et al. (1994) Anterior rectocele: assessment with radiographic defecography, dynamic magnetic resonance imaging, and physical examination. Dis Colon Rectum 37:249–259
7. Dvorkin L, Hetzer F, Scott S, et al. (2004) Open-magnet MR defaecography compared with evacuation proctography in the diagnosis and management of patients with rectal intussusception. Colorectal Dis 6:45–53
8. Fielding JR (2002) Practical MR imaging of female pelvic floor weakness. Radiographics 22:295–304
9. Fielding JR (2003) MR imaging of pelvic floor relaxation. Radiol Clin North Am 41:747–756
10. Fielding JR, Griffiths DJ, Versi E, et al. (1998) MR imaging of pelvic floor continence mechanisms in the supine and sitting positions. AJR Am J Roentgenol 171:1607–1610
11. Frohlich B, Hotzinger H, Fritsch H (1997) Tomographical anatomy of the pelvis, pelvic floor, and related structures. Clin Anat 10:223–230
12. Goh V, Halligan S, Kaplan G, et al. (2000) Dynamic MR imaging of the pelvic floor in asymptomatic subjects. AJR Am J Roentgenol 174:661–666
13. Goodrich MA, Webb MJ, King BF, et al. (1993) Magnetic resonance imaging of pelvic floor relaxation: dynamic analysis and evaluation of patients before and after surgical repair. Obstet Gynecol 82:883–891
14. Gufler H, Laubenberger J, DeGregorio G, et al. (1999) Pelvic floor descent: dynamic MR imaging using a half-Fourier RARE sequence. J Magn Reson Imaging 9:378–383
15. Gufler H, Ohde A, Grau G, et al. (2004) Colpocystoproctography in the upright and supine positions correlated with dynamic MRI of the pelvic floor. Eur J Radiol 51:41–47
16. Handa V, Pannu H, Siddique S, et al. (2003) Architectural differences in the bony pelvis of women with and without pelvic floor disorders. Obstet Gynecol 102:1283–1290
17. Healy JC, Halligan S, Reznek RH, et al. (1997a) Magnetic resonance imaging of the pelvic floor in patients with obstructed defaecation. Br J Surg 84:1555–1558
18. Healy JC, Halligan S, Reznek RH, et al. (1997b) Dynamic MR imaging compared with evacuation proctography when evaluating anorectal configuration and pelvic floor movement. AJR Am J Roentgenol 169:775–779
19. Hilfiker PR, Debatin JF, Schwizer W, et al. (1998) MR defecography: depiction of anorectal anatomy and pathology. J Comput Assist Tomogr 22:749–755

20. Hjartardottir S, Nilsson J, Petersen C, et al. (1997) The female pelvic floor: a dome – not a basin. Acta Obstet Gynecol Scand 76:567–571

21. Hodroff MA, Stolpen AH, Denson MA, et al. (2002) Dynamic magnetic resonance imaging of the female pelvis: the relationship with the pelvic organ prolapse quantification staging system. J Urol 167:1353–1355

22. Hoyte L, Ratiu P (2001) Linear measurements in 2-dimensional pelvic floor imaging: the impact of slice tilt angles on measurement reproducibility. Am J Obstet Gynecol 185:537–544

23. Huddleston HT, Dunnihoo DR, Huddleston PM, 3rd, et al. (1995) Magnetic resonance imaging of defects in DeLancey's vaginal support levels I, II, and III. Am J Obstet Gynecol 172:1778–1782; discussion 1782-1784

24. Kelvin FM, Maglinte DD, Hale DS, et al. (2000) Female pelvic organ prolapse: a comparison of triphasic dynamic MR imaging and triphasic fluoroscopic cystocolpoproctography. AJR Am J Roentgenol 174:81–88

25. Kruyt RH, Delemarre JB, Doornbos J, et al. (1991) Normal anorectum: dynamic MR imaging anatomy. Radiology 179:159–163

26. Kuhn RJ, Hollyock VE (1982) Observations on the anatomy of the rectovaginal pouch and septum. Obstet Gynecol 59:445–447

27. Lazarevski M (1974) Morphotopographic, static and dynamic changes in small pelvis with genital prolapse and urinary stress incontinence. MD thesis, Medical Faculty Skopje

28. Lienemann A (1998) An easy approach to functional magnetic resonance imaging of pelvic floor disorders. Tech Coloproctol 2:131–134

29. Lienemann A, Anthuber C, Baron A, et al. (1996) MR colpocystorectography: a new dynamic method for assessing pelvic floor descent and prolapse in women. Akt Radiol 6:182–186

30. Lienemann A, Anthuber C, Baron A, et al. (1997) Dynamic MR colpocystorectography assessing pelvic-floor descent. Eur Radiol 7:1309–1317

31. Lienemann A, Anthuber C, Baron A, et al. (2000a) Diagnosing enteroceles using dynamic magnetic resonance imaging. Dis Colon Rectum 43:205–212; discussion 212–213

32. Lienemann A, Sprenger D, Janssen U, et al. (2000b) [Functional MRI of the pelvic floor. The methods and reference values]. Radiologe 40:458–464

33. Lienemann A, Sprenger D, Anthuber C, et al. (2001) Functional cine magnetic resonance imaging in women after abdominal sacrocolpopexy. Obstet Gynecol 97:81–85

34. Pannu HK, Kaufman HS, Cundiff GW, et al. (2000) Dynamic MR imaging of pelvic organ prolapse: spectrum of abnormalities. Radiographics 20:1567–1582

35. Paulsen RD, Call GA and Murtagh FR (1994) Prevalence and percutaneous drainage of cysts of the sacral nerve root sheath (Tarlov cysts). AJNR Am J Neuroradiol 15:293–297; discussion 298–299

36. Rentsch M, Paetzel C, Lenhart M, et al. (2001) Dynamic magnetic resonance imaging defecography: a diagnostic alternative in the assessment of pelvic floor disorders in proctology. Dis Colon Rectum 44:999–1007

37. Retzky SS, Rogers jr RM, Richardson AC (1996) Anatomy of female pelvic support. In: Brubaker LT, Saclarides TJ (eds) The female pelvic floor disorders of function and support. F.A. Davis Company, Philadelphia, pp 3–21

38. Roos JE, Weishaupt D, Wildermuth S, et al. (2002) Experience of 4 years with open MR defecography: pictorial review of anorectal anatomy and disease. Radiographics 22:817–832

39. Schoenenberger AW, Debatin JF, Guldenschuh I, et al. (1998) Dynamic MR defecography with a superconducting, open-configuration MR system. Radiology 206:641–646

40. Shorvon PJ, McHugh S, Diamant NE, et al. (1989) Defecography in normal volunteers: results and implications. Gut 30:1737–1749

41. Singh K, Reid WM, Berger LA (2001) Assessment and grading of pelvic organ prolapse by use of dynamic magnetic resonance imaging. Am J Obstet Gynecol 185:71–77

42. Singh K, Reid WM, Berger LA (2002) Magnetic resonance imaging of normal levator ani anatomy and function. Obstet Gynecol 99:433–438

43. Sprenger D, Lienemann A, Anthuber C, et al. (2000) [Functional MRI of the pelvic floor: its normal anatomy and pathological findings]. Radiologe 40:451–457

44. Strohbehn K, Ellis JH, Strohbehn JA, et al. (1996) Magnetic resonance imaging of the levator ani with anatomic correlation. Obstet Gynecol 87:277–285

45. Tan IL, Stoker J, Zwamborn AW, et al. (1998) Female pelvic floor: endovaginal MR imaging of normal anatomy. Radiology 206:777–783

46. Unterweger M, Marincek B, Gottstein-Aalame N, et al. (2001) Ultrafast MR imaging of the pelvic floor. AJR Am J Roentgenol 176:959–963

47. Vanbeckevoort D, Van Hoe L, Oyen R, et al. (1999) Pelvic floor descent in females: comparative study of colpocysto-defecography and dynamic fast MR imaging. J Magn Reson Imaging 9:373–377

48. Voyadzis JM, Bhargava P, Henderson FC (2001) Tarlov cysts: a study of 10 cases with review of the literature. J Neurosurg 95:25–32

49. Yang A, Mostwin JL, Rosenshein NB, et al. (1991) Pelvic floor descent in women: dynamic evaluation with fast MR imaging and cinematic display. Radiology 179:25–33

50. Yoshioka K, Matsui Y, Yamada O, et al. (1991) Physiologic and anatomic assessment of patients with rectocele. Dis Colon Rectum 34:704–708

MR Pelvimetry

Ernst Beinder and Rahel Kubik-Huch

14

CONTENTS

E. Beinder, MD
University Hospital of Zurich, Department of Obstetrics,
Frauenklinikstr. 10, 8091 Zürich, Switzerland
R. A. Kubik-Huch, PhD
MPH, Kantonsspital Baden AG, Department of Radiology,
5404 Baden, Switzerland

14.1
Clinical Background

Arrest of labor with the necessity of performing secondary cesarean section is a major cause of maternal morbidity and mortality. The fetus is likewise affected by prolonged labor. Pelvimetry is performed to identify those women in whom an attempt at vaginal delivery is likely to fail due to a narrow pelvis or pelvic anomaly. Hence, the clinical significance of pelvimetry depends on how the following questions are answered:

- Is primary cesarean section associated with a lower morbidity and mortality of mother and child than secondary cesarean section after arrested labor has been diagnosed?
- Can arrested labor be treated effectively?
- Is there a reproducible method of pelvimetry with few side effects?
- Is there evidence from randomized and controlled studies that pelvimetry improves maternal and/or fetal outcome?

14.1.1
Primary versus Secondary Cesarean Section

The aim of pelvimetry is to identify maternal pelvic deviations that preclude vaginal delivery or would considerably prolong labor. If the results of pelvimetry suggest that vaginal delivery would be very difficult, primary cesarean section should be suggested. Both the mother and infant can thus be spared secondary cesarean section after protracted labor. The clinical significance of pelvimetry crucially depends on whether primary cesarean section can reduce maternal and fetal morbidity as compared with secondary cesarean section.

Cesarean section is performed as a primary (scheduled) or secondary (non-scheduled, after failure of labor to progress) procedure. The total number of cesarean sections, i.e. the sum of primary and secondary interventions, is 15%–30% in western industrialized countries. The mortality risk associated with vaginal delivery and cesarean section was determined in a study in Bavaria by WELSCH [1].

Cesarean section mortality attributable to the intervention is defined as the number of deaths occurring per 1000 cesarean sections during or within 42 days of the intervention and that are due to surgical or anesthesia-related complications in women who were healthy before the operation and had no pregnancy-related risks. In the survey by WELSCH, the maternal mortality risk of vaginal delivery versus cesarean section was 1:2.3 for the period from 1995 to 2000. However, the mortality rates no longer differ if only elective cesarean sections are compared with vaginal deliveries.

These figures underline that secondary cesarean sections after protracted labor or arrest of labor account for the excessive mortality of women during delivery.

Prolonged labor or arrest may have further adverse effects on mother and child:

- Perinatal Morbidity and Mortality: The duration of labor, in particular of the second stage, correlates with a decrease in fetal pH and pO_2 and an increase in pCO_2. Although fetal death during delivery has become rare, asphyxia contributes to perinatal morbidity. Detachment of the placenta due to uterine hyperactivity occurs in 1% of all pregnancies. Protracted labor often ends in vaginal operative delivery with the risk of fetal injury.
- Maternal Morbidity: Protracted labor involves numerous complications for the mother. Rupture due to overextension of a uterus not operated on before is nearly always due to excessively prolonged labor. The higher need for vaginal operative delivery in women with protracted labor is associated with a higher rate of maternal injuries, pain, hematomas, urinary retention, and anemia as compared with spontaneous delivery [2]. Women with prolonged labor and secondary cesarean section have an increased risk of infection or puerperal fever. Atonic postpartum hemorrhage is a characteristic of long labor and again increases the risk of protracted recovery and infectious complications.
- Birth Experience: No adequate systematic data is available on the emotional stress associated with prolonged and traumatic labor with secondary cesarean section. However, many women have problems coping with such an experience and do not become pregnant again.

In summary, prolonged labor and secondary cesarean section bear a considerable risk of maternal morbidity and mortality and also increase fetal morbidity. Modern obstetrical management therefore aims to ensure uncomplicated and speedy spontaneous delivery or, in women where this goal seems unattainable (or is not the mother's preferred option), to plan elective primary cesarean section beforehand. Hence, techniques that can predict the probability of an uncomplicated vaginal delivery before the onset of labor are of the utmost clinical significance.

14.1.2
Can Arrested Labor Be Treated Effectively?

Normal delivery is based on the complex interaction of maternal factors, fetal properties, and adequate labor. If this interaction of "Passages, Passenger, and Powers" is disturbed, labor is protracted or even arrested. The failure of labor to progress is therefore not a diagnosis but a symptom that is amenable to treatment (e.g. when caused by inadequate uterine contractions) or not (e.g. absolute cephalopelvic disproportion). Isolated evaluation of either of the three factors, passages, passenger, and powers, is of limited value as, for instance, cephalopelvic disproportion can be diagnosed only if one looks at both the maternal pelvis and the fetus ("this pelvis is too small for this fetus").

14.1.3
Abnormal Length of Labor: Diagnosis and Causes

14.1.3.1
Diagnosis

The onset of delivery is most commonly defined as the occurrence of regular and painful uterine contractions that result in progressive dilatation and effacement of the cervix.

The course of delivery is determined by the following variables:

- Size and shape of the maternal pelvis
- Flexibility of the maternal soft tissues in the pelvis, adaptation of the ligaments and bony pelvis to the fetus
- Remodeling of the cervix
- Regular birth mechanism of the fetus
- Fetal head molding
- Efficient uterine contractions

The results reported by FRIEDMAN in the 1950s still serve as the basis for diagnosing delayed labor [3, 4]. Arrest of labor during the first stage (the stage of cervical dilatation) is the absence of any progression of labor over a period of 2 h. The second stage (complete dilatation of the cervix until the onset of expulsive contractions) should not exceed 2 h.

14.1.3.2
Inadequate Progression of Labor Due to Maternal Factors ("the Passage")

14.1.3.2.1
Cephalopelvic Disproportion

Failure of adequate progression of labor due to cephalopelvic disproportion with imminent fetal asphyxia is the most common reason to perform secondary cesarean section. Arrest is typically caused by a combination of a large infant, an abnormal birth mechanism, and a narrow maternal pelvis. Detectable abnormal narrowing with an absolute disproportion occurs in 0.5%–1% of all deliveries today (Fig. 14.1). The incidence of borderline pelvic findings in which the size of the child and the birth mechanism together decide whether spontaneous delivery will be possible is much higher (Table 14.1).

Other maternal factors that may prolong or arrest labor include cervical leiomyomas or scarring of the cervix after prior surgery (conization, cerclage). Rare causes that prevent fetal descent are pelvic tumors such as large ovarian cysts or a pelvic kidney.

14.1.3.3
Inadequate Progression of Labor Due to Fetal Factors ("the Passenger")

An abnormal birth mechanism (abnormal fetal presentation and position) prevents adequate progression of labor just as often as maternal factors. Other fetal causes are macrosomia or fetal anomalies asso-

Table 14.1. Features of different pelvic shapes in comparison with the gynecoid (normal) pelvis. An android pelvis is associated with a higher incidence of deep transverse arrest, an anthropoid pelvis with a higher incidence of dorsoposterior position, and a platypelloid pelvis with high longitudinal position. All three pelvic shapes are characterized by protracted labor

Pelvic shape	Pelvic inlet	Pelvic outlet	Obstetric conjugate
Android	Normal	Shorter	Normal
Anthropoid	Shorter	Normal	Longer
Platypelloid	Longer	Normal	Shorter

ciated with macrohydrocephalus or an abnormally large circumference of the fetal abdomen or rump (pronounced ascites, sacrococcygeal teratoma).

14.1.3.4
Inadequate Progression of Labor Due to Inefficient Contraction ("the Powers")

Weak uterine contractions as a cause of inadequate progression of labor are most amenable to treatment. Inefficiency may become manifest as hypoactive, hyperactive, or uncoordinated contractions and hypertonic motility. Both hypoactivity and hyperactivity may occur secondary to mechanical obstruction.

14.1.4
Interventional Management of Inadequate Progression of Labor

Of the three components involved in normal delivery ("Passages, Passenger, Powers"), only labor ("Powers") is easily amenable to treatment.

Assistance in women with hypoactive and uncoordinated contractions is recommended if progression is delayed and cephalopelvic disproportion has been excluded as the cause. Oxytocin is the drug of first choice [5].

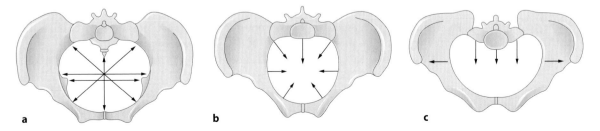

Fig. 14.1a–c. Pelvic shapes from *left* to *right*: Normal pelvic shape and width (cranial view). Generally narrow pelvis (all pelvic parameters are shortened). Platypelloid pelvis with a markedly shorter obstetric conjugate

In summary, arrested labor is often a multifactorial process resulting from the complex interaction of maternal pelvic size, size and presentation of the fetus, and labor activity. Effective therapeutic measures are only available for inadequate labor while no treatment is available for most other causes of arrested labor.

14.2
Clinical Methods of Pelvimetry

14.2.1
External Pelvimetry and Evaluation of Michaelis' Rhomboid

The normal values for the external pelvic measures are 25–26 cm for the interspinous distance, 28–29 cm for the intercrest distance, 31–32 cm for the intertrochanteric distance, and 20 cm for the external conjugate. The internal conjugate is calculated as the external conjugate minus 9 cm.

Michaelis's rhomboid is the rectangular area over the sacral bone formed by the dimple below the spinal processes of L3 to L4 (upper depression), the two posterior spines of the ilia (lateral depressions), and the groove at the distal end of the vertebral column (lower depression). The rhomboid is usually a square while its height increases considerably relative to its width in women with general narrowing of the pelvis. The lateral dimples are elevated in women with an android pelvis.

External pelvimetry will identify only pronounced deviations from the normal pelvic configuration that are rare in the European population.

14.2.2
Palpation of the Pelvis

The aim of palpation of the pelvis is to identify prominent bony structures that may obstruct labor. The examiner evaluates the angle of the pubic arch (> 90°), the promontory (cannot be reached), the anterior surface of the sacrum (smooth), the coccygis (not prominent and elastic), and the ischial spines (not prominent).

Palpation has the disadvantage that the results cannot be standardized. The examination is extremely uncomfortable for the patient.

14.3
MR Pelvimetry

Magnetic resonance (MR) pelvimetry was introduced in 1985 by STARK et al. [6]. MRI offers the benefit of accurate measurements of bony pelvic structures without exposure to ionizing radiation. The technique further allows imaging of soft-tissue structures, including the fetus, and has therefore replaced X-ray and computed tomography (CT) pelvimetry to become the modality of choice for obstetric pelvimetry [6–8].

14.3.1
Safety Issues and Contraindications

Whereas prenatal X-ray exposure has been associated with an increased risk of childhood cancer [9, 10], numerous studies of MRI in pregnant women have not revealed any experimental or clinical evidence of fetal harm. Thus, MRI is considered safe for both the mother and the developing fetus [11, 12].

MR pelvimetry has become a well-established clinical indication during pregnancy. Nevertheless, there is a general consensus that MRI should be performed in the first trimester of pregnancy only if there are clear medical indications since rapid organogenesis takes place at this time and the fetus is thus most susceptible to any potentially hazardous external influences.

In our institution, MR pelvimetry is performed either postpartum – in women whose delivery was complicated by protracted labor and who plan to become pregnant again – or in the last trimester of pregnancy.

Due to the lower energy deposition in tissue, gradient-echo sequences are preferred to spin-echo sequences for MR pelvimetry in pregnant women [13–15].

A substantial contraindication to MRI in general is claustrophobia; other contraindications such as pacemakers and metallic splinters are comparatively rare in the obstetric population.

It should however be kept in mind that many women referred for MR pelvimetry are unfamiliar with MRI and may be intimidated by the sheer bulk of the equipment. Despite current evidence that MRI has no adverse fetal effects and of which the women should be informed before MRI, the noise and claustrophobia of an MR exam may well induce fear for the fetus when imaging pregnant women and they should thus be especially well cared for during the exam by the staff of the MRI suite.

In women with physical effects like vena cava compression syndrome that may occur in late pregnancy, imaging can be performed in the lateral decubitus position.

14.3.2
MR Imaging Protocol

It has been shown in the literature that there are no significant differences in pelvimetric measurements between spin-echo and gradient-echo sequences [8, 14, 15]. Thus, gradient-echo sequences are favored over spin-echo sequences for MR pelvimetry due to the lower energy deposition already mentioned but also because of the shorter examination time [8, 13–15].

As mentioned above, MR pelvimetry is usually performed in the supine position. T1-weighted gradient-echo sequences of the maternal pelvis are acquired with the body coil in axial, sagittal, and oblique (in a plane through the symphysis and sacral promontory) orientation as shown in Fig. 14.2.

In our institution, MR pelvimetry is performed on a 1.5-Tesla Siemens Sonata MR scanner using a T1-weighted fast spoiled gradient-echo sequence (FSPGR) with the following parameters: repetition time (TR) 165 ms, echo time (TE) 10 ms, section thickness 6.0 mm, gap 20%, matrix 256×256, number of excitations (NEX) 2, anteroposterior phase-encoding direction. A large field of view (FOV), e.g. 380 mm, is used. Total examination time is only about 5–10 min.

14.3.3
Image Analysis

After the MR examination, pelvimetric measurements are performed on a workstation using the exterior surface of the appropriate bony cortex as the measuring point (Figs. 14.3, 14.4). The following pelvic distances are measured:

- The obstetric conjugate from the sacral promontory to the top inner cortex of the pubic bone at the symphysis is assessed in the midsagittal plane.
- The sagittal outlet, from the end of the sacrum to the bottom of the inner cortex of the symphysis, is also determined in the midsagittal plane.

- The interspinous distance represents the narrowest distance between the ischial spine some millimeters below or in the plane through the fovea capitis. It is measured in the axial plane.
- The intertuberous distance is the widest distance between the ischial tuberosities and is also measured in the axial plane.
- The transverse diameter represents the largest transverse distance in the oblique (through the promontory and the symphysis) axial plane [8, 16].

In our institution, all radiology suite technologists have been trained to select the appropriate images and measure the distances. Measurement is supervised by the radiologist writing the final report.

14.3.4
Reference Values for MR Pelvimetry

The groundwork in pelvimetry was laid using conventional radiography. Parameters were measured on lateral and anteroposterior views using various techniques to correct the distortion resulting from different distances from the film. These methods have since been superseded by cross-sectional imaging using computed tomography and, in particular, MRI. Nevertheless, values determined by plain radiography were still often used for guidance in the routine clinical setting. Yet studies comparing plain radiography and MR pelvimetry in the same population have described differences in some parameters, e.g. in intertuberous diameter [14, 17].

MR pelvimetric reference values in a large study population, stratified by delivery modality, have been established by our own group [8]. Results are shown in Table 14.2.

Table 14.2. Reference values for MR pelvimetry [8] based on 100 women undergoing spontaneous vaginal delivery

	Reference values ± SD (cm)
Obstetric conjugate	12.2 ± 0.9
Sagittal outlet	11.6 ± 1.0
Interspinous diameter	11.2 ± 0.8
Intertuberous diameter	12.1 ± 1.1
Transverse diameter	13.0 ± 0.9

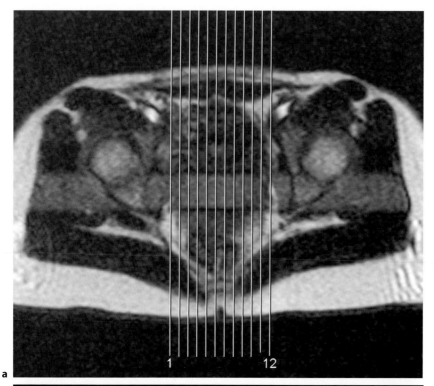

a

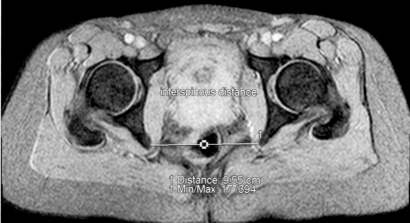

b

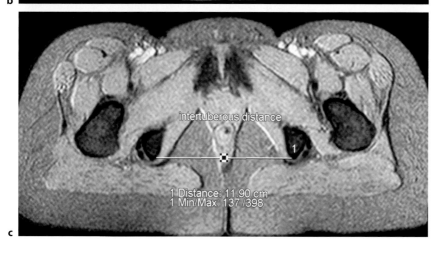

c

◁   ▷

Fig. 14.2a-g. Imaging protocol for MR pelvimetry. A 34-year-old woman with a history of secondary cesarean section; retroverted uterus with susceptibility artifacts from surgical incision. **a** Axial localizing image for the midsagittal plane (Flash; TR 1110 ms, TE 3.37 ms, NEX 1, FOV 400 mm). **b** Sagittal T1-weighted gradient-echo sequence (Flash; TR 165 ms, TE 10 ms, NEX 2, FOV 380 mm): The obstetric conjugate and sagittal outlet are measured in the midsagittal plane. **c** Coronal localizing image for the interspinous and intertuberous distances (for parameters see **a**). **d** Axial T1-weighted gradient-echo sequence at the level of the fovea capitis (for parameters see **b**): The interspinous distance represents the narrowest distance between the ischial spines. **e** Axial T1-weighted gradient-echo sequence (for parameters see **b**): The intertuberous distance represents the widest distance between the ischial tuberosities. **f** Sagittal localizing image for the transverse diameter (for parameters see **a**). **g** Axial oblique T1-weighted gradient-echo sequence (for parameters see **b**): The transverse diameter represents the largest transverse distance

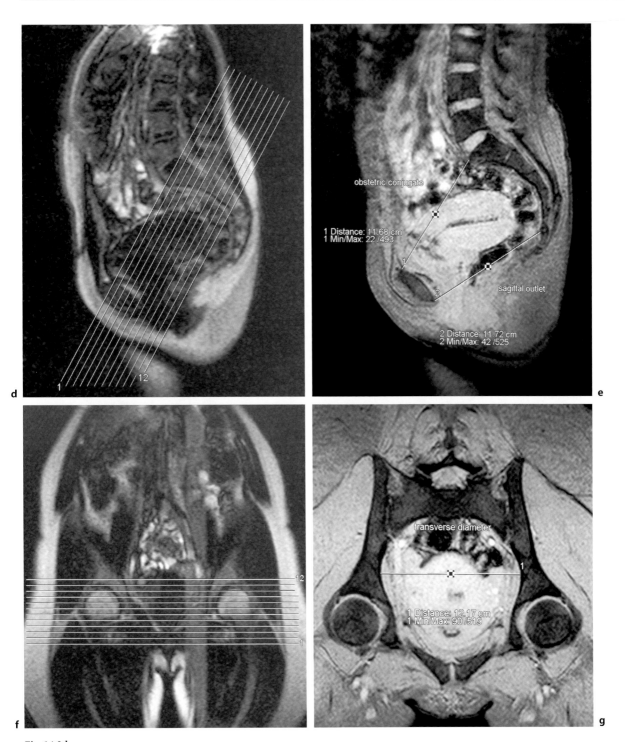

Fig. 14.2d-g.

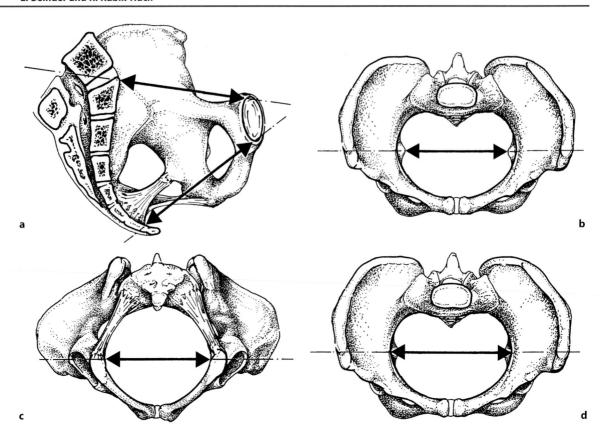

Fig. 14.3a-d. Pelvimetric diameters (drawings by G. Roth). **a** Obstetric conjugate and sagittal outlet. **b** Interspinous diameter. **c** Intertuberous diameter. **d** Transverse diameter (from [16])

It was demonstrated that the pelvimetric parameters associated with the largest intra- and interobserver error and intraindividual variability are the intertuberous distance and sagittal outlet. Obstetric decision-makers should therefore treat them with caution [8].

14.4
Can Pelvimetry Improve Maternal and/or Fetal Outcome?

Only few published studies have investigated the role of external pelvimetry. A prospective cohort study of primiparous African women showed that a combination of maternal height measurement and clinical external pelvimetry can identify a subgroup of patients with a high likelihood of cephalopelvic disproportion [18]. Comparable studies that present recent and robust data for western countries are not available.

A Cochrane Review lists four randomized controlled trials (RCT) on pelvimetry for fetal cephalic presentation [19]. All of these studies were performed using radiographic pelvimetry. The pelvimetry group had a higher rate of cesarean sections while fetal asphyxia and perinatal mortality tended to be lower but the difference did not reach significance (OR 0.61, CI 0.34–1.11 and OR 0.51, CI 0.18–1.42, respectively). Due to the small number of patients investigated and the poor quality of the studies quoted, the Cochrane Review concludes that the available evidence is not sufficient to prove a significant fetal benefit of radiographic pelvimetry in cephalic presentation.

One RCT has investigated pelvimetry in breech presentation [20]. In this study, van Loon et al. [20] demonstrate that pelvimetry significantly reduces the rate of emergency cesarean sections. More recent studies in smaller patient populations show promising results using pelvimetry (mostly performed by MRI) in combination with sonographic weight measurement of the fetus [21–23] but these findings must be confirmed by RCTs.

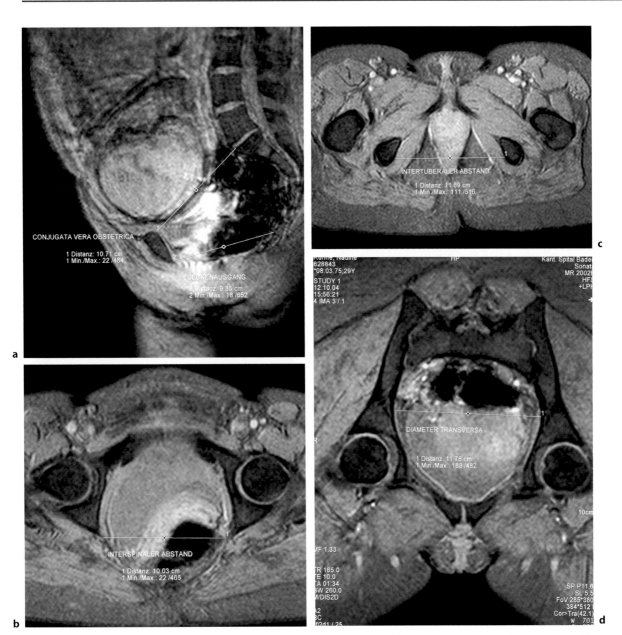

Fig. 14.4a–d. MR pelvimetry (T1-weighted gradient-echo imaging) in a 29-year-old pregnant woman in the last trimester with small pelvic dimensions. Vaginal delivery was attempted but failed and secondary cesarean section became necessary. The mid-sagittal section shows (**a**) the obstetric conjugate (10.7 cm) and sagittal outlet (9.8 cm). Axial sections show (**b**) the interspinous distance (10.0 cm), measured at the level of the foveae of the femoral heads, and (**c**) the intertuberous distance (11.7 cm). The oblique section (**d**) shows the transverse diameter (11.8 cm)

14.5
Indications for Pelvimetry

14.5.1
Breech Presentation and Maternal Preference for Spontaneous Delivery

Breech presentation is a common obstetric abnormality occurring in 3%–5% of single pregnancies and 10%–15% of multiple pregnancies but there is no agreement about its most suitable obstetric management. The Canadian Medical Research Council (MRC) initiated an international randomized multicenter trial of planned vaginal birth versus planned cesarean section for breech presentation at term after an uncomplicated pregnancy [24]. The results show that planned cesarean section reduces the fetal complication rate while not affecting the maternal complication rate and the authors conclude that planned cesarean section is the optimal method of delivery for a fetus in breech presentation.

Following publication of these results, the rate of primary cesarean sections for breech presentations increased to up to 80%. Nevertheless, spontaneous delivery in breech presentation may be the preferred option of the mother. In such cases it is particularly important to exclude cephalopelvic disproportion.

14.5.2
After Cesarean Section Due to Arrest of Labor

The probability of secondary cesarean section after spontaneous onset of labor is about 10% in women without prior cesarean section as opposed to 40%–50% in women having had a cesarean section before. In order to reduce the rate of secondary cesarean section, we perform postpartum pelvimetry and recommend primary cesarean section for future pregnancies in those women who are found to have a narrow pelvis because they are at high risk of renewed arrest of labor.

14.5.3
Clinically Conspicuous Abnormalities of Pelvic Shape and Status Post Pelvic Fracture

Only 0.5%–1% of all pregnant women have such obvious pelvic anomalies that absolute cephalopelvic disproportion is highly likely. The risk of abso-lute disproportion is especially high in women after pelvic fracture or with diseases that alter pelvic shape (osteochondroplasia, osteomalacia). In these cases, pelvimetry is mandatory.

References

1. Welsch H. Müttersterblichkeit (2004) In: Schneider H, Husslein P, Schneider KTM (eds) Die Geburtshilfe, 2nd edition. Springer-Verlag, Berlin Heidelberg New York
2. Angioli R, Gomez-Marin O, Cantuaria G, O›Sullivan JM (2000) Severe perineal lacerations during vaginal delivery: the University of Miami experience. Am J Obstet Gynecol 182:1083–1085
3. Friedman EA (1955) Primigravid labor. Obstet Gynecol 6:567–589
4. Friedman EA (1956) Labor in multiparae. Obstet Gynecol 8:691–703
5. Cardozo LD, Gibb DM, Studd JW et al. (1982) Predictive value of cervimetric labour patterns in primigravidae. Br J Obstet Gynaecol 82:33–38
6. Stark DD, McCarthy SM, Filly RA, Parer JT, Hricak H, Callen PW (1985) Pelvimetry by magnetic resonance imaging. AJR Am J Roentgenol 144:947–950
7. Pfammatter T, Marincek B, von Schulthess GK, Dudenhausen JW (1990) [MR pelvimetric reference values]. Rofo Fortschr Geb Rontgenstr Neuen Bildgeb Verfahr 153:706–710
8. Keller TM, Rake A, Michel SCA, Seifert B, Efe G, Treiber K, Huch R, Marincek B, Kubik-Huch R (2003) Obstetric MR pelvimetry: reference values and evaluation of inter- and intraobserver error and intraindividual variability. Radiology 227:37–43
9. Stewart A, Kneale GW (1968) Changes in the cancer risk associated with obstetric radiography. Lancet 1:104–107
10. Doll R, Wakeford R (1997) Risk of childhood cancer from fetal irradiation. Br J Radiol 70:130–139
11. Kanal E, Gillen J, Evans JA, Savitz DA, Shellock FG (1993) Survey of reproductive health among female MR workers. Radiology 187:395–399
12. Baker PN, Johnson IR, Harvey PR, Gowland PA, Mansfield P (1994) A three-year follow-up of children imaged in utero with echo-planar magnetic resonance. Am J Obstet Gynecol 170:32–33
13. Wright AR, English PT, Cameron HM, Wilsdon JB (1992) MR pelvimetry – a practical alternative. Acta Radiol 33:582–587
14. Wentz KU, Lehmann KJ, Wischnik A, et al. (1994) [Pelvimetry using various magnetic resonance tomography techniques vs. digital image enhancement radiography: accuracy, time requirement and energy exposure]. Geburtshilfe Frauenheilkd 54:204–212
15. Urhahn R, Lehnen H, Drobnitzky M, Klose KC, Gunther RW (1991) [Ultrafast pelvimetry using Snapshot-FLASH-MRT – a comparison with the Spinecho and FLASH techniques]. Rofo Fortschr Geb Rontgenstr Neuen Bildgeb Verfahr 155:432–435
16. Michel SC, Rake A, Treiber K, Seifert B, Chaoui R, Huch R, Marincek M, Kubik-Huch RA (2002) MR obstetric pelvime-

try: effect of birthing position on pelvic bony dimensions. AJR Am J Roentgenol 179:1063-1067

17. van Loon AJ, Mantingh A, Thijn CJ, Mooyaart EL (1990) Pelvimetry by magnetic resonance imaging in breech presentation. Am J Obstet Gynecol 163:1256–1260

18. Liselele HB, Boulvain M, Tshibangu KC, Meuris S (2000) Maternal height and external pelvimetry to predict cephalopelvic disproportion in nulliparous African women: a cohort study. Br J Obstet Gynecol 107:947–952

19. Pattinson RC, Farrell E (2005) Pelvimetry for fetal cephalic presentations at or near term. The Cochrane Library, vol. 2

20. Van Loon AJ, Mantingh A, Serlier EK, Kroon G, Mooyaart EL, Huisjes HJ (1997) Randomised controlled trial of magnetic-resonance pelvimetry in breech presentation at term. Lancet 350:1799-1804

21. Spörri S, Thoeny HC, Raio L, Lachat R, Vock P, Schneider H (2002) MR imaging pelvimetry: a useful adjunct in the treatment of women at risk for dystocia. AJR Am J Roentgenol 179:137–144

22. Fox LK, Huerta-Enochian GS, Hamlin JA, Katz VL (2004) The magnetic resonance imaging-based fetal-pelvic index: a pilot study in the community hospital. Am J Obstet Gynecol 190:1679–1688

23. O'Brien K, Rode M, Macones G (2002) Postpartum X-ray pelvimetry. Its use in calculating the fetal-pelvic index and predicting fetal-pelvic disproportion. J Reprod Med 47:845–848

24. Hannah ME, Hannah WJ, Hewson SA, et al. (2000) Planned caesarean section versus planned vaginal birth for breech presentation at term: a randomised multicentre trial. Term Breech Trial Collaborative Group. Lancet 356:1375–1483

Imaging of Lymph Nodes – MRI and CT

15

Matthias Taupitz

15.1
Background

In patients with cancer, the demonstration or exclusion of lymph node metastases is an important component of tumor staging besides evaluation of local tumor extent and has crucial implications for the patient's prognosis and therapeutic strategy, especially when deciding on curative versus palliative treatment. CT, with its limited contrast resolution, cannot differentiate metastasis from normal lymph node tissue. Unfortunately, MRI is also not able to distinguish between benign and malignant lymph

M. TAUPITZ, MD
Institut für Radiologie (Campus Mitte), Charité – Universitätsmedizin Berlin, Charitéplatz 1, 10117 Berlin, Germany

node enlargement despite its proverbial high soft tissue contrast. This limitation of MRI is due to the fact that lymphatic tissue and tumor have similar T1 and T2 relaxation times, as well as proton densities [3]. For these reasons, both CT and MRI rely on size as the only criterion for identifying metastatic lymph nodes. In general, a transverse diameter of 10 mm or greater is considered to indicate nodal metastasis. With currently available CT and MRI technology, it is not possible to identify metastases in lymph nodes of normal size. Although these limitations apply to both CT and MRI, MRI has some advantages over CT. These are not primarily due to the higher soft tissue contrast or the free selection of imaging planes but result from the superiority in local staging of pelvic tumors. It has been shown, for example, that in case of an early stage tumor the probability that lymph node metastases are present is very low, while a tumor invading beyond the organ is typically associated with lymph node metastases. For this reason, lymph node staging by MRI should always take into account the local tumor stage. Non-invasive lymph node imaging may be improved in the future by the use of a specific intravenous contrast agent on the basis of iron oxide nanoparticles [2, 6]. These agents have completed the clinical trial phase and are expected to be approved for clinical use in the near future.

15.2
Indications

There is no absolute indication for abdominal MRI or CT for lymph node imaging alone. Lymph node evaluation is always done in conjunction with imaging performed for the evaluation of the local tumor stage and metastatic spread in general.

What is discussed here, therefore, applies to those lymph node stations seen on MR or CT images acquired for diagnostic evaluation of a primary pelvic tumor. Of particular interest are gynecologic tumors of the true pelvis. Here, MRI is superior to CT for local tumor evaluation.

In the future, however, a lymphotrophic IV contrast agent might lead to new indications for MRI of the lymph nodes. As mentioned above, applications for clinical approval of such agents have been filed.

15.3
Technique

15.3.1
MRI

The body phased-array coils available today allow imaging of the entire abdomen with high resolution and should be used whenever available to assess retroperitoneal lymph nodes in addition to evaluating the regional pelvic lymph nodes in all MRI examinations of a primary pelvic tumor. In patients with cervical or endometrial cancer, the demonstration of suspicious retroperitoneal lymph nodes is important for therapeutic planning in patients scheduled for postoperative radiotherapy.

Transverse images enable good initial evaluation of abdominal and pelvic lymph nodes. These images may be supplemented by coronal images for evalua-

tion of the retroperitoneal lymph nodes or angulated coronal slices for lymph nodes along the external iliac vessels to assess their topographic relationship to the great vessels, but also to estimate the short-to-long axis ratio of the lymph nodes. Coronal slices are also highly suitable for assessing mesenteric and omental lymph nodes. Alternatively, slices in different orientations for lymph node assessment can be reconstructed from a 3D volume slab. In very rare cases it may become necessary to obtain double-angulated images for improved evaluation of a suspicious lymph node. What is important for lymph node imaging is to administer a spasmolytic agent to eliminate motion artifacts due to peristalsis (e.g. Buscopan or glucagon in patients with contraindications to Buscopan).

15.3.2
Pulse Sequences

Table 15.1 gives an overview of the sequences most suitable for lymph node assessment in different body regions (see also Chap. 1). As a rule, it is not necessary to obtain both T1- and T2-weighted images for identifying enlarged lymph nodes. Instead, choosing the sequence that provides the best anatomic detail resolution is recommended. Breath-hold imaging should be performed without fat suppression in order to achieve a high signal-to-noise ratio. When T2-weighted sequences with multiple signal averag-

Table 15.1. Pulse sequences recommended for MRI of abdominal lymph nodes. (Modified from [16])

Weighting	Plane	Sequence	TR (ms)	TE (ms)	Flip angle (°)	ETL (e.g.)	FS	Matrix ($N_{phase} \times N_{frequ}$)	FOV (mm)	N_{SL}	N_{AC}	SD (mm)	T_{AC} (min)	Breath-hold
PD/T1[a]	tra	TSE	~1500	10–15	–	3	No	228×512	320 (6/8)	23	3	8	about 5	no
T1 (fast)	tra (sag/cor)	GRE	165	4–5	90	–	Yes/no	128×256	320 (6/8)	19–23	1	8	0.3	yes
T2[b]	tra	TSE respiratory triggering	2500	80	–	7–15	Yes	168×320	300 (6/8)	48	2	4	5-7	no
T2 (fast)	tra (sag/cor)	single-shot TSE (e.g. HASTE), preset parameters						128×256	320 (6/8)	21	1	8	0.3	yes

Interslice gap always 20% of slice thickness (distance factor, 0.2).
Note: A body phased-array coil is recommended for acquisition of high-resolution TSE/FSE sequences and breath-hold sequences.
[a]Recommended for high-resolution imaging of pelvic lymph nodes (with administration of spasmolytic agent)
[b]Recommended for high-resolution imaging of retroperitoneal lymph nodes (with administration of spasmolytic agent)

ing are used, fat suppression (either spectral saturation or inversion prepulse) improves the demarcation of lymph nodes by depicting them with high signal intensity. For imaging of the female pelvis, a high-resolution T1- or proton density-weighted sequence should be acquired extending from the region of the aortic bifurcation to the pelvic floor, which will allow excellent evaluation of the pelvic lymph nodes when the sequence is obtained with administration of a spasmolytic agent. If available, the sequence should be acquired as a fast or turbo SE sequence with a rather short effective echo time (about 10–15 ms). Additional T1- or T2-weighted transverse images, preferably acquired during breath-hold, typically allow good evaluation of enlarged retroperitoneal lymph nodes (T1w GRE, T2w single-shot TSE, both during breath-hold). Alternatively, T2-weighted sequences with respiratory triggering (e.g. respiratory belt or cushion, navigator imaging [9]) in combination with spasmolysis provide images of the upper and middle abdomen with excellent image quality and good detail resolution. Additional imaging in coronal or sagittal planes should ideally be performed using sequences that can be acquired during breath-hold, which are not only faster but also provide an adequate image quality in coronal orientation, which is highly susceptible to degradation by motion artifacts when acquisition times are long (e.g. T1w GRE, T2w single-shot TSE).

15.3.3
Intravenous Unspecific Contrast Agents

There is no indication for administration of an unspecific Gd-based MR contrast agent with distribution in the extracellular space (e.g. Magnevist or Omniscan) for lymph node imaging. However, on T1w images, an unspecific contrast agent can improve the differentiation of lymph nodes from vessels. If an IV contrast agent is administered for evaluation of the primary tumor, necrosis in metastatic lymph nodes may be seen better.

15.3.4
Intravenous Tissue-Specific Contrast Agents

Tissue-specific contrast agents with accumulation in healthy lymph node tissue have been extensively investigated in clinical trials but still await approval for clinical use (Sinerem, Guerbet, Paris). This is why

only an outlook can be given here. Tissue-specific contrast agents are based on very small superparamagnetic iron oxide nanoparticles with a diameter of about 20 nm (ultrasmall superparamagnetic iron oxide particles – USPIO). Following peripheral venous administration, they extravasate from the capillary vascular bed into the interstitial spaces in all body regions and reach the draining nodes with the lymphatic fluid [12, 14, 15]. In intact lymph nodes, USPIO are taken up by macrophages and their strong T2-relaxation-time-shortening effect produces a signal loss that is best appreciated on T2*w GRE sequences. Metastatic lymph nodes do not accumulate the particles and hence show unchanged signal intensity. Once USPIO-based preparations have been approved and ongoing analysis of clinical trials confirm available results, these agents will be indicated for MRI of abdominal and pelvic lymph nodes, and there will be an indication for MRI in the diagnostic evaluation of lymph nodes.

15.3.5
CT

There are no specific technical requirements for CT of the lymph nodes. The reader is referred to the protocols presented in Chapter 1.

15.4
Imaging of Normal Lymph Nodes – MRI/CT

With conventional MR imaging techniques, lymph nodes are visualized when they have a size of at least 1.0–1.5 cm [10]. Optimized imaging techniques (body phased-array coil, 512 matrix, 3D acquisition) or state-of-the-art spiral or multislice CT scanners depict lymph nodes as small at about 3–5 mm [7, 8]. These techniques usually allow good evaluation of the lymph nodes adjacent to the straight great vessels (Fig. 15.1).

Nonactivated lymph nodes or lymph nodes not enlarged by metastasis have a mean diameter of only a few millimeters (abdominal lymph nodes 3–5 mm, pelvic lymph nodes about 3 mm, determined by CT [4, 13]) and are usually not visualized on MR images. If they are seen, normal lymph nodes are markedly hypointense relative to surrounding fat on T1-weighted images, moderately

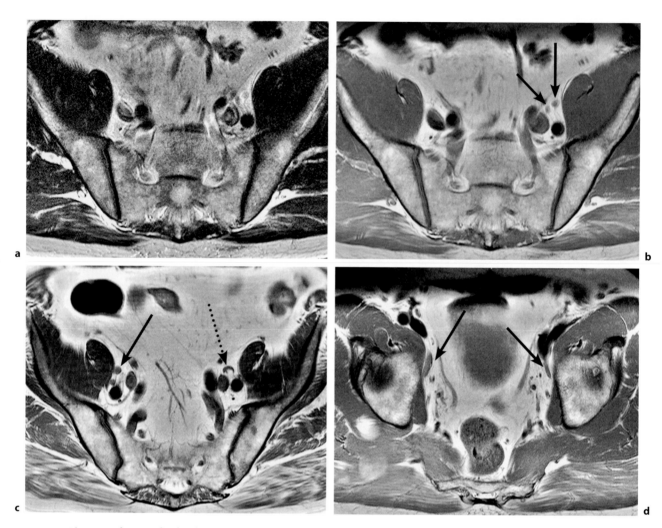

Fig. 15.1a–d. Normal pelvic lymph nodes. Axial MR images acquired with (**a**) T2w TSE sequence and (**b-c**) T1w TSE sequence at different levels (**a** and **b** are from the same level) (1.5 T). Small lymph nodes with a rounded appearance (**a–c**, *straight arrows* in **b** and **c**) are seen. They have low signal intensity on T1 and are nearly isointense to surrounding fat on T2. In addition, a lymph node on the left (*curved arrow*) is depicted with good visualization of the fatty hilus (fibrolipomatous degeneration, *dotted arrow* in **c**). Elongated lymph nodes on both sides at the pelvic wall (*arrows*, **d**)

hypointense on PD images, and isointense to fat or slightly hyperintense on T2-weighted images. At times, the fatty hilus can be differentiated from the stroma in a normal lymph node (Fig. 15.1c). Typical retroperitoneal lymph nodes are oval, while lymph nodes along the pelvic walls (internal iliac nodes, obturator nodes) may appear as elongated structures several centimeters in length (Fig. 15.1d). A schematic representation for referring to the different abdominal and pelvic lymph node stations is presented in Figure 15.2.

In the pelvic region, lymph nodes may be difficult to distinguish from elongated iliac vessels on nonan-

gulated axial images. This applies especially to T1w images, which depict both lymph nodes and vessels with low signal intensity. Differentiation is improved after intravenous contrast administration. On TSE images, vessels have low signal intensity. The differentiation between vessels and lymph nodes is optimal on PDw sequences which depict vessels as signal voids and lymph nodes with intermediate signal (compare Fig 15.1).

In patients without a known primary tumor, lymph nodes with a transverse diameter of 5–10 mm should be mentioned in the report without comment as their size is above the mean value for "normal"

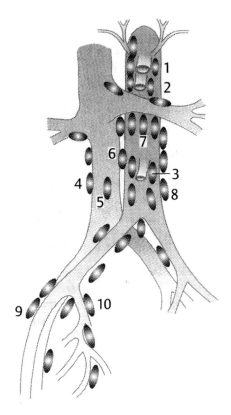

Fig. 15.2. Retroperitoneal lymph nodes. *1*, coelical lymph nodes; *2* and *3*, mesenterial lymph nodes; *4*, paracaval lymph nodes; *5*, precaval lymph nodes; *6*, interaortocaval lymph nodes; *7*, preaortic lymph nodes; *8*, paraaortic lymph nodes; *9*, external iliac lymph nodes; *10*, internal iliac lymph nodes

lymph nodes [1, 4, 13]. In general, lymph nodes with a transverse diameter of 10 mm or greater are considered suspicious for metastasis.

15.5
Imaging of Abnormal Lymph Nodes – MRI/CT

For lymph node staging, the reader should consult one of a standard reference (e.g. [11]). In general, the lymph node stage determined from MRI or CT findings plays only a small role in therapeutic decision making. If imaging demonstrates enlarged lymph nodes at sites that do not correspond to the first site of lymphatic spread of the patient's primary tumor, this is an important finding because

these lymph nodes should then be removed, not least for histologic examination.

Most abdominal tumors initially metastasize along the draining lymphatic pathways, first invading the regional nodes and later also the distal lymph node stations. Rarely, metastatic occlusion of lymphatic drainage can give rise to an atypical pattern of metastatic spread with primary distal or contralateral lymph node metastases. Pelvic tumors (uterus, cervix, upper third of vagina, urinary bladder) typically first spread to the lymph nodes of the pelvic wall (obturator nodes, external and internal iliac nodes). In patients with a primary tumor in one of these locations which is confined to the organ or appears as an early-stage tumor on MR imaging, visible but not pathologically enlarged lymph nodes (5–10 mm) are typically not considered suspicious. If, however, the primary tumor invades adjacent structures, such slight lymph node sizes can be considered suspicious for metastasis (Figs. 15.3–15.7).

When images in axial and coronal or sagittal planes are available, the radiologist can assess the configuration of enlarged lymph nodes. Nodal metastasis is more likely when an enlarged lymph node has a spherical shape. In X-ray lymphography this phenomenon is referred to as spherical transformation. In contrast, reactive hyperplasia is more likely when an enlarged lymph node has an elongated oval shape. The use of high-resolution 3D pulse sequences improves the evaluation of individual lymph nodes compared to conventional 2D sequences and makes it easier to measure the short and long axes and determine the short-to-long axis ratio (S/L ratio). Using a 3D MP RAGE sequence with a voxel size of 1.0×1.3×1.6 mm, JAGER and coworkers [8] were able to identify pelvic lymph nodes as small as 3 mm. In this study, the authors used a short axis diameter greater than 8 mm and an S/L ratio of over 0.8 (rounded lymph node) as criteria for malignancy. However, despite optimal morphologic resolution, the sensitivity for detecting metastatic nodes was only 60% (prostate cancer) and 83% (bladder cancer), while specificity was high at 98% for both tumors. In a study of pelvic lymph nodes in patients with cervical cancer, MRI had a sensitivity of 75% and specificity of 88% using a threshold of 1.5 cm for pelvic lymph nodes. Even lateral differences in the size of pelvic lymph nodes are not a reliable criterion as long as the lymph nodes are less than 10 mm in diameter [10]. The poor sensitivities are due to the fact that

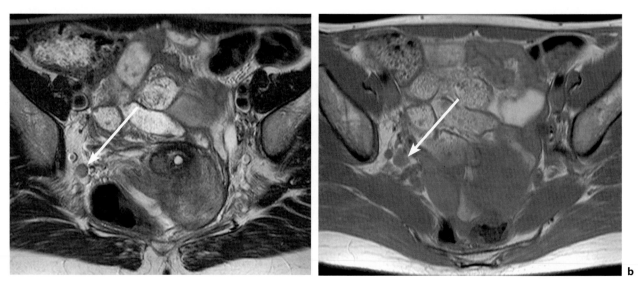

Fig. 15.3a,b. Slightly enlarged metastatic lymph node in the area of the internal iliac artery (*arrow*). Axial images obtained with (**a**) T2w TSE sequence and (**b**) T1w TSE sequence in a patient with advanced cervical cancer

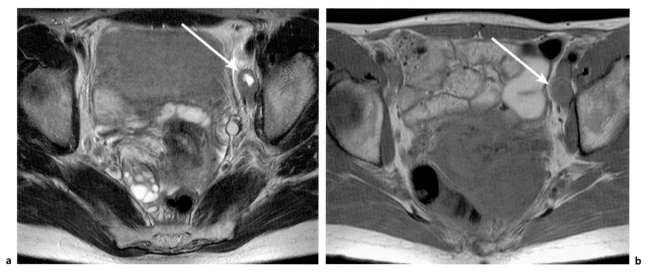

Fig. 15.4a,b. Abnormally enlarged metastatic lymph node on the left immediately posterior to the external iliac vein (*arrow*). Axial images obtained with (**a**) T2w TSE sequence and (**b**) T1w TSE sequence in a patient with advanced cervical cancer. The T2w image depicts the central necrosis with fluid signal intensity

the size criterion is rather unspecific because small metastases in normal-sized lymph nodes are quite common and nonmetastatic lymph nodes may show reactive enlargement. A histopathologic study of 310 pelvic lymphadenectomies identified lymph node metastases in 40 patients (12.9%) [5]. The nodal metastases were apparent on gross inspection in only six cases, while only histology identified the metastases in the other 34 cases.

Another major factor contributing to the poor performance of MRI in lymph node assessment is the fact that the signal intensities of lymph nodes on either T1- or T2-weighted images do not allow differentiation of normal and metastatic lymph nodes [3]. Both reactively enlarged nodes and metastatic nodes have low signal intensity on T1 and high signal intensity on T2 relative to surrounding fatty tissue. More reliable criteria are only avail-

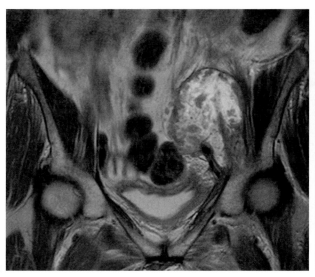 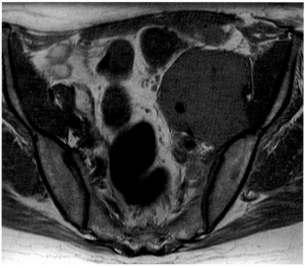

a   b

Fig. 15.5a,b. Large lymph node metastasis at the left pelvic wall with encasement of the external iliac vessels. (**a**) Coronal T2w TSE image and (**b**) axial T1w TSE image in a patient with advanced cervical cancer

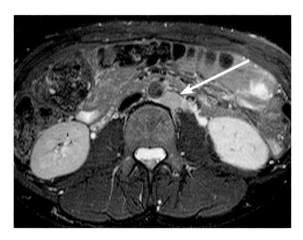

Fig. 15.6. Retroperitoneal (para-aortic) lymph node metastasis in a patient with endometrial cancer (*arrow*). Axial T2w TSE image obtained with respiratory triggering using the navigator technique

15.5.1
Contrast Administration

The standard unspecific contrast agents used in MRI and CT lead to an increase in signal intensity or density of both reactively enlarged and metastatic lymph nodes following IV administration and do not improve the differentiation of reactive and metastatic nodes [7]. The visualization of central necrosis in a metastatic node is improved after contrast administration.

Superparamagnetic iron oxide particles, on the other hand, are a promising new approach for improving MR imaging of lymph nodes (Fig 14.8). One USPIO preparation (Sinerem – Guerbet, Paris) has been investigated for lymph node imaging in different body regions (pelvis, abdomen, mediastinum, head and neck, axilla). Final analysis of these studies is under way, and approval for clinical application is expected in the near future. In a study of 58 patients with urinary bladder cancer, DESERNO and coworkers showed that USPIO improved sensitivity to 96% compared with 76% for the size criterion, while specificity decreased only slightly from 99% to 95% [2]. It is noteworthy that MRI in this study demonstrated metastases in 10 of 12 lymph nodes that were not enlarged (< 10 mm). In a study of patients with prostate cancer, HARISINGHANI and coworkers showed that USPIO-enhanced MRI had a sensitivity of 90% compared to 35% for the size criterion when analyzing individual lymph nodes [6].

able for advanced nodal metastasis, for example, central necrosis, which is clearly identified as a hyperintensity within a metastatic node on T2-weighted images. Moreover, lymph node conglomeration and multiple enlarged lymph nodes are highly indicative of nodal metastasis, especially in patients with a primary known to metastasize to the affected nodes.

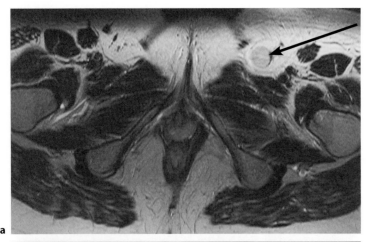

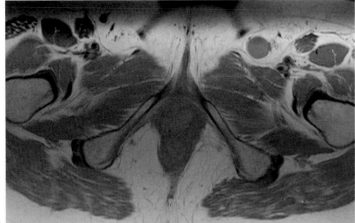

Fig. 15.7a,b. Abnormally enlarged metastatic inguinal lymph node on the left (*arrow*). Axial images obtained with (**a**) T2w TSE sequence and (**b**) T1w TSE sequence in a patient with vulvar cancer

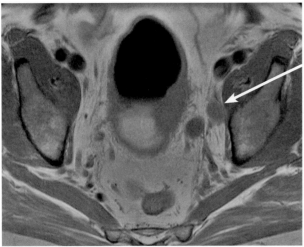

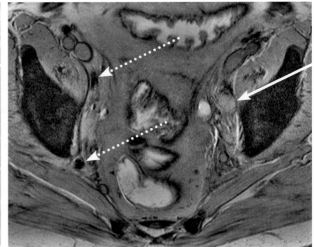

Fig. 15.8a,b. MR lymphography following intravenous administration of ultrasmall iron oxide particles (USPIO) in a patient with metastatic lymph nodes. Axial images obtained with (**a**) T1w SE sequence and (**b**) T2*w GRE sequence 24 h after intravenous injection of USPIO. Slightly enlarged lymph node at the left pelvic wall (*arrow*) with muscle signal intensity on T1 and unchanged signal on USPIO-enhanced image indicating nodal metastasis, which prevents uptake of the particles. Widening of the distal ureter due to infiltration of the left ureteral orifice. In nonmetastatic pelvic lymph nodes homogeneous signal due to contrast agent uptake of on the right (*dotted arrows*). (USPIO for MR lymphography are at the clinical trial stage)

References

1. Delorme S, van Kaick G (1996) Imaging of abdominal nodal spread in malignant disease. Eur Radiol 6:262–274
2. Deserno WM, Harisinghani MG, Taupitz M, Jager GJ, Witjes JA, Mulders PF, Hulsbergen Van De Kaa CA, Kaufmann D, Barentsz JO (2004) Urinary bladder cancer: preoperative nodal staging with Ferumoxtran-10-enhanced MR Imaging. Radiology
3. Dooms GC, Hricak H, Moseley ME, Bottles K, Fisher M, Higgins CB (1985) Characterization of lymphadenopathy by magnetic resonance relaxation times: preliminary results. Radiology 155:691–697
4. Dorfman RE, Alpern MB, Gross BH, Sandler MA (1991) Upper abdominal lymph nodes: criteria for normal size determined with CT. Radiology 180:319–322
5. Epstein JI, Oesterling JE, Eggleston JC, Walsh PC (1986) Frozen section detection of lymph node metastases in prostatic carcinoma: accuracy in grossly uninvolved pelvic lymphadenectomy specimens. J Urol 136:1234–1237
6. Harisinghani MG, Barentsz J, Hahn PF, Deserno WM, Tabatabaei S, van de Kaa CH, de la Rosette J, Weissleder R (2003) Noninvasive detection of clinically occult lymph-node metastases in prostate cancer. N Engl J Med 348:2491–2499
7. Heuck A, Scheidler J, Kimmig R, Muller Lisse U, Steinborn M, Helmberger T, Reiser M (1997) Lymphknotenstaging beim Zervixkarzinom: Ergebnisse der hochauflosenden Magnetresonanztomographie (MRT) mit einer Phased-Array-Körperspule. Fortschr Röntgenstr 166:210–214
8. Jager GJ, Barentsz JO, Oosterhof GO, Witjes JA, Ruijs SJ (1996) Pelvic adenopathy in prostatic and urinary bladder carcinoma: MR imaging with a three-dimensional TI-weighted magnetization-prepared-rapid gradient-echo sequence. Am J Roentgenol 167:1503–1507
9. Klessen C, Asbach P, Kroencke TJ, Fischer T, Warmuth C, Stemmer A, Hamm B, Taupitz M (2005) Magnetic resonance imaging of the upper abdomen using a free-breathing T2-weighted turbo spin echo sequence with navigator triggered prospective acquisition correction. J Magn Reson Imaging 21:576–582
10. Roy C, Le Bras Y, Mangold L, Saussine C, Tuchmann C, Pfleger D, Jacqmin D (1997) Small pelvic lymph node metastases: evaluation with MR imaging. Clin Radiol 52:437–440
11. Sobin LH, WC, (eds) (2002) TNM classification of malignant tumours. Wiley, 2002
12. Taupitz M, Wagner S, Hamm B (1996) Kontrastmittel für die magnetresonanztomographische Lymphknotendiagnostik (MR-Lymphographie). Radiologe 36:134–140
13. Vinnicombe SJ, Norman AR, Nicolson V, Husband JE (1995) Normal pelvic lymph nodes: evaluation with CT after bipedal lymphangiography. Radiology 194:349–355
14. Wagner S, Pfefferer D, Ebert W, Kresse M, Taupitz M, Hamm B, Lawaczeck R, Wolf K (1995) Intravenous MR lymphography with superparamagnetic iron oxide particles: experimental studies in rats and rabbits. Eur Radiol 5:640–646
15. Weissleder R, Elizondo G, Wittenberg J, Lee AS, Josephson L, Brady TJ (1990) Ultrasmall superparamagnetic iron oxide: an intravenous contrast agent for assessing lymph nodes with MR imaging. Radiology 175:494–498
16. Leppert A (1998) Lymphknoten. In: Galanski M, Prokop M (eds) Ganzkörper-Computertomographie. Thieme, Stuttgart

Evaluation of Infertility

16

Gertraud Heinz-Peer

G. Heinz-Peer, MD
Department of Radiology, Medical University of Vienna,
Währinger Gürtel 18–20, 1090 Vienna, Austria

16.1
Introduction

Infertility is defined as 1 year of unprotected intercourse that does not result in pregnancy [1]. Infertility is estimated to affect up to 10% of women of reproductive age [2]. Although uterine pathology accounts for less than 10% of cases, uterine imaging is important not only for establishing a specific diagnosis, but also for directing corrective therapy [3, 4]. Knowledge of structural abnormalities may indicate potential pregnancy complications including spontaneous abortion, intrauterine growth retardation, preterm delivery, malpresentation, and retained products of conception.

An imaging study to evaluate female infertility and uterine anomalies should necessarily exhibit many characteristics, such as a noninvasive nature, low cost, and high accuracy, among other qualities. Imaging modalities currently used to evaluate infertile women include hysterosalpingography, ultrasound, and magnetic resonance imaging. In this chapter, the use of these modalities to assess the various causes of infertility in females will be reviewed and specific attention will be drawn to anatomic and physiologic uterine abnormalities.

16.2
Imaging Techniques

16.2.1
Hysterosalpingography

Hysterosalpingography (HSG) uses fluoroscopic control to introduce radiographic contrast material into the uterine cavity and fallopian tubes. While today HSG is used primarily to assess tubal patency, this technique also provides indirect evidence for uterine pathology through depiction of abnormal uterine cavity contours.

16.2.1.1
Cycle Considerations

HSG should not be performed if there is a possibility of a normal intrauterine pregnancy. To avoid irradiating an early pregnancy, the "10-day rule" can be used. That means the procedure should not be performed if the interval of time from the start of the last menses is greater than 10–12 days. If the patient has cycles that are longer than 28 days (menses start usually 14 days after ovulation), the 10-day rule can be stretched to 13–15 days. If the patient has irregular cycles or absent menses, a pregnancy test before performing HSG is recommended.

16.2.1.2
Technical Considerations

The patient is placed supine with her knees flexed and heels apart. Stirrups on the table to support the feet can be used. The cervix is exposed with a speculum. Visualization of the cervix may be helped by elevating the patient's pelvis, particularly in thin women. The cervix and vagina are copiously swabbed with a cleansing solution such as Betadine and the HSG cannula is placed. A variety of cannulas can be used for HSG [5–7]. Once correct placement of the cannula is confirmed, the speculum should be removed. Leaving the speculum in is uncomfortable for the patient and a metal speculum obscures findings. Using fluoroscopic guidance, contrast agent at room temperature is slowly injected, usually 5–10 ml over 1 min, and radiographs are obtained. Injection of contrast agent is halted when adequate free spill into the peritoneal cavity is documented, when myometrial or venous intravasation occurs, or when the patient complains of increased cramping, which usually occurs when the tubes are blocked.

16.2.1.3
Side Effects and Complications

Mild discomfort or pain is commonly experienced by women undergoing HSG [8]. Routine analgesia is not necessary, although oral ibuprofen is a reasonable preprocedure medication. Reassurance and rapid and skillful completion of the examination are the best approach. Mild vaginal bleeding is common after HSG. Severe bleeding requiring curettage is unusual

and is presumably related to underlying pathology such as endometrial polyps. Other side effects such as vasovagal reactions and hyperventilation may occur and their prevalence may be reduced if the examiner is experienced and calming.

Pelvic infection is a serious complication of HSG, causing tubal damage. In a private practice setting, the overall incidence of post-HSG pelvic infection was 1.4%, occurring predominantly in women with dilated tubes [9]. For this reason, if dilated tubes are noted during the HSG procedure, particularly if there is a dilated tube with free spill, prophylactic antibiotics (e.g., doxycycline 200 mg orally) should be given before the patient leaves the department and a prescription for 5 days should be given to the patient.

An allergic or idiosyncratic reaction related to the contrast medium can occur after HSG, although the incidence is unknown and is presumably quite low.

Radiation exposure is a side effect not shared by sono-HSG. It is a concern, because the women being examined are of reproductive age. The incidence of irradiating an early pregnancy is quite low when HSG is routinely performed in the follicular phase of the cycle. Although cases are few, there is nothing to suggest that inadvertent performance of HSG in early pregnancy is harmful to the fetus [10]. Radiation exposure to the ovaries is minimal and can be further reduced by using good fluoroscopic technique and obtaining only the number of radiographs necessary to make an accurate diagnosis.

16.2.1.4
Anatomy and Physiology of Fallopian Tubes

The fallopian tubes connect the peritoneal cavity to the extraperitoneal world. Their function and anatomy is complex and includes conduction of sperm from the uterine end toward the ampulla, conduction of ova in the other direction from the fimbriated end to the ampulla, and support as well as conduction of the early embryo from the ampulla into the uterus for implantation. The normal fallopian tube ranges in length from 7 cm to 16 cm, with an average length of 12 cm (Fig. 16.1a). The tube is divided into four regions: (a) the intramural or interstitial portion, in the wall of the uterine fundus and 1 cm to 2 cm long, (b) the isthmic portion, which is about 2–3 cm long, (c) the ampullary portion, 5–8 cm long, and (d) the infundibulum, which is the trumpet-shaped distal end of the tube terminating in the fimbria. Patency of the fallopian tubes is established when contrast

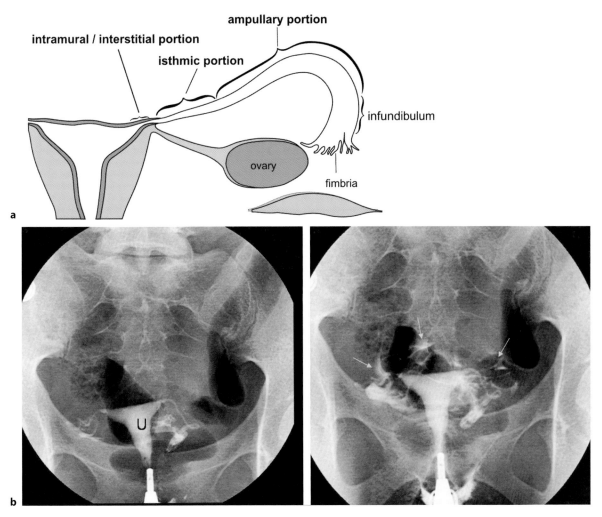

Fig. 16.1. a Scheme of normal fallopian tubes. The normal fallopian tube ranges in length from 7–16 cm (average, 12 cm). The tube is divided into four regions: (I) intramural or interstitial portion (1–2 cm), (II) isthmic portion, (2–3 cm), (III) ampullary portion (5–8 cm), and (IV) infundibulum terminating into the fimbria. **b** Normal hysterosalpingogram. The uterus (*U*) has a normal contour and shape. The fallopian tubes fill bilaterally with evidence of free spill into the pelvic peritoneum (*arrows*)

medium flows through them and freely around the ovary and loops of bowel at the time of salpingography, using either fluoroscopic or sonographic guidance (Fig. 16.1b).

16.2.1.5
Pathological Findings

Diverticula in the isthmic segment of the tube are caused by salpingitis isthmica nodosa (SIN) (Fig. 16.2). These would be difficult to appreciate by sonography. SIN was described more than 100 years ago as irregular benign extensions of the tubal epithelium into the myosalpinx, associated with reactive myohypertrophia and sometimes inflammation. There is an association between SIN and pelvic inflammatory disease; however, it is not clear whether SIN is caused by pelvic inflammation or is congenital and predisposes to inflammation.

Obstruction of the tubes can occur anywhere along their length (Fig. 16.3). Obstruction of the midisthmic portion may be missed by sonography, because of the small caliber of the tube and the absence of dilation when there is obstruction at this level.

Polyps are small, smooth, filling defects, which can be single or multiple, and do not distort the overall size and shape of the uterine cavity (Fig. 16.4). Leiomyomas are usually single, larger lobulated masses, which only partially project into the cavity, and often enlarge and distort the cavity (Fig. 16.5).

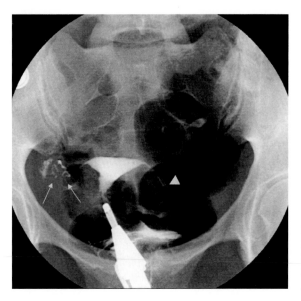

Fig. 16.2. Salpingitis isthmica nodosa: Multiple tiny diverticula in the right isthmic portion (*arrows*) caused by mucosal proliferation and muscular hypertrophy with mucosal invasion into the muscularis; partial tubectomy on the left side (*arrow head*)

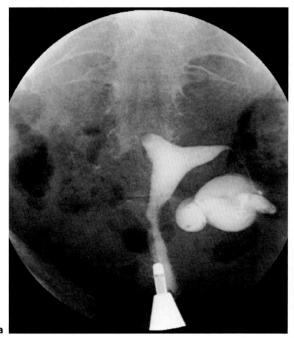

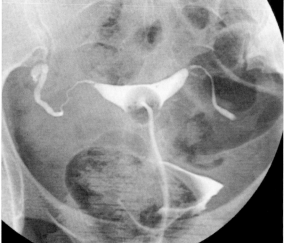

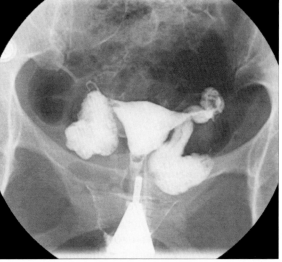

Fig. 16.3a–c. Bilateral fallopian tube obstruction (three different patients). There is dilated, obstructed tube on the left (hydrosalpinx) and obstruction of the right intramural portion (**a**), nondilated obstruction on both sides at the isthmic/ampullary portion (**b**), and huge bilateral dilatation without spill into the peritoneum–bilateral hydrosalpinx (**c**)

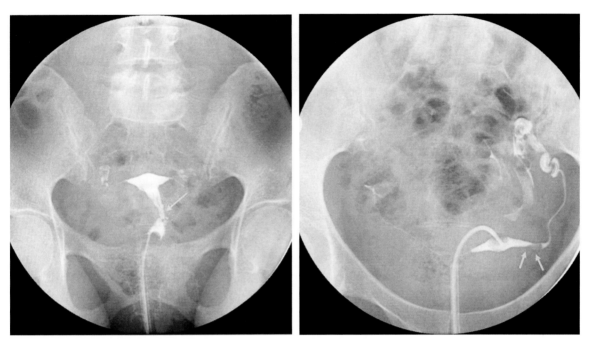

Fig. 16.4a,b. Endometrial polyps. Stalked filling defect within the endometrial cavity probably arising from the cervical canal (*arrow*). Note normal filling of the fallopian tubes and free spill into the peritoneum (**a**). In a different patient, the hysterosalpingogram shows a filling defect in the intramural portion of the left tube (*arrows*) causing narrowing but no obstruction; normal filling of the fallopian tubes (**b**)

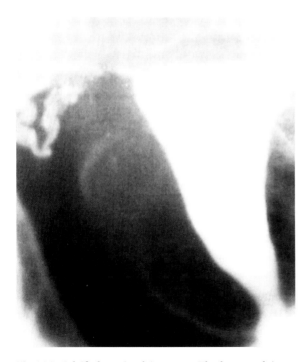

Fig. 16.5. Calcified uterine leiomyoma. The hysterosalpingogram shows that the uterine cavity is compressed and enlarged by a large partially calcified mass

Synechiae are scars that result from uterine trauma such as complications of pregnancy, curettage, uterine surgery, or uterine infection. Synechiae are generally linear and irregular (Fig. 16.6a) and extend from one wall to the opposite wall allowing contrast agent to flow around them only in one dimension. For this reason, they are more easily defined than the above mentioned masses, which in general allow contrast agent to flow around them in two dimensions. Synechiae may also manifest as absence of filling of the entire uterus or part of it, and can be confused with a müllerian defect (Fig. 16.6b)

Asherman syndrome is defined by the combination of infertility, hypomenorrhea or amenorrhea, and a history of uterine curettage. It is estimated to occur in 68% of infertile women who have undergone two or more curettages [11]. The pathophysiology consists of intrauterine adhesions (synechiae) that develop after traumatic endometrial injury, such as postpartum or postabortion uterine curettage. Less commonly, it results from endometritis [12]. It is hypothesized that infertility occurs because uterine adhesions and scarring interfere with sperm migration and embryo implantation.

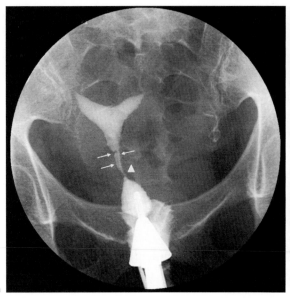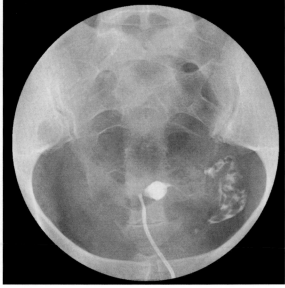

Fig. 16.6a,b. Synechiae. On hysterosalpingogram, irregular borders (*arrows*) and narrowing of the cervical canal (*arrowhead*) are depicted (**a**). In a different patient, HSG shows synechiae causing partial obstruction of the endometrial cavity and occlusion of the right fallopian tube (**b**). Note: HSG may not rule out müllerian duct anomaly with certainty in this particular case

16.2.1.6
Limitations of HSG

HSG should not be performed when there is active vaginal bleeding. This is to prevent the flushing of clots into the peritoneal cavity. HSG should also not be performed if there is active pelvic infection, because it could exacerbate the infection. The procedure should not be performed within 6 weeks of pregnancy, uterine surgery, tubal surgery, or uterine curettage because the defects in the endometrial or tubal lining predispose to venous intravasation of contrast material. The major limitations of the procedure are the ability to characterize only patent canals and the inability to evaluate the external uterine contour adequately. HSG also entails exposure to ionizing radiation in these typically young women.

16.2.2
Sonohysterography and Sonohysterosalpingography

Sonography is frequently used to evaluate uterine pathology because of its excellent diagnostic accuracy, minimal patient discomfort, low cost, and widespread availability. With the addition of transvaginal sonography, color Doppler imaging, and sonohys-terography, ultrasound has become a sensitive technique for detecting endometrial and myometrial pathology.

Sonosalpingography (SSG) is a technique that uses transvaginal sonography to evaluate tubal patency and morphology. It involves the use of either saline and/or contrast medium for assessment of tubal patency.

16.2.2.1
Cycle Considerations

Sonography should be performed during the secretory phase of the menstrual cycle, when the endometrial thickness and echo complex are better characterized [13] (Fig. 16.7a). However, for congenital anomaly evaluation, the timing of the sonography examination is not critical (Fig. 16.7b). For SSG, cycle considerations of conventional HSG should be considered.

16.2.2.2
Technical Considerations

Imaging should not only focus on conventional sagittal and transverse imaging of the pelvis but also include orthogonal images along the long axis of the uterus to characterize the external uterine contour. Transabdominal ultrasound is usually best performed with a 2- to 6-MHz transducer. Transvaginal ultrasound should be performed with an 5- to 8-MHz transducer. Transvaginal sonography has the advantage of improved spatial resolution, although at the expense of a decreased field of view.

SSG utilizes transvaginal sonography during instillation of either saline or contrast medium into the uterine lumen. It is best performed after sonohysterography, since sonohysterography is vital in delineating the endometrial surfaces for presence of synechiae or intraluminal lesions such as polyps or submucosal fibroids.

The examiner is encouraged to apply gentle pressure with the probe while sonographically assessing the mobility of the uterus, ovary, and tube.

Saline can be used initially for assessment of tubal patency. However, if there is any doubt about tubal spill, contrast should be used. It is necessary to have a ballooned catheter to block egress of fluid from the uterine lumen during injection. After sonohysterography has been performed, the saline should be removed prior to instillation of positive contrast.

Some investigators advocate the use of color Doppler sonography with saline instillation in order to best depict tubal patency [14–16]. This technique can also be used with contrast.

Microbubble contrast agents provide an echogenic contrast to document tubal patency and spillage. The safety of this contrast agent has been established in multiple studies, but its cost makes selected use necessary.

If there is pain during injection, this may be sign of tubal obstruction, either intrinsic or extrinsic from adhesions. Spasm may be present and may cause transitory lack of filling of the proximal portion of the tube

16.2.2.2.1
Normal and Abnormal Anatomy

With the use of saline or contrast, the normal tubal lumen is easily identified as thin serpentine adnexal structures.

Hydrosalpinges appear as fusiform cystic structures on TVS. The contrast may dilute or bubbles may come out of suspension, making complete delineation difficult to recognize.

16.2.2.3
Accuracy

Sonography has a reported accuracy of approximately 90%–92% [13–15]. SSG, with infusion of saline into the endometrial canal, provides improved delineation of the endometrium and internal uterine morphology. Three-dimensional ultrasound with surface- and transparent-mode reconstructions of the uterus has reported advantages over conventional two-dimensional scanning. In experienced hands, a sensitivity of 93% and a specificity of 100% have been achieved [16].

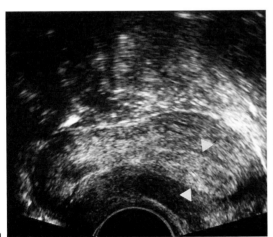
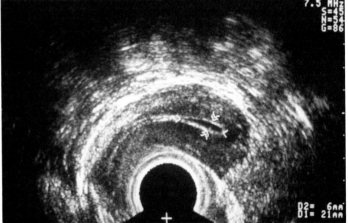

Fig. 16.7a,b. Normal TVUS. Clear demarcation of the relatively thick and hyperechoic endometrium (*arrowheads*) during the secretory phase (**a**), minimal fluid retention during the proliferation phase of the cycle (**b**)

16.2.2.4
Side Effects and Complications

The side effects and complications of sono-HSG are for the most part the same as for conventional HSG.

16.2.2.5
Limitations of Sono-HSG

Sono-HSG shares limitations similar to those of conventional transvaginal ultrasound and can only help evaluate patent endometrial canals [17].

The major drawback of this modality is its operator dependency. Additional limitations include factors that contribute to an unfavorable ultrasound image, such as a large body habitus and/or the presence of large fibroids (Fig. 16.8).

16.2.3
Magnetic Resonance Imaging

16.2.3.1
Indications

Magnetic resonance (MR) imaging is suitable for assessing female infertility, as infertility typically results from benign processes in women of reproductive age. The causes of female infertility include ovulatory disorders (i.e., pituitary adenoma and polycystic ovarian syndrome), disorders of the fallopian tubes (i.e., hydrosalpinx and pelvic inflammatory disease), uterine disorders (i.e., müllerian duct anomaly, adenomyosis, and leiomyoma), and pelvic endometriosis.

The applications of MR imaging include evaluation of the functioning uterus and ovaries, visualization of pituitary adenomas, differentiation of müllerian duct anomalies, and accurate noninvasive diagnosis of adenomyosis, leiomyoma, and endometriosis. In addition, MR imaging helps predict the outcome of conservative treatment for adenomyosis, leiomyoma, and endometriosis and may lead to selection of better treatment plans and management.

MR imaging provides clear delineation of internal and external uterine anatomy in multiple imaging planes, although it is not able to assess tubal patency or subtle, peritubular adhesion. The excellent tissue contrast of MR imaging allows specific diagnosis for many gynecological diseases.

As laparoscopic surgery is frequently the modality of choice to treat patients suffering from infertility, an accurate preoperative diagnosis is especially important for planning appropriate surgical intervention.

16.2.3.2
Technical Considerations

Patients are best imaged with a phased array MR surface coil. Current standard imaging protocols for infertility evaluation include axial, sagittal, and coronal fast spin echo sequence images of the uterus, which can be supplemented by oblique views to obtain true coronal and axial images of the uterus. Large field of view images to look for associated renal anomalies should be obtained. Further imaging of the pelvis with a transverse T1-weighted sequence should be performed. Gd-enhanced MR imaging is important for diagnosis of complex adn-

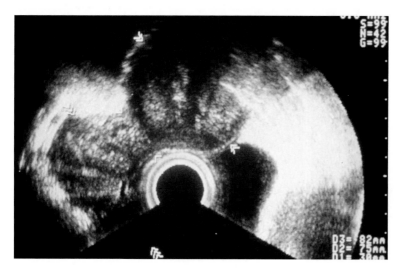

Fig. 16.8. TVUS. Unfavorable ultrasound image caused by a large fibroid

exal masses and distinguishing them from malignant processes.

Some authors recommend that an antiperistaltic (1 unit of glucagons or 20 mg of scopolamine butylbromide) be administered intramuscularly or intravenously before examination.

16.2.3.3
Limitations

As drawbacks of MRI are its higher cost, limited availability, and longer scanning time than ultrasound, MR imaging is often used as a problem solving modality when sonography findings are inconclusive [14, 18].

16.2.3.4
Normal MR Anatomy in Reproductive-Age Women

Uterine zonal anatomy is best demonstrated on T2-weighted images (Fig. 16.9). The endometrium has high signal intensity. The junctional zone, which corresponds to the innermost myometrium, appears as a band of low signal intensity. The peripheral myometrium has intermediate signal intensity that is higher than that of the striated muscle. The width of the endometrium and the junctional zone vary through the menstrual cycle; they are widest and most clearly visible in the late secretory phase. The uterine corpus is larger than the cervix throughout the reproductive-age period. In general the corpus measures 6–8 cm in length by 5–6 cm in transverse and anteroposterior dimensions [19].

The cervix also shows zonal architecture on T2-weighted images. The central area of high signal intensity represents epithelium and mucus, the middle area of low signal intensity represents fibrous stroma, and the outer area of medium signal intensity represents peripheral myometrium. The vaginal wall has low signal intensity on T2-weighted images. The texture of the ovaries is clearly imaged in women of reproductive age with hypointense stroma and hyperintense follicles on T2-weighted images.

Normal fallopian tubes are not routinely imaged because of their small diameter and tortuous course.

16.2.3.5
Normal MR Anatomy of Postmenopausal Women

After menopause, the uterine corpus becomes smaller and approximately equal in size to the cervix. The zonal anatomy is indistinct when women are not receiving exogenous hormones (Fig. 16.10). Although

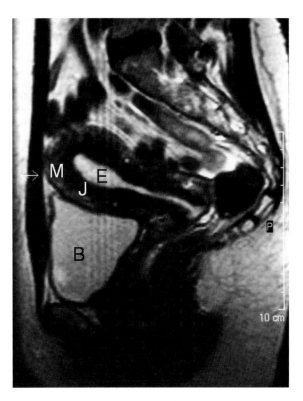

Fig. 16.9. Normal anatomy in reproductive-age women. Sagittal T2w MR image clearly demonstrates uterine zonal anatomy with high signal intensity of the endometrium (*E*), low signal of junction zone (*J*), and intermediate signal of the myometrium (*M*). *B* urinary bladder

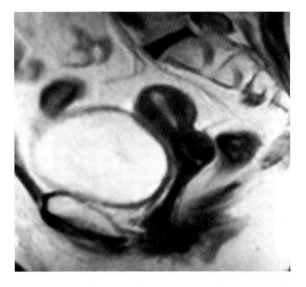

Fig. 16.10. Normal anatomy in postmenopausal women. Sagittal T2w MR images show a smaller uterine corpus with poor delineation of uterine zonal anatomy

the cervix does not atrophy significantly, the peripheral myometrium is usually unclear. Ovaries may be undetected at MR imaging since they seldom have follicles.

When a woman of reproductive age has a small uterus with indistinct zonal anatomy or undetectable ovaries, as seen in postmenopausal women, the possibility of a disorder related to insufficient hormone secretion should be considered [20].

16.3
Ovulatory Dysfunction

Disorders affecting ovulation account for 30%–40% of cases of female infertility [1]. Measures of ovarian function include measurement of basal body temperature, endometrial biopsy, measurement of serum progesterone level, endocrine tests, and monitoring of follicle growth with US. Thus the role of MR imaging is limited to assessment of whether a pituitary adenoma is present [20].

16.4
Pituitary Adenoma

Prolactin-producing hypophyseal adenoma (prolactinoma) is the most common functional pituitary adenoma. Its prevalence peaks in women between 20 and 30 years of age. Hyperprolactinemia can be a cause of infertility and is associated with diminished gonadotropin secretion, secondary amenorrhea, and galactorrhea. The patient should first be examined for drug-induced hyperprolactinemia before any infertility work-up is initiated. For example, antidepressants, cimetidine, dopamine antagonists, reserpine, sulpiride, verapamil, methyldopa, and estrogen therapy are known to interface with prolactin secretion.

When a patient is suspected of having hyperprolactinemia not associated with drugs, MR imaging is the imaging technique of choice. It can depict a pituitary microadenoma (≤1 cm) (Fig. 16.11). Most microadenomas have lower signal intensity than the normal pituitary gland on T1-weighted images. A convex outline of the pituitary gland or deviation of the pituitary stalk can also be detected. Dynamic

study with intravenous bolus injection of contrast medium is the preferred technique for assessing microadenomas, as it allows excellent delineation between the tumor and the normal pituitary gland. In the dynamic study, the normal pituitary gland and stalk show strong enhancement in the early phase of dynamic imaging, whereas microadenomas show relatively weak enhancement [21, 22].

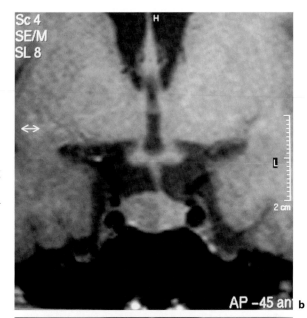

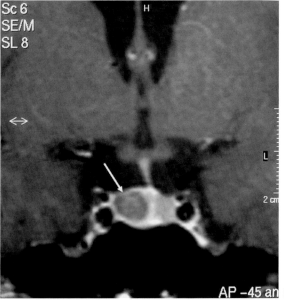

Fig. 16.11a,b. Pituitary adenoma. Unenhanced (**a**) and contrast-enhanced (**b**) T1w MR images show a small right-sided pituitary prolactinoma (*arrow*) leading to hyperprolactinemia with consecutive infertility

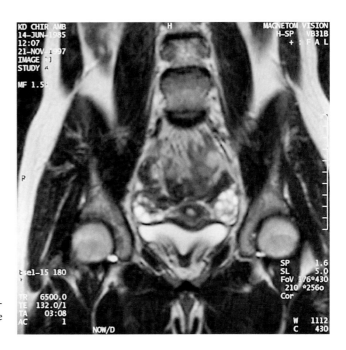

Fig. 16.12. Polycystic ovarian syndrome. On T2w coronal MR image, both ovaries are studded with multiple small cystic lesions

Macroadenomas (>1 cm) occupy the pituitary fossa and may cause visual abnormalities when they put pressure on the optic chiasm. Macroadenomas also tend to invade the cavernous sinus and erode the bony floor. The extent of the tumor can be determined by means of contrast-enhanced MR imaging.

16.5
Polycystic Ovarian Syndrome

The diagnosis of polycystic ovarian syndrome is based on hormone imbalance and laboratory findings. Patients with this syndrome often demonstrate an abnormal ratio of luteinizing hormone to follicle-stimulating hormone. The clinical manifestations include hirsutism, anovulation, and infertility. At gross pathologic analysis, the morphologic findings in the ovaries consist of multiple small follicular cysts surrounded by thickened and luteinized theca.

Follicle growth is usually monitored with US, and the usefulness of MR imaging is not proved. On T2-weighted images, polycystic ovarian syndrome appears as multiple tiny hyperintense peripheral cysts with hypointense central stroma [23, 24] (Fig. 16.12). However, MR imaging findings are nonspecific and serve only as supportive evidence of polycystic ovar-

ian syndrome. Multiple tiny, hyperintense peripheral cysts have been seen in patients with anovulation, medication-stimulated ovulation, or vaginal agenesis [24].

16.6
Disorders of the Fallopian Tubes

Disorders of the fallopian tubes are a common cause of female infertility, accounting for 30%–40% of cases [1]. Tubal disorders include damage to or obstruction of the fallopian tube and peritubal adhesions. HSG is the mainstay of evaluation of tubal patency, whereas laparoscopy is preferred for assessment of the peritubal environment. MR imaging aids in noninvasive assessment of tubal dilatation and peritubal disease. Dilated fallopian tubes manifest as fluid-filled ducts, which appear as retort-, sausage-, C-, or S-shaped cystic masses at MR imaging (Fig. 16.13). Thin, longitudinally oriented folds along the interior of the tube represent incompletely effaced mucosal or submucosal plicae [25]. Pelvic inflammatory disease is one of the most common causes of tubal or peritubal damage. The diagnosis is usually based on clinical or transvaginal US findings. MR imaging can also be helpful in assessment of pelvic inflammatory

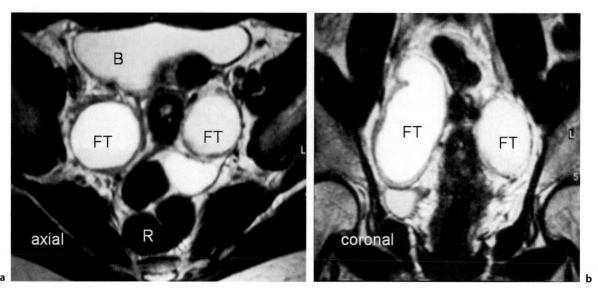

Fig. 16.13a,b. Bilateral hydrosalpinx. Sausage-, C-, or S-shaped cystic masses in the small pelvis as shown by these axial (**a**) and coronal (**b**) T2w MR images are clearly indicative of dilated fallopian tubes (*FT*). *B*, bladder; *R*, rectum

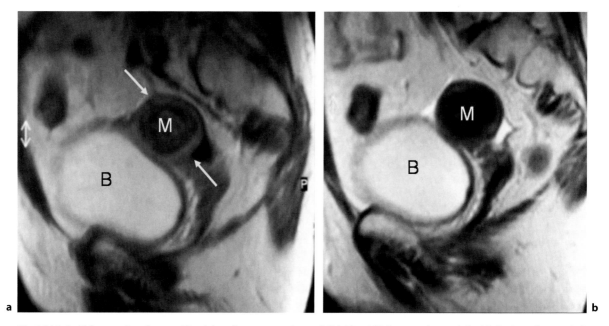

Fig. 16.14a,b. Tubo-ovarian abscess. T2w (**a**) and contrast-enhanced (**b**) T1w MR images show a left-sided adnexal mass (*M*) with rim-like enhancement (*arrows*) on contrast T1WI, which proved to be an abscess. *B*, bladder

disease (Fig. 16.14). Tubo-ovarian abscesses, dilated fluid-filled tubes, and free pelvic fluid can be depicted [26].

Endometriosis also causes peritubal adhesions. MR imaging is the most sensitive imaging tech-nique for evaluation of endometriosis. Moreover, dilated fallopian tubes with high signal intensity on T1-weighted images, which correspond to hematos-alpinx, reportedly correlate with one of the effects of endometriosis [25].

16.7
Uterine Disorders

16.7.1
Müllerian Duct Anomalies

If other causes of infertility are excluded, uterine anomalies may be suggested as a cause of infertility. On the other hand, unknown numbers of uterine anomalies may escape detection since reproductive ability is often unaffected or not noticeably affected [27].

Müllerian duct anomalies (MDAs) exhibit a prevalence of approximately 3%. Infertility issues are encountered in 25% of such women. Presenting symptoms vary depending on the specific anomaly. Amenorrhea is seen with imperforate hymen, vaginal atresia, uterine anomalies, Mayer-Rokitansky-Küster-Hauser syndrome, and Wünderlich syndrome. In the first two conditions, primary amenorrhea presents as cryptomenorrhea, in which menstrual blood cannot be extruded and patients commonly complain of periodic abdominal pain. MR imaging clearly demonstrates the point of obstruction, as well as the presence or absence of toceles, which includes hematometra, hematosalpinx, or blood in the rudimentary uterus [18, 28]. In addition, MR imaging allows evaluation of urinary tract abnormalities that are commonly associated, since embryologically, the müllerian and mesonephric ducts are closely related.

Müllerian duct anomalies may be depicted by HSG; however, the complex situation of the various classes of anomalies seem to be better defined by sonography or MR imaging.

Classification of MDAs according to the system adapted by the AMERICAN FERTILITY SOCIETY can be readily achieved based on MR findings [29]. In one comparative study, MR imaging attained 100% accuracy for diagnosis of uterine anomalies, as compared with 92% for ultrasound and less than 20% for HSG [14]. In the evaluation of uterine cavity deformation, highly accurate diagnosis of submucosal leiomyomas is easily established on MR imaging, readily differentiating the lesions from adenomyosis and endometrial polyps.

The most basic classification of müllerian duct defects consists of agenesis and hypoplasia, defects of vertical fusion, and defects of lateral fusion. In 1979, BUTTRAM and GIBBONS [30] proposed a classification of müllerian duct anomalies that was based on the degree of failure or normal development, and

they separated these anomalies into classes that demonstrate similar clinical manifestations, treatment, and prognosis for fetal salvage. Modified in 1988 by the AMERICAN SOCIETY OF REPRODUCTIVE MEDICINE [31], the classification remains the most widely accepted schematization and addresses uterovaginal anomalies (Fig. 16.15).

16.7.1.1
Class I: Hypoplasia or Agenesis

Failure of normal development of the müllerian ducts causes uterine agenesis or hypoplasia. Patients present with primary amenorrhea in adolescence. Agenesis or hypoplasia of any part of the genital tract (vagina, cervix, uterus, tubes) may occur either in isolation or, more, commonly, in combination. This relatively uncommon class of anomalies accounts for approximately 5% of müllerian duct anomalies. Vaginal agenesis is the most common subtype, and is often accompanied by uterine agenesis.

It is necessary to document whether a functioning uterine corpus and cervix are present.

Mayer-Rokitansky-Küster-Hauser syndrome is a combined anomaly that belongs to this entity. The typical form of this syndrome is characterized by congenital absence of the uterus and upper vagina. The ovaries and fallopian tubes are usually normal. The atypical form of the syndrome includes associated abnormalities of the ovaries and fallopian tubes and renal anomalies [32] (Fig. 16.16).

Women with acquired uterine hypoplasia due to drugs, pelvic irradiation, or ovarian failure may have a disproportionately small uterine corpus. In these patients, the ratio of the uterine body to the cervix is reduced to less than the normal 2:1, similar to a premenarchal uterus.

16.7.1.2
Class II: Unicornuate

This MDA consists of one normally developed müllerian duct, with the contralateral duct either hypoplastic (subtypes 2a–c) or absent (subtype 2d). Types 2a–c comprise approximately 90% of cases [2, 29] (Fig. 16.17).

Agenesis of a unilateral müllerian duct causes a single banana-shaped uterus with a single fallopian tube. If the rudimentary horn is either noncommunicating or lacks a cavity, it will not be detected by HSG. Sonographic findings, which are often subtle and easily overlooked, include a small uterine cavity, an

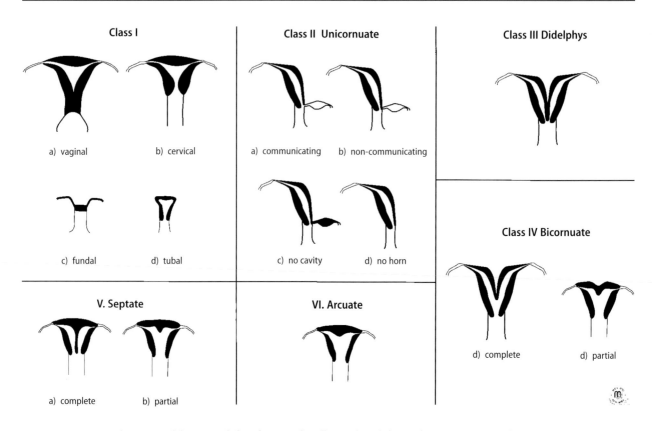

Fig. 16.15. The most widely accepted classification of müllerian duct defects, adressinguterovaginal anomalies

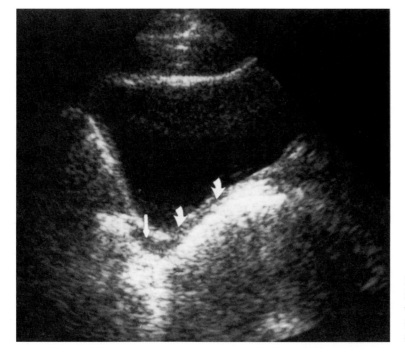

Fig. 16.16. Class I. Uterine agenesis. Sagittal midline sonogram shows normal vagina, small (*curved arrows*) cervix (*straight arrow*), and absent uterine corpus

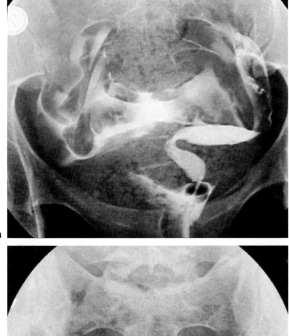

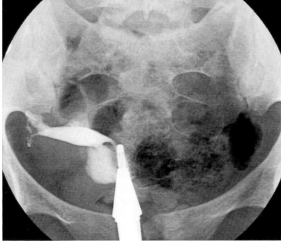

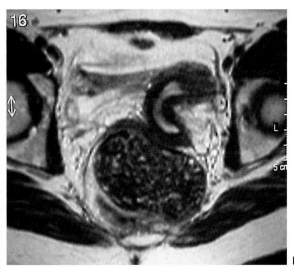

Fig. 16.17a–c. Class II. Left unicornuate uterus. HSG shows uterine cavity deviated toward left side with patent left fallopian tube (**a**). Axial T2w MRI in this patient shows no rudimentary horn on the right side (**b**). In another patient, HSG shows right unicornuate uterus with hydrosalpinx (**c**)

asymmetric ellipsoid fundal shape, and lateral deviation of the uterus. If the rudimentary horn is present without a cavity, it may be mistaken for a fibroid or the broad ligament.

MRI findings are similar to those seen with ultrasound, but cavity detection in the rudimentary horn can be facilitated by using heavily T2-weighted imaging sequences. Normal zonal anatomy is observed in a small uterus.

If the rudimentary horn is noncommunicating endometrial tissue expelled retrogradely through the fallopian tube during menstruation results in an increased frequency of endometriosis [33].

Spontaneous abortion and premature labor may occur in pregnancies with unicornuate uterus, and the poorest fetal survival among all uterine anomalies has been reported [27]. A potentially lethal complication is uterine rupture, which can occur if a pregnancy implants in a rudimentary horn.

16.7.1.3
Class III: Didelphys

Complete failure of fusion of the two müllerian ducts results in two complete uteri, each with its own cervix (Fig. 16.18). A longitudinal sagittal vaginal septum is usually, but not always, observed. Among all uterine anomalies, uterus didelphys is associated with the highest successful pregnancy rate, except for arcuate uterus [27]. Uterus didelphys is the least common of uterine duplication anomalies. HSG will clearly delineate the two separate uterine cavities if each cervix can be cannulated. In a small percentage of cases, the vaginal

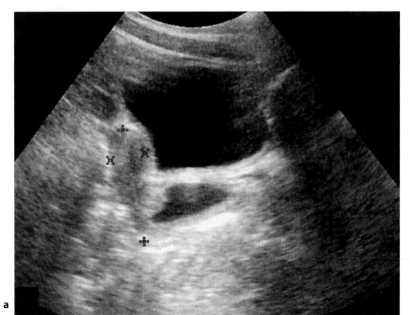

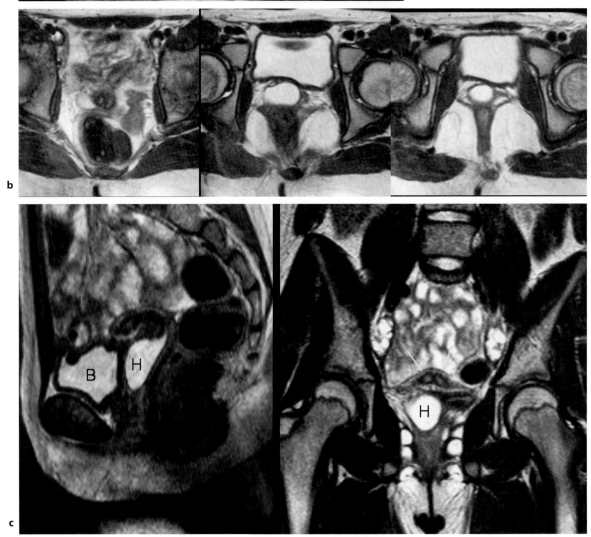

Fig. 16.18a–c. Class III: Wünderlich syndrome. On ultrasound (**a**) an obstructed hemivagina is seen in an 11-year old girl presenting with unilateral renal agenesis (not documented). Axial T2w MR images at different levels (**b**) as well as coronal and sagittal images (**c**) show two separate uteri (*arrows*) and two cervices, all of which have normal zonal anatomy indicating an uterus didelphys. In addition, a hematocele (*H*) due to obstruction of the right hemivagina is depicted. *B* (urinary bladder)

septum may prevent cannulation of one cervical canal, leading to the appearance of a unicornuate uterus.

Sonographic images reveal two widely spaced uterine fundi with myometrium and a deep cleft separating the two endometrial cavities. Two separate cervices may not be visible, since endocervical echoes are less prominent than endometrial echoes, but transvaginal imaging can demonstrate these findings better. Sonography is also useful for demonstrating hematocolpos, hematometra, and endometriosis in cases missed by HSG owing to an obstructing vaginal septum. Uterus didelphys with an obstructed hemivagina is termed Wünderlich syndrome (Fig. 16.18) and is usually associated with ipsilateral renal agenesis. Several series have noted a tendency for the right hemi-uterus to obstruct, in association with right renal agenesis [20].

MRI is best performed with multiplanar scans. To improve visualization of the fundal contour, coronal images should be obtained in a plane parallel to the tubal ostia and internal os. MR findings are similar to those of sonography, with a deep separating cleft (>3 cm) between the two uterine fundi. The widely spaced uterine horns have an obtuse intercornual angle (>110°), although occasional overlap with a bicornuate anomaly exists. Separate cervices and a vaginal septum (if present) can be demonstrated by caudal axial T2-weighted sections.

16.7.1.4
Class IV: Bicornuate

Partial fusion of two müllerian ducts results in a bicornuate uterus with one cervix. The uterine horns are widely divergent, the uteri fundi joined either at the uterine corpus (bicornis unicollis subtype) (Fig. 16.19a) or lower uterine segment (bicornis bicollis subtype) (Fig. 16.19b). In most cases, there is a single cervix; however, there may be two cervical openings, creating an appearance similar to septate uterus. Of all classes of MDAs, it is the bicornuate uterus that has the strongest association with cervical incompetence [34]. It is crucial to differentiate between a bicornuate and septate uterus because surgical correction of a bicornuate uterus is not generally warranted, since it is the cervical incompetence and not the cavity malformation that is the cause of the high spontaneous abortion rate with this anomaly. In addition, an abdominal metroplasty must be performed if surgical repair of a bicornuate uterus is undertaken, as opposed to hysteroscopic septoplasty, which is performed for a septate uterus [35].

HSG of a bicornuate uterus will demonstrate separate uterine cavities with an intercornual angle that usually exceeds 105°. With this imaging modality, however, the outer uterine contour cannot be evaluated, and overlap with the appearance of a septate uterus can occur.

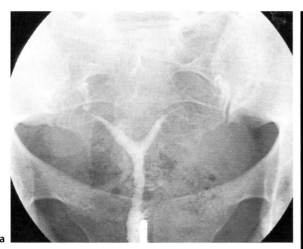
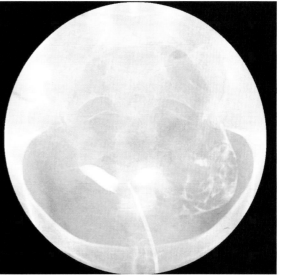

Fig. 16.19a,b. Class IV. HSG shows widely splayed uterine horns with an intercornual angle greater than 100° and with uterine fundi joined at the lower uterine segment, indicating a bicornis unicollis subtype (**a**). HSG in a different patient shows uterine fundi joined at the level of the cervix, suggesting a bicornis bicollis subtype (**b**)

Sonographic diagnosis of a bicornuate uterus is made by analysis of both the outer fundal contour as well as visualization of a separate endometrial stripe in each horn. However, sonographic differentiation of a bicornuate uterus from a septate uterus may be difficult.

MRI diagnostic criteria are similar to those described for sonography. Imaging should be performed during the secretory phase to maximize contrast between the T2 signal of endometrium, the junctional zone, and the myometrium. On transaxial images, the intercornual distance exceeds 4 cm, and the tissue dividing the endometrial cavities is isointense with normal myometrium. On coronal images of the fundus, obtained in the plane of the tubal ostia, the serosal concavity exceeds 1 cm [14].

16.7.1.5
Class V: Septate

Septate uterus results from failure of resorption of a septum after complete fusion of the müllerian ducts. In the majority of cases the midline, septum is partial and extends for a variable distance from the fundus into the corpus or lower uterus segment (subseptate uterus). Less commonly the septum extends to the level of the cervix, forming a complete septate uterus. With a complete septate uterus, there may be two cervical openings, but this results from division of one canal, and not two separate cervices as occurs with a uterus didelphys (Fig. 16.20).

Most patients evaluated for repeated abortions and found to have a uterine anomaly will have a septate uterus [27]. Avascular fibrous septa can be safely resected hysteroscopically, whereas vascularized myometrial tissue within the septum requires metroplasty as a surgical procedure for treatment of this anomaly and may enhance fetal survival, with one report indicating that 95% of patients became pregnant, 73% carried to term, and 77% delivered a liveborn baby [36].

HSG of a septate uterus demonstrates two narrowly diverging cavities, yielding a V-shape configuration with relatively straight medial borders. The angle formed by the medial borders of the two uterine hemi-cavities is usually greater than 75°. Diagno-

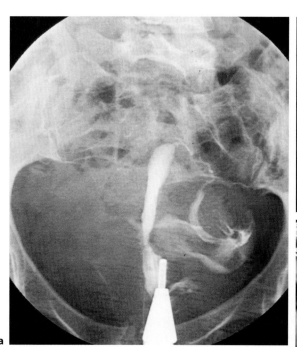

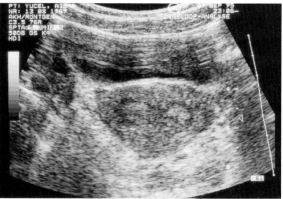

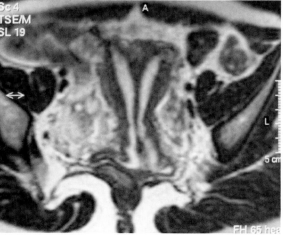

Fig. 16.20a–c. Class V. Complete septate uterus. On HSG one cervical opening was missed; only one uterine cavity was spilled with contrast media; a unicornuate uterus was assumed (**a**). Sonography (**b**) and coronal T2 w MRI (**c**) clearly demonstrate the uterine cavity divided by a thick septum extending to the level of the cervix. The angle formed by the medial borders of the two uterine hemi-cavities is greater than 75°

sis of a septate uterus is often not possible by HSG because the outer uterine contour cannot be imaged, and angle measurement may be difficult.

Sonography and MRI are each superior to HSG. The external uterine contour is normally convex, flat, or minimally indented by less than 1 cm [14], in contrast to that of a bicornuate uterus. Coronal MRI allows the characteristic fundal changes of a septate uterus to be identified.

In addition to fundal contour, a second sonographic feature of a septate uterus is splitting of the endometrial echo by a hypoechoic band, most easily seen in the fundus.

16.7.1.6
Class VI: Arcuate

Formerly this MDA was classified as the mildest form of either a bicornuate or septate uterus. In 1988, the American Fertility Society issued a separate classification of arcuate uterus. Arcuate uterus should be considered a normal variant and it has no effect on fertility.

HSG of the arcuate uterus reveals a broad smooth indentation into the fundal cavity, which causes a saddle-shaped appearance (Fig. 16.21). The indentation is approximately one-fifth the height of the uterus.

Both MRI and sonography reveal a smooth outer contour, associated with a subtle broad-based shallow indentation impressing the endometrial stripe.

16.7.1.7
Class VII: Diethylstilbestrol-Related

These anomalies comprise sequelae of in utero diethylstilbestrol (DES) exposure. DES was used to prevent miscarriage from the 1940s to the 1970s [35]. Most likely as a result of DES disrupting vaginal plate development and stromal differentiation, structural anomalies occurred in the fetal vagina, cervix, uterus, and tubes. Because of the variability and overlap of features of associated cervical and vaginal malformations, these changes generally are not incorporated into the basic schematics and are reported as a subset of the primary uterine defect.

Structural anomalies encountered at physical examination are vaginal adenosis and the presence of an anterior cervical ridge or hood. Uterine cavity anomalies associated with DES exposure include hypoplasia, focal constrictions, bulbous dilatation of the lower uterine segment, and a T-shaped

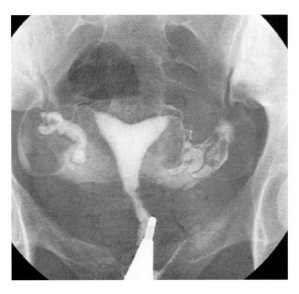

Fig. 16.21. Class VI. HSG shows minor indentation of the fundal uterine cavity indicating an arcuate uterus. Note normal filling of the fallopian tubes with evidence of free spill into the pelvic peritoneum

uterine configuration. These uterine anomalies are associated with an increased incidence of spontaneous abortion, preterm labor, and ectopic pregnancy [34].

HSG is an excellent imaging modality for diagnosing DES-related uterine anomalies. Typical cavity contour changes seen include scalloping and constriction bands, while uterine shape abnormalities are hypoplasia, T-configuration, and a bulbous lower uterine segment (Fig. 16.22).

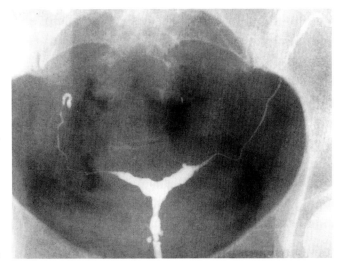

Fig. 16.22. Class VII. Hypoplastic T-shaped deformity of the uterus with filling of dilated glands in the cervix in a proven DES uterus

To date, there has been a paucity of reported ultrasound or MRI studies to detect DES-related uterine changes. Most likely, this reflects relatively subtle findings on these examinations.

16.7.2
Adenomyosis

Adenomyosis is not a common cause of infertility. The frequency of symptomatic adenomyosis peaks between the ages of 35 and 50 years, and it is most often found in parous women [37]. However, nulligravid women are sometimes affected and experience infertility. The exact reasons for infertility in patients with adenomyosis remain unclear, although an enlarged uterus may be associated with reduced uterine or endometrial receptivity (Fig. 16.23).

16.7.3
Leiomyoma

Uterine leiomyoma, especially submucous leiomyoma, may be associated with pregnancy loss rather than infertility. Although leiomyoma is an infrequent cause of infertility, there may be some interference with sperm transport or implantation as a result of distortion, an increased surface area within the uterine cavity, or impingement by the leiomyoma on the endocervical canal or interstitial portion of the fallopian tubes [38] (Fig. 16.24).

Both transvaginal ultrasound and MRI are reliable methods for identification of leiomyomas. Sonohysterography can clearly demonstrate the relationship between the endometrium and submucosal leiomyomas and thus serves as an important adjunct to transvaginal US [39].

16.7.4
Endometriosis

Endometriosis is found in 25%–50% of infertile women, and 30%–50% of women with endometriosis are infertile [40].

Laparoscopy is the mainstay for diagnosis, staging, and treatment of the disease. Transvaginal US is the preferred imaging technique to identify ovarian endometrioma. However, US has limited usefulness in identifying peritoneal implants. MR imaging has also proved to be a useful modality for establishing an accurate diagnosis of endometriosis (Fig. 16.25).

In conclusion, the various causes of infertility in women need to be carefully evaluated by use of the appropriate imaging techniques. The conventional HSG is still a widely available, rather safe, and rapid as well as easy performable technique to assess tubal patency. HSG is minimally invasive and also entails exposure to low ionizing radiation. Sonohysterogra-

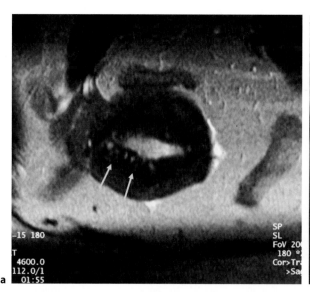
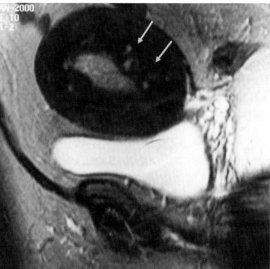

Fig. 16.23a,b. Adenomyosis. Multiple high-signal foci predominantly in the posterior aspect of the uterus on these axial (**a**) and sagittal (**b**) T2w MR images, indicating a more focal adenomyosis. Poor delineation of the junctional zone is shown

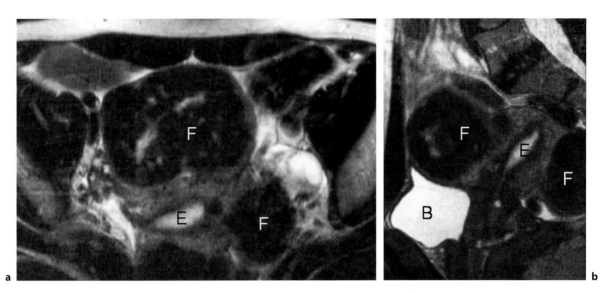

Fig. 16.24a,b. Leiomyoma. Enlarged uterus with large fibroids (*F*) in the anterior and posterior aspect of the uterus being of typical low signal intensity on this axial (**a**) and sagittal (**b**) T2w MR images. *B* (urinary bladder), *E* (endometrial cavity)

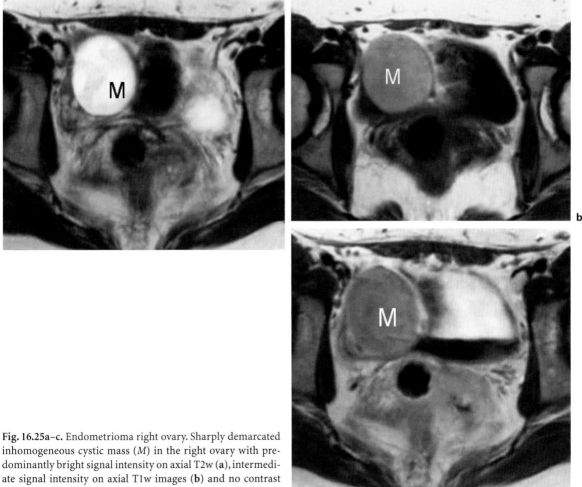

Fig. 16.25a–c. Endometrioma right ovary. Sharply demarcated inhomogeneous cystic mass (*M*) in the right ovary with predominantly bright signal intensity on axial T2w (**a**), intermediate signal intensity on axial T1w images (**b**) and no contrast uptake after i.v. Gd-DTPA (**c**)

phy and sono-HSG allow both evaluation of tubal patency and uterine pathology. MR imaging is a useful modality as an adjunct for routine infertility workups. It is valuable for detection of pituitary adenoma when patients are suspected of having a disorder of the hypothalamic–pituitary–ovarian axis. The role of MR imaging in assessing the pelvic cavity in patients with infertility includes evaluation of the functioning uterus and ovaries, differentiation of müllerian duct anomalies, and accurate noninvasive diagnosis of adenomyosis, leiomyoma, and endometriosis. MR imaging also helps to predict the outcome of conservative treatment of adenomyosis, leiomyoma, and endometriosis.

References

1. Hornstein MD, Schust D (1996) Infertility. In: Berek JS, Adashi EY, Hillard PA (eds) Novak's gynecology, 12th edn. Williams and Wilkins, Baltimore, pp 915–962
2. Heinonen PK, Saarikoski S, Pystynen P (1982) Reproductive performance of women with uterine anomalies: an evaluation of 182 cases. Acta Obstet Gynecol Scand 61:157–162
3. Collins JI, Woodward PJ (1995) Radiological evaluation of infertility. Semin Ultrasound CT MR 16:304–316
4. Lev-Toaff AS (1996) Sonohysterography: evaluation of endometrial and myometrial abnormalities. Semin Roentgenol 31:288–298
5. Margolin FR (1988) A new cannula for hysterosalpingography. AJR Am J Roentgenol 151:729–730
6. Sholkoff SD (1987) Balloon hysterosalpingography catheter. AJR Am J Roentgenol 149:995–996
7. Thurmond AS, Uchida BT, Rosch J (1990) Device for hysterosalpingography and fallopian tuber catherization. Radiology 174:571–572
8. Soules MR, Spadoni LR (1982) Oil versus aqueous media for hysterosalpingography: a continuing debate based on many options and few facts. Fertil Steril 38:1–11
9. Pittaway DE, Winfield AC, Maxson W, Daniell J, Herbert C, Wentz AC (1983) Prevention of acute pelvic inflammatory disease after hysterosalpingography: efficacy of doxycycline prophylaxis. Am J Obstet Gynecol 147:623–626
10. Justesen P, Rasmussen F, Anderson PE Jr (1986) Inadvertently performed hysterosalpingography during early pregnancy. Acta Radiol Diag 27:711–713
11. Bacelar AC, Wilcock D, Powell M, Worthington BS (1995) The value of MRI in the assessment of traumatic intra-uterine adhesions (Asherman syndrome). Clin Radiol 50:80–83
12. Kurman RJ, Mazur MT (1987) Benign diseases of the endometrium. In: Kurman RJ (ed) Blaustein's Pathology of the female genital tract, 3rd edn. Springer-Verlag, Berlin Heidelberg New York, pp 292–321
13. Nicolini U, Bellotti M, Bonazzi B, Zamberletti D, Candiani GB (1987) Can ultrasound be used to screen uterine malformations? Fertil Steril 47:89–93
14. Pellerito JS, McCarthy SM, Doyle MB et al (1992) Diagnosis of uterine anomalies: relative accuracy of MR imaging, endovaginal sonography, and hysterosalpingography. Radiology 183:795–800
15. Fedele I, Ferrazzi E, Dorta M, Verzellini P, Candiani GB (1988) Ultrasonography in the differential diagnosis of "double" uteri. Fertil Steril 50:361–364
16. Kupesic S, Kurjak A (2000) Ultrasound and Doppler assessment of uterine anomalies. In: Kupesic S, de Ziegler D (eds) Ultrasound and infertility. Parthenon, Pearl River, NY, pp 147–153
17. Goldberg JM, Falcone T, Attaran M (1997) Sonohysterographic evaluation of uterine anomalies noted on hysterosalpingography. Hum Reprod 12:1251–1253
18. Javitt MC (1997) Magnetic resonance imaging in the diagnosis of congenital uterine anomalies. In: Fleischer AC, Javitt MC, Jeffresy RB Jr, Jones HW Jr (eds) Clinical gynecologic imaging. Lippincott-Raven, Philadelphia, pp 299–310
19. Fleischer AC, Kepple DM (1997) Normal pelvic anatomy as depicted by various sonographic techniques. In: Fleischer AC, Javitt HC, Jeffrey RB Jr, Jones HW III (eds) Clinical gynecologic imaging. Lippincott-Raven, Philadelphia, pp 10–22
20. Imaoka I, Wada A, Matsuo M, Yoshida M, Kitagaki H, Sugimura K (2003) MR imaging of disorders associated with female infertility: use in diagnosis, treatment, and management. Radiographics 23:1401–1421
21. Miki Y, Matsuo M, Nishizawa S et al (1990) Pituitary adenomas and normal pituitary tissue: enhancement patterns on gadopentate-enhanced MR imaging. Radiology 177:35–38
22. Bartynski WS, Lin L (1997) Dynamic and conventional spin-echo MR of pituitary microlesions. AJNR Am J Neuroradiol 18:965–972
23. Mitchell DG, Gefter WB, Spritzer CE et al (1986) Polycystic ovaries: MR imaging. Radiology 160:425–429
24. Kimura I, Togashi K, Kawakami S et al (1996) Polycystic ovaries: implications of diagnosis with MR imaging. Radiology 201:549–552
25. Outwater EK, Siegelman ES, Chiowanich P, Kilger AM, Dunton CJ, Talerman A (1998) Dilated fallopian tubes: MR imaging characteristics. Radiology 208:463–469
26. Tukeva TA, Aronen HJ, Karjalainen PT, Molander P, Paavonen T, Paavonen J (1999) MR imaging in pelvic inflammatory disease: comparison with laparoscopy and US. Radiology 210:209–216
27. Rock JA (1997) Surgery for anomalies of the müllerian ducts. In: Rock JA, Thompson JD (eds) Te Linde's operative gynecology, 8th edn. Lippincott-Raven, Philadelphia, pp 687–729
28. Togashi K, Nishimura K, Itoh K, Fujisawa I, Nakano Y, Torizuka K, Ozasa H, Ohshima M (1987) Vaginal agenesis: classification by MR imaging. Radiology 162:675–677
29. Carrington BM, Hricak H, Nuruddin RN, Secaf E, Laros RK Jr, Hill EC (1990) Müllerian duct anomalies: MR imaging evaluation. Radiology 176:715–720
30. Buttram VC, Gibbons WE (1979) Müllerian anomalies: a proposed classification (an analysis of 144 cases). Fertil Steril 32:40–46
31. Anonymous (1988) The American Fertility Society clas-

sifications of adnexal adhesions, distal tubal obstruction, tubal occlusion secondary to tubal ligation, tubal pregnancies, müllerian anomalies and intrauterine adhesions. Fertil Steril 49:944–955

32. Strübbe EH, Willemsen WNP, Lemmens JAM, Thijn CJP, Rolland R (1993) Mayer-Rokitansky-Küster-Hauser syndrome: distinction between two forms based on excretory urographic, sonographic, and laparoscopic findings. AJR Am J Roentgenol 160:331–334

33. Brody JM, Koelliker SL, Fishman GN (1998) Unicornuate uterus: imaging appearance, associated anomalies and clinical implications. AJR Am J Roentgenol 171:1341–1347

34. Patton PE (1994) Anatomic uterine defects. Clin Obstet Gynecol 37:705–721

35. Fielding JR (1996) MR imaging of müllerian anomalies: impact on therapy. AJR Am J Roentgenol 167:1491–1495

36. Rock JA, Jones HW Jr (1977). The clinical management of the double uterus. Fertil Steril 28:798–806

37. Braly PS (1999) Disease of the uterus. In: Scott JR, Di-Saia PJ, Hammond CB, Spellacy WN (eds) Danforth's obstetrics and gynecology, 8th edn. Lippincott Williams & Wilkins, Philadelphia, pp 837–855

38. Thompson JD, Rock JA (1997) Leiomyoma uteri and myomectomy. In: Rock JA, Thompson JD (eds) Te Linde's operative gynecology, 8th edn. Lippincott-Raven, Philadelphia, pp 731–770

39. Becker E Jr, Lev-Toaff AS, Kaufman EP, Halpern EJ, Edelweiss MI, Kurtz AB (2002) The additional value of transvaginal sonohysterography over transvaginal sonography alone in women with known or suspected leiomyoma. J Ultrasound Med 21:237–247

40. Schenken RS (1999) Endometriosis. In: Scott JR, Di-Saia PJ, Hammond CB, Spellacy WN (eds) Danforth's obstetrics and gynecology, 8th edn. Lippincott Williams & Wilkins, Philadelphia, pp 669–675

Acute and Chronic Pelvic Pain Disorders

17

Rosemarie Forstner and Astrid Schneider

17.1
Introduction

One of the most challenging problems in clinical routine is discerning the cause of pelvic pain. From a practical point of view, it seems useful to classify pelvic pain as acute or chronic, because these presentations differ in their differential diagnoses and therefore different imaging strategies for their evaluation may be appropriate. Pelvic pain that has been present for 6 months or longer is defined as chronic pelvic pain.

The differential diagnosis of lower abdominal and pelvic pain is long, and encompasses gynecological, pregnancy-related, gastrointestinal, urological, neurological, and abdominal wall causes. Furthermore, psychological factors have been attributed to play an important role in women suffering especially from chronic pelvic pain.

The single most important laboratory test in assessing pelvic pain in a woman of reproductive age is a pregnancy test, because ectopic pregnancy should be ruled out in any women in this age group presenting with the symptoms of abdominal pain. The top diagnoses of gynecological emergencies account for the vast majority of referrals and include ectopic pregnancy, corpus luteum cyst rupture, and pelvic infection. Appendicitis accounts for most of nongynecological emergencies.

R. Forstner, MD, A. Schneider, MD
PD, Department of Radiology, Landeskliniken Salzburg, Paracelsus Private Medical University, Müllner Hauptstrasse 48, 5020 Salzburg, Austria

Sonography plays a pivotal role as the primary imaging modality in gynecologic disorders causing pelvic pain. CT and MRI allow complementary assessment of the pelvis and abdomen including the gastrointestinal and urologic system.

In this chapter, common gynecological and nongynecological causes of acute and chronic pelvic pain will be covered. Their relative frequency of imaging by MRI or CT is listed in Table 17.1. Gynecologic disorders highly associated with chronic pelvic pain such as endometriosis uterine fibroids and adenomyosis are discussed in previous chapters in this book.

Table 17.1. Relative frequency of imaging for pelvic pain in clinical routine

Gynecological pathologies	Frequency	Nongynecological pathologies	Frequency
PID	+	Pelvic congestion syndrome	+
Tuboovarian abscess	++	Appendicitis	+++
Hydropyosalpinx	++	Diverticulitis	+++
Ovarian torsion	+	Appendagitis epiploica	+
Ovarian vein thrombosis	+	Crohn disease	++
Endometriosis	++	Rectus sheath hematoma	+
Uterine fibroids	++		

+, Low frequency; ++, medium frequency; +++, high frequency.

17.2
Gynecological Causes of Pelvic Pain

17.2.1
Pelvic Inflammatory Disease

Pelvic inflammatory disease (PID) refers to an acute infection of the upper genital tract in women in the reproductive age, involving the uterus, fallopian tubes, and ovaries. Per definition, PID should be distinguished from pelvic infections caused by medical procedures, pregnancy, and other primary abdominal processes. PID usually results from sexually transmitted ascending infections typically by *Neisseria gonorrhoeae* or *Chlamydia trachomatis*, although 30%–40% of cases are polymicrobial. Actinomyces and tuberculosis account for rare causes of PID and may cause tubo-

ovarian abscesses [1]. If PID is untreated or incompletely treated, there is a sixfold risk of ectopic pregnancy. Twenty percent of the patients may complain about pelvic pain, and infertility is seen in 25%–60% of women with more than one series of PID [2]. Occasionally patients with PID may develop Fritz-Hugh-Curtis syndrome due to peritonitis of the right upper quadrant surfaces and the of right lobe of the liver caused by bacterial spread along the paracolic gutters [3].

17.2.1.1
Imaging Findings

Imaging findings in early PID are typically subtle and their interpretation is based on the clinical findings. Findings on CT and MRI may include mild pelvic edema that results in thickening of the uterosacral ligaments and haziness of the pelvic fat. Contrast enhancement and thickening of the fallopian tube may be signs of salpingitis. Enlarged and abnormally enhancing ovaries, which may demonstrate a polycystic appearance, also present inflammatory changes (Fig. 17.1). Periovarian stranding and enhancement of the adjacent peritoneum are common associated findings. In cases of endometritis, an abnormal endometrial enhancement and fluid within the endocervical canal, which displays similar imaging characteristics as fluid in the cul-de-sac, may be observed. (Fig. 17.1) The uterine cervix may be enlarged with an abnormally enhancing endocervical canal in cases with associated cervicitis. Especially the uterine changes are better assessed on MRI than on CT [3].

17.2.2
Hydropyosalpinx

Salpingitis is the most important cause for obliteration of the fimbriated end of the tube, which leads to hydrosalpinx. Other etiologies include fallopian tube tumors, endometriosis, and adhesions from prior surgery. Serous fluid, blood, or pus may accumulate and cause distension of the fallopian tube.

17.2.2.1
Imaging Findings

Dilated fallopian tubes appear as fluid-filled tubular structures arising from the uterine fundus, separated from the ipsilateral ovary. The typical finding is a tubular tortuous cystic structure with interdigitating mural septa (Fig. 17.2) These septa are thin and display low

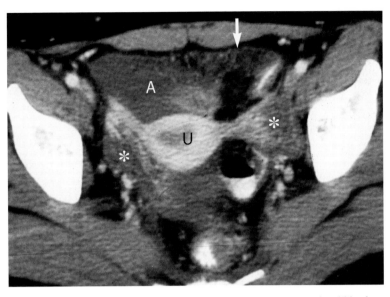

Fig. 17.1. CT findings in PID in a 29-year-old woman. Haziness and weblike fatty infiltration of pelvic fat (*arrow*), free fluid (*A*), marked swelling of the left ovary, and mild dilatation of the uterine cavity (*U*) are demonstrated in infection by *Chlamydia trachomatis*. The ovaries (*) are difficult to discriminate from ascites due to their polycystic appearance in oophoritis

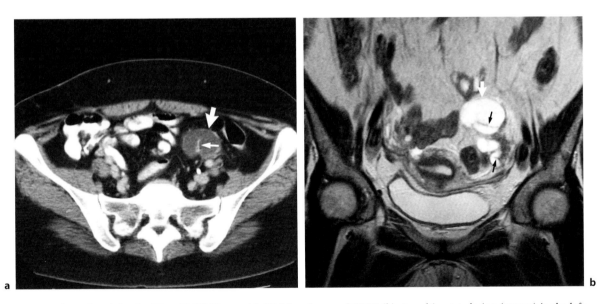

Fig. 17.2a,b. Hydrosalpinx in CT and MRI. Transaxial CT (**a**) and coronal T2WI (**b**). A multiseptate lesion (*arrows*) in the left adnexal region is demonstrated in CT (**a**) and MRI (**b**): Its tubular structure with widening at the cephalad end is demonstrated on MRI (**b**). The thin incomplete, interdigitating septa (*small arrows*) are a typical finding of a dilated fallopian tube in CT and MRI

signal intensity on T2-weighted images. Distinct septal enhancement on contrast-enhanced T1WI or CT may support the diagnosis of pyosalpinx (Fig. 17.3) [4]. The nature of fluid within a dilated salpinx can be best evaluated by MRI. The signal intensity on the T1 and T2WI varies in accordance with the contents, which ranges from water-like fluid to proteinaceous or hemorrhagic components. Multiplanar imaging and bowel opacification facilitates depiction of the tubal origin and differentiation from dilated bowel loops.

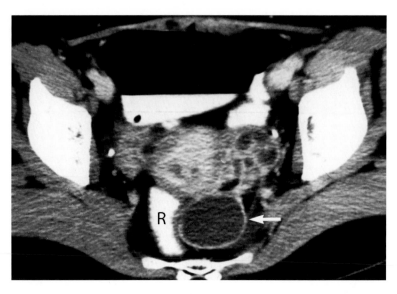

Fig. 17.3. Pyosalpinx in CT. A pedunculated cystic lesion (*arrow*) is identified adjacent to the retroflected uterus. It extends from the left adnexal region posteriorly and displaces the opacified rectum (*R*). The distinct wall enhancement is indicative of a pyosalpinx

17.2.2.2
Differential diagnosis

Pyosalpinx can often not be reliably differentiated from hydrosalpinx. As diameters up to 10 cm are not uncommon, hydrosalpinx may mimic multiloculated ovarian tumors, especially cystadenomas. Identification of the ovary separate from the lesion and multiplanar imaging aids in differentiation. Any enhancing component within a dilated tube should suggest the possibility of fallopian tube carcinoma or ectopic pregnancy [5].

17.2.3
Tuboovarian Abscess

In the majority of cases, tuboovarian abscesses (TOA) result from pelvic inflammatory disease. It is reported to complicate PID in up to one-third of patients hospitalized for treatment [6]. Other etiologies include complications of surgery or intra-abdominal inflammatory bowel diseases, such as appendicitis, diverticulitis, or Crohn disease. In most cases, TOA is caused by a polymicrobial infection with a high prevalence of anaerobes. IUD users, especially in the first few months after insertion, are also under a higher risk of PID. Pelvic actinomycosis is considered to be highly associated with the use of IUD [1].

TOA most commonly occurs in women in the reproductive ages. Tuboovarian abscesses in post-menopausal women are rare, and encountered in patients with diabetes or previous radiation therapy [7]. Because of the significant association with malignancies in postmenopausal women presenting with TOAs, a concomitant pelvic malignancy should be excluded [8].

The pathway of the inflammatory disease includes direct extension along the fallopian tubes. A hematogenous or lymphatic spread is found in the rare tuberculous involvement of the genital tract [1].

The vast majority of tuboovarian abscesses are multilocular masses with thick walls and necrotic areas. Bowel, uterus, parietal peritoneum, and omentum usually become adherent. The abscess may enlarge and fill the cul-de-sac or leak and produce metastatic abscesses and cause local peritonitis.

17.2.3.1
Imaging Findings

In CT and MRI, tuboovarian abscesses are thick-walled, complex heterogenous fluid-containing adnexal masses that are found unilaterally or bilaterally (Fig. 17.4) They may contain irregular inner contours, internal septa, gas, fluid, or a fluid-debris level [3]. Necrosis or loculated liquid areas may resemble serous fluid, but also be proteinaceous or hemorrhagic with T1 shortening. On T2WI, tuboovarian abscesses display most commonly a heterogeneously hyperintense signal on T2-weighted images [2]. They are surrounded by thick, well-enhancing outer borders. Because of dense pelvic adhesions or fibrosis, mesh-like strands in the pelvic fat planes are almost always found and are well enhanced on CT or contrast-enhanced T1WI, and display a low signal on T2WI.

Involvement of adjacent structures includes thickening of bowel loops and/or dilatation due to paralysis. Peritoneal enhancement, especially in the lesser pelvis, and small amounts of ascites are signs of associated peritonitis (Fig. 17.5). Obstruction of the ureters may also be observed. Internal gas bubbles are

the most specific radiologic sign of an abscess but are unusual in tuboovarian abscesses [9]. In cases of tuberculous TOAs, large amounts of ascites have been described [1].

17.2.3.2
Differential diagnosis

Endometriomas may sometimes display similar imaging characteristics with a thick rim; however, the clinical background is different. Ovarian cancer and especially metastases often present also as multiseptate ovarian masses. In ovarian cancers, well-enhanced septa and solid intralesional compo-

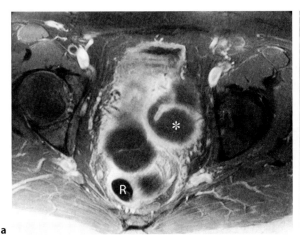
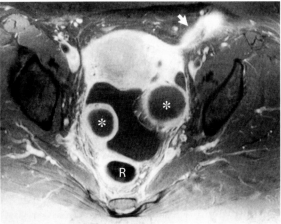

Fig. 17.4a,b. Bilateral tuboovarian abscesses. Consecutive transaxial FS T1WI (**a, b**) at the level of the acetabulum. Bilateral centrally cystic thick-walled adnexal lesions (*) show ill-defined margins toward the surrounding fat. Excessive contrast enhancement along the uterosacral ligaments, rectal wall, mesorectal fat tissue and the left round ligament (*arrow*) is also noted (**b**). *R*, rectum. Courtesy of Dr A. Heuck, Munich

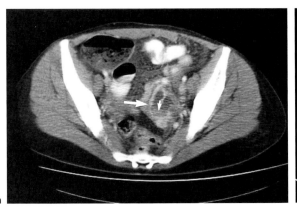
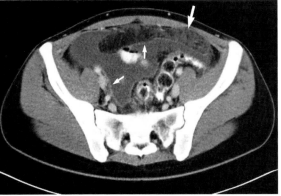

Fig. 17.5a,b. Peritonitis in tuboovarian abscess. Transaxial CT sans in the mid pelvis (**a, b**). A left-sided tuboovarian abscess is located adjacent to the pelvic sidewall (*arrow*) between internal and external iliac vessels (**a**). It presents as a cystic peripherally enhancing lesion with a fluid–fluid level (*arrowhead*) presenting debris (**a**). Associated findings include ascites, linear peritoneal enhancement (*small arrows*), and a netlike involvement of the pelvic fat and the omentum (*arrow*) (**b**)

nents are typically found. Signs of inflammation of the pelvic fat are missing in ovarian cancers. Furthermore, ovarian cancer is usually not associated with tubal dilatation. However, in postmenopausal women with TOA, malignancy is a special concern [8]. If tuboovarian abscesses involve adjacent pelvic organs, the site of origin often cannot be reliably defined (Fig. 17.6). Tuberculous peritonitis involving the adnexa mimics peritoneal carcinomatosis with nodularities along tuboovarian surfaces, and large amounts of ascites [1].

17.2.3.3
Value of Imaging

The diagnosis of PID is based on laboratory studies, assessment of vaginal secretions in combination with the clinical examination, and sonographic findings. In case of nonspecific findings or suspected complications of PID, especially tuboovarian abscess or peritonitis, CT or MRI serve as adjunct imaging modalities. CT is commonly used to assess complications of PID, especially when a tuboovarian abscess or peritonitis is suspected. Furthermore, it aids in defining the origin of the tuboovarian abscess and differentiates it from inflammatory bowel disease. It is also especially useful as a guidance for surgery or a CT drainage. MRI and CT are both useful in differentiation between an adnexal tumor and an abscess. The imaging findings, however, can only be interpreted in context with the clinical background. MRI is more useful than CT in differentiating a hydrosalpinx from a cystic ovarian tumor.

17.2.4
Ovarian Torsion

Ovarian torsion is most commonly associated with tubal torsion. Two age groups tend to be affected: children and women in their first three decades, and postmenopausal women.

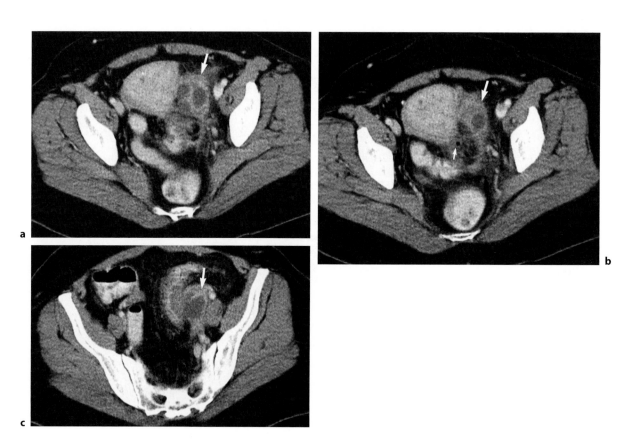

Fig. 17.6a–c. Abscess involving ovaries and sigmoid colon. Three consecutive CT scans (**a–c**) in and above the acetabular level in a 36-year-old woman with pelvic pain and leukocytosis. A multiseptate cystic lesion (*arrow*) with perilesional fat stranding is identified lateral of the uterus (**a, b**) involving the left adnexa and sigmoid colon. The tiny spot of free air (*small arrow*) is highly specific of the inflammatory nature of this process (**b**)

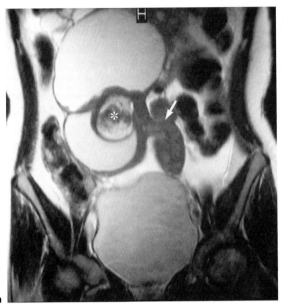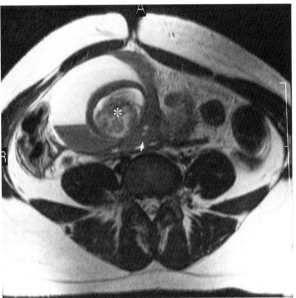

a   b

Fig. 17.7a,b. Twisted ovarian dermoid. Coronal (**a**) and transaxial T2WI (**b**). A large lesion with a fluid–fat level (**b**) and a Rokitansky nodule (*) typical for a dermoid is seen in the right midabdomen. Twisting (*arrow*) of the thickened pedicle, which leads from the uterus to the lesion, is seen on the coronal plane (**a**). The ovarian origin of the lesion can be identified because of the small peripheral ovarian follicles (*small arrows*) (**b**).Courtesy of Dr. K. Kinkel, Geneva

Ovarian torsion is caused by partial or complete rotation of the ovarian vascular pedicle. While venous flow is initially compromised, causing swelling and edema, arterial flow usually maintains until late in the course, which is attributed to the dual blood supply of the ovary [10]. Finally, hemorrhagic infarction leads to irreversible loss of the ovary. Predisposing factors for ovarian torsion include an underlying unilateral ovarian tumor (50%–60%), most likely dermoids (Fig. 17.7), and cystic ovarian lesions including paratubal cysts. Lesion size of more than 6 cm seems a higher risk for torsion [11]. Especially in children, torsion may also be encountered in normal-sized ovaries [12]. Furthermore, hypermobile adnexa or elongated fallopian tubes and increased abdominal pressure have been reported to be responsible for ovarian torsion. Women in their first three decades have the highest incidence of ovarian torsion, which is related to the higher frequency of physiological cysts and benign cystic tumors, infertility therapy, and pregnancy. Approximately 20% of torsions occur during pregnancy, typically during the first and second trimesters. In postmenopausal women, torsion typically affects a benign adnexal tumor, most commonly serous cystadenomas, whereas malignant tumors tend not to undergo a torsion [13].

Massive edema of the ovary is a rare disorder found in the second and third decades of life and considered a variant of ovarian torsion. It results from partial or intermittent torsion and is characterized by an excessively enlarged edematous ovary [10].

The right ovary is more likely to twist than the left, suggesting that the sigmoid colon may help to prevent torsion.

17.2.4.1
Imaging Findings

The finding of a cystic ovarian tumor, especially a dermoid cyst in young women who present with acute pain and vomiting is highly suspicious of adnexal torsion.

The imaging findings depend on the degree and duration of torsion. Thickening of the fallopian tube with hemorrhage is suggestive of torsion, especially when associated with an adnexal cystic mass. Torsed adnexal masses are often located midline, cranial to the uterine fundus. A twisted edematous pedicle can be observed arising from the lesion to the uterus with mixed signal intensity on all sequences on MRI (Fig. 17.7) [14]. Sometimes when tracking down the ovarian vascular pedicle, a coiled vascular pedicle may produce the whirl pool sign [15]. In prepubertal and pubertal girls where torsion of a normal ovary occurs in 50%, a unilateral solid mass with peripheral small cysts is indicative of a torsed ovary (Fig. 17.8). In case of hemorrhagic infarction, the enlarged ovary may show low signal intensity on T2WI due to interstitial hemorrhage, and no wall enhancement of the displaced follicles is observed [14].

In adults, most commonly a mass with hyperintense signal on T1 and T2 due to hemorrhage has been described [16]. Smooth wall thickening of the twisted adnexal cystic mass and a thin hyperintense rim at the periphery of the lesion on T1-weighted images are further signs in ovarian torsion.

A tubular or comma-like structure partially covering the ovary represents the fallopian tube and may also display hemorrhagic contents. CT studies have reported a diameter of the fallopian tube of 2–4 cm [17].

Contrast enhancement on CT and MRI depends on the degree of vitality [16]. MR findings in hemorrhagic infarction include lack of enhancement, engorged vessels surrounding the lesion and signal intensity of hematoma with high SI on T1 and T2 WI [18]. Nonspecific findings include deviation of the uterus to the twisted side, ascites, and obliteration of pelvic fat.

17.2.4.2
Differential diagnosis

Clinically, ruptured ovarian cysts may resemble ovarian torsion. In a patient with acute pelvic pain, a hemorrhagic lesion within a normal size ovary is typically a ruptured ovarian cyst. Furthermore, unlike in most cases of ovarian torsion, clotted blood may be detected in the lesser pelvis. Wall edema of an adnexal mass, engorged adnexal vessels or dilatation of the fallopian tube are missing. Tuboovarian abscess and hydrosalpinx may resemble advanced adnexal torsion. Lack of enhancement supports the diagnosis of ovarian torsion. In children, sonography usually allows the diagnosis of appendicitis as a cause of acute pelvic pain. In case of a suspected abscess or an ovarian mass, MRI may aid in further assessment of the adnexa. Rarely, a calcified mass may result from chronic infarction which cannot reliably be differentiated from a calcified ovarian tumor [19].

17.2.4.3
Diagnostic Value

Early diagnosis is crucial to prevent irreversible ovarian damage and prevent infectious complications.

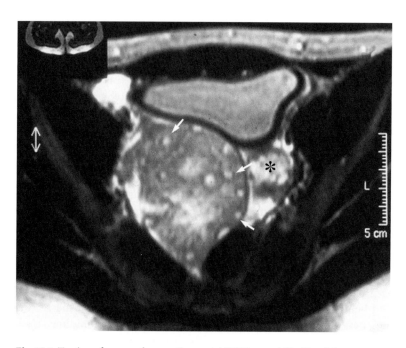

Fig. 17.8. Torsion of a normal ovary. Transaxial T2WI at umbilical level. In a 14-year-old girl with excessive intermittent pelvic pain for several days, sonography detected an indeterminate solid right adnexal mass. MRI shows a predominantly low-signal-intensity mass with numerous small peripheral cysts (*small arrows*), representing displaced follicles. Normal left ovary(*) At surgery, the right ovary had undergone complete hemorrhagic infarction. Courtesy of Dr. K. Kinkel, Geneva

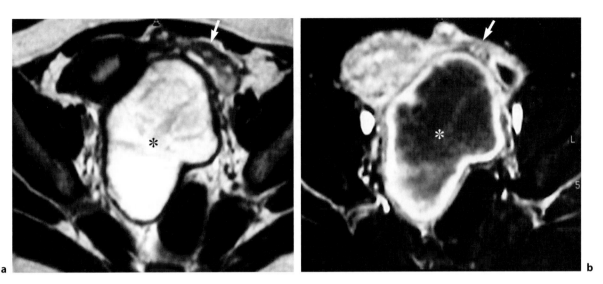

a   b

Fig. 17.9a,b. Hematosalpinx in ectopic tubal pregnancy. Transaxial T2WI (**a**) and contrast-enhanced T1WI with fat saturation (FS) (**b**). In a 27-year-old woman with a positive pregnancy test, a cystic adnexal mass (*) displaces the uterus, which displays widening of the endometrial cavity. The adnexal lesion is separated from the adjacent left ovary (*arrow*) and displays inhomogenous signal intensity with areas of high and low SI on T2WI (**a**) indicative of hemorrhage. The cystic contents of the fallopian tube and distinct homogenous tubal wall enhancement is demonstrated following contrast media administration (**b**). Courtesy of Dr. T.M. Cunha, Lisbon

This is why in most cases patients with suspected torsion on sonography will immediately undergo surgical untwisting. MRI and CT are often used in clinically not so typical cases, especially in chronic torsion. Particularly in early torsion, the imaging signs may be indicative but not specific of ovarian torsion. MRI and CT are particularly useful in detecting twisted lesions displaced outside the pelvis, where sonography may be limited. In pregnancy and in children, MRI is the modality of choice to further assess suspected ovarian torsion.

17.2.5
Ectopic Pregnancy

Ectopic pregnancy describes implantation and growth of the fertilized ovum at any site other than the endometrial cavity. The fallopian tube accounts for the vast majority of all ectopic gestations (95%), with 75% found in the ampulla and the remainder about equally occurring in the fimbrial and isthmic portions [20]. Rarely, ectopic pregnancy may occur within the ovary (3.2%), or within the peritoneal cavity (1.3%). Ectopic cervical pregnancy is more commonly found in pregnancies achieved through in-vitro fertilization technologies [21]. The major cause of ectopic pregnancy is disruption of normal tubal patency due to infection, surgery, müllerian

anomalies, or tumors. The rise of ectopic pregnancies within the last decades is highly associated with the increased incidence of pelvic inflammatory disease. A history of PID with chronic salpingitis is found in 35%–50% of patients with ectopic pregnancy.

17.2.5.1
Imaging Findings

Tubal wall enhancement and fresh tubal hematoma are described as specific findings for ectopic tubal pregnancy [22] (Fig. 17.9). The gestational sac is a cystic, centrally fluid-filled structure that is surrounded by a thick-walled peripheral rim. The latter displays inhomogeneous signal intensity on T2WI and medium signal intensity on T1WI, which may contain small areas of high signal intensity suggestive of blood [23]. When such a gestational sac-like structure is found separated from the uterus without tubal structures, this finding is equivocal, due to the differential diagnostic problems of cystic ovarian masses [22]. Identification of the uterine junctional zone between the gestational sac surrounded by myometrium and the uterine cavity is highly suggestive of a rare type of ectopic pregnancy, interstitial pregnancy [24]. In suspected ectopic pregnancy, the combination of an adnexal mass and intraperitoneal hemorrhage is suggestive of tubal rupture.

17.2.5.2
Differential Diagnosis

In women of reproductive age presenting with elevated human chorionic gonadotropin levels, demonstration of a gestational sac-like structure is highly suggestive of ectopic pregnancy. However, ovarian cancer may rarely be detected during early pregnancy and be misdiagnosed as ectopic pregnancy [25]. Based on the MRI findings alone, ectopic pregnancy may be misdiagnosed as an ovarian mass, e.g., ovarian cancer or endometriosis. Interstitial ectopic pregnancy may resemble cystic adenomyomas or necrotic fibroids [24].

17.2.5.3
Value of imaging

The diagnosis of ectopic pregnancy is usually established by the combination of beta hCG levels and transvaginal sonography. The role of MRI has not been defined. It may, however, provide additional information in case of unequivocal sonography, especially to better determine the exact site of origin of ectopic pregnancy [24].

17.3
Nongynecological Causes of Pelvic Pain

17.3.1
Pelvic Congestion Syndrome

Pelvic congestion syndrome or pelvic venous incompetence is a common cause of chronic noncyclical pelvic pain that affects most often multiparous women of reproductive age. The symptoms of chronic dull pelvic pain, pressure, and heaviness have been attributed to dilated, tortuous, and congested veins that are produced by retrograde flow through incompetent valves in ovarian veins. Patients with pelvic congestion syndrome may also suffer from dyspareunia (71%), dysmenorrhea (66%), and postcoital ache (65%) [26]. The prevalence of pelvic congestion syndrome is closely related to the frequency of ovarian varices, which occur in 10% of the general population of women. Within this group of patients, up to 60% may develop pelvic congestion syndrome [27]. The pathogenesis of pelvic congestion syndrome is most likely multifactorial and influenced by hormonal effects, multiparity, and previous surgeries.

Pelvic congestion syndrome may also result from obstructing anatomic anomalies such as a retroaortic left renal vein or right common iliac vein compression [26]. It may also be associated with asymptomatic hematuria in the nutcracker phenomenon, which is caused by left ovarian vein congestion secondary to compression of the left renal vein by the superior mesenteric artery [28]. Dilated veins involved include veins in the broad ligaments, ovarian plexus, in the pelvic sidewalls. Varices within the paravaginal plexus, vulva, or the lower extremities may also be found [28]. Polycystic changes in ovaries are associated in approximately 40% of cases [29].

17.3.1.1
Imaging Findings

The typical imaging findings are dilated and tortuous vascular structures engorging the uterus and ovaries, which may extend to the pelvic sidewalls or communicate with paravaginal veins. CT as well as MR imaging are noninvasive methods used to diagnose pelvic varices. The diagnosis of pelvic varicosities in CT is established by the demonstration of at least four ipsilateral dilated parauterine veins of varying caliber, with a width of at least one vein larger than 4 mm or a diameter of the ovarian vein of more than 8 mm (Fig. 17.10) [30]. On T1-weighted MR images, pelvic varices display low signal intensity because of flow-void artifacts. On T2WI, the signal intensity depends on the velocity of blood flow. Contrast-enhanced MRA displays enhancing veins with maximal opacification in a venous phase. On gradient-echo MR images, the varices typically display high signal intensities.

17.3.1.2
Differential Diagnosis

Incompetent and dilated ovarian veins are frequently seen on CT in asymptomatic parous women (Fig. 17.11) [31]. Congenital or acquired vascular malformations of the uterus or parametria present also as vascular lesions. Contrast-enhanced CT or MRI may aid in the differentiation by the early enhancement of arteriovenous malformations in contrast to a more delayed enhancement in varicosities [32]. Adnexal masses with torsion or rare uterine tumors, especially choriocarcinomas may also be surrounded by thick, tortuous, well-enhanced vessels. The clinical background and imaging findings of an adnexal or uterine mass aid in the differential diagnosis.

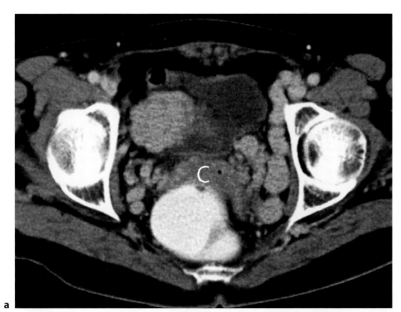

Fig. 17.10a–c. Pelvic congestion syndrome. Transaxial CT at the level of the cervix uteri (**a**) and coronal scans in the pelvis and retroperitoneum (**b, c**). Multiple dilated tortuous pelvic vascular structures are demonstrated within the parametria and pelvic sidewalls (**a**). The coronal images demonstrate engulfment of the uterus (*U*) by these vascular structures (**b, c**). Dilatation of both ovarian veins (*arrows*), which display a diameter of more than 8 mm, is shown in **c**. *U*, uterine corpus, *C*, cervix

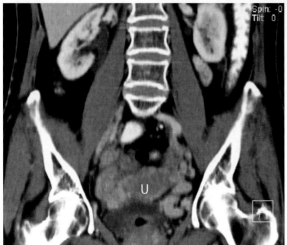

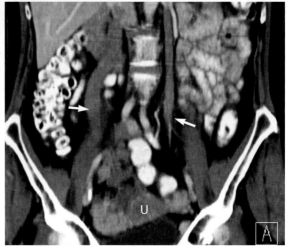

17.3.1.3
Value of Imaging

The diagnosis of ovarian and pelvic varices is established by sonography. CT or MRI are used to confirm the diagnosis and to aid in therapy guidance. However, these cross-sectional imaging techniques, which are not performed in an upright position may underestimate the venous pathology.

Several treatment options for pelvic congestion syndrome, including laparoscopic transperitoneal ligation of ovarian veins are currently under investigation. Percutaneous coil embolization of the gonadal vein seems to be a safe technique that relieves pelvic pain in many patients with pelvic congestion syndrome [27].

17.3.2
Ovarian Vein Thrombosis

Ovarian vein thrombosis typically presents a complication in the postpartum period and is encountered most frequently after caesarean section. It is caused by venous stasis and hypercoagulability. The incidence of puerperal vein thrombosis (POVT) is approximately 1 in 2,000 deliveries [33]. Other conditions such as infection, recent surgery, malignancy, and Crohn disease increase the risk for ovarian vein thrombosis [34]. Although a rare entity, ovarian vein thrombosis presents a differential diagnostic problem because of the unspecific clinical symptoms, including fever, and the potential of fatal complications due to uterine necrosis

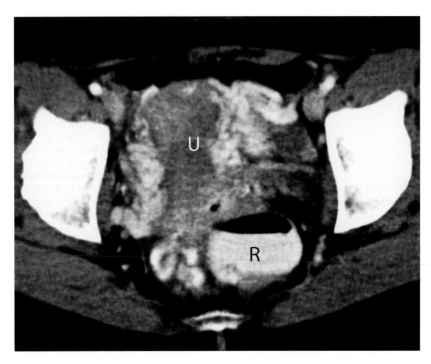

Fig. 17.11. Pelvic varices in an asymptomatic woman. CT shows numerous dilated para-uterine veins of varying diameter in an asymptomatic 37-year-old multiparous woman. *U*, uterus. *R*, rectum

or septic emboli [35]. As the majority (80%–90%) of ovarian vein thromboses occur in the right ovarian vein, right-sided pain is a typical clinical presentation.

17.3.2.1
Imaging Findings

Ovarian vein thrombosis is usually well depicted as a dilated tubular structure extending from the adnexa to the para-aortal region near the renal hilum. Contrast-enhanced CT allows direct visualization of the low attenuating central thrombus surrounded by vascular contrast-enhancement (Fig. 17.12) [36]. In MRI, the thrombus may display high SI on T1 and T2WI. Transaxial gradient-echo images or contrast-enhanced T1WI images aid in differentiation of flow artifacts from thrombosis. Imaging in the coronal plane demonstrates the full extent of ovarian vein involvement.

17.3.2.2
Differential diagnosis

The differential diagnosis includes other causes of right-sided pelvic pain such as appendicitis, adnexal

torsion, pelvic abscess, pyelonephritis, and endometritis [37].

17.3.2.3
Value of Imaging

Color Doppler ultrasound is the primary imaging modality in patients with suspected ovarian vein thrombosis. Especially in the postpartal period, its performance is often limited due to uterine enlargement, postoperative changes, or obesity. This is why CT or MRI are commonly performed to rule out ovarian vein thrombosis.

17.3.3
Appendicitis

Appendicitis affects all age groups; it peaks in the early twenties and then gradually declines toward the senium. Appendicitis is found 1.4 times more frequently in men than in women. In the majority of cases, appendicitis results as a development from obstruction of the lumen by fecaliths, lymphoid follicle hyperplasia, foreign bodies, and tumors. Variations in the appendiceal location make the clinical assessment of appendicitis difficult. The position of the appendix is retroperitoneal in about 30% of cases. Intraperitoneal location includes retrocecal, retroileal, deep pelvic, and rarely right upper quadrant location.

Acute appendicitis is the most common cause of emergency abdominal surgery. Since clinical diagnosis is difficult, appendectomy after false-positive diagnosis of appendicitis is still performed in up to 20% of cases [38]. In women of fertile age, the error rate reaches up to 40%, because acute gynecological processes tend to clinically simulate acute appendicitis [39].

Patients with appendicitis have a significantly shorter duration of pain than patients with other disorders.

Perforation and abscess formation complicated appendicitis in 38%–55%, with the highest rates occurring in children and in elderly patients.

17.3.3.1
Imaging Findings

On CT the normal appendix appears as a tubular structure with a diameter of less than 6 mm that often contains air or contrast media. CT findings of acute appendicitis include enlargement of the appendix (>6 mm in outer diameter), enhancement of the thickened appendiceal wall, and fat stranding of the periappendiceal region (Fig. 17.13) [40]. Signs indicative of perforation include extraluminal air, extraluminal appendicolith, a defect in the enhancing appendiceal wall, and an abscess or phlegmon [41]. A phlegmon is characterized by diffuse inflammation of the periappendiceal fat with no or small, ill-defined fluid collections. An abscess is a well-delineated fluid collection with rim enhancement [41]. Focal thickening of

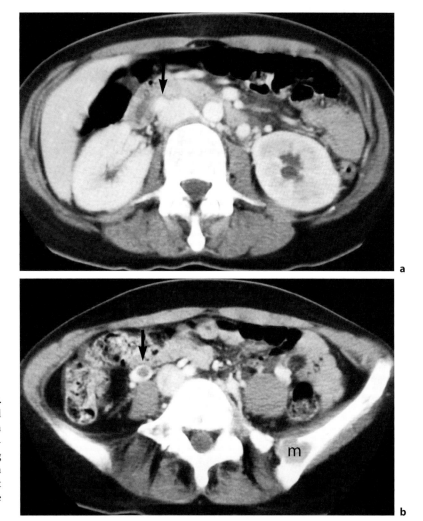

Fig. 17.12a,b. ovarian vein thrombosis. CT scans at the level below the renal hilum (**a**) and lower lumbar region (**b**). In a patient with bony metastasizing breast cancer (*m*), a nonoccluding thrombus (*arrow*) is identified within the dilated right ovarian vein (**b**). At the level just below the renal hilum, the renal vein (*arrowhead*) is patent (**a**)

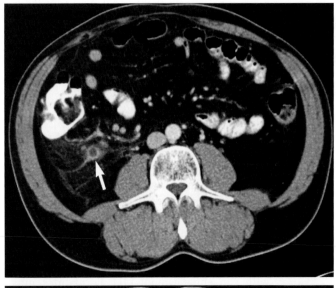

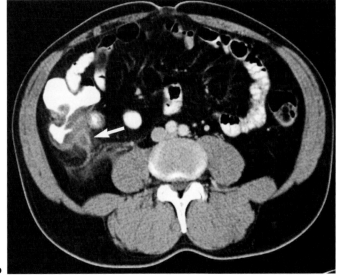

Fig. 17.13a,b. CT findings in acute appendicitis . Transaxial scans in right lower quadrant (**a, b**). The tubular enhancing structure with a diameter of 9 mm represents the dilated appendix (*arrow*). It is surrounded by marked fat stranding of the pericecal fat and adjacent facial thickening.. At the base of the appendix (*arrow*), thickening of the cecum can be observed, which presents the arrowhead sign (**b**). A small fluid collection is seen along the surface of the psoas muscle (**b**)

the cecum due to the inflammatory process can be observed and has been described as the arrowhead sign [40]. MR criteria suggesting acute appendicitis do not differ from those as described in CT. They include thickening of the appendiceal wall, a dilated fluid-filled lumen, and increased intensity of peri-appendiceal tissue on T2-weighted imaging or contrast-enhanced images (Fig. 17.14) [42]. Extraintestinal fluid-filled hyperintense lesions with walls that are hypointense on T2-weighted images and thick on the contrast-enhanced images are indicative of abscesses. Demonstration of air within such a lesion on MRI or CT allows the definite diagnosis of an abscess [43].

17.3.3.2
Value of Imaging

In children and women of childbearing age, sonography is the primary imaging modality to assess a patient with suspected acute appendicitis. However, due to its inability to visualize the normal appendix, and due to variations in location, CT is warranted in a negative US study [38]. It is regarded as the imaging modality of choice in the diagnosis of appendicitis, with excellent performance (sensitivity and specificity rates of 90%–95% and 95%–100%, respectively). Due to its lack of ionization, MR is an alternative, highly useful imaging tool in the assessment of acute

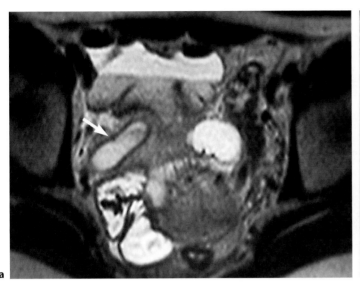
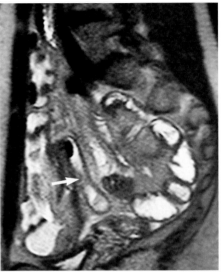

a   b

Fig. 17.14a,b. Appendicitis in MRI. Transaxial (**a**) and sagittal T2WI (**b**). A tubular fingerlike lesion (*arrow*), characteristic of the dilated fluid-filled appendix is seen in the right lower quadrant. The low-signal-intensity structure at the base of the appendix seen in the sagittal plane (**b**) presents an appendicolith (*). Appendicoliths are a highly specific sign of appendicitis; however, they are found in only 12% of cases. Courtesy of Dr. M. Umschaden, Wolfsberg

right-lower-quadrant pain, especially in children and pregnant women [44, 45].

17.3.4
Diverticulitis

Colonic diverticulosis is a very common condition in Western society, affecting 5%–10% of the population over 45 years, and 80% over 85 years of age [46].

Diverticula are small sacculations of mucosa and submucosa through the muscularis of the colonic wall. They develop where the nerve and blood vessel penetrate the muscularis between the teniae coli and mesentery [47]. The most common location for diverticula is the sigmoid colon. Acute diverticulitis occurs when the neck of a diverticulum is occluded by food particles, stool, or inflammation, resulting in microperforation of the diverticulum and surrounding mild pericolic inflammation, which is usually contained by pericolonic fat and mesentery. This may lead to a localized abscess or, if adjacent organs are involved, a fistula. Poor containment results in free perforation and peritonitis [48]. The leading clinical symptom is left-lower-quadrant pain and tenderness, which is often present for several days before admission. Low-grade fever and mild leukocytosis are common but their absence does not exclude diverticulitis.

Right-sided diverticulitis occurs in only 1.5% of patients in Western countries but is more common in Asians and tends to affect younger patients (Fig. 17.15) [49]. Diverticulitis of small intestine or transverse colon is rare [50].

17.3.4.1
Imaging Findings

At CT, diverticulosis appears as small, air-filled outpouchings of the colonic wall, most commonly in the sigmoid colon. In MRI on T1WI diverticula appear as hypointense against the high-signal-intense pericolonic fat. The most common imaging finding in diverticulitis is paracolic fat stranding, which is characteristically more severe than the focal colonic wall thickening (Fig. 17.16.) The key to distinguishing diverticulitis from other inflammatory conditions affecting the colon is the presence of diverticula in the involved segment [50]. Contrast-enhanced CT or fat-suppressed T1-weighted image contrast provides the best assessment of thickening of the colonic wall and the pericolonic fat stranding. Other common imaging findings are thickening of the lateral conal fascia and small amounts of ascites in the cul-de-sac. Accumulation of fluid in the root of the sigmoid mesentery is called the comma sign and engorgement of the mesenteric vessels is called the "centipede sign" [51].

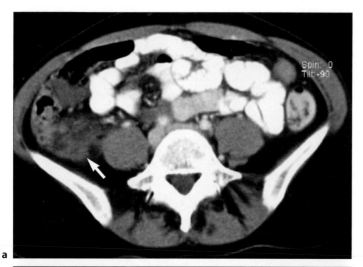

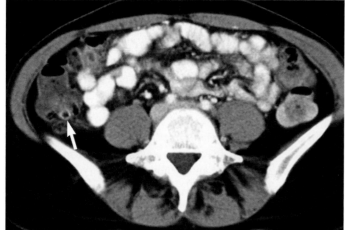

Fig. 17.15a,b. Right-sided diverticulitis. Transaxial CT scans at the level of the pelvic crest at the initial presentation (a) and after 3 weeks (b). In a 33-year-old woman who presented with acute right quadrant pain and laboratory signs of inflammation, a diffuse inflammatory process (*arrow*) in the pericecal region is demonstrated. It was diagnosed as acute retrocecal appendicitis (a). At surgery, there was no evidence of inflammatory changes of the appendix. The follow-up 3 weeks later demonstrated complete resolution of the inflammatory reaction and revealed several diverticula (*arrow*) of the cecum (b)

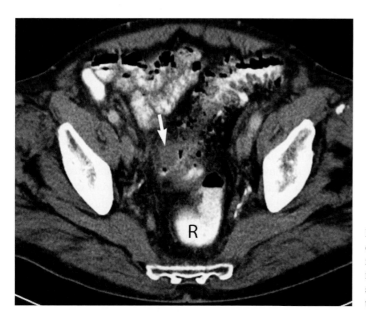

Fig. 17.16 Sigmoid diverticulitis. Multiple air-containing diverticula are found along the sigmoid colon. In this patient with acute pelvic pain, focal wall thickening, stenosis, and paracolic fat stranding (*arrow*) are signs of acute diverticulitis involving the distal sigmoid colon. *R*, rectum

Complications of diverticulitis include diverticular abscess, colovesical fistula, and perforation. An abscess that occurs in up to 30% of cases appears as a hypodense fluid collection with a contrast-enhancing rim and surrounding inflammatory changes. It may contain air or air–fluid levels [47]. A colovesical fistula is suspected when air is seen in the bladder and there is thickening of the bladder wall adjacent to a diseased segment of bowel [52]. Another complication of diverticulitis can be focal contained perforations. They appear as small extraluminal deposits of air or extravasation of oral contrast material. Pneumoperitoneum is a rare finding in patients with diverticulitis [47].

17.3.4.2
Differential Diagnosis

The most important differential diagnosis is colon carcinoma. The presence of pericolic lymph nodes suggests the diagnosis of colon cancer rather than diverticulitis [53]. The length of the involved segment (>10 cm), engorgement of adjacent sigmoid mesenteric vasculature, and the presence of fluid in the root of the sigmoid mesentery favors the diagnosis of diverticulitis [47, 54]. However, in some cases it may not be possible to distinguish diverticulitis from colon cancer and concomitant diseases may be found in 3%–18% [54].

17.3.4.3
Value of Imaging

The role of imaging in diverticulitis is to rule out complications of diverticulitis and the necessity for emergent surgery. If an abscess is detected CT guided percutaneous drainage may be perfumed. MR imaging can be useful in the diagnosis of right sided diverticulitis in young or pregnant patients with suspected appendicitis.

17.3.5
Epiploic Appendagitis

Appendices epiploicae are pedunculated fat filled structures protruding from the external surface of the colon into the peritoneal cavity. They vary considerably in size, shape, and contour. In obese persons and people who have recently lost weight, they are largest. The average length is 3 cm, although they are occasionally up to 15 cm in size [55]. They are presumed to serve a protective cushion during peristalsis. Epiploic appendagitis, also known as hemorrhagic epiploitis or appendicitis epiploica, is a rare benign self-limiting pathology secondary to torsion or spontaneous venous thrombosis of a draining vein. It occurs most commonly in the second to fifth decades of life, with a similar incidence among men and women [55].

Patients most commonly present with sudden onset of abdominal pain without leukocytosis and fever [56].

17.3.5.1
Imaging Findings

Normal appendices epiploicae are usually not seen on CT or MRI unless they are surrounded by a sufficient amount of intraperitoneal fluid such as ascites or hemoperitoneum (Fig. 17.17). Imaging findings of epiploic appendagitis include an oval-shaped finger-like paracolic mass with the attenuation of fat and periappendiceal fat stranding [57]. In CT, the density tends to be higher than uninvolved fat. A well circumscribed hyperattenuating rim that surrounds the mass and represents the inflamed visceral peritoneal lining is a characteristic finding (Fig. 17.18). Adjacent colonic wall thickening and compression may also be seen [56]. Sometimes a high attenuation central dot representing thrombosed central vessels or central areas of hemorrhage can be seen [57]. Rarely, dystrophic calcification from a previously infarcted appendage may be evident [58].

17.3.5.2
Differential Diagnosis

Segmental omental infarction, which is often localized on the right side of the omentum, occurs similarly to appendagitis epiploica from torsion or spontaneous venous thrombosis. Imaging findings range from subtle focal hazy soft-tissue infiltration of the omentum to a tumor-like inflammatory processes that may or may not lie immediately adjacent to the colon [57,58]. As features may also overlap with those of appendagitis epiploica, the term "focal fat infarction" has been suggested by some authors for both entities [57].

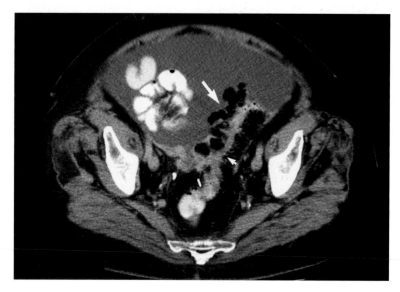

Fig. 17.17. Normal appendices epiploicae in CT. Appendices epiploicae of the sigmoid colon present pedunculated fat structures, which protrude from the sigmoid surface into the peritoneal cavity (*arrow*). They are easily visualized because of ascites in this woman with peritoneal carcinomatosis. Small sigmoid diverticula which present air-containing mural outpouchings into the perisigmoid fat tissue are also demonstrated (*arrowhead*)

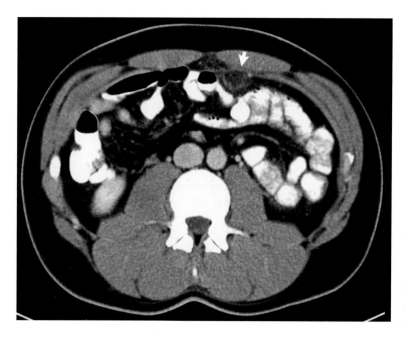

Fig. 17.18. Appendagitis epiploica. In a 29-year-old patient with acute pain, a tender 2.5-cm soft-tissue infiltration (*arrow*) with adjacent reticular fatty infiltration at the umbilical level is demonstrated. Because of its well-circumscribed hyper-attenuating rim, it presents more likely appendagitis epiploica than omental infarction. The lesion vanished within a few days of conservative therapy

17.3.5.3
Value of Imaging

Epiploic appendagitis and omental infarction are causes of acute pelvic pain that are often misdiagnosed clinically as acute appendicitis or diverticulitis. Based on the imaging findings, especially CT allows a definite diagnosis in most cases and patients can be managed conservatively.

17.3.6
Crohn Disease

Crohn disease is a chronic granulomatous inflammatory intestinal disease with a mean age of presentation in the third and fourth decades. It can affect any part of the gastrointestinal tract from the mouth to the anus, often involving multiple discontinuous sites. The small intestine is involved in 80% of cases, most commonly at the terminal ileum. The colon is affected either with or without involvement of the small intestine [59]. Leading clinical manifestations are prolonged diarrhea with abdominal pain, weight loss, and fever. Because of transmural inflammation, bowel loops may adhere to each other and result in masses, fistulas, and obstruction. The development of sinus tracts can lead to serous penetration and bowel wall perforation. This complication may be associated with an acute presentation of localized peritonitis with fever, abdominal pain, and tenderness. Perianal disease such as anal fissures, fistulas, and abscesses occur in 22% of patients with Crohn disease, and are often the first clinical manifestation [60].

17.3.6.1
Imaging Findings

Bowel wall thickening, usually ranging from 1 to 2 cm, is the most consistent feature of Crohn disease in CT and MRI images [61]. Particularly after intravenous administration of contrast material, mural stratification (target appearance) is often seen in active lesions. An inflamed bowel wall displays marked enhancement after intravenous contrast media, and the intensity of enhancement correlates with the degree of inflammatory lesion activity [62]. Luminal narrowing, prestenotic dilatation, and fibrofatty proliferation of the mesentery, and mesenteric lymph nodes ranging from 3 to 8 mm in size are further common findings (Fig. 17.19). In

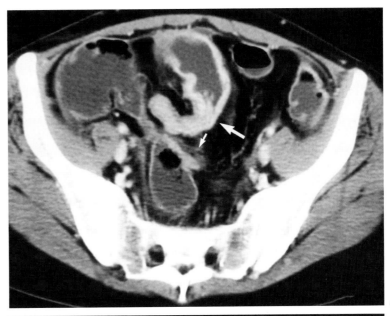

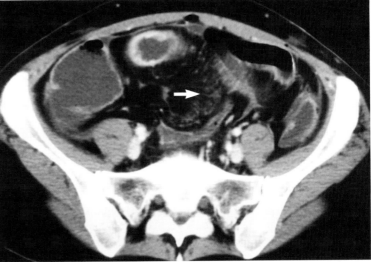

Fig. 17.19a,b. Crohn disease in CT. Small bowel loops with dilatation and stenoses are demonstrated in two pelvic CT scans (**a, b**). An ileum sling shows transmural wall thickening and intense contrast enhancement (*arrow*) (**a**). Adjacent mesenteric hypervascularity presents the comb sign (*long arrow*) and is another sign of inflammatory activity (**b**). Heterogeneity of surrounding fat with increased attenuation presents fibrofatty proliferation (*arrowhead*) (**a**)

CT, fibrofatty proliferation shows a slightly increased attenuation. In MRI, the signal intensity is decreased compared with normal fat separating the bowel loops. Phlegmon and abscesses can occur in the small bowel mesentery, abdominal wall, or psoas muscle or perianally. They are well demonstrated on CT and fat-saturated T1W MR imaging [59]. Fistulas and sinus tracts are also depicted; however, the reported sensitivity of MR imaging for depicting sinus tracts is 50%–75% compared to a conventional enteroclysis study [63].

17.3.6.2
Differential Diagnosis

Ulcerative colitis is a mucosal disease that primarily affects the rectum. It is typically left-sided or diffuse, and only rarely involves the right colon exclusively [64]. The mean wall thickness in Crohn disease is usually greater than in ulcerative colitis [65]. The halo sign, a low-attenuation ring in the bowel wall caused by deposition of submucosal fat, is seen more commonly in ulcerative colitis than in Crohn disease. Proliferation of mesenteric fat is almost exclusively seen in Crohn disease, whereas proliferation of peri-rectal fat is nonspecific and can result from Crohn disease, ulcerative colitis, pseudomembranous colitis, or radiation colitis [64]. Abscesses are almost exclusively found in Crohn disease and not in ulcerative colitis [62].

17.3.6.3
Value of Imaging

Cross-sectional imaging is able to demonstrate transmural extent, skip lesions beyond severe luminal stenoses, and intraperitoneal extraintestinal complications. However, CT and MR imaging are inferior compared to enteroclysis in the depiction of early disease manifestations and of fistulas and sinus tracts [59].

17.3.7
Rectus Sheath Hematoma

Rectus sheath hematoma is an uncommon and often misdiagnosed condition resulting from either rupture of the epigastric vessels or the rectus muscle itself. The hematoma may be caused by coagulation disorders, trauma, or anticoagulation therapy [65]. Clinically, most patients present with acute abdominal pain, a peri- or infraumbilical mass, and anemic syndrome. Some patients also have a history of severe coughing episodes due to bronchial infection.

17.3.7.1
Imaging Findings

The shape of rectus sheath hematomas depends on the relationship to the arcuate line, which is 3.5–5 cm below the umbilical level [66]. Above this level, they usually appear as spindle-shaped due to encasement by firm aponeurotic sheaths (Fig. 17.20). Below the arcuate line, hematomas tend to appear spherical and may communicate with extraperitoneal pelvic and perivascular pelvic spaces [66]. In CT, hematomas present as homogeneous hyperdense lesions with thin circumferential halos of low density. Clot resorption leads to diminution of density and fluid–fluid levels because a hematocrit effect may be found within hematomas [67, 68]. Additional findings of rectus sheath hematoma include increased density of the adjacent subcutaneous fat and enlargement of the anterolateral muscles [66]. On MRI, rectus sheath hematomas demonstrate heterogeneous signal intensities with areas of high signal intensity on T1-weighted and T2-weighted images. Fluid–fluid levels and a concentric ring sign can also be noted [69].

17.3.7.2
Differential Diagnosis

The acute clinical onset in a patient under anticoagulation supports the diagnosis of a rectus sheath hematoma. MR imaging may be useful in differentiation of chronic rectus sheath hematomas from anterior abdominal wall masses such as lipoma, hemangioma, neurofibroma, desmoid tumor, soft-tissue sarcoma, lymphoma, or metastatic lesions. Although bleeding into neoplasm may occur, hyperintense regions are rarely observed in tumors [66].

17.3.7.3
Value of Imaging

In the presence of a clinically suspected rectus sheath hematoma or equivocal findings in sonography, CT should be performed. CT usually allows the correct diagnosis and obviates unnecessary surgical interventions [67].

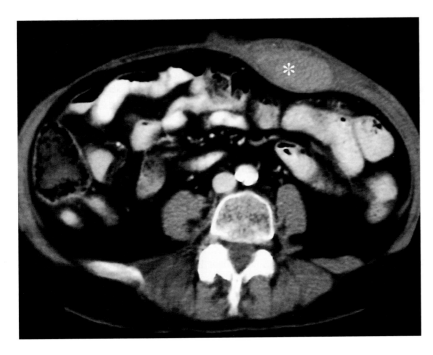

Fig. 17.20. Rectus sheath hematoma in CT. At the umbilical level, a spindle-shaped lesion is seen in the left rectus muscle (*arrow*). It shows homogenous high density and is surrounded at its anterior periphery by a minimal hypodense rim. Only minimal thickening of the adjacent lateral abdominal muscles can be noted

References

1. Kim SH, Kim SH, Yang DM et al (2004) Unusual causes of tubo-ovarian abscess. CT and MR imaging findings. Radiographics 24:1575–1589
2. Ghiatas AA (2004) The spectrum of pelvic inflammatory disease. Eur Radiol 14:E184–E192
3. Sam JW, Jacobs JE, Birnbaum BA (2002) Spectrum of CT findings in acute pyogenic pelvic inflammatory disease. Radiographics 22:1327–1334
4. Tukeva TA, Aronen HJ, Karjalainen PT et al (1999) MR imaging in pelvic inflammatory disease: comparison with laparoscopy and US. Radiology 210:209–216
5. Kawakami S, Togashi K, Kimura I et al (1993) Primary malignant tumor of the fallopian tube: appearance at CT and MR imaging. Radiology 196:503–508
6. Livengood CHH (2005) Tuboovarian abscess. www.uptodate.com. Cited 21 April 2006
7. Rodriguez-de Valesques A, Yoder CI, Velasquez PA et al (1995) Imaging effects of diabetes on the genitourinary system. Radiographics 15:1051–1068
8. Protopapas AG, Diakomanolis ES, Milingos SD et al (2004) Tubo-ovarian abscesses in postmenopausal women:gynaecological malignancy until proven otherwise? Eur J Obstet Gynecol Reprod Biol 15:114:203–209
9. Bennett GL, Slywotzky CM, Giovanniello G et al (2002) Gynecologic causes of acute pelvic pain: spectrum of CT findings. Radiographics 22:785–801
10. Lee EJ, Kwon HC, Joo HJ et al (1998) Diagnosis of ovarian torsion with color Doppler sonography: depiction of twisted vascular pedicle. J Ultrasound Med 17:83–89
11. Sherard GB, Hodson CA, Williams HJ et al (2003) Adnexal masses and pregnancy: a 12-year experience. Am J Obstet Gynecol 189:358–362
12. Graif M, Itzach Y (1988) Sonographic evaluation of ovarian torsion in childhood and adolescence. AJR Am J Roentgenol 150:647–649
13. Koonings PP, Grimes DA (1989) Adnexal torsion in postmenopausal women. Obstet Gynecol 73:11–12
14. Haque TL, Togashi K, Kobayashi H et al (2000) Adnexal torsion: MR findings of viable ovary. Eur Radiol 10:1954–1957
15. Lee AR, Kim KHK, Lee BH, Chin SY(1993) Massive edema of the ovary: imaging findings. AJR Am J Roentgenol 161:343–344
16. Kimura I, Togashi K, Kawakami S et al (1994) Ovarian torsion: CT and MRI appearances. Radiology 190:337–341
17. Ghossain MA, Buy JN, Bazot M et al (1994) CT in adnexal torsion with emphasis on tubal findings: correlation with US. J Comput Assist Tomogr 18:619–625
18. Rha SE, Byun JY, Jung SE et al (2003) CT and MR imaging features of adnexal torsion. Radiographics 22:283–294
19. Currarino G, Rutledge JC (1989) Ovarian torsion and amputation resulting in partially calcified, pedunculated cystic mass. Pediatr Radiol 19:395–399
20. Bouyer J, Coste J, Fernandez H et al (2002) Sites of ectopic pregnancy: a 10 year population based study of 1,800 cases. Human Reprod 17:3224–3230
21. Ushakov FB, Elchalal U, Aceman PJ et al (1997) Cervical pregnancy: past and future. Obstet Gynecol Surv 52:45–59

22. Kataoka ML, Togashi K, Kobayashi H et al (1999) Evaluation of ectopic pregnancy by magnetic resonance imaging. Human Reprod 14:2644–2650

23. Nishino M, Hayakawa K, Kawamata K et al (2002) MRI of early unruptured pregnancy: detection of gestational sac. J Comput Assist Tomogr 26:134–137

24. Filhastre M, Dechaud H, Lesnik A et al (2005) Interstitial pregnancy: role of MRI. Europ Radiol 15:93–95

25. Riley GM, Babcook C, Jain K (1996) Ruptured malignant ovarian tumor mimicking ectopic pregnancy. J Ultrasound Med 15:871–873

26. Kuligowska E, Deeds L Lu K (2005) Pelvic pain: overlooked and underdiagnosed gynaecologic conditions. Radiographics 25:3–20

27. Mathias SD, Kuppermann M, Liberman RF et al (1996) Chronic pelvic pain: prevalence, health-related quality of life, and economic correlates. Obstet Gynecol 87:321–327

28. Umeoka S, Koyama T, Togashi K et al (2004) Vascular dilatation in the pelvis: identification with CT and MR imaging. Radiographics 24:193–208

29. Park SJ, Lim JW, Ko YT et al (2004) Diagnosis of pelvic congestion syndrome using transabdominal and transvaginal sonography. AJR Am J Roentgenol 182:683–688

30. Hricak H, Reinhold C, Ascher SM (2004) Ovarian dysgerminomas. In: Hricak H, Reinhold C, Ascher SM (eds) Gynecology top 100 diagnoses. WB Saunders Company, Amirsys, Salt Lake City, pp 274–275

31. Rozenblit AM, Ricci ZJ, Tuvia J et al (2001) Incompetent and dilated ovarian veins: a common CT finding in asymptomatic parous women. AJR Am J Roentgenol 176:119–122

32. Gulati MS, Paul SB, Batra A et al (2000) Uterine arteriovenous malformations: the role of intravenous "dual phase" CT angiography. Clin Imaging 24:10–14

33. Witlin AG, Mercer BM, Sibai BM (1996) Septic pelvic thrombophlebitis or refractory postpartum fever of undetermined etiology. J Matern Fetal Med 5:355–358

34. Dunnihoo DR, Gallaspy JW, Wise RB et al (1991) Postpartum ovarian vein thrombophlebitis: a review. Obstet Gynecol Surv 46:415–427

35. Savader S, Otero RR, Savader BL (1988) Puerperal ovarian vein thrombosis: evaluation with CT, US, and MR imaging. Radiology 167:637–639

36. Quane LK, Kidney DD, Cohen AJ (1998) Unusual causes of ovarian vein thrombosis as revealed by CT and sonography. AJR Am J Roentgenol 171:487–490

37. Kubik-Huch RA, Hebisch G, Huch R et al (1999) Role of duplex color Doppler ultrasound, computed tomography, and MR angiography in the diagnosis of septic puerperal ovarian vein thrombosis. Abdom Imaging 24:85–91

38. Paulson EK, Kalady MF, Pappas TN (2003) Suspected appendicitis. N Engl J Med 348:236–242

39. Andersson RE, Hugander A, Thulin AJ (1992) Diagnostic accuracy and perforation rate in appendicitis: association with age and sex of the patient and with appendectomy rate. Eur J Surg 158:37–41

40. Rao PM, Rhea JT, Novelline RA (1997) Sensitivity and specificity of the individual CT signs: experience with 200 helical appendiceal CT examinations. J Comput Assist Tomogr 21:686–692

41. Horrow M, White DS, Horrow JC (2003) Differentiation of perforated from nonperforated appendicitis at CT. Radiology 227:46–51

42. Nitta N, Takahashi M, Furukawa A et al (2005) MR imaging of the normal appendix and acute appendicitis. J Magn Reson Imaging 21:156–165

43. Oto A, Ernst R, Shah R et al (2005) Right-lower-quadrant pain and suspected appendicitis in pregnant women: evaluation with MR imaging – initial experience. Radiology 234:445–451

44. Cobben LP, Groot I, Haans L et al (2004) MRI for clinically suspected appendicitis during pregnancy. AJR Am J Roentgenol 183:671–675

45. Birchard KR, Brown MA, Hyslop WB et al (2005) MRI of acute abdominal and pelvic pain in pregnant patients. AJR Am J Roentgenol 184:452–458

46. Ferzoco LB, Raptopoulos V, Silen W(1998) Acute diverticulitis. N Engl J Med 338:1521–1526

47. Horton KM, Corl MF, Fishman EK (2000) CT evaluation of the colon: inflammatory disease. Radiographics. 20:399–418

48. Young-Fadok T, Pemberton JH (2005) Clinical manifestations and diagnosis of colonic diverticular disease. www.UpToDate.com. Cited 21 April 2006

49. Kang JY, Melville D, Maxwell JD (2004) Epidemiology and management of diverticular disease of the colon. Drugs Aging. 21:211–228

50. Pereira JM, Sirlin CB, Pinto PA et al (2004) Disproportionate fat stranding: a helpful CT sign in patients with acute abdominal pain. Radiographics 24:703–715

51. Rao PM (1999) CT of diverticulitis and alternative conditions. Semin Ultrasound CT MR 20:86–93

52. Labs JD, Sarr MG, Fishman EK et al (1988) Complications of acute diverticulitis of the colon: improved early diagnosis with computerized tomography. Am J Surg 155:331–336

53. Cintapalli KN, Chopra S, Ghiatas AA et al (1999) Diverticulitis versus colon cancer: differentiation with helical CT findings. Radiology 210:429–435

54. Cobben LP, Groot I, Blickman JG et al (2003) Right colonic diverticulitis: MR appearance. Abdom Imaging 28:794–798

55. Gelrud A, Cardenas A, Chopra A (2005) Epiploic appendagitis. www.uptodate.com. Cited 21 April 2006

56. Rao PM, Novelline RA (1999) Case 6: primary epiploic appendagitis. Radiology 210:145–148

57. Pereira JM, Sirlin CB, Pinto P et al (2005) CT and MR imaging of extrahepatic fatty masses of the abdomen and pelvis: techniques, diagnosis, differential diagnosis and pitfalls. Radiographics 25:69–85

58. Pickhardt PJ, Bhalla S (2005) Unusual nonneoplastic peritoneal and subperitoneal conditions: CT findings. Radiographics 25:719–730

59. Furukawa A, Saotome T, Yamasaki M et al (2004) Cross-sectional imaging in Crohn disease. Radiographics 24:689–702

60. Williams DR, Coller JA, Corman ML et al (1981) Anal complications in Crohn's disease. Dis Colon Rectum 24:22–24

61. Rollandi GA, Curone PF, Bisalde E et al (1999) Spiral CT of the abdomen after distension of small bowel loops with transparent enema in patients with Crohn's disease. Abdom Imaging 24:544–549

62. Gore RM, Balthazar EJ, Ghahremani GG et al (1996) CT

features of ulcerative colitis and Crohn's disease. AJR Am J Roentgenol 167:3–15

63. Gourtsoyiannis N, Papanikolaou N, Grammatikakis J et al (2002) MR enteroclysis: technical considerations and clinical applications. Eur Radiol 12:2651–2658
64. Philpotts LE, Heiken JP, Westcott MA et al (1994) Colitis: use of CT findings in differential diagnosis. Radiology 190:445–449
65. Fishman EK, Wolf EJ, Jones B et al (1987) CT evaluation of Crohn's disease: effect on patient management. AJR Am J Roentgenol 148:537–540
66. Fukuda T, Sakamoto I, Kohzaki S et al (1996) Spontane-

ous rectus sheath hematomas: clinical and radiological features. Abdom Imaging 21:58–61
67. Berná JD, Garcia-Medina V, Guirao J et al (1996) Rectus sheath hematoma: diagnostic classification by CT. Abdom Imaging 21:62–64
68. Wolverson MK, Crepps LF, Sundaram M et al (1983) Hyperdensity of recent hemorrhage at body computed tomography: incidence and morphologic variation. Radiology 148:779–784
69. Blum A, Bui P, Boccaccini H et al (1995) Imaging of severe forms of hematoma in the rectus abdominis under anticoagulants. J Radiol 76:267–273

Subject Index

V

W

X

Y

Z

List of Contributors

ERNST BEINDER, MD
PD, University Hospital of Zurich
Department of Obstetrics
Frauenklinikstrasse 10
8091 Zürich
Switzerland

DIDIER CHARDONNENS, MD
PD, Hôpital de la Tour
Meyrins
Switzerland

TANJA FISCHER, MD
Institut für Klinische Radiologie
Universitätsklinikum München – Innenstadt
Brustzentrum 1
Maistrasse 11
80337 München
Germany

ROSEMARIE FORSTNER, MD
PD, Department of Radiology
Landeskliniken Salzburg
Paracelsus Private Medical University
Müllner Hauptstrasse 48
5020 Salzburg
Austria

KATHRIN A. FREI BONEL, MD
Department of Obstetrics and Gynecology
University Hospital Bern, Inselspital
Effingerstrasse 102
3010 Bern
Switzerland

HELGA FRITSCH, MD
Professor
Division of Clinical and Functional Anatomy
Department of Anatomy, Histology
und Embryology
Medical University of Innsbruck
Müllerstrasse 59
6020 Innsbruck
Austria

BERND HAMM, MD
Professor and Chairman
Instituts für Radiologie (Campus Mitte)
Klinik für Strahlenheilkunde (Campus Virchow-Klinikum
und Campus Buch)
Charité – Universitätsmedizin Berlin
Charitéplatz 1
10117 Berlin
Germany

GERTRAUD HEINZ-PEER, MD
Professor, Department of Radiology
Medical University of Vienna
Währinger Gürtel 18 – 20
10090 Wien
Austria

KAREN KINKEL, MD
PD, Institut de radiologie
Clinique des Grangettes
chemin des Grangettes 7
1224 Chêne-Bougeries
Switzerland

CLAUDIA KLÜNER, MD
Institut für Radiologie (Campus Mitte)
Charité – Universitätsmedizin Berlin
Charitéplatz 1
10117 Berlin
Germany

THOMAS J. KRÖNCKE, MD
Institut für Radiologie (Campus Mitte)
Charité – Universitätsmedizin Berlin
Charitéplatz 1
10117 Berlin
Germany

RAHEL KUBIK-HUCH, MD, MPH
PD, Kantonsspital Baden AG
Department of Radiology
5404 Baden
Switzerland

ANDREAS LIENEMANN, MD
HELIOS Kliniken Schwerin
Institut für Röntgendiagnostik
Wismarsche Strasse 393–397
19049 Schwerin
Germany

PATRIK ROGALLA, MD
Institut für Radiologie (Campus Mitte)
Charité – Universitätsmedizin Berlin
Charitéplatz 1
10117 Berlin
Germany

JUSTUS ROOS, MD
Department of Radiology
Medical Center Stanford University
300 Pasteur Drive, Room S-072
Stanford, CA 94305
USA

ASTRID SCHNEIDER, MD
Department of Radiology
Landeskliniken Salzburg
Paracelsus Private Medical University
Müllner Hauptstrasse 48
5020 Salzburg
Austria

MATTHIAS TAUPITZ, MD
Institut für Radiologie (Campus Mitte)
Charité – Universitätsmedizin Berlin
Charitéplatz 1
10117 Berlin
Germany

UTA ZASPEL, MD
Institut für Radiologie (Campus Mitte)
Charité – Universitätsmedizin Berlin
Charitéplatz 1
10117 Berlin
Germany

MEDICAL RADIOLOGY Diagnostic Imaging and Radiation Oncology

Titles in the series already published

DIAGNOSTIC IMAGING

Innovations in Diagnostic Imaging
Edited by J. H. Anderson

Radiology of the Upper Urinary Tract
Edited by E. K. Lang

The Thymus - Diagnostic Imaging, Functions, and Pathologic Anatomy
Edited by E. Walter, E. Willich, and W. R. Webb

Interventional Neuroradiology
Edited by A. Valavanis

Radiology of the Pancreas
Edited by A. L. Baert, co-edited by G. Delorme

Radiology of the Lower Urinary Tract
Edited by E. K. Lang

Magnetic Resonance Angiography
Edited by I. P. Arlart, G. M. Bongartz, and G. Marchal

Contrast-Enhanced MRI of the Breast
S. Heywang-Köbrunner and R. Beck

Spiral CT of the Chest
Edited by M. Rémy-Jardin and J. Rémy

Radiological Diagnosis of Breast Diseases
Edited by M. Friedrich and E.A. Sickles

Radiology of the Trauma
Edited by M. Heller and A. Fink

Biliary Tract Radiology
Edited by P. Rossi, co-edited by M. Brezi

Radiological Imaging of Sports Injuries
Edited by C. Masciocchi

Modern Imaging of the Alimentary Tube
Edited by A. R. Margulis

Diagnosis and Therapy of Spinal Tumors
Edited by P. R. Algra, J. Valk, and J. J. Heimans

Interventional Magnetic Resonance Imaging
Edited by J. F. Debatin and G. Adam

Abdominal and Pelvic MRI
Edited by A. Heuck and M. Reiser

Orthopedic Imaging
Techniques and Applications
Edited by A. M. Davies and H. Pettersson

Radiology of the Female Pelvic Organs
Edited by E. K.Lang

Magnetic Resonance of the Heart and Great Vessels
Clinical Applications
Edited by J. Bogaert, A.J. Duerinckx, and F. E. Rademakers

Modern Head and Neck Imaging
Edited by S. K. Mukherji and J. A. Castelijns

Radiological Imaging of Endocrine Diseases
Edited by J. N. Bruneton in collaboration with B. Padovani and M.-Y. Mourou

Trends in Contrast Media
Edited by H. S. Thomsen, R. N. Muller, and R. F. Mattrey

Functional MRI
Edited by C. T. W. Moonen and P. A. Bandettini

Radiology of the Pancreas
2nd Revised Edition
Edited by A. L. Baert. Co-edited by G. Delorme and L. Van Hoe

Emergency Pediatric Radiology
Edited by H. Carty

Spiral CT of the Abdomen
Edited by F. Terrier, M. Grossholz, and C. D. Becker

Liver Malignancies
Diagnostic and Interventional Radiology
Edited by C. Bartolozzi and R. Lencioni

Medical Imaging of the Spleen
Edited by A. M. De Schepper and F. Vanhoenacker

Radiology of Peripheral Vascular Diseases
Edited by E. Zeitler

Diagnostic Nuclear Medicine
Edited by C. Schiepers

Radiology of Blunt Trauma of the Chest
P. Schnyder and M. Wintermark

Portal Hypertension
Diagnostic Imaging-Guided Therapy
Edited by P. Rossi
Co-edited by P. Ricci and L. Broglia

Recent Advances in Diagnostic Neuroradiology
Edited by Ph. Demaerel

Virtual Endoscopy and Related 3D Techniques
Edited by P. Rogalla, J. Terwisscha Van Scheltinga, and B. Hamm

Multislice CT
Edited by M. F. Reiser, M. Takahashi, M. Modic, and R. Bruening

Pediatric Uroradiology
Edited by R. Fotter

Transfontanellar Doppler Imaging in Neonates
A. Couture and C. Veyrac

Radiology of AIDS
A Practical Approach
Edited by J.W.A.J. Reeders and P.C. Goodman

CT of the Peritoneum
Armando Rossi and Giorgio Rossi

Magnetic Resonance Angiography
2nd Revised Edition
Edited by I. P. Arlart, G. M. Bongratz, and G. Marchal

Pediatric Chest Imaging
Edited by Javier Lucaya and Janet L. Strife

Applications of Sonography in Head and Neck Pathology
Edited by J. N. Bruneton in collaboration with C. Raffaelli and O. Dassonville

Imaging of the Larynx
Edited by R. Hermans

3D Image Processing
Techniques and Clinical Applications
Edited by D. Caramella and C. Bartolozzi

Imaging of Orbital and Visual Pathway Pathology
Edited by W. S. Müller-Forell

Pediatric ENT Radiology
Edited by S. J. King and A. E. Boothroyd

Radiological Imaging of the Small Intestine
Edited by N. C. Gourtsoyiannis

Imaging of the Knee
Techniques and Applications
Edited by A. M. Davies and V. N. Cassar-Pullicino

Perinatal Imaging
From Ultrasound to MR Imaging
Edited by Fred E. Avni

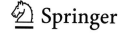

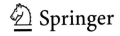

Printing and Binding: Stürtz GmbH, Würzburg